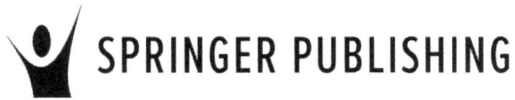

GET THE MOST FROM YOUR BOOK

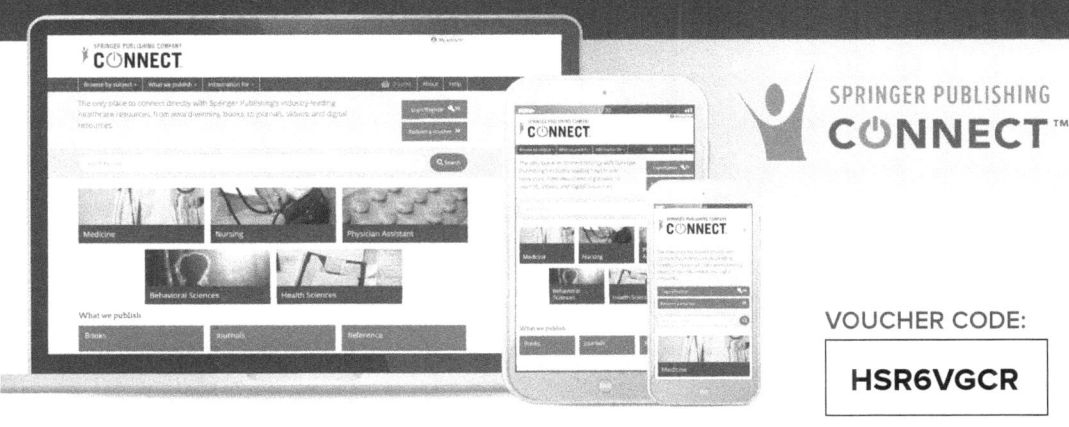

VOUCHER CODE:

HSR6VGCR

Online Access

Your print purchase of *Child and Adolescent Psychopathology for School Psychology* includes **online access via Springer Publishing Connect™** to increase accessibility, portability, and searchability.

Insert the code at http://connect.springerpub.com/content/book/978-0-8261-3587-2 today!

Having trouble? Contact our customer service department at cs@springerpub.com

Instructor Resource Access for Adopters

Let us do some of the heavy lifting to create an engaging classroom experience with a variety of instructor resources included in most textbooks SUCH AS:

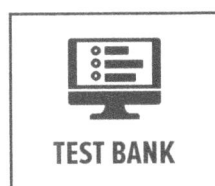

Visit **https://connect.springerpub.com/** and look for the **"Show Supplementary"** button on your **book homepage** to see what is available to instructors! First time using Springer Publishing Connect?

Email **textbook@springerpub.com** to create an account and start unlocking valuable resources.

Child and Adolescent Psychopathology for School Psychology

Terry Diamanduros, PhD, completed her doctoral studies at New York University, earning a PhD in school psychology. Dr. Diamanduros has several years of experience working with children and adolescents in school and clinical settings in New York City. She is currently a professor in the school psychology program at Georgia Southern University and has been a faculty member in the program since 2004. Her research interests focus on childhood trauma, cyberbullying, and the influence of technology on child development. She currently teaches courses in child psychopathology, developmental diagnosis, personality and behavioral assessment, assessment in academic achievement, and practicum in school psychology. Dr. Diamanduros is a member of the National Association of School Psychologists (NASP) and served as an NASP delegate for the state of Georgia. She is an active member of the Georgia Association of School Psychologists (GASP) and has served on its executive board. Dr. Diamanduros also serves on the editorial boards for the *Journal of Aggression, Maltreatment and Trauma*; *School Psychology Review*; *Psychology in the Schools*; and *Journal of Child Sexual Abuse*.

P. Dawn Tysinger, PhD, NCSP, earned a doctorate in pychology with a concentration in school psychology and a subspecialization in counseling interventions from the University of Memphis in Memphis, Tennessee. Dr. Tysinger has also earned the Nationally Certified School Psychologist credential from the National Association of School Psychologists (NASP). Dr. Tysinger is a full professor and program director in the nationally recognized and NASP-approved school psychology program at Georgia Southern University. Before coming to Georgia Southern University, she practiced in the public schools in both Louisiana and Kansas and served as an adjunct faculty member for Emporia State University in Emporia, Kansas. Dr. Tysinger has contributed to her field through active participation in NASP, publications in school psychology journals, and presentations given at the local, state, regional, national, and international levels. She currently serves as a reviewer for the NASP program review board and is a member of the editorial boards of *Psychology in the Schools*, *School Psychology Training and Pedagogy*, *National Youth-At-Risk Journal*, and *Journal of Online Learning Research*.

Jeffrey A. Tysinger, PhD, NCSP, is a professor at Georgia Southern University. From 2003 to 2007, he was a member of the faculty at Emporia State University, in the nationally accredited school psychology program. He has worked as a school psychologist in Anchorage, Alaska, and in Lafourche Parish, Louisiana. He obtained his doctorate in school psychology with an emphasis in counseling and interventions from the University of Memphis. Working at all levels of the profession (specialist, doctoral practitioner, and now a trainer) has given him a unique perspective and influenced his philosophy of school psychology. He regularly presents at local, state, regional, national, and international conferences. He has been the president of the Kansas Association of School Psychologists (KASP), editor of the KASP Newsletter, a committee member of KASP Futures, and a KASP National Certification in School Psychology (NCSP) committee member. He has been a member of the National Association of School Psychologists (NASP) since 1997 and has been a nationally certified school psychologist since 1997. He has also been an NASP program reviewer, an NCSP portfolio reviewer, and a member of Georgia Association of School Psychologists.

Pamela A. Fenning, PhD, ABPP, is a professor and co-director of the school psychology program at Loyola University Chicago. She is a licensed clinical and school psychologist in Illinois and holds board certification in school psychology. Her research and clinical work focus on multitiered academic and behavioral interventions at the high school level, racial bias in exclusionary discipline and entry to the juvenile justice system, inequities in school discipline policy, evaluation of state-level discipline reform, and professional development of school personnel in creating more equitable and inclusive school environments as well as school-based supports of military youth. She has published widely in these areas. She is the immediate past-president of the Trainers of School Psychologists, the chair of the National Association of School Psychologists (NASP) Professional Positions Committee, and a member of the NASP [Graduate] Program Accreditation Board.

Child and Adolescent Psychopathology for School Psychology

A Practical Approach

Terry Diamanduros, PhD
P. Dawn Tysinger, PhD, NCSP
Jeffrey A. Tysinger, PhD, NCSP
Pamela A. Fenning, PhD, ABPP

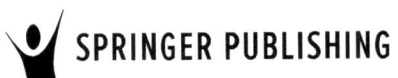

Copyright © 2023 Springer Publishing Company, LLC
All rights reserved.

No part of this publication may be reproduced, stored in a retrieval system, or transmitted in any form or by any means, electronic, mechanical, photocopying, recording, or otherwise, without the prior permission of Springer Publishing Company, LLC, or authorization through payment of the appropriate fees to the Copyright Clearance Center, Inc., 222 Rosewood Drive, Danvers, MA 01923, 978-750-8400, fax 978-646-8600, info@copyright.com or at www.copyright.com.

Springer Publishing Company, LLC
11 West 42nd Street, New York, NY 10036
www.springerpub.com
connect.springerpub.com/

Acquisitions Editor: Rhonda Dearborn
Compositor: S4Carlisle Publishing Services

ISBN: 978-0-8261-3578-0
ebook ISBN: 978-0-8261-3587-2
DOI: 10.1891/9780826135872

SUPPLEMENTS:
Instructor materials:

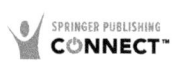

A robust set of instructor resources designed to supplement this text is located at http://connect.springerpub.com/content/book/978-0-8261-3587-2. Qualifying instructors may request access by emailing textbook@springerpub.com.

Instructor Manual ISBN: 978-0-8261-3723-4
Instructor PowerPoints ISBN: 978-0-8261-3724-1
Instructor Test Bank ISBN: 978-0-8261-3722-7

22 23 24 25 26 / 5 4 3 2 1

The author and the publisher of this Work have made every effort to use sources believed to be reliable to provide information that is accurate and compatible with the standards generally accepted at the time of publication. The author and publisher shall not be liable for any special, consequential, or exemplary damages resulting, in whole or in part, from the readers' use of, or reliance on, the information contained in this book. The publisher has no responsibility for the persistence or accuracy of URLs for external or third-party Internet websites referred to in this publication and does not guarantee that any content on such websites is, or will remain, accurate or appropriate.

Library of Congress Cataloging-in-Publication Data

Names: Diamanduros, Terry, author. | Tysinger, P. Dawn, author. | Tysinger,
   Jeffrey A., author. | Fenning, Pamela, author.
Title: Child and adolescent psychopathology for school psychology : a
   practical approach / Terry Diamanduros, P. Dawn Tysinger, Jeffrey A.
   Tysinger, Pamela A. Fenning.
Identifiers: LCCN 2021060484 (print) | LCCN 2021060485 (ebook) | ISBN
   9780826135780 (cloth) | ISBN 9780826135872 (ebook)
Subjects: LCSH: Child psychopathology–Textbooks. | Adolescent
   psychopathology–Textbooks. | School children–Mental health–Textbooks.
   | School psychology–Textbooks.
Classification: LCC RJ499 .D497 2023 (print) | LCC RJ499 (ebook) | DDC
   618.92/89–dc23/eng/20220211
LC record available at https://lccn.loc.gov/2021060484
LC ebook record available at https://lccn.loc.gov/2021060485

Contact sales@springerpub.com to receive discount rates on bulk purchases.

Publisher's Note: New and used products purchased from third-party sellers are not guaranteed for quality, authenticity, or access to any included digital components.

Printed in the United States of America.

Contents

Preface xi
Instructor Resources xv

UNIT 1: ADDRESSING CHILD AND ADOLESCENT MENTAL HEALTH DISORDERS IN SCHOOLS

1. Child and Adolescent Mental Health 3
   Introduction 3
   Addressing Child and Adolescent Mental Health in the Schools:
      The Role of School Psychologists 6
   Identification of Mental Health Problems in Schools:
      Diagnostic and Statistical Manual of Mental Disorders
      Versus Individuals With Disabilities Education Improvement Act 9
   Concluding Remarks 11
   Summary Points 11

UNIT 2: MENTAL HEALTH DISORDERS IN CHILDREN AND ADOLESCENTS: NEURODEVELOPMENTAL DISORDERS

2. Attention Deficit Hyperactivity Disorder 17
   Introduction 17
   Diagnostic Issues: DSM-5 and School-Based Services 17
   Cultural Issues Related to Attention Deficit Hyperactivity Disorder in Youth 22
   Impact of Attention Deficit Hyperactivity Disorder on Social–Emotional
      and Behavioral Functioning in School and Home Environments 24
   Impact of Attention Deficit Hyperactivity Disorder on Learning
      in the Classroom 26
   Implications for School Psychologists 28
   Educational Supports 30
   School-Based Mental Health Interventions and Supports 32
   Summary Points 35

3. Intellectual Disabilities 39
   Introduction 39
   Diagnostic Issues: DSM-5 and IDEA 40
   Cultural Issues Related to Intellectual Disability in Youth 42
   Impact of Intellectual Disability on Social–Emotional and Behavioral Functioning in School
      and Home Environments 46
   Impact of Intellectual Disability on Learning in the Classroom 49
   Implications for School Psychologists 50
   Educational Supports 52
   School-Based Mental Health Interventions and Supports 53
   Summary Points 57

4. Autism Spectrum Disorder   61
   Introduction   61
   Diagnostic Issues Related to Autism Spectrum Disorder   61
   Cultural Issues Related to Autism Spectrum Disorder in Youth   64
   Impact of Autism Spectrum Disorder on Social–Emotional
         and Behavioral Functioning in School and Home Environments   65
   Impact of Autism Spectrum Disorder on Learning in the Classroom   66
   Implications for School Psychologists   67
   Educational Supports   69
   School-Based Mental Health Interventions and Supports   70
   Summary Points   72

UNIT 3: MENTAL HEALTH DISORDERS IN CHILDREN AND ADOLESCENTS: DISRUPTIVE, IMPULSE-CONTROL, AND CONDUCT DISORDERS

5. Conduct Disorder   79
   Introduction   79
   Diagnostic Issues: DSM-5 and School-Based Services   79
   Cultural Issues Related to Conduct Disorder in Youth   84
   Impact of Conduct Disorder on Social–Emotional and Behavioral
         Functioning in School and Home Environments   85
   Impact of Conduct Disorder on Learning in the Classroom   87
   Implications for School Psychologists   88
   Educational Supports   91
   School-Based Mental Health Interventions and Supports   92
   Summary Points   96

6. Oppositional Defiant Disorder   99
   Introduction   99
   Diagnostic Issues: DSM-5 and School-Based Services   99
   Cultural Issues Related to Oppositional Defiant Disorder in Youth   104
   Impact of Oppositional Defiant Disorder on Social–Emotional
         and Behavioral Functioning in School and Home Environments   105
   Impact of Oppositional Defiant Disorder on Learning in the Classroom   107
   Implications for School Psychologists   108
   Educational Supports   110
   School-Based Mental Health Interventions and Supports   111
   Summary Points   114

7. Intermittent Explosive Disorder   117
   Introduction   117
   Diagnostic Issues: DSM-5 and School-Based Services   117
   Cultural Issues Related to Intermittent Explosive Disorder in Youth   121
   Impact of Intermittent Explosive Disorder on Social–Emotional
         and Behavioral Functioning in School and Home Environments   123
   Impact of Intermittent Explosive Disorder on Learning in the Classroom   125
   Implications for School Psychologists   126
   Educational Supports   128
   School-Based Mental Health Interventions and Supports   129
   Summary Points   132

UNIT 4: MENTAL HEALTH DISORDERS IN CHILDREN AND ADOLESCENTS: ANXIETY DISORDERS

8. Generalized Anxiety Disorder   137
   Introduction   137
   Diagnostic Issues: DSM-5 and School-Based Services   137
   Cultural Issues Related to Generalized Anxiety Disorder in Youth   140
   Impact of Generalized Anxiety Disorder on Social–Emotional
      and Behavioral Functioning in School and Home Environments   142
   Impact of Generalized Anxiety Disorder on Learning in the Classroom   143
   Implications for School Psychologists   144
   Educational Supports   146
   School-Based Mental Health Interventions and Supports   146
   Summary Points   149

9. Separation Anxiety Disorder   153
   Introduction   153
   Diagnostic Issues: DSM-5 and School-Based Services   153
   Cultural Issues Related to Separation Anxiety Disorder in Youth   161
   Impact of Separation Anxiety Disorder on Social–Emotional
      and Behavioral Functioning in School and Home Environments   162
   Impact of Separation Anxiety Disorder on Learning in the Classroom   164
   Implications for School Psychologists   164
   Educational Supports   166
   School-Based Mental Health Interventions and Supports   166
   Summary Points   170

10. Social Anxiety Disorder   173
    Introduction   173
    Diagnostic Issues: DSM-5 and School-Based Services   174
    Cultural Issues Related to Social Anxiety Disorder in Youth   181
    Impact of Social Anxiety Disorder on Social–Emotional and Behavioral
       Functioning in School and Home Environments   182
    Impact of Social Anxiety Disorder on Learning in the Classroom   183
    Implications for School Psychologists   184
    Educational Supports   185
    School-Based Mental Health Interventions and Supports   186
    Summary Points   189

11. Selective Mutism   193
    Introduction   193
    Diagnostic Issues: DSM-5 and School-Based Services   193
    Cultural Issues Related to Selective Mutism in Youth   196
    Impact of Selective Mutism on Social–Emotional and Behavioral
       Functioning in School and Home Environments   197
    Impact of Selective Mutism on Learning in the Classroom   198
    Implications for School Psychologists   199
    Educational Supports   201
    School-Based Mental Health Interventions and Supports   202
    Summary Points   205

UNIT 5: MENTAL HEALTH DISORDERS IN CHILDREN AND ADOLESCENTS: MOOD DISORDERS

12. Major Depressive Disorder   211
    Introduction   211
    Diagnostic Issues: DSM-5 and School-Based Services   211
    Cultural Issues Related to Major Depressive Disorder in Youth   215
    *Impact of Major Depressive Disorder on Social–Emotional
        and Behavioral Functioning in School and Home Environments*   217
    Impact of Major Depressive Disorder on Learning in the Classroom   218
    Implications for School Psychologists   219
    Educational Supports   221
    School-Based Mental Health Interventions and Supports   221
    Summary Points   224

13. Disruptive Mood Dysregulation Disorder   227
    Introduction   227
    Diagnostic Issues: DSM-5 and School-Based Services   227
    Cultural Issues Related to Disruptive Mood Dysregulation Disorder in Youth   231
    *Impact of Disruptive Mood Dysregulation Disorder on Social–Emotional and Behavioral
        Functioning in School and Home Environments*   232
    *Impact of Disruptive Mood Dysregulation Disorder on Learning
        in the Classroom*   233
    Implications for School Psychologists   233
    Educational Supports   235
    School-Based Mental Health Interventions and Supports   236
    Summary Points   239

14. Persistent Depressive Disorder   243
    Introduction   243
    Diagnostic Issues: DSM-5 and School-Based Services   243
    Cultural Issues Related to Persistent Depressive Disorder in Youth   246
    *Impact of Persistent Depressive Disorder on Social–Emotional
        and Behavioral Functioning in School and Home Environments*   247
    Impact of Persistent Depressive Disorder on Learning in the Classroom   248
    Implications for School Psychologists   249
    Educational Supports   251
    School-Based Mental Health Interventions and Supports   251
    Summary Points   253

UNIT 6: MENTAL HEALTH DISORDERS IN CHILDREN AND ADOLESCENTS: OBSESSIVE-COMPULSIVE DISORDERS

15. Obsessive-Compulsive Disorder   259
    Introduction   259
    Diagnostic Issues Related to Obsessive-Compulsive Disorder   260
    Cultural Issues Related to Obsessive-Compulsive Disorder in Youth   265
    *Impact of Obsessive-Compulsive Disorder on Social–Emotional
        and Behavioral Functioning in School and Home Environments*   267
    Impact of Obsessive-Compulsive Disorder on Learning in the Classroom   272
    Implications for School Psychologists   274
    Educational and Social–Emotional Supports   279
    School-Based Mental Health Interventions for Obsessive-Compulsive Disorder   281
    Summary Points   284

16. Hoarding Disorder   289
    Introduction   289
    Diagnostic Issues: DSM-5 and School-Based Services   290
    Cultural Issues Related to Hoarding in Youth   293
    Impact of Hoarding on Social–Emotional and Behavioral Functioning
        in School and Home Environments   294
    Impact of Hoarding on Learning in the Classroom   295
    Implications for School Psychologists   296
    Educational Supports   299
    School-Based Mental Health Interventions and Supports   299
    Summary Points   302

UNIT 7: MENTAL HEALTH DISORDERS IN CHILDREN AND ADOLESCENTS: TRAUMA- AND STRESSOR-RELATED DISORDERS

17. Posttraumatic Stress Disorder   307
    Introduction   307
    Diagnostic Issues: PTSD and Developmental Trauma Disorder   308
    Cultural Issues Related to Posttraumatic Stress in Childhood   310
    Impact of Child Trauma on Social–Emotional and Behavioral
        Functioning in School and Home Environments   311
    Impact on Learning in the Classroom   314
    Implications for School Psychologists   315
    Educational and Social–Emotional Supports   320
    School-Based Mental Health Interventions   321
    Summary Points   324

18. Reactive Attachment Disorder   329
    Introduction   329
    Diagnostic Issues Related to Reactive Attachment Disorder   330
    Cultural Issues Related to Reactive Attachment Disorder in Youth   335
    Impact of Reactive Attachment Disorder on Social–Emotional
        and Behavioral Functioning in School and Home Environments   336
    Impact of Reactive Attachment Disorder on Learning in the Classroom   341
    Implications for School Psychologists   342
    Educational and Social–Emotional Supports   345
    School-Based Mental Health Interventions and Supports   347
    Summary Points   350

19. Disinhibited Social Engagement Disorder   355
    Introduction   355
    Diagnostic Issues Related to Disinhibited Social Engagement Disorder   355
    Cultural Issues Related to Disinhibited Social Engagement Disorder in Youth   359
    Impact on Disinhibited Social Engagement Disorder on Social–Emotional
        and Behavioral Functioning in School and Home Environments   359
    Impact of Disinhibited Social Engagement Disorder on Learning in the Classroom   363
    Implications for School Psychologists   363
    Educational Supports   366
    School-Based Mental Health Interventions and Supports   366
    Summary Points   369

Index   373

Preface

Child and Adolescent Psychopathology for School Psychology: A Practical Approach is designed as a textbook for school psychology graduate students enrolled in child and adolescent psychopathology courses. This textbook provides a comprehensive view of mental health disorders in children and adolescents that incorporates a school psychological approach in addressing issues related to diagnosis based on criteria of the *Diagnostic and Statistical Manual of Mental Disorders* (5th ed.; *DSM-5*; American Psychiatric Association, 2013) and educational disability determination under the federal legislation of the Individuals with Disabilities Education Improvement Act (IDEA) of 2004 (U.S. Department of Education, n.d.). It also examines culturally related issues associated with specific disorders and the social, emotional, and behavioral needs of youth with mental health conditions. Implications for school psychologists and ways in which they can have a pivotal role in helping schools meet the mental health and learning needs of children and adolescents are addressed. Furthermore, evidence-based educational and mental health supports and interventions applicable to schools are offered. In this preface, we provide information on (a) the overall goal of this textbook and our reasons for developing it, (b) tools created to support school psychology graduate students' learning of the content covered in the chapters, (c) instructor resources, (d) the intended audience, and (e) content covered in the major sections of the textbook.

OVERALL GOAL OF THE BOOK

Our overall goal in writing *Child and Adolescent Psychopathology for School Psychology: A Practical Approach* was to create a textbook for school psychology graduate students that provides training about child and adolescent mental health disorders from the viewpoint of a school psychologist. As experienced graduate educators in school psychology, we have found it challenging to find a child and adolescent psychopathology textbook that gives consideration to a school psychological perspective in identifying mental health problems in children and adolescents. Most child and adolescent psychopathology textbooks are written from a clinical psychology perspective and do not focus on ways in which children's and adolescents' mental health and educational needs can be addressed in schools through the work of school psychologists. We wanted to create a textbook that was specifically designed for school psychology graduate students that addressed issues beyond *DSM-5* criteria, focusing on how mental health conditions in youth can be addressed by the provision of school psychological services. We aimed to provide a comprehensive view of identifying mental health disorders in children and adolescents using *DSM-5* diagnostic features and examining disability categories under IDEA that multidisciplinary teams in schools may consider when determining eligibility for special education services. By addressing both types of classification systems (*DSM-5* and IDEA disability categories), school psychology graduate students gain knowledge of *DSM-5* criteria and eligibility criteria of possible educational disabilities. We also sought to guide school psychology graduate students in considering cultural issues that may be related to specific mental health disorders and the impact that a disorder may have on the child's or adolescent's social–emotional and behavioral functioning in school and at home. *Child and Adolescent Psychopathology for School Psychology: A Practical Approach* further advances the knowledge of school psychology graduate students by examining how learning is affected by a child's mental health struggles and how school psychologists can work with teachers to address the educational needs of students. Furthermore, it was our goal to guide future school psychologists in considering the multiple aspects of a child or adolescent's functioning to help them better recognize and understand the social–emotional and behavioral needs of youth with specific mental health disorders and the potential roles that they, as future school psychologists, can have in providing school-based mental health services. It is our hope that school psychology graduate educators who teach child and adolescent psychopathology courses and their students will find the textbook to be an effective, yet practical approach in which mental health conditions in youth can be addressed from a school psychological perspective.

LEARNING TOOLS

Child and Adolescent Psychopathology for School Psychology: A Practical Approach includes several learning tools that will be helpful to school psychology graduate students as they progress through the chapters on various mental health disorders. The *Quick Facts* feature in each chapter highlights major points about a particular disorder such as diagnostic issues, cultural considerations, impact on social–emotional and behavioral functioning, learning difficulties that might be experienced by the child or adolescent with mental health conditions, implications for school psychologists, and types of educational and mental health supports that could be applied in a school setting. Each chapter covering a specific mental health disorder includes a case study that discusses diagnostic features and challenges that the child and family may encounter and possible ways in which the school may respond. In addition, each chapter has a *Test Your Knowledge* feature, which includes multiple-choice and true–false questions as well as discussion questions. We have also included a list of resources in each chapter that may be helpful to school psychology graduate students in their future work with students, parents, and school personnel.

RESOURCES FOR INSTRUCTORS

In our textbook, *Child and Adolescent Psychopathology for School Psychology: A Practical Approach*, we have provided resources that may be helpful for instructors. Within each chapter, learning objectives as well as a few test questions and discussion questions are provided. Each chapter also has a case study that can be an effective tool for instructors in helping students conceptualize a case and learn how educational and mental health needs may be addressed in the school.

Ancillary materials are also provided for course instructors. These include an *Instructor's Manual*, which offers (a) National Association of School Psychologists (NASP) domains (2020), (b) learning objectives, (c) chapter summary, (d) discussion questions with suggested main points that need to be covered in the response, and (e) useful resources to consider for each chapter. As an instructional tool, a *PowerPoint presentation* has been created for each chapter that highlights the main points covered. Instructors can easily add more content to the PowerPoints. In addition, a *test bank* of 10 multiple-choice questions covering material from each chapter is also included in the ancillary materials for instructors.

INTENDED AUDIENCE

The audience for *Child and Adolescent Psychopathology for School Psychology: A Practical Approach* is intended to be school psychology graduate students enrolled in a school psychology training program. We hope that school psychology graduate educators will find the book useful in helping graduate students in their programs to understand the differences between *DSM-5* diagnostic and educational disability (i.e., IDEA) criteria and the ways in which mental health conditions can affect a child's or adolescent's functioning across social, emotional, behavioral, and learning domains. Examples of titles of graduate-level courses for which this book is intended include the following:

- Child psychopathology,
- Child and adolescent psychopathology,
- Psychopathology of childhood and adolescence,
- Developmental psychopathology in educational settings,
- Developmental psychopathology of childhood,

- Advanced child and adolescent psychopathology, and
- Child and adolescent abnormal psychology.

ORGANIZATION OF THE TEXTBOOK CONTENT

The content of the book is organized into seven parts. In the first part of the book, mental health disorders in youth and the need for school-based mental health services are addressed. The remaining parts of the book include Chapters 2 through 19, which focus on specific categories of mental health disorders. Each chapter is organized into the following sections:

- Introduction,
- Diagnostic Issues,
- Cultural Issues,
- Impact on Social–Emotional and Behavioral Functioning in School and Home Environments,
- Impact on Learning in the Classroom,
- Implications for School Psychologists,
- Educational Supports,
- School-Based Mental Health Interventions and Supports,
- Case Study: Background and Discussion, and
- Chapter Resources.

Unit I: Addressing Child and Adolescent Mental Health Disorders in Schools

The first part of the book includes a chapter that provides the audience with an introduction to child and adolescent mental health. The first chapter includes information on the prevalence of mental health disorders in youth; stress-related challenges that impact mental health such as poverty, racial stress, social media, and cyberbullying; risk factors; and protective factors. The role of school psychologists in addressing mental health conditions in youth at school and the importance of school-based mental health services are discussed. The chapter also examines the identification of mental health problems in schools and compares the *DSM-5* diagnosis of mental health disorders and educational disabilities classified under IDEA.

Unit 2: Mental Health Disorders in Children and Adolescents: Neurodevelopmental Disorders

Chapters 2 through 4 focus on neurodevelopmental disorders. Specific disorders covered in this section include attention deficit hyperactivity disorder (ADHD), intellectual disabilities, and autism spectrum disorder.

Unit 3: Mental Health Disorders in Children and Adolescents: Disruptive, Impulse-Control, and Conduct Disorders

The third part of the textbook includes Chapters 5 through 7, which examine conduct disorder, oppositional defiant disorder, and intermittent explosive disorder.

Unit 4: Mental Health Disorders in Children and Adolescents: Anxiety Disorders

Chapters 8 through 11 focus on anxiety disorders in youth. Specific disorders examined in this part of the textbook include generalized anxiety disorder, separation anxiety, social anxiety, and selective mutism.

Unit 5: Mental Health Disorders in Children and Adolescents: Mood Disorders

Part 5 of the textbook includes chapters that examine three mood disorders in youth: major depressive disorder, disruptive mood dysregulation disorder, and persistent depressive disorder (formerly referred to as *dysthymia*).

Unit 6: Mental Health Disorders in Children and Adolescents: Obsessive-Compulsive Disorders

This part of the textbook includes Chapters 15 and 16, which focus on obsessive-compulsive disorder (OCD) and hoarding disorder.

Unit 7: Mental Health Disorders in Children and Adolescents: Trauma- and Stressor-Related Disorders

The content in Part 7 of the textbook focuses on trauma- and stressor-related disorders. Chapters 17 through 19 examine posttraumatic stress disorder (PTSD), reactive attachment disorder (RAD), and disinhibited social engagement disorder (DSED).

Terry Diamanduros
P. Dawn Tysinger
Jeffrey A. Tysinger
Pamela A. Fenning

REFERENCES

American Psychiatric Association. (2013). *Diagnostic and statistical manual of mental disorders* (5th ed.). https://doi.org/10.1176/appi.books.9780890425596

National Association of School Psychologists. (2020). *The professional standards of the National Association of School Psychologists*. Author.

U.S. Department of Education. (n.d.). *Individuals with Disabilities Education Improvement Act*. https://sites.ed.gov/idea/

Instructor Resources

Child and Adolescent Psychopathology for School Psychology includes quality resources for the instructor. Faculty who have adopted the text may gain access to these resources by emailing textbook@springerpub.com.

Instructor resources include:
- **Instructor's Manual**
    o NASP (2020) Domains
    o Learning Objectives
    o Chapter Summaries
    o Discussion Questions
    o Useful Resources for Instructors
- **Test Bank**
    o Multiple-Choice Questions With Answers/Rationales
- **Chapter-Based PowerPoint Presentations**

UNIT 1

ADDRESSING CHILD AND ADOLESCENT MENTAL HEALTH DISORDERS IN SCHOOLS

CHAPTER 1

Child and Adolescent Mental Health

LEARNING OBJECTIVES

- Gain an understanding of the current status of child and adolescent mental health.
- Describe current stress-related events that may impact a child's mental health.
- Discuss the need for school-based mental health services.
- Discuss the role of school psychologists in the provision of mental health services.
- Compare the use of the *Diagnostic and Statistical Manual of Mental Disorders* (5th ed.; *DSM-5*; American Psychiatric Association, 2013) in diagnosing mental health disorders in medical/clinical settings and the Individuals with Disabilities Education Improvement Act (IDEA) in identifying disability categories in schools.

INTRODUCTION

Mental Health in Children and Adolescents

Social–emotional development provides a child with the skills needed to interact socially with others and to express their feelings in appropriate ways. Children who are mentally healthy have effective coping skills, view themselves positively, interact appropriately in social situations, and are able to regulate their emotions. However, some children struggle in managing their emotions and behaviors and may become overwhelmed in social situations. They may begin to exhibit behavioral outbursts, or "meltdowns," because they cannot manage their emotions and begin to socially isolate themselves because it is too overwhelming to be around others. In the United States, concern about the mental health status of infants, children, and adolescents has been growing for over 20 years and was even considered a public health crisis two decades ago (U.S. Department of Health and Human Services, 2000). Specific concerns included inaccurate diagnoses, limited availability of research-based treatments and services, limited access to available services, and unidentified/untreated mental health problems in youth. In response to the need for a call to action, the U.S. Surgeon General held a conference in 2000 titled "Children's Mental Health: Developing a National Action Agenda" (U.S. Department of Health and Human Services, 2000). Although that conference took place over 20 years ago, the same concerns about children's mental health persist today.

According to the American Psychological Association (n.d.), it is estimated that approximately 15 million children and adolescents have diagnosable mental health disorders. Although this number is alarming, it is equally, if not more concerning that only 7% of children who are in need of psychological services actually receive therapeutic services from a mental health provider. Scholars have examined the impact of adverse childhood experiences (ACEs) on a child's mental and physical health. This type of experience is one that is stressful and potentially traumatic and includes events such as abuse or living in environments that may be emotionally or physically harmful (Boullier & Blair, 2018). It is estimated that almost 35 million children in the United States have experienced at least one ACE (Child and Adolescent Health Measurement Initiative, 2013). Children in our country today face several psychosocial challenges that can perhaps be viewed as ACEs that affect their lives on a daily basis. These stress-related challenges include poverty, racial stress, school violence, and social media and cyberbullying.

It is estimated that approximately 15 million children and adolescents have diagnosable mental health disorders.

POVERTY

The Children's Defense Fund *State of America's Children 2021* report indicated that children in the United States are the "poorest age group in America, with children of color and young children suffering the highest poverty rates" (2021, p. 10). The report found that one in seven children, or 10.5 million children, live in poverty. The findings of the report also indicated that approximately 71% of children living in poverty were children of color and almost one in six children under the age of 6 were poor, with approximately half of the children living in extreme poverty (Children's Defense Fund, 2021).

Scholars have reported that children living in poverty experience difficulties in self-regulation (regulating one's emotions and behaviors), executive functioning (cognitive skills such as working memory and planning), impulsivity, inattention, poor peer relationships, and defiance (American Academy of Pediatrics [AAP], 2016). These types of problems render a child vulnerable to the onset of mental health disorders such as attention deficit hyperactivity disorder (ADHD). The AAP (2016) reports that stress associated with poverty, such as inadequate food, energy, housing, and transportation, can influence parenting. Poverty is also associated with poor developmental and psychosocial outcomes (AAP, 2016).

RACIAL STRESS

Scholars have examined the impact of racism on the social–emotional well-being of minority youth. Evidence in the literature indicates that continued racial discrimination against Black adolescents results in increased symptoms of anxiety, depression, and trauma (Priest et al., 2013). Graham and colleagues (2017) have noted that boys of color may experience at least five ACEs prior to their 18th birthday. Other scholars have found that, on average, Black adolescents experience race-related acts five times per day (English et al., 2020). Examples of race-related acts included being teased because of one's race or being told an offensive joke. Community violence against youth of color has been found to be associated with symptoms of posttraumatic stress (Deane et al., 2020). The social–emotional well-being of youth of color can be negatively influenced by community violence (Lanier et al., 2017), and some scholars contend that the impact of this violence may be intensified by racial stress (Saleem et al., 2020). Over time, race-related acts can have a cumulative effect on a child or adolescent that makes them sensitive to situations in which a threat might be experienced (National Child Traumatic Stress Network [NCTSN], Justice Consortium, Schools Committee, and Culture Consortium, 2017). Racial stress may be exhibited as anxiety, depression, and hypervigilance as well as maladaptive behaviors such as aggression (NCTSN, Justice Consortium, Schools Committee, and Culture Consortium, 2017). According to some scholars, race-related events can be perceived as chronic violence that can make a young child or adolescent of color vulnerable emotionally and at risk for posttraumatic stress disorder (PTSD; Tynes et al., 2019). It is important to keep in mind that media coverage of high-profile cases involving violent acts against an ethnic group may be traumatic triggers for a child (Proctor et al., 2020).

SCHOOL VIOLENCE

School violence, unfortunately, is not a new occurrence. In fact, scholars consider it a public health concern (Janosz et al., 2008). The Centers for Disease Control and Prevention's (CDC) Youth Risk Behavior Survey (2019) reports that one in five high school students acknowledges being bullied at school, and about 8% of high school students have been in a fight at school. A study conducted by Flannery et al. (2004) examined exposure of violence to children in grades 3 through 12. Approximately 56% of children had witnessed another child being beaten up, and 87% watched someone else being slapped or hit (Flannery et al., 2004). The study also revealed that about 44% of students had been threatened when they were at school. The authors found that students with exposure to high levels of violence at school tended to experience more clinical levels of trauma than students exposed to low levels of violence at school (Flannery et al., 2004). Other scholars have found that school violence victimization was positively linked to depressive symptoms (Estévez et al., 2005) and observing violence at school was a better predictor of subsequent externalizing behaviors than actual victimization (Janosz et al., 2008). Based on the results of the CDC's Youth Risk Behavior Survey (2019), more than 7% of high school students surveyed indicated that they had been threatened or harmed with a weapon at school and approximately 9% of students had not attended school because they felt that they would not be safe while at school. Mental health outcomes of youth exposed to mass shootings include depression, anxiety, traumatic stress, suicide, and substance abuse (Cimolai et al., 2021). One concerning line of research proposes that the internet could provide a support group for male shooters if they decide to shoot peers at their school (Markward et al., 2001).

SOCIAL MEDIA AND CYBERBULLYING

Although social media may serve as a way for people to connect and maintain friendships, its use as a tool to cyberbully others can have a concerning impact on the social–emotional and behavioral well-being of youths. For example, Richards and colleagues (2015) reviewed studies to examine the impact of cyberbullying on the health of children and adolescents. The findings revealed the greatest impact was on their mental health. Specifically, the findings indicated an association between social media use and self-esteem and body image. The authors emphasize that cause and effect is difficult to determine and suggest that more research is needed. Other studies have found that cyberbullying was associated with an increase in depression. Some scholars have conducted longitudinal studies to examine the relationship between cyberbullying and symptoms of depression and anxiety. Rose and Tynes (2015) followed a sample of youth between grades 6 and 12. The study was done over a 3-year period. The results of the study revealed a reciprocal relationship between cyber-victimization and depression and cyber-victimization and anxiety (Rose & Tynes, 2015). Overall, these findings revealed that cyberbullying may have adverse impacts on the mental well-being of children and adolescents.

Prevalence

As noted earlier, concern has been expressed by professionals about the number of youth with mental health problems. The CDC (n.d.-a) reports data from the National Survey of Student Health on the prevalence of mental health disorders. According to the CDC (n.d.-b), approximately 13% to 20% (one out of five) have a mental health condition. Among externalizing behaviors, ADHD occurred most frequently, whereas anxiety disorders occurred more often than other internalizing disorders.

EXTERNALIZING DISORDERS: ATTENTION DEFICIT HYPERACTIVITY DISORDER AND BEHAVIORAL PROBLEMS

ADHD occurs more frequently than other disorders. Among children between the ages of two and 17, approximately 9.4%, or 6.1 million, are diagnosed with ADHD (CDC, n.d.-a). With regard to emotional–behavioral types of referrals, most school psychologists are likely to get more referrals regarding issues related to ADHD than any other disorder. Among children between three and 17, disruptive behaviors are diagnosed in about 7.4% of children in this age range, which is about 4.5 million children (CDC, n.d.-a). It should be noted that boys are more likely to be diagnosed with ADHD than are girls (CDC, n.d.-b). In addition, behavior problems are reportedly more common in children between the ages of six and 11 compared to either younger or older children (CDC, n.d.-a).

INTERNALIZING DISORDERS: ANXIETY AND DEPRESSION

Among internalizing disorders, anxiety disorders occur most frequently in the general population. Based on the data reported by the CDC (n.d.-a), anxiety disorders occur in 7.1% of children between the ages of three and seventeen, or 4.4 million. It occurs more frequently than depression, which is diagnosed in 3.2% of children and adolescents between the ages of three and 17, or 1.9 million children. It should be noted that anxiety and depression become more common with increased age.

Comorbidity

When disorders coexist with each other, this is referred to as *comorbidity*, which is associated with worse outcomes. According to the CDC (n.d.-a), about three in four children (73.8%) with depression between the ages of three and 17 will most likely be diagnosed with anxiety. Also, about one in two children (47.2%) with depression between the ages of three and 17 will be diagnosed with a disruptive behavior disorder. Among children ages three and 17 who are diagnosed with anxiety, more than one in three (37.9%) will also have behavior problems and about one in three (32.3%) will also be diagnosed with depression. With regard to comorbidity among children ages three to 17 with behavior problems, more than one in three (36.6%) will also be diagnosed with an anxiety disorder and approximately one in five (20.3%) will also be diagnosed with depression.

Risk Factors and Protective Factors

Vulnerability to the effects of a mental health disorder is influenced by the presence of risk and protective factors. It is helpful for the school psychologist to have a thorough developmental history and background information on the student to determine whether there are factors that make the child more at risk to the influence of mental health problems or whether there are factors in the background that protect them. According to a report by the U.S. Surgeon General (U.S. Public Health Service et al., 2009), risk factors are linked with a higher chance of developing some negative outcome. For example, risk factors may be biological, resulting from genetics, or familial, such as having a family member with a mental illness. Common risk factors for developing mental health problems include low self-esteem, negative family home environment, stressful events, peer rejection, etc. (U.S. Public Health Service et al., 2009). On the other hand, there are factors known as *protective factors that* help protect the child from the adverse effects of mental illness. Examples of protective factors include having good coping skills, high self-esteem, supportive relationships, and so on (U.S. Public Health Service et al., 2009).

> Common risk factors for developing mental health problems include low self-esteem, a negative home environment, stressful events, and peer rejection.

ADDRESSING CHILD AND ADOLESCENT MENTAL HEALTH IN THE SCHOOLS: THE ROLE OF SCHOOL PSYCHOLOGISTS

The Need to Address Child and Adolescent Mental Health in the Schools

In 2004, the Committee on School Health of the American Pediatrics Association published a policy statement on the need for school-based mental health services. The statement noted that, at that time, more than 20% of youth experienced mental health problems. The statement acknowledged the responsibility of the healthcare profession to inform interdisciplinary professionals who work with children and adolescents about the adverse impact that mental health problems may have on children and the need for school-based mental health services. According to the policy, the need for mental health services is evident in the rising number of children struggling with mental health conditions who are seen by pediatricians. In a 20-year span, the percentage of children with psychiatric problems seen in pediatric clinics increased from 7% to 19% (Kelleher et al., 2000, as cited in American Pediatric Association Committee on School Health, 2004). School violence, bullying, and suicides among youth were commonly reported events at that time. Concern was expressed regarding the outcomes of untreated mental health disorders among the young such as increased school dropout rates, juvenile incarceration rates, and family dysfunction. With regard to the types of mental health disorders experienced by youths, it was reported that 13% experienced anxiety, 6.2% had a mood disorder, 10.3% had disruptive behaviors, and 2% experienced substance use (American Pediatric Association Committee on School Health, 2004). The policy also noted barriers that are associated with the provision of mental health services in settings outside the school. These barriers included financial constraints for services not covered by insurance, transportation issues in getting to facilities, and the stigma associated with mental health problems. Barriers such as these can lead to premature termination of therapeutic services. On the other hand, benefits of school-based mental health programs noted in the policy included identifying mental health problems early, which can lead to children and adolescents obtaining therapeutic services. It is interesting to note that the policy statement strongly advocated for collaboration between school mental health providers and the pediatric community and endorsed the use of a system of service support within schools.

Others have also recognized the need for school-based mental health services to address the emotional and behavioral needs in children and adolescents. Davis and colleagues (2006) point out that much attention has been given to documenting prevalence rates of mental health problems in this population, yet in the literature, less attention has been given to provision of school-based mental health services. Davis et al. also note that the problem of untreated mental health problems in youth had, however, been acknowledged at the federal level by the President's New Freedom Commission on Mental Health (2003), which acknowledged that services could be provided in schools to address the mental health needs of youth. Perfect and Morris (2011) note prevalence rates indicate that as many as 20% of youth experience emotional and behavioral problems, including anxiety, obsessive-compulsive disorder, and disruptive behaviors. The authors contend that untreated mental health conditions can lead to school-related problems such as absenteeism, discipline problems, poor grades, grade retention, and juvenile delinquency (Perfect & Morris, 2011). Perfect and Morris (2011) emphasize the need for the provision of school-based mental health services and encourage support for school psychologists as providers of mental health services in schools. Similarly, the National Association of School Psychologists (NASP; 2015) points out the connection between emotional and behavioral wellness and positive gains in achievement and graduation rates, safe school environments, reduced disciplinary actions, and prevention of risk-taking behaviors. In addition, these factors are important to the future lives of students in regard to interpersonal relationships, higher salaries, higher employment stability, and decreased likelihood of being involved in criminal acts (NASP, 2015).

Although these studies support the provision of school-based mental health services, one must also examine the results of studies investigating the effectiveness of such services. Salerno (2016) reviewed research studies investigating mental health awareness interventions that were targeted to improve emotional and behavioral outcomes in K-12 students in the United States. The findings of the study revealed that there was improvement in knowledge about mental health in all studies and most studies revealed improvement in attitudes toward mental health and help-seeking behaviors. The authors concluded improvement existed in regard to mental health, but more research is needed because there were methodological problems in some of the research studies reviewed. O'Connor et al. (2018) also conducted a systematic review of studies that investigated the effectiveness of school-based mental health services. Their analysis revealed three themes of effectiveness related to school-based mental health interventions that include help-seeking and coping, social–emotional well-being, and psychoeducational effectiveness. Overall, the authors concluded that the findings were promising, but more robust research is needed.

National Association of School Psychologists Practice Model and School Psychologists as Mental Health Providers

School psychologists are in a unique position to advocate for provision of mental health services in the school and to deliver school-based mental health services. The role of school psychologists as mental health providers is endorsed by NASP (2020) as evident in its Model for Comprehensive and Integrative School Psychological Services, which is often referred to as the *NASP Practice Model* (NASP, 2021).

The NASP endorses the role of school psychologists as mental health providers in schools.

The model (NASP, 2020) consists of 10 domains: Domain 1: Data-Based Decision-Making; Domain 2: Consultation and Collaboration; Domain 3: Academic Interventions and Instructional

Supports; Domain 4: Mental and Behavioral Health Services and Interventions; Domain 5: School-Wide Practices to Promote Learning; Domain 6: Services to Promote Safe and Supportive Schools; Domain 7: Family, School, and Community Collaboration; Domain 8: Equitable Practices for Diverse Student Populations; Domain 9: Research and Evidence-Based Practices; and Domain 10: Legal, Ethical, and Professional Practice.

Domain 4 of the NASP Practice Model, Mental and Behavioral Health Services and Interventions (NASP, 2020), acknowledges the unique training preparation of school psychologists, their knowledge of factors that influence a child's mental health and behavior, and their understanding of supports needed. NASP encourages school psychologists in their role as mental health providers in the school and in their collaborative work with other school professionals to evaluate student need. NASP states:

> *School psychologists understand the biological, cultural, developmental, and social influences on mental and behavioral health; behavioral and emotional impacts on learning; and evidence-based strategies to promote social-emotional functioning. School psychologists, in collaboration with others, design, implement, and evaluate services that promote resilience and positive behavior, support socialization and adaptive skills, and enhance mental and behavioral health.* (2020, p. 5)

Moreover, comprehensive mental health services should be suitable for the learning environment. School psychologists understand how children's social–emotional and behavioral well-being, learning, and family lives combine to affect behavior in the classroom, as well as how teaching that occurs in the classroom and the context of the school all interact together to guide children's and adolescents' development and well-being (NASP, 2021).

In providing comprehensive school-based mental health services, there are specific roles that school psychologists can have to ensure the social–emotional and behavioral well-being of the children with whom they work. NASP (2021) has identified school psychologists as being leaders in the implementation of Multi-Tiered Systems of Support (MTSS) in schools. MTSS typically consist of three tiers that are used to deliver supports and services of increasing intensity to meet the needs of students. The first tier provides universal social–emotional wellness and behavioral supports to all students. The second tier provides services that are targeted for students identified as needing additional social–emotional and/or behavioral services beyond those provided in Tier 1 that could be provided in a small group. The third tier provides more intensive mental health supports and interventions to individual students (NASP, 2016). Through the use of a framework, such as MTSS, that provides academic, social–emotional, and behavioral supports, children's mental health needs can be identified and addressed before they fully manifest (as in the case of universal prevention), worsen, or become long-lasting. MTSS can also provide services that are data driven and increasingly intensive for individual children (NASP, 2021). NASP (2021) has proposed a continuum of comprehensive school-based mental and behavioral services that consists of the following levels: (a) universal wellness promotion and prevention services such as social–emotional learning programs and universal screening for all students, (b) early identification of and support for mental and behavioral health concerns which could include services such as trauma-informed services, (c) targeted school mental and behavioral interventions such as group counseling and functional behavioral assessments, (d) intensive school interventions such as direct therapeutic interventions for individual students, and (e) intensive community services such as psychiatric services or family counseling.

NASP (2016) has aligned this comprehensive school-based mental health model with federal legislation, the Every Student Succeeds Act (ESSA), which recognizes the importance of comprehensive and integrative mental and behavioral health services. ESSA acknowledges school psychologists are qualified mental health professionals and specialized instructional support personnel who are instrumental in (a) school and district assessment and accountability, (b) provision of supports that are targeted toward school improvement, (c) efforts to enhance school climate and school safety, and (d) ensuring access to high-quality comprehensive learning and mental-health–related supports (Every Student Succeeds Act, 2015). NASP (2016) contends that, in addition to providing direct services to children and adolescents, school psychologists can be instrumental in (a) establishing and delivering system-wide prevention supports delivered in MTSS; (b) understanding and interpreting data for program-planning purposes; (c) creating and monitoring program services; (d) consulting with professionals at the system-wide, classroom, and individual case levels; (e) creating crisis prevention and response protocols; as well as (f) planning and coordinating services with community providers (NASP, 2016). Moreover, NASP (2016) contends that school psychologists can effectively support decision-making across levels that will lead to improved MTSS services.

The framework for the comprehensive school-based mental health services proposed by NASP (2021) includes a continuum of school and community services. Community services that some children may need may go beyond the capability of the school. Hence, community resources and support may become involved in the tiered system at the point when the intensity of the support increases. Integrating both school and community services requires much planning and coordination between school and community professionals. School psychologists could be involved in these efforts and effectively guide them by establishing partnerships with community sources such as mental health clinics or agencies that can provide more intensive services. In order to reduce an overlap or redundancy in services and to avoid creating stress for the family, clear communication between the school and community agency regarding the contribution of each group is essential. Each group must understand what its role will be in this partnership. As part of this partnership, school psychologists would play a pivotal role as a liaison between the school and community mental health providers (NASP, 2021).

IDENTIFICATION OF MENTAL HEALTH PROBLEMS IN SCHOOLS: *DIAGNOSTIC AND STATISTICAL MANUAL OF MENTAL DISORDERS* VERSUS INDIVIDUALS WITH DISABILITIES EDUCATION IMPROVEMENT ACT

As mental health providers in schools, it is important for school psychologists to understand the classification system used by the community resources or agencies providing more intensive mental health services as well as the classification system used in the schools to identify a child as having a disability. Knowledge of *Diagnostic and Statistical Manual of Mental Disorders* (5th ed.; *DSM-5*; American Psychiatric Association, 2013) disorders provides school psychologists with an understanding of symptoms associated with a particular disorder and how symptoms may manifest in the classroom and impact the child or adolescent in the school setting. Differences in the medical and educational models are described in the next section.

Medical Model: The Use of the *DSM-5* Classification

In medical or clinical settings, such as a child psychiatric outpatient clinic or a community-based mental health agency, mental health disorders are diagnosed using the *DSM-5* (American Psychiatric Association, 2013). The first version of the *DSM* was published in 1844 as a "statistical classification of institutionalized mental patients" (American Psychiatric Association, 2013, p. 6). Its purpose was to enhance communication about the various types of clients served in hospital settings. As noted by the American Psychiatric Association (2013), the *DSM* underwent major revisions to evolve into a system that allowed psychiatrists, clinical psychologists, and other mental health professions to use a common language to describe the primary features of a mental disorder. In the current edition, *DSM-5* (American Psychiatric Association, 2013), diagnostic criteria are presented and based on these, the mental health professional determines whether diagnostic criteria are met for a particular disorder. The *DSM-5* indicates that it is designed to help guide medical and clinical practitioners in decisions regarding treatment and management of disorders. Within the *DSM-5*, disorders are classified by major groups that share a common characteristic. For example, neurodevelopmental disorders, such as an intellectual disability, ADHD, or autism spectrum disorder (ASD), all have a neurodevelopmental basis. There were major revisions from the previous version that are described in the manual (American Psychiatric Association, 2013). (For those who would like more information about these changes, please see American Psychiatric Association, 2013.)

In the medical or clinical setting, a child or adolescent may be referred to a clinical or medical professional who evaluates the child to determine whether a mental disorder is present. Although comprehensive psychiatric or psychological evaluations may differ, they share some common elements. During this evaluation, the practitioner will ask the parent and child (if developmentally appropriate) to describe the symptoms or behaviors that the child or adolescent is experiencing (John Hopkins, n.d.). Questions will attempt to ascertain when the behavior began, the duration of the behavior, how often it occurs, the types of conditions in which it occurs, and so on. The evaluation also attempts to determine the effect that the behaviors have had on the child (John Hopkins, n.d.). A criterion for many disorders within the *DSM-5* is whether the symptoms have had a significant impact on the child's or adolescent's functioning. For example, a medical or clinical professional evaluating a child for suspected ADHD will ask questions that are related to symptoms of inattentiveness and hyperactivity/impulsivity and how the child's behavior has affected school functioning, such as whether there are indications that the child has a difficulty time staying seated, listening to the teacher, organizing material, and so forth. Information is gathered regarding whether these types of behaviors have impacted the child's functioning, such as a decline in grades or disciplinary action for disruptive behaviors. There may be other components to the evaluation depending on the professional conducting the evaluation. For example, a licensed clinical psychologist may also do a psychological assessment using norm-referenced standardized tests, whereas a psychiatrist, who is a medical doctor, may assess the need for medication to manage the presenting symptoms. Following the evaluation, the clinical or medical professional will determine whether the child or adolescent meets the criteria for a *DSM-5* diagnosis. Based on all of the information gathered during the evaluation, a treatment plan will be developed if applicable.

Educational Model: The Use of the IDEA Disability Classification

In school, the classification of disabilities is based on the Individuals with Disabilities Education Improvement Act (IDEA) of 2004. This federal legislation originated from the Education for All Handicapped Children Act (Public Law 94-142), which stipulated that students with disabilities have the right to a free, appropriate public education (FAPE; Salvia et al., 2016). This law also stipulated that students with disabilities must be educated in the least restrictive environment possible, have an Individual Education Program (IEP), and be assessed with instruments and practices that are fair and unbiased. It also indicates that parents of students with disabilities have the right to inspect their child's school record and to challenge changes in the child's placement. In 1986, amendments were made to the law to ensure that the law extended to preschoolers with disabilities and that every school district "conduct a multidisciplinary assessment and develop an individualized family service plan for every preschooler with a disability" (Salvia et al., 2016, p. 26). Four years later, the law was reauthorized in 1990 and became known as *IDEA* (U.S. Department of Education, n.d.). IDEA was reauthorized again in 1997 and in 2004. IDEA of 2004 includes 13 disability categories. These are Autism, Deaf-Blindness, Developmental Delay, Emotional Disturbance, Hearing Impairment, Intellectual Disability, Multiple Disabilities, Orthopedic Impairment, Other Health Impairment, Specific Learning Disability, Speech–Language Impairment, Traumatic Brain Injury, and Visual Impairment (U.S. Department of Education, n.d.). Each of the 13 disability categories has a set of eligibility criteria that must be met.

Teachers make many of the referrals for an evaluation, although parents may request an evaluation. Prior to getting a referral, students will have received supports or interventions to address any social–emotional, behavioral, or learning problems that were evident in the classroom. Students who fail to respond to these supports or interventions may be referred for an evaluation to determine eligibility for special education services. Once parental consent is obtained, hearing and vision tests are conducted by the school nurse. The school psychologists and other members of the multidisciplinary team will have 60 days to conduct an evaluation (U.S. Department of Education, n.d.). Once the evaluation is completed, a multidisciplinary team reviews all of the assessment data collected from multiple sources and determines whether the child is considered a student with a disability under IDEA. To be determined to be a student with a disability, eligibility criteria for one of the 13 disability categories must be met and a need demonstrated for special education services and/or related services for the child to be successful in the classroom (Salvia et al., 2016). Hence, the child's disability is found to have an adverse impact on the child's classroom performance. If a child is found to be eligible for special education services, the team has 30 days to develop an IEP, which is a legal written plan that identifies the specific special education services the child will receive (Salvia et al., 2016).

If the multidisciplinary team determines that the child is not in need of special education services, consideration may be given to developing a 504 plan, which determines accommodations needed for the child to succeed. This plan is provided through Section 504 of the Rehabilitation Act of 1973, which is civil rights legislation. It provides students with any type of disability equal access to services if their disability limits an area of daily life functioning.

CONCLUDING REMARKS

As future school psychologists, the services that you provide to the school will play a major role in the decisions made about the children's education. These decisions can influence their time spent in the educational system and affect their future career/vocational choices.

SUMMARY POINTS

- The prevalence of mental health disorders in children and adolescents is high.
- School-based mental health services are needed to address the social–emotional and behavioral needs of youth.
- Domain 4 of the NASP Practice Model applies to the role of school psychologists in regard to the provision of school-based mental health services.
- While IDEA classification of disabilities is used in schools to identify children in need of special education services, the *DSM-5* classification of mental health disorders is used to make a medical diagnosis.

TEST YOUR KNOWLEDGE

1. Which of the following domains of the NASP Practice Model supports the role of school psychologists as mental health providers?
   a. Domain 2
   b. Domain 3
   c. Domain 4
   d. Domain 5

2. Protective factors help protect, or decrease the likelihood of, the child developing a mental health condition.
   a. True
   b. False

3. The *DSM-5* is the classification system used to identify disability categories for special education services.
   a. True
   b. False

4. Common risk factors for developing mental health problems include low self-esteem, a negative home environment, stressful events, and peer rejection.
   a. True
   b. False

5. Which of the following disorders is the most common among children and adolescents?
   a. ADHD
   b. Anxiety disorders
   c. Depressive disorder
   d. Disruptive behavior problems

Answers: (1) c, (2) a, (3) b, (4) a, (5) a.

DISCUSSION QUESTIONS

1. Describe the differences between the medical model used to classify disorders with the *DSM-5* and the education model, which uses IDEA disability categories.

2. Identify three risk factors and three protective factors that are associated with mental health problems.

3. Discuss how racial stress can impact a child's mental health.

4. Discuss the need for school-based mental health services.

5. Discuss the role of school psychologists as providers of mental health services in schools.

CHAPTER RESOURCES

National Association of School Psychologists *Comprehensive School-Based Mental and Behavioral Health Services and School Psychologists*: www.nasponline.org/resources-and-publications/resources-and-podcasts/mental-health/school-psychology-and-mental-health/comprehensive-school-based-mental-and-behavioral-health-services-and-school-psychologists

National Association of School Psychologists *Practice Model: Improving Outcomes for Students and Schools*: www.nasponline.org/standards-and-certification/nasp-practice-model

National Association of School Psychologists *Position Statement: Ensuring High-Quality, Comprehensive, and Integrated Student Supports*: http://www.nasponline.org/research-and-policy/policy-priorities/position-statements

National Association of School Psychologists *The Professional Standards of the National Association of School Psychologists*: www.nasponline.org/standards-and-certification/nasp-2020-professional-standards-adopted

KEY REFERENCES

Only key references appear in the print edition. The full reference list appears in the digital product on Springer Publishing Connect: connect.springerpub.com/content/book/978-0-8261-3587-2/part/part01/chapter/ch01

American Pediatric Association Committee on School Health. (2004). School-based mental health services. *Pediatrics, 113*(6), 1839–1845. https://doi.org/10.1542/peds.113.6.1839

American Psychological Association. (n.d.). *Children's mental health*. https://www.apa.org/pi/families/children-mental-health

Child and Adolescent Health Measurement Initiative. (2013). *Overview of adverse child and family experiences among US children*. Data Resource Center, supported by Cooperative Agreement 1-U59-MC06980-01 from the U.S. Department of Health and Human Services, Health Resources and Services Administration, Maternal and Child Health Bureau. https://www.childhealthdata.org

Deane, K., Richards, M., & Santiago, C. D. (2020). Violence exposure, posttraumatic stress, and affect variability among African American youth: A time sampling approach. *Development and Psychopathology, 33*(3), 1085–1096. https://doi.org/10.1017/S095457942000036X

English, D., Lambert, S. F., Tynes, B. M., Bowleg, L., Zea, M. C., & Howard, L. C. (2020). Daily multidimensional racial discrimination among Black U.S. American adolescents. *Journal of Applied Developmental Psychology, 66*. https://doi.org/10.1016/j.appdev.2019.101068

Individuals with Disabilities Education Improvement Act. (2004). 20 U.S.C. § 1400.

National Association of School Psychologists. (2015). *School psychologists: Qualified health professionals providing child and adolescent mental and behavioral health services* [White paper]. Author.

National Association of School Psychologists. (2016). *Ensuring high quality, comprehensive, and integrated specialized instructional support services* [Position statement]. Author.

National Association of School Psychologists. (2021). *Comprehensive school-based mental and behavioral health services and school psychologists* [Handout]. Author.

Perfect, M. M., & Morris, R. J. (2011). Delivering school-based mental health services by school psychologists: Education, training, and ethical issues. *Psychology in the Schools, 48*(10), 1049–1063. https://doi.org/10.1002/pits.20612

UNIT 2

MENTAL HEALTH DISORDERS IN CHILDREN AND ADOLESCENTS: NEURODEVELOPMENTAL DISORDERS

CHAPTER 2

Attention Deficit Hyperactivity Disorder

LEARNING OBJECTIVES

- Summarize the diagnostic features for the *Diagnostic and Statistical Manual of Mental Disorders* (5th ed.; *DSM-5*; American Psychiatric Association [APA], 2013) diagnosis of attention deficit hyperactivity disorder (ADHD).
- Highlight the risk factors for ADHD in children and adolescents.
- Describe common social–emotional and behavioral concerns for children with ADHD.
- Understand the classroom implications for students with ADHD.
- Identify effective social, emotional, and behavioral interventions for students with ADHD.

INTRODUCTION

According to the *Diagnostic and Statistical Manual of Mental Disorders,* Fifth Edition (*DSM-5*; American Psychiatric Association [APA], 2013), Attention Deficit Hyperactivity Disorder (ADHD) is categorized as a Neurodevelopmental Disorder. Neurodevelopmental Disorders feature onset primarily during childhood. Though they have an early age of onset, the issues associated with these conditions frequently persist into adulthood. These disorders are characterized by broad deficits across a number of domains, including academic, social, and emotional concerns. Some examples of other Neurodevelopmental Disorders include intellectual disability and autism spectrum disorder (APA, 2013). The inclusion of ADHD under this umbrella is new to the *DSM-5*; it was previously included in the category of Disorders Usually Diagnosed in Infancy, Childhood, and Adolescence (Carlew & Zartman, 2017) in the prior edition, the *DSM-IV-TR* (APA, 2000).

DIAGNOSTIC ISSUES: *DSM-5* AND SCHOOL-BASED SERVICES

DSM-5 Diagnosis

The *DSM-5* outlines five criteria for the diagnosis of individuals with ADHD. The first criterion describes the inattentive and hyperactive/impulsive behaviors typically associated with ADHD. This criterion is subdivided into two parts. The first part outlines nine symptoms of inattention. These symptoms are inattention to details, challenges with maintaining attention to tasks, appearing distracted when addressed, failure to finish activities, disorganization, avoidance of tasks that require focus, issues with losing items or possessions, concerns with distractibility, and forgetfulness. The second part of the first ADHD diagnostic criterion addresses symptoms related to hyperactivity and impulsivity. This subpart also consists of nine symptoms. They are frequent fidgeting or squirming, out-of-seat behavior when remaining seated is the expectation, inappropriate running or climbing, inability to engage in quiet activities, perpetual movements in most situations, excessive talking, interrupting during conversation or blurting inappropriately, impatience with waiting, and intrusive behaviors. Across the two subparts of the first criterion, a child (younger than age 17) must demonstrate six symptoms (of either subpart—inattention or hyperactivity/impulsivity) over a course of 6 months to meet this criterion, and an individual older than 17 years must exhibit five symptoms over the same period of time. In addition, in order to meet the first criterion, the aforementioned symptoms must not be the result of purposeful defiance or lack of understanding. The second criterion for diagnosis relates to the onset of symptoms. The *DSM-5* notes that several of the symptoms of inattention or hyperactivity should have been noted prior to the age of 12 (APA, 2013). This age-of-onset criterion represents a change in the *DSM-5* as previous versions dictated symptom onset by the age of 7. According to Chandra et al. (2021), this change was supported by research that found that later-onset cases were just as consistent with ADHD symptoms and impairment as earlier detection of symptoms, and those researchers further validated the change through consistency in symptoms, functioning, quality of life, and psychiatric comorbidity between those who report later (less than 12 years of age) versus those who report earlier (less than 7 years of age) symptom onset. The third criterion for ADHD prescribes that several of the symptoms must be present in two or more settings. The fourth criterion for diagnosis of ADHD indicates that the symptoms impair the individual's functioning in at least one domain of daily life, and the final criterion states that the symptoms do not occur solely during psychotic episodes or in relation to another psychiatric condition (APA, 2013).

Beyond the criteria for diagnosis, the *DSM-5* also stipulates three different specifiers that may be applied to the diagnosis of ADHD. The first specifier relates to the presentation of symptoms. A child or adolescent may be diagnosed with combined presentation if they meet the required number of symptoms for both inattention and hyperactivity/impulsivity within the 6 months prior to diagnosis. If that is not the case, then the youth can be described as having either predominantly inattentive presentation or predominantly hyperactive/impulsive presentation based on symptom expression (APA, 2013). Prior versions of the *DSM* referred to these as *subtypes*, so the notion of presentations is new to the *DSM-5* and reflects that symptomatology of an individual may vary across the life span (Woolraich et al., 2019). Of note, some research suggests that there may be underdiagnosis of ADHD among individuals who have predominantly inattentive symptomatology (Mowlem et al., 2019). The second specifier is noted when one is in partial remission from symptoms. This specifier is applied when the individual previously met criteria but has not demonstrated the required number of symptoms in the past 6 months. Yet, the individual with this specifier must continue to struggle with issues related to remaining symptoms in at least one area of life functioning (APA, 2013). In fact, research has found that as individuals age, they often struggle with fewer ADHD symptoms even when their impairment in daily life remains high (Ramtekkar et al, 2010). Finally, the third specifier is indicative of the determination of severity. With mild severity, there are few symptoms beyond the number required for diagnosis and impairment in life functioning is considered minimal. On the other end of the continuum, the individual's severity is considered severe when the person exhibits numerous symptoms beyond the minimal criteria for diagnosis, and many of the symptoms are significant in nature and lead to serious impairment in at least one domain. Last, moderate severity is noted when the expressed symptomatology and level of impairment are between the descriptors noted for mild and severe impairment (APA, 2013). The severity specifier represents a new addition to the ADHD diagnostic criteria with the *DSM-5* (Carlew & Zartman, 2017).

> Some research suggests that ADHD may be underdiagnosed among individuals who have predominantly inattentive symptomatology (Mowlem et al., 2019).

Although the name may have changed over time, Woolraich et al. (2019) note that descriptions of ADHD-like symptoms and behaviors were discussed among professionals as early as 1902. These symptoms and behaviors were commonly thought to be associated with brain damage until evidence suggested otherwise. When the *DSM-II* was published in 1968, diagnostic criteria were included for a mental health condition called *hyperkinetic reaction of childhood disorder* (Carlew & Zartman, 2017; Woolraich et al., 2019). The name *attention deficit disorder with or without hyperactivity* first appeared in the *DSM-III* in 1980 after the focus on the issues with functioning evolved from those related to hyperactivity to those associated with inattention, and the name *ADHD* emerged with the publication of *DSM-IV* in 1994 (Carlew & Zartman, 2017).

Although some researchers suggest that the *DSM* criteria for ADHD have become more research based over time, others indicate that they continue to fall short of where they should be in terms of specificity, empirical evidence, and ability to discriminate (Carlew & Zartman, 2017; Fabiano & Haslam,

2020). In fact, research by Fabiano and Haslam (2020) found evidence of diagnostic inflation for ADHD based on decreased stringency in the criteria for diagnosis over time. Their study revealed that diagnoses of ADHD increased 18% from *DSM-III* (APA, 1980) to *DSM-III-R* (APA, 1987), 33% from *DSM-III-R* to *DSM-IV*, and another 17% from *DSM-IV* to *DSM-5* (Fabiano & Haslam, 2020). Similarly, Fairman et al. (2020) found that from 2008 to 2013, diagnoses of ADHD climbed by 36% in adults and 18% in children (22% for girls and 17% for boys), whereas the National Institute of Mental Health (NIMH; n.d.) indicates an increase in diagnosis of 42% from 2003 to 2007 based on the National Survey of Children's Health (NSCH). Finally, statistics from the Centers for Disease Control and Prevention (CDC; n.d.) and Xu et al. (2018) also reflect increasing rates of diagnosis among children and adolescents in the United States. In their comprehensive study of data from 1997 to 2016, Xu et al. (2018) found increases in prevalence of ADHD across all subgroups related to age, gender, race/ethnicity, family income, and geographic region within the United States. Perhaps related, Martinhago et al. (2019) warn that over time, diagnostic criteria have shifted in a way that has begun to pathologize normal behaviors of childhood, and this can be seen in the criteria for ADHD. Regardless of the cause of diagnostic inflation, this certainly warrants clinicians to be cautious to ensure accuracy in diagnosis so as to prevent overdiagnosis of ADHD among children and adolescents.

At the time of publication, the *DSM-5* noted the prevalence of ADHD to be approximately 5% among children and adolescents around the globe (APA, 2013). This is consistent with research by Chung et al. (2019), who found a prevalence of 4.78% from 2007 to 2016 in their large U.S. clinical sample; however, they also noted an increase in prevalence of 26.4% during that same time span. This would provide further support for the diagnostic inflation in ADHD noted previously by Fabiano and Haslam (2020). According to the CDC (n.d.), approximately 6.1 million children in the United States have been diagnosed with ADHD at some point in their lives. This includes 388,500 children aged 2 to 5, and 2,400,000 and 3,300,000 from ages 6 to 11 and 12 to 17, respectively. As would be expected given the psychosocial difficulties of individuals with ADHD, Baggio et al. (2018) found a staggering prevalence of ADHD (26.2%) among people living in detention (including psychiatric facilities), but the retrospective prevalence from childhood was estimated at 41.1%. Finally, for every 1,000 physician office visits in the United States in 2012 and 2013, 52.05 resulted in ADHD diagnoses among children (Fairman et al., 2020).

A relationship has been noted between the severity of children's ADHD and their age of onset of symptoms and subsequent diagnosis. Data from the NSCH indicates that the median age of onset across all children is 6 years. However, children with mild severity have a median age of diagnosis at age 7, and children with moderate severity are typically diagnosed by age 6. Finally, for those children who demonstrate symptomatology consistent with the specifier of severe ADHD, the median age of diagnosis is merely 4 years old. According to the *DSM-5*, the primary characteristic of ADHD at preschool ages is hyperactivity (APA, 2013).

Consistent with these age-based findings related to severity, Manfro et al. (2019) found that childhood onset of ADHD is associated with a higher number of psychiatric symptoms based on both parent and teacher report as compared with adolescent or adult onset of this mental health condition. With regard to age of referral, research supports that girls are referred at younger ages than boys when they demonstrate externalizing behavioral issues that are similar to those that are more common in boys (Arcia & Conners, 1998). Similarly, qualitative research with teachers also supports that they find the behaviors of children and adolescents with ADHD to be more acceptable among boys than among girls (Lawrence et al., 2017). Despite the generally early age of onset of ADHD and the diagnostic criterion requiring symptom presence prior to age 12, a growing body of research is supporting a form of later-onset ADHD with emergence of symptoms in adolescence or even adulthood (Asherson & Agnew-Blaise, 2019; Lin & Gau, 2020; Moffitt et al., 2015; Shaw & Polanczyk, 2017).

With regard to gender, the *DSM-5* notes that the diagnosis of ADHD in males is twice as common as in females during childhood and adolescence. Recent data from Davis et al. (2021) also indicate that in one state, twice as many males as females were diagnosed with ADHD in 2017, but Mowlem et al. (2019) suggests a ratio of 2.5:1 male-to-female children with ADHD among their large sample of youth. However, data from the National Comorbidity Survey Replication Adolescent Supplement records a discrepancy of 3 to 1 in diagnosis of males to females aged 13 to 18 in the United States (NIMH, n.d.).

Not surprising, research by Mowlem et al. (2019) indicates that greater symptom severity increases the probability of diagnosis in both male and females. They further noted that in population-based samples, males exhibit higher symptom severity than females across all domains under study, and that females may be underdiagnosed with ADHD unless they demonstrate externalizing concerns. In fact, hyperactivity/impulsivity and conduct problems were significantly greater predictors of diagnosis in females as compared to their male counterparts. They state that their data "may indicate a greater symptom threshold requirement for referral and diagnosis in females" (Mowlem et al., 2019, p. 486).

With regard to comorbidity, the *DSM-5* indicates significant co-occurrence of the following disorders with ADHD: oppositional defiant disorder, conduct disorder, disruptive mood dysregulation disorder, specific learning disorder, anxiety disorders, major depressive disorder, intermittent explosive disorder, substance abuse disorders, antisocial personality disorder, obsessive-compulsive disorder, tic disorders, and autism spectrum disorder. Most of the aforementioned mental health conditions occur with greater frequency among children and adults with ADHD than they do within the general population (APA, 2013). Larson et al. (2011) report that approximately 67% of children with ADHD have at least one other co-occurring psychiatric diagnosis. This is comparable to the 60% reported by the CDC (CDC, n.d.). According to recent research by Sun et al. (2019), the combined subtype of ADHD in childhood is related to greater comorbidities than the inattentive type alone, particularly in relation to oppositional defiant disorder, conduct disorder, and sleep disorders. In reference to those comorbidities most common in childhood and adolescence, Gnanavel et al. (2019) report a co-occurrence of 30% to 50% between externalizing disorders (oppositional defiant disorder and conduct disorder) and 70% between ADHD and learning disorders (with challenges with writing being the most common difficulty). Comorbidity with depression ranges from 12% to 50% and from 15% to 35% for anxiety among youth with ADHD, depending on the research and its methodology (Gnanavel et al., 2019). The CDC reports comorbid depression and anxiety among children and adolescents with ADHD at 17% and 33%, respectively. Research further documents significant comorbidity between ADHD and autism spectrum disorder despite the fact that they were not able to be diagnosed together prior to the *DSM-5* (Antshel et al., 2016; Gnanavel et al., 2019), and comorbid ADHD and autism spectrum disorder often lead to greater symptom expression and severity for both disorders (Gargaro et al., 2014). Gnanavel et al. (2019) report the comorbidity between the two to be at 42%, and they highlight the symptom overlap between these two neurodevelopmental disorders. However, the CDC reports this figure at a much lower rate of 14% (CDC, n.d.). Ramtekkar (2017) also found a struggle with sleep disturbances to be common within both diagnoses. The sleep disturbances for children and adolescents with ADHD include anxiety or resistance at bedtime, difficulty falling asleep, challenges with staying asleep, and daytime sleepiness (Cortese et al., 2009). Research by Walsh et al. (2020) suggests that ADHD may even serve as a precursor to bipolar disorder.

Beyond comorbidity with other psychiatric diagnoses, ADHD is also associated with other health and psychosocial issues. A number of individual studies and meta-analyses have documented the co-occurrence of ADHD and obesity (Hanc & Cortese, 2018; Inoue et al., 2019). ADHD is also associated with delinquent and criminal behavior, and individuals with ADHD often engage in these behaviors at significantly younger ages than their non-ADHD counterparts (Philipp-Wiegmann et al., 2017). In addition, when incarcerated for their criminal acts, people with ADHD are more likely to engage in verbal and physical aggression with peers and staff (Gordon et al., 2012), and they are more likely to return to incarceration for subsequent convictions following release (Gonzalez et al., 2016). Finally, and alarmingly, ADHD is associated with an overall greater number of hospitalizations and hospitalizations from injury (Fleming et al., 2017), and an increased likelihood of premature death, including suicide and accidents (Dalsgaard et al., 2015; Sun et al., 2019). Also very alarming, Chen et al. (2019) found suicidality to be 3 times higher among children with ADHD in Taiwan in relation to children without this diagnosis. In the research of Sun et al. (2019), a later age of onset of psychiatric comorbidities appears to be especially related to untimely deaths among individuals with ADHD. They noted that inattention, impulsivity, and risk-taking behaviors may be the reason for the significantly elevated risk of unexpected death for people with this mental health condition. Beyond these issues, comorbidities with ADHD are a concern because of the increased likelihood of impairment they cause in children's and adolescents' social and educational functioning (Larson et al., 2011).

School-Based Eligibility

The federal legislation that eventually became the Individuals with Disabilities Education Improvement Act (IDEA) was initially passed through Congress and enacted into law in 1975. IDEA applies to all organizations and entities (including public schools) that receive any form of federal funding. IDEA requires that schools provide a free and appropriate public education in the least restrictive environment for any student found to be eligible under one of its 13 disability categories (U.S. Department of Education, n.d.). To determine eligibility, the student is subject to an evaluation by a multidisciplinary team that includes the child's parents, a general education teacher, a special education teacher, an administrative representative for the school, and someone who is able to interpret test results. This is often the school psychologist. The team is charged with assessing the child in all areas of suspected disability in order to answer two questions that determine eligibility under IDEA. The first question is whether the student meets criteria for one of the disability categories, and the second question is whether the student demonstrates a need for special services in order to sufficiently progress in the curriculum (U.S. Department of Education, n.d.).

In the case of a child or adolescent with ADHD, the majority of these evaluations for special education services are associated with the disability category called *Other Health Impairment*. According to IDEA, an individual who is eligible under this category is noted as "having limited strength, vitality, or alertness, including a heightened alertness to environmental stimuli that results in limited alertness with respect to the educational environment" (U.S. Department of Education, n.d., Section 300.8 (c) (9)). The tenets of Other Health Impairment specify ADHD may apply. Other conditions listed for application to Other Health Impairment are asthma, diabetes, epilepsy, a heart condition, hemophilia, lead poisoning, leukemia, nephritis, rheumatic fever, sickle cell anemia, and Tourette syndrome. Although ADHD is noted in the criteria, the diagnosis alone is not a sufficient determinant of eligibility. Consistent with the two eligibility questions noted previously, the criteria further state that the health condition must also impair the student's educational performance in order to qualify for services (U.S. Department of Education, n.d.).

If the multidisciplinary team determines (through thorough and appropriate evaluation) that the child or adolescent with ADHD does not meet the IDEA criteria for Other Health Impairment, the student may be eligible to receive other services and supports under another federal law. Section 504 of the Rehabilitation Act of 1973 is civil rights legislation to protect individuals with disabilities. This law is intended to provide equal access to services and activities that receive federal funding (like public schools). Similar to the IDEA evaluation, a multidisciplinary team must conduct an evaluation to determine whether the child or adolescent exhibits an impairment that inhibits a major life function like caring for oneself, performing manual tasks, walking, hearing, seeing, speaking, breathing, learning, or working. In addition, Section 504 notes that other life functions may be considered as deemed appropriate by the team. With regard to the functional impairments listed for 504 eligibility, the Office of Civil Rights (OCR; n.d.) states that the following may apply: "physiological disease or condition, cosmetic disfigurement, or anatomical loss affecting one or more of the following body systems: neurological; musculoskeletal; special sense organs respiratory including speech organs; cardiovascular; reproductive; digestive; genito-urinary; hemic and lymphatic, skin; and endocrine; or any mental or psychological disorder, such as mental retardation, organic brain syndrome, emotional or mental illness and specific learning disabilities" (Section 104.3 (2) (i)).

In the case of eligibility under IDEA or Section 504, the child or adolescent may receive a number of specialized services to meet their needs in order to allow them to function and progress in the curriculum. Although special education services are often unique to IDEA eligibility, the school is legally bound to provide other supports as deemed necessary by the multidisciplinary team (OCR, n.d.). For a child or adolescent with ADHD, these are likely to include both academic and behavioral accommodations and modifications. Some common accommodations for students with ADHD include providing extra time for exams, utilizing technology to assist with learning, allowing more frequent breaks from instruction or tasks, limiting distractions in the classroom, and directing school personnel to provide individualized instruction. Beyond these supports, the student with ADHD may also benefit from medication management services from the school nurse and/or counseling/therapy services from the school psychologist.

Some common accommodations for students with ADHD include providing extra time for exams, utilizing technology to assist with learning, allowing more frequent breaks from instruction or tasks, limiting distractions in the classroom, and directing school personnel to provide individualized instruction.

CULTURAL ISSUES RELATED TO ATTENTION DEFICIT HYPERACTIVITY DISORDER IN YOUTH

Risk Factors for Attention Deficit Hyperactivity Disorder

The heritability of ADHD has been estimated as high as 80% (Polanczyk et al., 2007) with parental ADHD serving as a significant risk factor in the development of ADHD in children (Noordermeer et al., 2017). However, research suggests that this heritability may be significantly more pronounced in females as opposed to males. Studies indicate that there are much higher rates of ADHD within families when a female first-degree relative has been diagnosed with the condition as opposed to a male relative (Rhee & Waldman, 2004; Taylor et al., 2016). Yet, the research also indicates a female protective factor exists in that females require greater exposure to both genetic and environmental risk factors to demonstrate expression of ADHD symptomatology (Martin et al., 2018).

Other potential genetic factors include issues in the frontal lobe and thalamus that have been demonstrated to be related to the development of ADHD. Reduced volume in the frontal lobe has been found in a number of neurological studies of individuals with ADHD, including children and adolescents. Gene studies have also highlighted multiple genes that likely contribute to the onset of this mental health condition, although the research lacks consistency in this area. Researchers suggest that small sample sizes across studies and the heterogeneity of the disorder itself contribute to the lack of clarity with regard to genetic etiology and ADHD (Luo et al., 2019).

Beyond genetic factors, research points to some environmental conditions impacting the probability of developing ADHD symptomatology as well. One such risk factor is hailing from a home of lower socioeconomic status (SES). Across very large research studies in a variety of countries, researchers have found a greater probability of ADHD diagnosis among children and adolescents from less affluent homes (Larsson et al., 2014; Russell et al., 2014; Zablotsky & Alford, 2020). Data reported by the CDC (n.d.) also reflects that among children in the United States aged 2 to 5, those who receive government-funded health insurance were twice as likely to be treated for ADHD as those children who were a part of employer-funded health insurance plans. In addition, poverty may be related to ADHD comorbidity, as Larson et al. (2011) found that children from families living below the poverty line in the United States were 4 times more likely to have three or more comorbid conditions as compared to children from families of higher socioeconomic status.

Although a number of studies have found lower socioeconomic status to be a risk factor for the diagnosis of ADHD among children and adolescents (Larson et al., 2011; Russell et al., 2014), Rowland et al. (2018) note that the association may not be strictly due to family income. In their very large empirical study, they found a complex interaction between the level of a family's socioeconomic status, the parental history of ADHD, and the child's probability for ADHD diagnosis. To be specific, children from low SES families were 6.2 times more likely to be diagnosed with ADHD than their higher income counterparts when there was no parental history of ADHD diagnosis. When there is a parent-reported history of ADHD, then those children from low income families have a 10 times greater probability of diagnosis of this mental health condition than children from high-income families with no parental history. In addition, when comparing all children whose parents have experienced ADHD, those from low-income families are 16.7 times more likely to eventually have a diagnosis of ADHD as compared to 12.0 times higher likelihood of diagnosis in children from more affluent families. Thus, the researchers concluded that both SES and parental history of diagnosis represent familial risk factors for diagnosis of ADHD among offspring (Rowland et al., 2018). Assari and Caldwell (2019) also found interactions between SES and race. Their data suggest that higher family income serves as a protective factor against ADHD for White children and adolescents;

however, this finding did not hold true for Black youth. According to Assari and Caldwell (2019), societal barriers in the form of marginalization and stigmatization of racial minorities may result in an inability to benefit from economic advantage in the same manner as the majority culture.

Another environmental condition related to the development of ADHD among children and adolescents is experiencing adverse life events (Brown et al., 2017; Jimenez et al., 2017; Noordermeer et al., 2017). According to Noordermeer et al. (2017), parental divorce and family conflict are both predictive of ADHD in children. Likewise, conflict and hostility between parents and the child and early deprivation are also linked with the development of ADHD in children and adolescents (Pheula et al., 2011). Brown et al. (2017) found associations between ADHD diagnosis and moderate to severe levels of ADHD with the following factors: poverty, parental divorce, familial mental illness, neighborhood violence, domestic violence, and familial incarceration. Similarly, research by Sharp et al. (2021) found an interaction between affluence of children's neighborhoods, their family's SES, family conflict, and the progression of ADHD symptoms. They noted that children with ADHD in less affluent neighborhoods tend to show a worsening of symptomatology when their parents are also of low income and the family has a high level of conflict. With regard to adverse life experiences and ADHD, Jimenez et al. (2017) offer that more research is needed to ascertain whether trauma symptoms are being misinterpreted as ADHD or whether there is, in fact, a causal relationship between adverse life experiences and the development of ADHD in young people.

> With regard to adverse life experiences and ADHD, Jimenez et al. (2017) offer that more research is needed to ascertain whether trauma symptoms are being misinterpreted as ADHD or whether there is, in fact, a causal relationship between adverse life experiences and the development of ADHD in young people.

According to the *DSM-5*, there are also other factors that may contribute to the development of ADHD although the research is largely inconclusive. Maternal smoking during pregnancy has been consistently shown to be related to ADHD in children though researchers are uncertain whether that relationship is merely correlational in nature or causal (APA, 2013; Huang et al., 2018). Relatedly, very low birth weight (which can also be associated with maternal smoking) has been shown as an ADHD risk factor. Environmental toxins and diet issues may contribute to a small number of ADHD cases as well (APA, 2013).

Overall, the etiology of ADHD in children and adolescents is confusing at best and conflicting at worst. Many genetic and environmental variables contribute small variances to the development of ADHD, and they may interact with one another for greater developmental impact. According to Luo et al. (2019), it is these small contributions and their interactions that lead to both the development of ADHD and the heterogeneity seen in its expression.

Cultural Considerations

Findings by Fairman et al. (2020) support some differential diagnoses based on age and race. Among adults, Black people were 77% less likely to be diagnosed with ADHD as compared to their White peers. However, the inverse was true across youth samples; Black youth were 24% more likely to be diagnosed with ADHD than White youth. Youths who identified as belonging to other races were significantly less likely than White children to receive ADHD diagnoses. In addition, when participants in the study were Black and diagnosed with conduct disorder, then they were 3.78 times more likely to receive an ADHD diagnosis than White peers (Fairman et al., 2020). Among a sample of youth in 2017, prevalence of diagnosis was similar across Black and White children aged 6 to 17 at 14% and 15%, respectively. However, much lower prevalence of 6% was noted for Hispanic youth (Davis et al., 2021).

Kang and Harvey (2020) found other issues of racial disparity with regard to the perceptions of ADHD symptoms in children. Both teachers' and parents' reports of behavior are frequently critical to the initial assessment and diagnosis of ADHD among young people. Yet, the researchers found significant discrepancies in their perceptions of the symptoms and behaviors of children as related to race and ADHD. According to Kang and Harvey (2020), White teachers were more likely than

Black parents to endorse higher levels of ADHD behaviors in Black boys as opposed to Black girls or White children. They also indicated greater confidence that the Black boys may meet criteria for ADHD than all other children would. This was particularly true among teachers who reported more negative attitudes toward Black people. However, the researchers note that their study does not offer conclusive evidence as to whether White teachers overestimate the ADHD behaviors of Black boys or whether Black parents underestimate those same symptoms. Finally, another interesting result of this study was that, for Black parents, those who reported experiencing higher levels of racial discrimination themselves were more likely to indicate higher ADHD behavioral symptomatology across all children regardless of race (Kang & Harvey, 2020).

Research by Cummings et al. (2017) highlighted some disparities in ADHD treatment for racial and ethnic minority youth as compared to White adolescents with ADHD as well. They found that after diagnosis and medication prescription, African American young people are less likely to receive follow-up care than their White peers, but Hispanic youth were more likely to receive follow-up care than White youth with ADHD. However, both African American and Hispanic children and adolescents were significantly more likely to prematurely discontinue ADHD medication therapy in comparison to White youth. Cummings et al. (2017) suggest that treatment disengagement by children from minority groups may be due to cultural beliefs about health or concerns related to the ADHD treatment itself. This notion may be supported by other research among African American families that indicated that they are less likely than White families to believe that ADHD is a condition in need of treatment (Bussing et al., 2003).

IMPACT OF ATTENTION DEFICIT HYPERACTIVITY DISORDER ON SOCIAL–EMOTIONAL AND BEHAVIORAL FUNCTIONING IN SCHOOL AND HOME ENVIRONMENTS

Social–Emotional and Behavioral Functioning in School

According to Manfro et al. (2019), students with childhood-onset ADHD report experiencing a significantly greater number of adverse school experiences as compared to their typically developing peers, and overall, youth with ADHD purport having up to 500,000 negative interactions per year (Hoza et al., 2005). Children and adolescents with ADHD struggle with a plethora of peer relationship issues as explained in the research literature. In fact, Thorsen et al. (2018) found that peer problems in the preadolescent stage are reliably predicted by ADHD symptoms in the preceding 3 to 4 years. Peer relationship issues also partly mediate the development of depression among adolescents with ADHD (Powell et al., 2020).

Hoza et al. (2005) note that, among young people who have ADHD, approximately 50% report feeling socially rejected. The literature indicates that youth with ADHD are less liked by peers (Forner et al., 2017; Hoza et al., 2005), perceive themselves as different from peers (Shea & Wiener, 2003; Wiener, 2020a), engage in more frequent peer conflict, and experience greater peer rejection (Strine et al., 2006) as compared to non-ADHD youth. This peer rejection is particularly associated with the more highly aggressive behaviors of children and adolescents with the combined type of ADHD (Thorsen et al., 2018). Fogleman et al. (2019) found evidence to support that the emotion regulation issues of youth with ADHD often lead them to be victimized by peers. The relationship between the two is direct in that increases in emotional dysregulation lead to subsequent increases in peer victimization. Emotional dysregulation has been associated with social skill deficits among those with ADHD, and those deficits further impair social development and relationships for these students. The authors suggest that the issues with emotion regulation may impair the child's ability to use effective prosocial techniques and problem-solving skills in social situations (Fogleman et al., 2019). Emotion regulation is a central component of executive functioning, and Forner et al. (2017) also found a relationship between executive functioning deficits and peer relationship issues for children and adolescents with ADHD. Children with predominantly inattentive ADHD also struggle with being socially withdrawn, and researchers suggest that this may be the result of their inability to follow and remember content of conversations as related to processing-speed deficits often noted in these youth (Thorsen et al., 2018). When the youth with ADHD do engage in friendships, those relationships are often of poor quality and marked by less reciprocity than the friendships of their typically developing peers (Normand et al., 2011). Finally, Tseng et al. (2014) note that social relationships may decline over time for children and adolescents with ADHD. They explain that the social issues and the ADHD symptoms serve to magnify each other over the course of the life span.

> The literature indicates that youth with ADHD are less liked by peers (Forner et al., 2017; Hoza et al., 2005), perceive themselves as different from peers (Shea & Wiener, 2003; Wiener, 2020a), engage in more frequent peer conflict, and experience greater peer rejection (Strine et al., 2006) as compared to non-ADHD youth.

Beyond their struggles with peer relationships in the school setting, teacher relationships may also be a source of distress for children and adolescents with ADHD (Rogers et al., 2015). The symptomatology inherent in the diagnosis of ADHD often serves as a strain on teacher–student interactions and relationships due to the additional attention, support, and structure required of teachers in relation to students with ADHD. Qualitative research highlights the emotional toll that teachers experience in working with their students with ADHD (Lawrence et al., 2017). The behavioral components alone can negatively impact overall classroom and individual student functioning (Rogers et al., 2015; Rushton et al., 2020). According to Rushton et al. (2020), the student–teacher relationship for boys and girls with ADHD is a critical factor in the student's overall emotional engagement with school. Yet, they found that higher expression of ADHD symptoms was associated with greater conflict between teachers and students with ADHD, and this negatively impacted the students' engagement with school. This is of particular concern given that school engagement is related to improved academic achievement, successful school completion, and personal well-being for students (Fredricks et al., 2016). Research with teachers by Moore et al. (2017) found that teachers strongly endorse the idea that it is relationships within the school setting (as opposed to other supports or strategies) that are critical to successful adjustment within that environment for students with ADHD. Thus, interventions within the school setting should focus on the relationships between students with both their peers and teachers to increase the probability of positive school outcomes for children and adolescents with ADHD.

Social–Emotional and Behavioral Functioning at Home

The significant heritability of ADHD often results in multiple family members within the same household struggling with this condition, including parents and siblings. Research further indicates that, due to genetic factors, siblings of females with ADHD have an increased likelihood of being diagnosed with ADHD themselves than do siblings of males with ADHD (Martin et al., 2018). Multiple children would represent a strain on the home; however, the picture becomes even more complicated when the parents themselves experience ADHD symptoms. Evidence suggests that parents with ADHD may struggle with using effective parenting strategies and that struggle increases the probability of the children and adolescents exhibiting behavioral issues (Johnston et al., 2012). This has been found to be especially the case with fathers who evidence ADHD symptoms (Williamson et al., 2017). Children's ADHD symptoms are also associated with more child-rearing disagreements as reported by both mothers and fathers with ADHD (Williamson et al., 2017). In addition, Williamson et al. (2017) found that inattentive symptoms in fathers with ADHD was especially predictive of parenting difficulties, but mothers' inattentive symptoms only related to parenting issues when the fathers also exhibited symptoms of inattention. Finally, they suggest that the most challenging combination of symptoms for parenting occurs when fathers have higher levels of hyperactivity/impulsivity, and mothers have lowered hyperactive/impulsive symptomatology. This combination is most likely to result in negative parenting styles within the family (Williamson et al., 2017).

Addressing ADHD symptoms across the family unit is vital to improved outcomes for children and adolescents with ADHD as research supports that children are less likely to benefit from treatment when their mothers have higher levels of ADHD symptomatology (Jensen et al., 2007). For their children with ADHD, Johnston et al. (2012) suggest that parents with ADHD may have difficulty with treatment adherence. For example, the parent with ADHD may be unable to administer their child's or adolescent's dose of medication according to schedule and/or accurately collaborate with service providers regarding effectiveness or side effects. Lawrence et al. (2017) further explains that parents with ADHD may be less capable than unaffected parents in modeling effective strategies for organization and social interactions. When the intervention regimen for the child or adolescent includes behavioral parent training, Johnston et al. (2012) advocate for less focus on psychoeducation and more intense practice and rehearsal of skills. They also recommend that parents with ADHD may need more individualized instruction with emphasis on hands-on activities and an increased number of breaks in order to benefit from the trainings. Finally, they indicate a need for more frequent and explicit reinforcement of positive parenting techniques for parents with ADHD (Johnston et al., 2012).

These parenting issues may relate to the findings by Larson et al. (2011) that denote high parent–child communication problems and reported parental aggravation with children with ADHD, and research by Markel and Wiener (2014) that evidenced higher levels of conflict between parents and their children with ADHD than between parents and their typically developing children. These conflicts often revolve around school-related issues like grades and work completion. On the issue of familial communication, the *DSM-5* notes that interactional styles are not known to be a direct cause for the development of ADHD; they may exacerbate symptomatology and lead to other conduct-related challenges for the child or adolescent.

Perhaps adding to strain within the home of children and adolescents with ADHD, Chang et al. (2020) found significant levels of affiliate stigma among some caregivers for youth with ADHD. They found that mothers with higher levels of education experience greater affiliate stigma. The authors suggest that as females, they may be more likely to be judged for their child's behavior, and their higher education level may result in more unmet academic expectations for their child as well. These perceptions of judgment are also supported through qualitative research with teachers. According to Lawrence et al. (2017), teachers have expressed beliefs that ADHD behaviors may be created or exacerbated by home environments. Specifically, they have endorsed beliefs that the parents are lacking in discipline, involvement, and/or encouragement with their children with ADHD. Chang et al. (2020) further noted that affiliate stigma is associated with negative attitudes toward the diagnosis and available treatment options. Regardless of the cause of the stigma, its presence in the caregiver is likely to result in strained relationships within the family and may even lead to withdrawal from social relationships outside the nuclear family (Chang et al., 2020).

IMPACT OF ATTENTION DEFICIT HYPERACTIVITY DISORDER ON LEARNING IN THE CLASSROOM

Children with ADHD have not been found to differ from their typically developing peers with regard to their overall cognitive ability as measured by IQ tests (Roy et al., 2016); however, data does demonstrate lower academic achievement among people who were diagnosed as having ADHD in childhood (Barbaresi et al., 2007; Rigoni et al., 2020). Manfro et al. (2019) also note that individuals with childhood onset of ADHD demonstrate poorer overall academic performance as well as lower scores on reading and writing assessments as compared to typically developing peers. This is consistent with Rigoni et al. (2020), who found that all of the *DSM* symptoms of inattention were associated with impaired achievement in reading, written expression, and handwriting, and six out of the nine symptoms of inattention were related to challenges in mathematics achievement. They noted that children with the inattentive type of ADHD were significantly more likely to qualify for special school services than children with other types of ADHD (Rigoni et al., 2020). Further, de Zeeuw et al. (2017) suggest a causal hypothesis with relation to ADHD and academic achievement. After controlling for genetic and environmental factors, these researchers found that children with ADHD demonstrated significantly lowered educational progress. Taken together, these factors suggest that the symptoms of ADHD impair the classroom performance of students with this mental health condition. Likewise, Larson et al. (2011) found that among children with ADHD and comorbid psychiatric diagnoses, it was reported that 81% experience school problems, with approximately 46% having been retained in at least one grade.

Research regarding ADHD, gender, and school performance has produced conflicting results. Some studies suggest that males with ADHD are more likely than females with ADHD to experience learning and school adjustment difficulties (Biederman et al., 2002), whereas other research has found equivalence between male and female students with ADHD and their level of school-based concerns (Mowlem et al., 2019). Yet, CDC data (n.d.) reflect that 90% of children and adolescents in the United States (regardless of gender) with ADHD are receiving some form of support for their condition within the school setting.

Many students with ADHD are prescribed stimulant medications primarily for their benefit in curbing behavioral concerns. Although these medications may be important in improving focus and compliance in the classroom, the evidence for their impact on the academic achievement of children and adolescents with ADHD is unclear. Some researchers have found improved academic outcomes for students with ADHD who are on stimulant medication (Barbaresi et al., 2007; de Zeeuw et al., 2017), whereas other studies have not demonstrated a positive association between the use of stimulant medication in the treatment of ADHD and the acquisition of academic content (Voight et al., 2017). Likewise, qualitative research with teachers indicates mixed feelings concerning the effectiveness of medication in improving classroom functioning for children and adolescents with ADHD (Moore et al., 2017). A large study across schoolchildren in Scotland evidenced that educational outcomes are bleak for youth with ADHD even when under pharmacologic treatment (Fleming et al., 2017). Compared to typically developing peers, medicated students with ADHD have greater numbers of unexcused absences and absences due to disciplinary infractions. They are also more likely than their peers to be in need of special education services, have lowered educational attainment, drop out of school, and experience future unemployment (Fleming et al., 2017).

> Some researchers have found improved academic outcomes for students with ADHD who are on stimulant medication with ADHD (Barbaresi et al., 2007; de Zeeuw et al., 2017), whereas other studies have not demonstrated a positive association between the use of stimulant medication in the treatment of ADHD and the acquisition of academic content (Voight et al., 2017).

Further, researchers have found executive functioning deficits among adults and children with ADHD even when controlling for variables, including age, sex, and ethnicity (Forner et al., 2017; Graham, 2017; Luo et al., 2019; Manfro et al. 2019; Silverstein et al., 2020). Research also indicates that the inattentive symptoms of ADHD have a higher association with executive function deficits than hyperactive/impulsive symptoms do. This may be related to research that suggests an association between inattention and issues with working memory (Barkley et al., 2008). Manfro et al. (2019) found that executive functioning deficits are more pronounced in individuals who are diagnosed with ADHD in childhood versus those who experience adolescent- or adult-onset ADHD. Research by Barnett et al. (2001) revealed other evidence of spatial working memory issues in children with ADHD but noted that their research indicated that those deficits may be mediated through the use of stimulant medication. Neurological research has also documented the presence of deficits in spatial working memory, sustained attention, reaction times, and planning ability in adults who were diagnosed with ADHD as children (Lin & Gau, 2020). Working memory issues have also been evidenced in functional magnetic resonance imaging and positron emission tomography research with children and adolescents with ADHD (Fassbender et al., 2011). In addition, other executive functioning components, like inhibition, have been found to be negatively correlated with ADHD symptomatology (Forner et al., 2017; Fried et al., 2016; McLuckie et al., 2021).

Overall, these executive functioning deficits are the likely reason that children and adolescents with ADHD consistently exhibit more off-task classroom behaviors and fewer on-task classroom behaviors than their typically developing peers (Imeraj et al., 2013; Steiner et al., 2014). Silverstein et al. (2020) described a number of practical concerns associated with executive functioning deficits that may impair the classroom performance of a child or adolescent with ADHD. They write, "failure in inhibition may result in one being more likely to interrupt, blurt out answers, and be easily distracted. Difficulties with planning make it challenging to complete tasks, follow instructions, and organize activities. Deficits in working memory can result in being easily forgetful and making careless mistakes" (p. 45). Thus, the symptomatology of ADHD frequently results in both academic and behavioral concerns that disrupt the functioning of the individual learner and the classroom environment as a whole.

IMPLICATIONS FOR SCHOOL PSYCHOLOGISTS

Assessment Role

As noted previously, multidisciplinary teams (that frequently include school psychologists) are tasked with conducting evaluations to determine eligibility of children for special services under the auspices of IDEA and Section 504. The role of the school psychologist is particularly critical in the assessment process for children and adolescents with ADHD. These evaluations are begun when the school has received parent permission for them to proceed, and they must be concluded (and appropriate services rendered) within 60 school days from the time the consent for evaluation was written.

Relevant data are collected from a variety of sources for the decision-making process. This often begins with a review of school-based extant documentation related to the child's functioning in that environment, including such products as attendance records, disciplinary files, academic grades, and prior standardized test results. Beyond the data from school sources, permission is frequently sought from the parents to access records from any external providers who have been involved in the child's care like pediatricians, psychologists, psychiatrists, and/or therapists. The evaluation and analysis of this information then leads to the collection of more current data. This information comes in the form of interviews with the student, the student's teacher(s), and the student's parent(s), as well as classroom observations. Classroom observations are conducted as a part of the process and may form the basis of a functional behavioral assessment when substantial behavioral concerns are noted. The functional behavioral assessment process investigates the antecedents that trigger a target behavior and the conditions that follow the behavior that serve to maintain it in the environment. These findings are used to design or identify an evidence-based intervention that fulfills the psychological need being met from the target behavior and provides reinforcement for the demonstration of a more socially acceptable or adaptive behavior that serves the same purpose for the student. Other manners of behavioral assessment are undertaken in these assessment processes as well. The completion of behavior rating scales is a near-universal component of evaluation for children and adolescents with ADHD, and Wiener (2020b) notes that adolescents should be included through use of self-reported ratings as research supports that adolescents' assessment of their functioning is equally accurate to that of parents and teachers. These rating scales should cover both general behavior and functioning for the child as well as symptomatology specific to ADHD. Finally, the school psychologist is likely to assess academic achievement and cognitive ability through the use of individually administered instruments appropriate to the purpose of determining possible educational impact of the student's ADHD.

> The completion of behavior rating scales is a near-universal component of evaluation for children and adolescents with ADHD, and Wiener (2020b) notes that adolescents should be included through use of self-reported ratings as research supports that adolescents' assessment of their functioning is equally accurate to that of parents and teachers.

Aside from their role in the evaluation of students for specialized services, school psychologists may conduct other assessment functions as well. Many schools routinely screen all students for the presence of social, emotional, and/or behavioral concerns in an effort to direct them toward appropriately structured interventions (see the section in this chapter titled "School-Based Mental Health Interventions and Supports"). The training of school psychologists allows them expertise and credibility in the selection of screening tools and interventions used to to meet the needs of children and adolescents with ADHD. School psychologists also routinely direct or assist in data-collection and interpretation processes aligned with these support frameworks within the school setting.

Advocacy Role

According to Woolraich et al. (2019), stimulant medications and behavioral interventions have been the primary methods of treatment for children and adolescents with ADHD symptomatology for over 45 years. Long-term research funded by the National Institute of Mental Health has found that pharmacological intervention is the most effective singular intervention, and behavioral methods are the most preferred by families (Jensen et al., 2001). The safety and effectiveness of long-acting stimulant medication in the treatment of ADHD in children and adolescents was also established in more recent, comprehensive research by Cortese et al. (2018) and in a review by Brown et al. (2018). In general, the greatest efficacy in symptom alleviation is achieved through the combination of these two interventions (Jensen et al., 2001), but scholars in this area recommend that treatment in preschool children should begin with behavioral intervention before proceeding to pharmacologic treatment (Brown et al., 2018; Davis et al., 2019). School psychologists should be aware of treatment options and their implications in order to effectively advocate for children and families within the school setting but also through use of community-based services.

Recent research has highlighted differential treatment effectiveness based on comorbidities with ADHD. According to Gnanavel et al. (2019), children and adolescents with ADHD and anxiety are especially amenable to behavioral therapy, but those with ADHD alone do not appear to have improved outcomes with this treatment alone. Likewise, youth with ADHD and oppositional defiant disorder or conduct disorder do not seem to benefit from behavioral therapy in isolation. Those children with ADHD, anxiety, and an externalizing disorder were more treatable with the combination of the two therapies (Gnanavel et al., 2019).

Based on data reported by the CDC (n.d.), among children and adolescents with ADHD in the United States, 77% receive some form of treatment. Across those treated children, 32% receive a combination of behavioral therapy and medication, 30% are treated with medication alone, and 15% are engaged in behavioral interventions in isolation (CDC, n.d.). Danielson et al. (2018) report that approximately two thirds of children in the United States are receiving either medication or school supports for the management of their ADHD symptoms. It appears that medication usage may be on the rise for children and adolescents with ADHD as well, as the NSCH data indicate an increase of 4% in prescription medications being used in the treatment of ADHD youths from 2007 to 2011 (NIMH, n.d.). However, it is important to note that the increase in medication use does not equate to the increase in diagnosis during that same period of time. Finally, research by Mowlem et al. (2019) found that females are less likely than males to be prescribed medication for the management of their ADHD symptomatology unless they exhibit externalizing behavioral concerns. This is consistent with findings from Davis et al. (2021), who also noted significantly fewer recommendations for treatment with medication for females aged 6 to 17 with ADHD as compared with their male peers with this mental health condition.

The community-based treatment options are critical for the school psychologist to understand in order to effectively advocate for all children and adolescents with ADHD (or those suspected of having ADHD) to receive safe, timely, and accurate diagnosis and treatment. School psychologists can serve as frontline workers in assisting families in understanding and accessing essential medical care for students with this mental health condition. However, it is also imperative that school psychologists are aware of potential limitations as well. And, as noted by Brown et al. (2018), "appropriate, individually tailored treatment plans, working with behavioral, medical, and educational providers around children and adolescents with ADHD can help each individual succeed" (p. 45).

Consultation Role

School psychologists may play a critical role in psychoeducation for teachers regarding ADHD (Wiener, 2020b). This may take the form of critical inservice trainings. Research by Lawrence et al. (2017) indicates that teachers within their study report having few formal learning opportunities about ADHD diagnoses and effective classroom strategies and have garnered the bulk of their knowledge about this mental health condition from inservice offerings, informal collaborations with colleagues, and personal experiences. Further, teachers in this study described their own knowledge as insufficient and noted eagerness to improve their comprehension and skills in this area (Lawrence et al., 2017). However, research also indicates that teachers are only willing to invest about half to 1 day of training on this topic (Gaastra et al., 2020). Therefore, school psychologists should design inservice opportunities that are targeted, concise, and practical for teachers of students with ADHD.

Aside from educating school personnel on ADHD, school psychologists have other opportunities to positively impact the school environment through both direct and indirect service provision. School-based behavioral interventions have demonstrated their efficacy for improving functioning for children and adolescents with ADHD across decades of research (Evans et al., 2016), and school psychologists have the knowledge, skills, and dispositions to serve as effective consultants in their design and implementation in the classroom. In support of teamwork in this regard, DuPaul et al. (2011) note, "One overlooked aspect of treatment of children with ADHD is the need to form partnerships among school professionals who can work collaboratively on interventions for children with ADHD" (p. 35). In this quote, the authors are referring specifically to the collaborative relationships forged between teachers and their school psychologist colleagues for the betterment of students with ADHD within the educational environment. Dort et al. (2020) suggest that teachers do not receive adequate support for implementing classroom management strategies for students with ADHD. Therefore, this is a natural gap for school psychologists to fill. Although this relationship has a high potential for success, it is also critical when broaching consultation with teachers that school psychologists are aware of, acknowledge, and address barriers to the implementation of any intervention borne out of the consultative relationship. According to Gaastra et al. (2020), teacher-reported barriers to implementation of interventions include large class sizes, the presence of students with diverse needs, and limited time. Thus, it behooves the school psychologist to be sensitive to these issues as they work toward designing academic or behavioral intervention programs with teachers for children and adolescents with ADHD.

Counseling/Therapy Role

According to Danielson et al. (2018), few children and adolescents receive psychosocial treatments in accordance with their ADHD diagnosis. Their data indicate that 39% of youth with the diagnosis have received some form of social skills training, 31% have had their parents involved in parent training, 30% have been a part of a peer intervention, and 20% have participated in cognitive behavioral therapy. However, school psychologists are uniquely suited to provide therapeutic intervention in the setting where significant issues (e.g., peer social struggles, academic issues, and behavioral challenges) occur, and Wiener (2020a) recommends the use of cognitive behavioral strategies for this purpose. She notes that it is particularly critical for school psychologists to target faulty beliefs among children and adolescents with ADHD that their behaviors and outcomes are beyond their control due to their diagnosis. In addition, school psychologists' presence within the setting is likely to benefit treatment adherence for children and adolescents with ADHD. Thus, school psychologists should engage in this direct service provision to students to allow for improved adjustment and outcomes in the arena where children and adolescents may spend the majority of their waking hours and which impacts their functioning and quality of life beyond its walls and into their futures.

EDUCATIONAL SUPPORTS

Research suggests that teachers readily engage in strategies designed to improve academic and behavioral functioning for children and adolescents with ADHD. However, Moore et al. (2017) surmise that the interventions most used by teachers are not those that are core to ADHD symptomatology, but rather strategies that target skill deficits as noted by the teachers. As such, it is critical that intervention efforts in the classroom be evidence based and relevant to the needs of students with ADHD.

One deficit often noted as impairing school functioning for children and adolescents with ADHD is behavioral inhibition. As previously indicated, issues with interrupting, blurting out, off-task behavior, task incompletion, and failure to follow directions may represent significant disruption in the classroom setting. As such, researchers suggest the use of behavioral intervention strategies to modify these challenges within the academic environment (DuPaul et al., 2011). According to the American Academy of Pediatrics (2011), behavioral interventions should be considered as first-line treatment for children and adolescents with ADHD. Simple strategies, such as posting and reiterating classroom rules and providing frequent positive feedback, have been shown to be effective in improving classroom behavior for students with ADHD. In addition, reducing the length of assignments, including engaging content within tasks, and providing assignment choices often improve engagement for children with ADHD and subsequently reduce disruptions to the learning situation (DuPaul et al., 2011). Finally, verbal and nonverbal techniques like adapting voice control (firm and calm), using shortened phrases, repeating instructions, using student names, and offering visual cues are effective for children and adolescents with ADHD in the learning environment (Geng, 2011).

When more directed behavioral intervention is necessary, the school psychologist is frequently called upon to work in concert with the teacher to design individual behavioral interventions for the student with ADHD. These interventions target the function (or cause) of the behavior. The educational personnel would work together to conduct observations, collect data, and analyze the data to determine any triggers or setting events that precipitate the behavior. Further, they use the data to make informed decisions about what psychological or environmental conditions are reinforcing the child to continue to engage in the behavior. The school psychologist and teacher collaborate to design an intervention that provides reinforcement for the child in exhibiting more adaptive behaviors for the setting (Chandler & Dahlquist, 2015). These interventions not only serve to alleviate problematic behaviors but also often lead to subsequent academic improvements as the challenging behaviors are curbed in favor of more adaptive classroom engagement.

Self-regulated interventions are often used with success in the classroom with students with ADHD. According to DuPaul et al. (2011), self-regulated interventions develop students' skills monitoring and reinforcing their own behaviors. When children are taught to rate their own behavioral performance, these ratings can be compared with teacher ratings and reinforced for accuracy and compliance. Thus, students practice self-monitoring and reflection on their own behaviors in a manner that is generalizable to a number of situations and settings. This type of self-regulation is effective in improving both academic and behavioral challenges for children and adolescents with ADHD (DuPaul et al., 2011). However, despite the evidence supporting their effectiveness, Gaastra et al. (2020) found that these interventions are the least likely to be used by teachers due to their perceptions that self-regulated interventions do not support improvements in behavior for children with ADHD. Given these findings, the authors suggest that teachers would benefit from further training (like the aforementioned inservice opportunities) to improve potential acceptability of evidence-based interventions for children and adolescents with ADHD (Gaastra et al., 2020).

Finally, classroom supports for students with ADHD should include academic intervention for skill deficits when necessary. Similar to the process for designing individual behavioral interventions, school psychologists and teachers can work together to collect and analyze data to identify specific academic content areas in need of intervention. In addition to direct instruction, the students may benefit from reinforcement to develop the skills needed to maintain engagement and focus in the intervention process (Peacock & Collett, 2009). Research by Gaastra et al. (2020) found that teachers perceive these types of interventions to be the most effective for students with ADHD.

Beyond strategies and supports that merely reside within the walls of the classroom, the evidence suggests the effectiveness of efforts that increase the frequency and effectiveness of communication between the teacher in the school and the parent in the home. One such program uses a daily report card. The daily report card is widely used for children and adolescents with ADHD, and its ability to improve outcomes for students has been demonstrated through meta-analysis of the empirical work done in this area (Pyle & Fabiano, 2017; Santos & Albuquerque, 2019). The daily report card is constructed of a list of narrowly defined target behaviors specific to the child on which the teacher can provide immediate behavioral feedback. Home-based rewards may also be associated with reaching specified behavioral goals.

Since the literature on ADHD and effective ADHD interventions has expanded exponentially over the preceding decades, school psychologists and school personnel have a variety of strategies, supports, and interventions from which to choose to promote better adjustment and higher quality functioning for students with ADHD within the educational environment. With an array of options, a willingness to intervene, and an effective collaborative relationship, there is a high likelihood of effecting long-lasting and positive change for children and adolescents with ADHD.

SCHOOL-BASED MENTAL HEALTH INTERVENTIONS AND SUPPORTS

Despite evidence suggesting the effectiveness of a number of psychosocial and therapeutic interventions in the treatment of ADHD, after extensive review of the existing literature on the etiology of ADHD, Luo et al. (2019) warns that more research is needed to truly guide appropriate interventions for individuals with this diagnosis. Yet, the literature does offer a variety of intervention strategies that have demonstrated effectiveness with this population of individuals, and many may be used in combination to meet the plethora of needs often indicated in children and adolescents with ADHD. In fact, DuPaul et al. (2011) state, "Multiple treatment strategies implemented in a consistent fashion across school years can optimize the school success of students with ADHD" (p. 35). This multimodal approach should encompass the child's psychological, behavioral, and educational needs (Dreschler et al., 2020). Although other portions of this chapter have addressed some aspects of the behavioral and educational supports indicated for children and adolescents with ADHD, this section focuses on their psychological needs.

For young children, parent training has been demonstrated as particularly effective in addressing behavioral and social–emotional needs of youth with ADHD diagnoses (Dreschler et al., 2020). These trainings could take place within the school setting by school psychologists to ease the burden of cost for families. Parent trainings should focus on positive parenting strategies and effective discipline techniques. Psychoeducation regarding the etiology and potential impact of ADHD on the child and family are also beneficial components of this type of intervention (Drescler et al., 2020). Although this is not a direct mental health support for children and adolescents with ADHD, the indirect influence of this intervention supports more positive adjustment and outcomes for youth.

> For young children, parent training has been demonstrated as particularly effective in addressing behavioral and social–emotional needs of youth with ADHD diagnoses (Dreschler et al., 2020).

Both person-centered and cognitive behavioral approaches have shown promise in reducing challenging behaviors often associated with ADHD and in demonstrating improvement in anger management for children and adolescents with ADHD (Santos & Albuquerque, 2019). According to Dreschler et al. (2020), "Cognitive behavioral therapy (CBT) is a form of behavior intervention which aims at reducing ADHD behaviors or associated problems by enhancing positive behaviors and creating situations in which desired behaviors may occur" (p. 326). Data on cognitive behavioral therapy suggests improvement in anger management skills in aggressive children (Miranda & Presentacion, 2000), fewer externalizing behaviors, and reduced symptoms of inattention (Antshel et al., 2012). Cognitive behavioral therapy typically encompasses the use of techniques like cognitive restructuring, problem-solving, role-play, and modeling of adaptive skills. Through their training and experiences, school psychologists should be well versed in the effective delivery of this type of therapeutic intervention.

Given the importance of relationships within the academic setting to overall engagement in school and the social challenges often experienced by children and adolescents with ADHD, social skills training (a type of cognitive behavioral intervention) may be implemented by school psychologists to target this area for progress and to improve outcomes of interactions with teachers and peers for the student with ADHD. In this regard, the literature supports that the most effective interventions are those that occur in a natural setting for the child (e.g., school) and incorporate parents or peers to improve maintenance and generalization of the skills addressed through the intervention (Barnes et al., 2017). Even the use of peers as social coaches for children and adolescents with ADHD has shown promise in improving behavior in academic and social settings (Ahmann, et al., 2017). For young children, Barnes et al. (2017) demonstrated the effectiveness of a play-based social skills training that incorporated aspects of empathy-building, engagement, modeling, and strengthening dyadic friendships. Sadly, Morris et al. (2021) indicates that the field is badly in need of more research on interventions targeting peer social functioning for adolescents with ADHD as their meta-analysis failed to find significant, positive outcomes across a variety of intervention methodologies.

Finally, mental health interventions and supports for children and adolescents with ADHD may occur within the framework of Multi-Tiered Systems of Support (MTSS). Within the MTSS structure, schools are committed to the regular screening of students within the environment for social, emotional, or behavioral issues and to providing progressively intensive interventions according to students' needs. At Tier 1, universal screening of all students occurs, and in this case, that would be screening for ADHD (Tobin et al., 2014). These screenings would normally take the form of rating scales. At this tier, preventative interventions are provided for all students, and students at risk for ADHD are identified. When at-risk students are noted through the screening process, then those students may move to Tier 2 for targeted group interventions. According to Tobin et al. (2014), these students should receive accommodations and modifications in the general education environment similar to the strategies noted in the "Educational Supports" section of this chapter. Over time, data is collected and monitored for behavioral change and should be communicated to parents. After the application of multiple targeted interventions, if the data do not demonstrate sufficient positive change, then the student may be moved to the most intensive level of support—Tier 3. At Tier 3, intensive, individual interventions are provided for the student. This may include some of the mental health supports noted earlier and/or referral for a special education evaluation. School psychologists should be involved throughout the process in data collection, data interpretation, and decision-making regarding the intervention process and movement through the tiers.

CASE STUDY 2.1 ELI: CASE OF A KINDERGARTENER WITH ADHD

Background

Eli is 6 years old and a kindergarten student in a suburban elementary school. He was born into a single-parent home. He lives with his mother and his 11-year-old brother, Peter. Eli's mother, Dana, works on an assembly line in a factory, and the family lives in a government-subsidized housing development. Eli and Peter's father left the home prior to Eli's second birthday, and the family has no contact with him. Dana has a history of academic difficulties. She struggled through the early years of school and was often in trouble for minor behavioral infractions like out-of-seat behavior, blurting out, and peer conflicts. After being retained once in elementary school and once in middle school, Dana dropped out of high school as a 16-year-old freshman. She had difficulty maintaining a job for a while because she would often forget tasks, leave work incomplete, have conflict with colleagues, and miss work due to confusion over her work schedule. However, she has held the factory job for nearly 3 years and seems to benefit from the structured schedule and repetitive nature of the work. Two years ago, school personnel started to express concerns about Peter's boisterous behavior and his inability to focus on his academic work. Dana took him to the pediatrician. After Dana completed some rating scales, the pediatrician diagnosed Peter with ADHD and prescribed a stimulant medication. Because Dana recognized some similarities between Peter's behavior and her own past and present functioning, Dana decided to visit her family practice physician. Upon collecting some information from Dana, the doctor determined that Dana's childhood, adolescent, and adult concerns with adaptation in school and work environments were likely due to ADHD. She was also given the diagnosis and a prescription for stimulant medication. When Dana and Peter are taking their medications consistently, they both exhibit improved functioning in their respective environments. However, Dana has difficulty remembering when or if she has dispensed their medications. They frequently miss taking it for several days at a time and take the medication at various times throughout the day whenever she does remember to give the pills. With the boys, Dana's parenting can be described as

(continued)

CASE STUDY 2.1 ELI: CASE OF A KINDERGARTENER WITH ADHD (continued)

inconsistent. On some days, she has very high expectations for them and expresses significant displeasure at even minor disappointments. On other days, her parenting is lax with few behavioral expectations or boundaries. Her discipline is nearly always reactive in nature and consequences vacillate between overly harsh and nonexistent. The family members engage in frequent conflict with one another. Although Dana recognizes some similar behaviors in Eli as she sees with Peter's ADHD symptomatology, she does not believe that she can manage more doctor's appointments or medication administration, so she has largely ignored her sense that Eli may also have ADHD.

Discussion

When Eli began school in the fall, his teacher was quick to notice that his behaviors differed from peers. He appears immature in comparison. Throughout the school day, Eli struggles with following directions. He rarely completes tasks. Eli is often out of his assigned area; he frequently wanders about the room and even left the classroom a couple of times during the first week of school. Eli is loud and impulsive in his verbalizations. In the classroom and on the playground, his energy is unmatched by his fellow kindergarteners. He climbs on furniture, throws items, snatches materials and toys from peers, and resists nearly all forms of redirection from his teacher. At the end of the first month of school, the educational personnel begin universal screenings for academic, social, emotional, and behavioral concerns as a part of their MTSS process. The screening measures completed for Eli indicate that he is at risk in all domains. The school psychologist and MTSS team reach out to Dana to convey the findings and recommend that Eli be placed in Tier 2 group interventions for academic, social, emotional, and behavioral support. Dana agrees with the needs that were identified for Eli, and she decides that she will now seek consultation with Eli's pediatrician. During the first 9 weeks of intervention, Eli makes slow but steady academic gains but fails to demonstrate increases in his social, emotional, and behavioral skills based on progress-monitoring data. In this same period of time, Dana takes Eli to the pediatrician and requests that the school psychologist share information with the physician about Eli's school functioning. The school psychologist attends the appointment via virtual means and collaborates with the doctor. Although the doctor's assessment indicates that Eli meets *DSM-5* criteria for ADHD, the pediatrician, the school psychologist, and Dana all agree that more psychosocial interventions should be attempted before trying stimulant medication due to Eli's young age. After this appointment, the MTSS team, the school psychologist, and Dana meet to discuss their options. The group concludes that Eli will remain at Tier 2 for academics but that he would benefit from Tier 3 support for social, emotional, and behavioral interventions. The team determines that the school psychologist will become more highly involved in Eli's support services at this individualized level. They decide that Eli may benefit from an interactive, computerized intervention that builds social skills, and the school psychologist will begin the functional behavioral assessment process to design and implement a behavioral intervention for the classroom. Finally, the school psychologist will begin individual counseling sessions with Eli. These sessions will be play based but use a cognitive behavioral orientation. The school psychologist will use role-playing and modeling to build empathy and emotional awareness. The team collaborates on objective goals for the various interventions. They will reconvene in another 9 weeks to review Eli's progress. If adequate progress is made, then the team may return him to Tier 2 interventions. If not, then they will discuss the possibility of conducting an evaluation for Oher Health Impairment under IDEA.

SUMMARY POINTS

- A child with ADHD may be described as having a combined presentation, inattentive presentation, or hyperactive/impulsive presentation.
- Diagnoses of ADHD are significantly increasing significantly in the United States.
- The significant heritability of ADHD increases the likelihood of more than one individual in the home having the diagnosis and often relates to increased strain on familial relationships.
- ADHD symptomatology often relates to both academic and behavioral concerns in the classroom.
- School psychologists can engage in many roles and functions to support the needs of students with ADHD, including assessment, advocacy, consultation, and counseling and/or therapy.
- Children and adolescents with ADHD often benefit from multimodal interventions.

TEST YOUR KNOWLEDGE

1. A student with ADHD may qualify for special education services under which IDEA category?
   a. Anxiety Disorders
   b. Other Health Impairment
   c. Specific Learning Disability
   d. Intellectual Disability

2. Adverse childhood experiences have been related to the development of ADHD.
   a. True
   b. False

3. ADHD is related to conflict and communication issues between parents and children.
   a. True
   b. False

4. Which of the following is NOT associated with the development of ADHD in children and adolescents?
   a. Adverse life events
   b. Low socioeconomic status
   c. Parental depression
   d. Reduced frontal lobe volume

5. Parent training should be the first-line intervention for preschoolers with ADHD.
   a. True
   b. False

Answers: (1) b, (2) a, (3) a, (4) c, (5) a.

DISCUSSION QUESTIONS

1. List some reasons why ADHD diagnoses are increasing.
2. Highlight the IDEA criteria for eligibility under the category of Other Health Impairment.
3. Explain why parents with ADHD may struggle with treatment adherence for their child with ADHD.
4. Describe how ADHD symptoms may inhibit classroom performance.
5. List some effective classroom strategies for students with ADHD.

CHAPTER RESOURCES

American Academy of Child and Adolescent Psychiatry *ADHD Resource Center:* www.aacap.org/aacap/Families_and_Youth/Resource_Centers/ADHD_Resource_Center/Home.aspx

American Academy of Pediatrics *Caring for Children With ADHD: A Practical Resource Toolkit for Clinicians*: https://publications.aap.org/toolkits/pages/ADHD-Toolkit

American Psychological Association *ADHD:* www.apa.org/topics/adhd

Centers for Disease Control and Prevention *Attention Deficit Hyperactivity Disorder:* www.cdc.gov/ncbddd/adhd/index.html

Children and Adults with Attention-Deficit/Hyperactivity Disorder *Assignment Accommodations:* https://chadd.org/for-educators/assignment-accomodations

Children and Adults with Attention-Deficit/Hyperactivity Disorder *Classroom Accommodations:* https://chadd.org/for-educators/classroom-accommodations

Children and Adults with Attention-Deficit/Hyperactivity Disorder *Instructional Process*: https://chadd.org/for-educators/instructional-process

Children and Adults with Attention-Deficit/Hyperactivity Disorder *Teacher Training and Video Series*: https://chadd.org/for-educators/teacher-training-video-series

Children and Adults with Attention-Deficit/Hyperactivity Disorder *Webinars for Early Childhood Educators*: https://chadd.org/for-educators/webinars-for-early-childhood-educators

National Federation of Families *ADHD Resources:* www.ffcmh.org/resources-add
National Institute of Mental Health *Shareable Resources on Attention Deficit Hyperactivity Disorder:* www.nimh.nih.gov/get-involved/education-awareness/shareable-resources-on-adhd

KEY REFERENCES

Only key references appear in the print edition. The full reference list appears in the digital product on Springer Publishing Connect: connect.springerpub.com/content/book/978-0-8261-3587-2/part/part02/chapter/ch02

American Psychiatric Association. (2013). *Diagnostic and statistical manual of mental disorders* (5th ed.). https://doi.org/10.1176/appi.books.9780890425596

Dreschler, R., Brem, S., Brandeis, D., Grunblatt, E., Berger, G., & Walitza, S. (2020). ADHD: Current concepts and treatments in children and adolescents. *Neuropediatrics, 51*, 315–335. https://doi.org/10.1055/s-0040-1701658

Fabiano, F., & Haslam, N. (2020). Diagnostic inflation in the *DSM*: A meta-analysis of changes in the stringency of psychiatric diagnosis from *DSM-III* to *DSM-5*. *Clinical Psychology Review, 80*, 101889. https://doi.org/10.1016/j.cpr.2020.101889

Gaastra, G. F., Groen, Y., & Tucha, L. (2020). Unknown, unloved? Teachers' reported use and effectiveness of classroom management strategies for students with symptoms of ADHD. *Child & Youth Care Forum, 49*, 1–22. https://doi.org/10.1007/s10566-019-09515-7

Gnanavel, S., Sharma, P., Kaushal, P., & Hussain, S. (2019). Attention deficit hyperactivity disorder and comorbidity: A review of literature. *World Journal of Clinical Cases, 7*(17), 2420–2426. https://doi.org/10.12998/wjcc.v7.i17.2420

Hoza, B., Mrug, S., Gerdes, A. C., Hinshaw, S. P., Bukowski, M. W., Gold, J. A., Kraemer, H. C., Pelham, W. E., Wigal, T., & Arnold, L. E. (2005). What aspects of peer relationships are impaired in children with attention-deficit/hyperactivity disorder? *Journal of Consulting and Clinical Psychology, 73*(3), 411–423. https://doi.org/10.1037/0022-006X.73.3.411

Johnston, C., Mash, E. J., Miller, N., & Ninowski, J. E. (2012). Parenting in adults with attention-deficit/hyperactivity disorder (ADHD). *Clinical Psychology Review, 32*(4), 215–228. https://doi.org/10.1016/j.cpr.2012.01.007

Lawrence, K., Estrada, R. D., & McCormick, J. (2017). Teachers' experiences with and perceptions of students with attention deficit/hyperactivity disorder. *Journal of Pediatric Nursing, 36*, 141–148. https://doi.org/10.1016/j.pedn.2017.06.010

Office of Civil Rights. (n.d.). *Protecting students with disabilities: Frequently asked questions about Section 504 and the education of children with disabilities*. https://www2.ed.gov/about/offices/list/ocr/504faq.html

Tobin, R. M., Schneider, W. J., & Landau, S. (2014). Best practices in the assessment of youth with attention deficit hyperactivity disorder within a multitiered services framework. In P. L. Harrison & A. Thomas (Eds.), *Best practices in school psychology: Student-level services*. National Association of School Psychologists.

U.S. Department of Education. (n.d.). *Individuals with Disabilities Education Improvement Act*. https://sites.ed.gov/idea/

CHAPTER 3

Intellectual Disabilities

LEARNING OBJECTIVES

- Summarize the diagnostic features for the *Diagnostic and Statistical Manual of Mental Disorders* (5th ed.; *DSM-5*; American Psychiatric Association [APA], 2013) diagnosis of Intellectual Disability.
- Outline the components of Individuals with Disabilities Education Improvement Act (IDEA) eligibility for Intellectual Disability.
- Highlight the cultural considerations for children and youth with intellectual disability.
- Describe common social–emotional and behavioral concerns for children with intellectual disability.
- Understand the classroom implications for a student with intellectual disability.
- Identify effective social, emotional, and behavioral interventions for students with intellectual disability.

INTRODUCTION

The *Diagnostic and Statistical Manual of Mental Disorders,* Fifth Edition (*DSM-5*; American Psychiatric Association [APA], 2013), classifies Intellectual Disability as one of a number of Neurodevelopmental Disorders. Intellectual Disability and the other disorders under the umbrella of Neurodevelopmental Disorders share this distinction due to their onset during the early-childhood period and their tendency to cause impairments across multiple domains related to the individual's functioning. Some examples of other Neurodevelopmental Disorders include Attention Deficit Hyperactivity Disorder (ADHD; discussed in Chapter 2) and Autism Spectrum Disorder (ASD; addressed in Chapter 4).

A prior and often derogatory term once used for *intellectual disability* was *mental retardation*. In 2010, the U.S. Congress passed Public Law 111-256 (also referred to as *Rosa's Law*), which changed all usage of *mental retardation* in federal law to *intellectual disability* and updated all occurrences of *mentally retarded individual* to *individual with intellectual disability* (GovInfo, n.d.; Rosa's Law, 2017). The change in terminology reflected a desire to bring more respect and dignity to individuals with intellectual disabilities and to remove a term that is often associated with bullying. Changes in federal law were made to the Rehabilitation Act of 1973, the Individuals with Disabilities Education Improvement Act (IDEA), the Higher Education Act of 1965, and the Elementary and Secondary Education Act of 1965 (Rosa's Law, 2017).

Previous editions of the *DSM* used the term *mental retardation* when referencing this disorder, including the *DSM-IV-TR*, which was published in 2000 (APA, 2000). Although the change to the term in the *DSM-5* was a critical step forward in bringing more respectful reference to individuals with intellectual disability, this most recent version of the *DSM* also made important updates regarding the diagnosis of intellectual disability.

DIAGNOSTIC ISSUES: *DSM-5* AND IDEA

DSM-5 Diagnosis

In the *DSM-5* (APA, 2013), three criteria are required to be met in order to determine a diagnosis of intellectual disability. Those criteria address deficits in the intellectual and adaptive functioning of the individual and also dictate that the developmental concerns arise during childhood or adolescence. Prior to the *DSM-5*, the diagnostic criteria specified particular IQ score ranges for the determination of intellectual disability. Although the current revision indicates that intellectual functioning must be assessed and that the resulting IQ scores should be approximately 2 standard deviations below the mean on a psychometrically sound and culturally appropriate cognitive assessment, the *DSM-5* acknowledges the importance of the clinician in using professional judgment as it relates to the intellectual assessment process. The clinician should determine aspects, such as validity of the test results, interpretation of the scores, appropriateness to the diagnostic situation, and limitations of the findings with respect to the overall functioning of the individual, during the diagnostic decision-making process. The instruments used for the measurement of cognitive functioning for a diagnosis of intellectual disability should be individually administered and assess areas such as memory, verbal abilities, processing speed, quantitative skills, and abstract thought. If a child is under the age of 5, exhibiting significant developmental delays, and cannot be assessed with a cognitive assessment tool to determine whether the intellectual functioning criterion is met (due to age or significant impairment), then the child can be given the diagnosis of *global developmental delay*. In this case, the child should be reassessed when they reach an age or skill level that allows for standardized assessment in this area (APA, 2013).

In addition to the evolution of criteria in intellectual functioning, more emphasis is placed on adaptive functioning in the *DSM-5* than in prior versions of the *DSM* (APA, 2013; Kaufmann, 2018). This shift reflects an awareness that IQ may not fully address a person's ability to reason and function in daily-life situations (Mahour & Panday, 2015). *Adaptive functioning* is described as an individual's ability to perform age-appropriate personal and daily-living skills across three domains. Those domains include the conceptual (academic) domain, the social domain, and the practical domain. The *DSM-5* criteria require greater impairment in daily-living skills to warrant a diagnosis of intellectual disability than was needed in the *DSM-IV-TR* (APA, 2000) as the focus shifted from adaptive skills to these adaptive domains (Kaufmann, 2018). However, the adaptive skills continue to play an important role in the diagnosis of intellectual disability in that each adaptive domain is made up of adaptive skills relevant to functioning in that area. For example, the conceptual domain includes skills like reading, writing, and problem-solving; the social domain encompasses abilities such as empathy, social judgment, and awareness of the feelings of others; and the practical domain covers functions like personal care, recreation, and self-management of behaviors (APA, 2013). Research by Papazoglou et al. (2014) found that the change in criteria related to adaptive behavior from the *DSM-IV-TR* (APA, 2000) to the *DSM-5* (APA, 2013) resulted in a 9% decrease in the number of children eligible for the diagnosis of intellectual disability.

> The change in criteria related to adaptive behavior from the *DSM-IV-TR* to the *DSM-5* resulted in a 9% decrease in the number of children eligible for the diagnosis of intellectual disability (Papazoglou et al., 2014).

In order to meet the criteria regarding adaptive functioning, any adaptive deficits must be associated with the intellectual functioning deficits and be significant enough in at least one of the aforementioned domains to warrant continuous support in order for the child to function in an age-appropriate manner in at least one life setting (school, work, home, and/or community). It is important to note that some researchers in this area stress that the link between intellectual functioning deficits and deficits in adaptive behavior are correlational not causal (Tasse et al., 2016). This means that intellectual functioning deficits and adaptive deficits often occur together, but one does not cause the other. Similar to the *DSM-5* intellectual functioning criteria (APA, 2013), a child's adaptive ability must be measured with a culturally appropriate standardized assessment possessing adequate psychometric properties. When appropriate, the child should participate in a self-evaluation of skills, but the participation of another familiar respondent is also required. The respondent is often a parent, educator, caretaker, or other professional involved in providing services to the child. If individual factors or setting constraints do not allow for the standardized assessment of adaptive skills, then an individual meeting the criteria related to intellectual functioning deficits and childhood/adolescent onset of those deficits may instead be diagnosed with unspecified intellectual disability if that child is also greater than 5 years of age. In addition to assessment through a standardized tool, adaptive behavior must also be assessed through a clinical evaluation of sources, such as interviews and educational, medical, or other existing records, in order to corroborate the reported deficits (APA, 2013).

The overall assessment of the child's adaptive functioning is necessary in determining whether the youth meets criteria as an individual with an intellectual disability, but it is also a determinant in the classification of severity. The *DSM-5* requires that the clinician provide an estimate of severity with each diagnosis of intellectual disability. The severity levels are *mild, moderate, severe,* and *profound*. The identified level of severity should be established based on the quality and quantity of external supports necessary for the individual to function in a variety of settings and across the conceptual, social, and practical domains (APA, 2013).

Finally, as previously mentioned, the third criteria for diagnosis with the *DSM-5* relates to the onset of the timing of deficits in cognitive functioning and adaptive behavior. The collected information through medical and/or educational record reviews and interviews should support the presence of the deficits during childhood or adolescence. The greater the severity of the deficits, the more likely they are to be detected early (APA, 2013). Those infants and young children with more severe deficits are also more likely to have a known and observable underlying cause (likely biological) for the intellectual disability, whereas those young children in the mild range of severity are less likely to have a known etiology (Patel et al., 2020).

The overall prevalence of intellectual disabilities across the global population is 1% to 3% with about twice as many males diagnosed with intellectual disability as females (Patel et al., 2020). Within that 1% to 3%, it is estimated that about 75% to 85% of individuals with intellectual disability are categorized as mild in severity with another 10% at the moderate level of severity (Patel et al., 2020; Saad & ElAdl, 2019). People in the severe category make up about 3% to 4% of all individuals diagnosed with intellectual disability, and individuals categorized as profound are less than 1% of the overall population of individuals with this diagnosis. The independence expected for individuals with intellectual disability ranges from the ability to function with minimal assistance in many settings and achievement of some level of academic attainment with support for students with mild intellectual disability to individuals needing full-time care (even for the most basic of needs) across all settings for children and adolescents with profound intellectual disability (Saad & ElAdl, 2019). Patel et al. (2020) indicate that that the frequency of mild intellectual disability within the global population is actually declining, but it is not noted why this might be the case.

About twice as many males are diagnosed with intellectual disability as females (Patel et al., 2020).

IDEA Eligibility

Given that school psychologists most frequently encounter, interact, and work with students in the school setting, it is important to also have an understanding of how intellectual disability is determined within the educational environment. A *DSM* diagnosis of intellectual disability is neither necessary nor sufficient for a student to be served within a special education setting for intellectual disability. The process for determining intellectual disability within schools is entirely separate from an evaluation provided in a medical or psychological setting. However, data from a source external to the school may be considered as a part of a school-based evaluation.

The process for determining intellectual disability within schools is entirely separate from those performed in a medical or psychological setting.

According to the U.S. Department of Education, IDEA is the federal law that provides for the free and appropriate public education in the least restrictive environment for children and adolescents who meet criteria for special education services and who demonstrate a need for those services in the public schools (U.S. Department of Education, n.d.). Based on the most recent data from the National Center of Education Statistics, approximately 14% of the public-school students in the United States are classified within one of the 13 disability categories of IDEA. Intellectual Disability is one such eligibility category. Within the population of all students with identified disabilities, 6% of children and adolescents were eligible for services under the category of Intellectual Disability during the 2018 to 2019 school year. This represents approximately 439,000 students aged 3 to 21 being served with intellectual disability in the United States (National Center for Education Statistics, n.d.).

In Section 300.8 (c) (6), IDEA defines *intellectual disability* in the following manner: "Intellectual Disability means significantly subaverage general intellectual functioning, existing concurrently with deficits in adaptive behavior and manifested during the developmental period, that adversely affects a child's educational performance" (U.S. Department of Education, n.d., Section 300.8 (c) (6)). There is an obvious and warranted similarity between the description of *intellectual disability* in *DSM-5* and IDEA.

Determination of eligibility for special education services begins with a request for an evaluation by the child's parent, an employee of the local education agency (LEA), or another state agency. If the parent was not the entity who requested the evaluation, then the LEA must seek parent consent to conduct the evaluation. When that consent is obtained, the school district has 60 school days to determine whether the child has a disability and the need for services. The child must be assessed in every area of suspected disability with psychometrically sound instruments that are reliable and valid for the purpose for which they are being used. The assessor or assessment team must use a variety of tools (no one instrument is sufficient for determining eligibility) to attain information regarding the child's cognitive, academic, and adaptive status (U.S. Department of Education, n.d.). Most state guidelines indicate that intellectual functioning should be measured with an IQ test and the resulting scores should be subaverage for qualification as a student with an intellectual disability. *Subaverage* is broadly interpreted as scores that are at least 2 standard deviations below the mean. However, other scientifically sound procedures can be used in place of an IQ test in some instances. Individually administered achievement tests and adaptive behavior assessments are typically used to measure a student's academic progress and adaptive functioning, respectively. Commensurate deficits should also be noted in the academic and adaptive areas in order to determine qualification under the category of Intellectual Disability (Jacob et al., 2016). When all relevant assessment information has been gathered, a team of individuals (including the child's parent/guardian, a general education teacher, a special education teacher, an individual qualified for interpreting results, and an LEA representative) determine whether the child meets criteria as a student with a disability and demonstrates a need for special education services (U.S. Department of Education, n.d.). Please visit sites.ed.gov/idea for a more detailed treatment of the evaluation process.

CULTURAL ISSUES RELATED TO INTELLECTUAL DISABILITY IN YOUTH

Risk Factors for Intellectual Disability

Children and adolescents with intellectual disability span all races, ethnic backgrounds, cultures, and geographic locations. The etiology of intellectual disability is often known in more severe cases where there is an associated biological cause such as a genetic syndrome, metabolic issue, or neurological abnormality (Patel et al., 2020). However, cultural issues may also play a role in etiology, assessment, and care of children and adolescents with intellectual disability.

In a meta-analysis of 17 studies involving over 55,000 participants, Huang et al. (2016) attempted to ascertain risk factors for an eventual diagnosis of intellectual disability across the prenatal, perinatal, and neonatal developmental stages. Through this extensive work, they found the greatest number of identifiable risk factors to be among prenatal factors. Those included the following characteristics of the mother: advanced age (defined as older than 35 years old), African American race, lower level of education, having given birth three or more times, alcohol use, tobacco use, diabetes, hypertension, epilepsy, and asthma. Among the aforementioned factors that were found to be significant, the most strongly associated factors were advanced maternal age, race, education, three or more births, alcohol use, and epilepsy. In addition to these prenatal factors, preterm birth, male sex, and low birth weight were also found to be risk factors that are strongly associated with intellectual disability. Other researchers have found advanced paternal age to be a risk factor for intellectual disability as well (Roeleveld et al., 1992). However, one should also note that several of the identified risk factors are also associated with poverty, including race, level of education, preterm birth, and low birth rate (Emerson, 2007). In addition, research has supported that children with intellectual disability are more likely to be born into poverty, and their families are more likely to remain in poverty than families who do not have a child with a disability (Emerson, 2007; Emerson et al., 2010). Thus, school psychologists should be aware of prenatal risk factors associated with intellectual disability but also consider the relationship between those factors and familial poverty for youths with intellectual disability.

Culturally Sensitive Assessment Considerations

With regard to assessment of individuals suspected of intellectual disability, the *DSM-5* (APA, 2013) cautions that care should be taken to ensure cultural sensitivity in the assessment process. Similarly, the National Association of School Psychologists (NASP; n.d.) espouses the need for cultural competence across all services engaged in by school psychologists, including assessment. Concerns over biased assessment practices in the United States date back many decades. For an overview of the key historical points in relation to fairness in testing, the reader is encouraged to explore Ortiz (2014).

The need for school psychologists to engage in culturally sensitive assessment processes is also addressed within the NASP's *Principles for Professional Ethics* (2020). Standards I.3.1 and I.3.2 describe a school psychologist's responsibility to avoid active participation in/passive acceptance of discriminatory practices and a duty to correct any such school practices, respectively. Even more specific to the assessment process for eligibility determination (including intellectual disability), Standard II.3.8 dictates that school psychologists must use nondiscriminatory means of assessing children and interpreting assessment results in relation to their overall life experiences, including culture and language. According to Standard II.3.9, these assessment processes may include the use of qualified translators when deemed to be appropriate according to the child's background (NASP, 2020). However, Ortiz (2014) challenges practitioners to accept that no assessment can ever be completely free from bias, but it is the responsibility of the school psychologist to recognize and minimize the impact of bias and discrimination on the assessment process to improve outcomes for children and adolescents. Bias can inhabit any element of the assessment though it is often most associated with testing. According to Ortiz (2014), "Bias is not a function of technical or psychometric deficiencies in a test but rather differences in experience between an individual taking the test and individuals on whom the test was normed" (p. 675). Engaging in nondiscriminatory assessment practices will help to ensure that children are not saddled with the life-altering diagnosis of intellectual disability if it is not correct to do so, but it will also help to accurately identify those students who should be identified as having a disability (Ortiz, 2014). When appropriately applied, a diagnosis of intellectual disability will help a child access medical and educational services, as well as legal protections (Luckasson & Schalock, 2013).

No assessment can ever be completely free of bias (Ortiz, 2014).

Diagnostic Stigma and Culture

The need for culturally sensitive and accurate assessment practices is especially relevant with intellectual disability. Many labels and diagnoses have negative connotations (even stigma or taboo) associated with them, and this seems particularly true with intellectual disability. Therefore, it behooves school psychologists to ensure that any eligibility for intellectual disability is conducted thoroughly, accurately, and with cultural sensitivity due to the social implications of that classification. Research supports that despite efforts to reduce stigma associated with intellectual disability, it still largely exists in many countries around the world (Scior et al., 2020). One of the most chilling and extreme examples of the ramifications of this stigma comes from West Africa, where the ritual abandonment and killing of children with intellectual disability has been reported even though the extent of the practice is unknown (Bayat, 2015). In the collectivist culture of China, the stigma of the intellectual disability often extends beyond the child or adolescent to the family as well. The intellectual disability of the child may even be viewed as punishment for some wrongful act by a family member, which then causes the entire family to "lose face" due to the presence of the disability (Chiu et al., 2013). In Canada, researchers found that men tend to have more negative attitudes toward individuals with disabilities than women, but overall adults tend to have more negative perceptions of individuals with intellectual disability when they are lower functioning (Morin et al., 2013). Finally, here in the United States, Gold and Richards (2012) assert that the stigma of labels (including intellectual disability) is especially problematic for African American youth. They assert that labeling any child with a disability leads to learned helplessness and issues with self-image, but labeling an African American child as having a disability is potentially of greater negative impact due to the long history of harmful labels assigned to African Americans in this country.

Stigma associated with intellectual disability still largely exists around the world.

Cultural Considerations in Caregiving

As with many physical and mental conditions and disabilities, a diagnosis for a family member reverberates through the entire family unit, and naturally, the same is true with intellectual disability. Families with a child with intellectual disability often experience strain beyond what occurs in families with typically developing children. Caregiving often falls primarily to the parents, who are faced with significant challenges, including a longer period of caregiving, a need for more intensive supports for the child, greater financial commitment to caregiving, and a lack of social support (McIntyre, 2016). The familial and/or parental stress of caring for a child with intellectual disability has been well documented in the literature (Baxter et al., 2000; Emerson, 2003; Masulani-Mwale et al., 2018; McIntyre, 2016; Patton et al., 2018; Totsika et al., 2011). In addition to the caregiving stress, there are unique cultural caregiving considerations for the school psychologist as well when working with the families of children with intellectual disability. Individual cultures may affect how families understand the disability and their caregiving approach. Dura-Vila et al. (2010) explained that, "Once identified, parents are faced with a process of meaning-making drawing on the available cultural models of normal and abnormal child development to build their understanding of their own child's delays" (p. 172).

In the Chinese culture, the family is often viewed as one body (a belief informed by Confucian teachings), and caregiving of a child with a disability is seen as a moral obligation of the family members (Chiu et al., 2013). Family members may also blame themselves for the onset of the disability (Chiu et al., 2015) and the stigma of the disability extends from the individual with the diagnosis (Chiu et al., 2013). Despite the challenges of caregiving under these circumstances, Yang et al. (2016) found that the parents report both positive and negative perceptions associated with caring for a child with intellectual disability. The researchers indicate that this ambivalence is rooted in a cultural context that values both collectivism and interdependence. The parents believe that it is their mission to care for the child but also experience few external supports for doing so. In fact, research demonstrates that Chinese families report a lack of support even when living in areas where community supports may be available to them (Wong et al., 2004). Chiu et al. (2013) note that it is important for professionals working with caregivers to recognize the shame, guilt, and anxiety that those caregivers are likely experiencing. This recommendation is sound for school psychologists who are engaging with Chinese families in relation to their child with intellectual disability.

As with the Chinese attributional beliefs described by Chiu et al. (2015), John et al. (2017) found that Indian families often initially ascribe blame to themselves regarding their child's intellectual disability. However, their understanding of etiology often progresses over time, particularly through interactions with the school system. Some Indian parents begin the journey with a child with intellectual disability with superstitious or religious beliefs (e.g., Hindu theory of Karma) regarding the cause of the disability but often come to a more scientific understanding through their work with professionals (John et al., 2017). This is critical for school psychologists who may find themselves in an educational role with caregiving parents. When frustration mounts with traditional, Western medicine approaches, John et al. (2017) also found that Indian families may be more likely to seek less common and/or nontraditional treatment options for the child with intellectual disability such as physical therapy, use of natural substances, and Ayurveda (an Indian approach for establishing mind–body balance). The input of extended family members is often sought in treatment and caregiving decisions.

Within Latino families, Cauce and Domenech-Rodriguez (2002) describe the concept of attitudinal familism whereby family members feel a strong sense of duty to one another. This belief focuses on the closeness of the family and the family members' responsibility to one another for the well-being of the entire family. Research has supported that Latino family members are significantly more likely to endorse the concepts of attitudinal familism than non-Latino families (Cortes, 1995). Cohen (2013) notes that this is why Latino families who are caring for a child with intellectual disability are more likely to expect support from extended family, which leads to greater caregiving self-efficacy for those parents. Lauderdale-Littin and Blacher (2017) found that Latino mothers of children with intellectual disability reported higher levels of stress than nonminority mothers of children with intellectual disability, but the Latino mothers also endorsed more positive perceptions about parenting than their nonminority counterparts. Research has additionally found that spirituality and faith (more than religion) are considered a positive source of support among many Latino families with children with intellectual disability (Dura-Vila et al., 2010).

Latino families who are caring for a child with intellectual disability are more likely to expect support from extended family, which leads to greater caregiving self-efficacy for those parents (Cohen, 2013).

Regarding child development expectations, Cohen also indicates that many Latino families believe in nurturing and pampering children. When the child has a disability, this may appear to some as reinforcing atypical behaviors for a child of a certain age when the parents allow the child to continue with behaviors or habits usually associated with younger children. Thus, Cohen (2013) recommends that non-Latino professionals respect this cultural aspect by focusing intervention efforts on social–emotional skills rather than self-help skills in deference to the family's culture. This recommendation is particularly useful for school psychologists as they work with Latino parents in educational and intervention planning and implementation for a child with an intellectual disability.

According to Terhune (2005), among African American families, the ideas regarding and communication about developmental disabilities (such as intellectual disability) are "influenced by assimilation, education, socioeconomic status, history, and other factors" (p. 19). Similar to the spiritual support found by Latino families, African American families also report that their faith and religious leaders are important resources in their parenting of a child with intellectual disability. Their faith and their fellow church members provide needed support during times of challenge (Rogers-Dulan, 1998). This faith-based support may be particularly important in the African American culture in which families of lower socioeconomic status have typically had less access to supportive services despite a greater proportion of African American youth being diagnosed with intellectual disability as compared to White families (Walker et al., 1996). In relation to caregiving, African American parents are more likely to use extended family for support than external agencies or resources (Yamaki & Fujiura, 2002).

For school psychologists engaging in practice with African American families, clear communication is vital for teaming with families and effective service delivery. Harry et al. (1995) reports that it is common for African American parents of young children with intellectual disability to believe that school-based services are intended to help the child "catch up" with their peers and disillusionment with the entire system can develop when they come to the realization that the disability is a permanent condition. Terhune's (2005) research suggests that African American families perceive that interactions with agencies regarding support for their children are rarely collaborative—rather the agency or the family is in control depending on the situation. Thus, for effective teaming, school psychologists should ensure that assessment results are delivered with accuracy, eligibility and placement determinations for special education are conducted collaboratively, and educational options are explained thoroughly to allow parents to offer informed opinions for the decision-making process. Terhune also indicates that, "They desire their family values to be respected, not drowned out by professionals claiming best practice" (p. 26). With regard to curriculum, it is also reported that African American families often value the teaching of social and relationship skills to individuals with intellectual disability over adaptive or functional living skills (Terhune, 2005). Therefore, the school psychologist should strive to understand the family's values, priorities, and expectations in order to engage them in the process and provide for better outcomes for the child.

Although the aforementioned cultural considerations are based in research, it is important for any school psychologist to remember that there are often more in-group differences than there are between-group differences regardless of the setting, circumstance, or individuals involved. Thus, the school psychologist should be cautioned against generalizing from cultural considerations to a child with intellectual disability or that child's family. Each individual should be approached with openness, empathy, and the expectation of a willingness to hear and learn in the context of advocacy for the best interests of the child.

IMPACT OF INTELLECTUAL DISABILITY ON SOCIAL–EMOTIONAL AND BEHAVIORAL FUNCTIONING IN SCHOOL AND HOME ENVIRONMENTS

Social–Emotional and Behavioral Functioning in School

According to the *DSM-5* (APA, 2013), intellectual disability commonly occurs in conjunction with a number of other diagnoses that impact the social–emotional and behavioral functioning of children and adolescents. The most common disorders comorbid with intellectual disability are ADHD, ASD, depressive and bipolar disorders, anxiety disorders, stereotypic movement disorder, impulse-control disorders, and major cognitive disorder. Similarly, Dekker et al. (2002) engaged in a large research project to compare children aged 6 to 18 with intellectual disability to a sample of children without intellectual disability on the basis of emotional and behavioral concerns. They found that the children with intellectual disability were more likely than children without intellectual disability to be rated by parents and teachers as exhibiting problems with attention, social concerns, aggression, isolation, and thought problems. Overall, the researchers determined that about 50% of their sample of children and adolescents with intellectual disability exhibited problematic social–emotional issues and behaviors. This prevalence was 3 to 4 times greater than in the sample of typically developing children. Other researchers have also found greater risk of depression and anxiety among children with intellectual disability as compared to their typically developing peers (Alimovic, 2013; Maiano et al., 2018; Whitney et al., 2019). It also seems that children with intellectual disability that is comorbid with either ADHD or ASD are at an especially high risk for symptoms of anxiety and depression as well as other behavioral concerns. On a more encouraging note, Hispanic children with intellectual disability and children who have comorbid intellectual disability and Down's syndrome are less likely to experience depressive symptoms than other children with intellectual disability (Whitney et al., 2019).

> Research suggests that about 50% of children and adolescents with intellectual disability exhibit problematic behavior (Dekker et al., 2002).

Given the at-risk nature of children with intellectual disability compounded with social–emotional concerns, behavioral challenges often arise in the school setting. Several research studies have highlighted the significantly higher rate of behavioral issues among children with intellectual disability as compared to their peers (Dekker et al., 2002; Emerson, 2003; Emerson & Einfield, 2010). The presence of disruptive behavior also appears to occur with equal frequency among both boys and girls with intellectual disability (Baker & Blacher, 2015). Disruptive behavior increases the probability that the individual will experience social exclusion (Emerson, 2001) and be placed in care outside of their familial home (Myrbakk & von Tetzchner, 2008). In some extreme cases, children and adolescents even become involved with the juvenile justice system, where youth with intellectual disability are overrepresented as compared to their peers without disabilities (Frize et al., 2008; van der Put et al., 2014). According to van der Put et al. (2014), a diagnosis of intellectual disability is actually a risk factor for delinquency and recidivism in juvenile detention centers.

In addition, within the school setting, research has demonstrated that African American students and White students with intellectual disability are significantly more likely to be suspended based on behavioral infractions than White students without disabilities (Krezmien et al., 2017). However, data analysis from 2003 in Maryland also found that African Americans students with intellectual disability were suspended at greater frequency than their non-disabled White peers, but White, Hispanic, Asian, and Native American students with intellectual disability were not suspended at greater rates than White students without a disability (Krezmien et al., 2006). According to Krezmien et al. (2017), students with intellectual disability may engage in verbal aggression toward others as well as physical aggression with individuals and/or property. These behaviors often lead to suspension although there is little research to support the effectiveness of suspension for students with intellectual disability and despite the fact that students who are eligible under the IDEA category of *intellectual disability* are provided with some disciplinary protections.

IDEA requires that positive interventions and supports should be provided for any child with a disability when the child's behavior interferes with their own learning or the learning of peers in the environment (U.S. Department of Education, n.d.). In fact, it is critical for school psychologists to understand that these positive behavior interventions that derive from a functional behavioral assessment are the most effective for preventing and modifying challenging behavior among students with intellectual disability (Wong et al., 2015). However, should the behavioral supports continue to be ineffective, the LEA can seek to remove a student with a disability (including intellectual disability) from the current school placement for no more than 10 days. This would include placement in an alternative setting and/or suspension.

If the LEA seeks a change in placement longer than 10 days, then they must conduct a manifestation determination (U.S. Department of Education, n.d.), and school psychologists often feature heavily in this course of action. With the manifestation determination, school personnel and the parent must review all available data to determine whether the behavioral incident was related to the disability and/or a result of the failure of the school to follow the student's Individual Education Program (IEP). If either of these conditions are met, then the behavior is considered to be a manifestation of the child's disability, and the team is required to conduct a new or review an existing functional behavioral assessment and behavior intervention plan. The child cannot be removed from the current placement. Alternatively, if neither condition is met, then the child may be disciplined in a way that is commensurate with what would be the expected punishment for a child without a disability. If that consequence includes a change of placement or suspension, then the LEA is required to continue providing educational services to make progress toward the goals of the child's IEP. These procedures are followed for all children with disabilities unless the behavioral infraction is related to on-campus incidents with weapons, drugs, or serious bodily harm of another individual (U.S. Department of Education, n.d.).

With regard to more prosocial behaviors among children and adolescents with intellectual disability, Brooks et al. (2015) has highlighted the need for participation in both structured and unstructured social activities for the development of well-rounded social skills despite the fact that children with intellectual disabilities engage in both types of activities with less frequency than their typically developing peers (Solish et al., 2010). Activities with predetermined expectations and rules (such as sports or dance lessons) that are often performed under adult supervision are considered structured activities. In contrast, unstructured activities (like playdates or recess) provide opportunities for social interaction with looser guidelines for behavior. Brooks et al. (2005) found that more time in unstructured activities was associated with greater social competence in children with intellectual disability. Research also supports that children and adolescents who participate in more activities are often perceived as having more strengths by their parents (Carter et al., 2015). Thus, in their advocacy role, school psychologists should explore, promote, and support the inclusion of children with intellectual disability in structured and unstructured activities.

Social–Emotional and Behavioral Functioning at Home

Social–emotional and behavioral concerns for children with intellectual disability are certainly not limited to the school environment. These issues often lead to significant stressors within the home as well. The parental stress associated with caring for a child or adolescent with intellectual disability is well documented in the literature (Baxter et al., 2000; Emerson, 2003; Masulani-Mwale et al., 2018; McIntyre, 2016; Patton et al., 2018; Totsika et al., 2011). Research also indicates that children with intellectual disability are 3 to 4 times more likely to suffer from physical abuse and neglect in their homes than children without disabilities (Jones et al., 2012; McDonnell et al., 2019) and are more likely to have the perpetrator be an immediate family member (McDonnell et al., 2019). McDonnell et al. (2019) also note that children with intellectual disability "are at risk for more frequent and complex maltreatment" (p. 582) even when compared to other abused or neglected children. Even when it does not reach the level of abuse, children with intellectual disability are more likely to be disciplined with physical punishment in the home (Kimura & Yamazaki, 2016).

Although it behooves school psychologists to be aware of these alarming statistics regarding violence directed at children and adolescents with intellectual disability, it is also important to recognize some protective factors for parental stress in the home. Patton et al. (2018) found that high social support served as a buffer to lower stress of parents of children with intellectual disability. Similarly, Kimura and Yamazaki (2016) propose that increasing parents' understanding and expectations of behavior as well as providing respite care may reduce parental levels of stress when caring for a child with intellectual disability.

Beyond their own stress associated with caregiving for a child with intellectual disability, another body of literature suggests that parents often feel conflicted about talking to their child about their disability. Although some research suggests that parents often avoid these conversations (Cunningham et al., 2000), more recent research indicates that about 66% of parents of adolescents with intellectual disability have held conversations with their child about their disability status (Jones et al., 2014). Parents who know and understand the etiology of their child's intellectual disability are more likely to discuss it with their child (Jones et al., 2014). However, it is reported that parents often avoid the conversations due to a belief that the child would not understand or would be distressed by the information; yet children with intellectual disabilities often report awareness of their disability even when parents have not spoken with them about it (Cunningham et al., 2000). When parents do choose to engage in conversations with their child regarding their intellectual disability, the conversation often results from issues related to social exclusion or bullying (Jones et al., 2014). In practice, it is critically important for the school psychologist to understand and respect the family's position on discussing the child's disability status while also intervening and advocating in situations of social, emotional, or behavioral consequence for the child.

> In practice, it is critically important for the school psychologist to understand and respect the family's position on discussing the child's disability status while also intervening and advocating in situations of social, emotional, or behavioral consequence for the child.

Another important concept in the parenting and home life of a child with intellectual disability relates to the parent's beliefs about the child's self-determination. The concept of self-determination includes aspects of self-advocacy, decision-making, and problem-solving for oneself. For many years, society believed that individuals with intellectual disability were unable to exhibit self-determination, but a focus in recent decades on positive psychology has highlighted the importance of using a strengths-based approach for children with intellectual disability. Research supports that the promotion of self-determination during adolescence is particularly important for a successful transition into adulthood (Wehmeyer, 2014). However, problem behaviors of the child often negatively impact the parents' perceptions of the child's ability to engage in self-determination and in ratings of overall strengths of the child (Carter et al., 2009, 2015). In addition, parents frequently report internal conflict regarding self-determination for their children as they want to give them some sense of autonomy while also protecting them from perceived harm (Arellano & Peralta, 2013). Somewhat startling, research has found that teachers often rate their students as having few skills related to self-determination, but parents of those same children rate them significantly lower than even the teachers. This may be due to the context in which the children are observed or the raters' perception and expectations for behavior (Grigal et al., 2011). Not surprising, parents' perceptions of the severity of their child's intellectual disability often relate to their assessment of their child's self-determination skills such that parents who perceive their child's disability as less severe rate the child's self-determination skills as higher than those parents who indicate that their child has a more severe form of intellectual disability (Carter et al., 2013).

School psychologists can play a critical role in helping families to foster self-determination skills in their children with intellectual disability. Carter et al. (2013) note that self-determination should be prioritized as a goal during transition services due to their link to more favorable outcomes regarding future employment (Cimera et al., 2014) and independent living. If the child is receiving special education services, then IDEA requires that a plan for transition (including goals and supports) for future education, training, employment, and independent living be devised and enacted (U.S. Department of Education, n.d.). School psychologists can and should assist with these determinations and their implementation in the school and/or home. Specific to the home setting, Wehmeyer (2014) suggests basic strategies that parents can use to increase these skills and promote more positive outcomes. Parents should be encouraged to allow the child to explore and take risks. They should spend quality time with the child and address questions regarding their intellectual disability. Finally, modeling goal setting with realistic expectations, providing explanations for the parents' decisions, and creating decision-making opportunities for the child are simple steps that parents can take to promote self-determination in children with intellectual disability. School psychologists are perfectly positioned as a liaison between the school and home to assist with providing knowledge to parents and/or home-based interventions for the development of self-determination skills.

IMPACT OF INTELLECTUAL DISABILITY ON LEARNING IN THE CLASSROOM

It is arguable that one of the most important educational decisions made on behalf of a student with an intellectual disability is the student's educational placement. The *placement* refers to the setting in which services and supports are provided in the school. The most inclusive educational placement for a child with intellectual disability is within the general education classroom. Although this was once considered progressive, it is now commonplace within school environments. Thus, teacher attitudes toward inclusion of children with disabilities within their classrooms is critical to the success (or failure) of the setting for the child. Some factors have emerged from the literature as supportive of positive attitudes of teachers toward students with intellectual disability. Dessemontet et al. (2014) found that providing teachers with inservice training specific to intellectual disability not only increased teachers' knowledge regarding the rights of children with intellectual disability but also improved their perceptions of the capabilities of students with intellectual disability. In addition, experience in teaching a child with intellectual disability increased the teachers' confidence in their ability to teach children with intellectual disability and their willingness to support inclusion of children with disabilities in their classrooms.

Similar to their teachers' attitudes, research has also supported that exposure to a student with a disability increases peers' attitudes toward and acceptance of children with disabilities in an inclusive classroom (Siperstein et al., 2007). Although some educators and parents are concerned about the educational impact on typically developing children resulting from including students with intellectual disability in the general education classroom, many studies support neutral or even positive academic outcomes for the typically developing students in inclusive classrooms (Demeris et al., 2007; Dessemontet & Bless, 2013; Kalambouka et al., 2007).

Of course, there is more to the classroom experience for children and adolescents with intellectual disability than teacher and peer acceptance. Each student's executive functioning plays a vital role in their ability to acclimate and prosper in the classroom. Memisevic and Sinanovic (2014) define *executive functioning* as "a set of higher cognitive skills responsible for many everyday activities and abilities such as planning, organizing, cognitive flexibility, working memory, monitoring, and self-regulation" (p. 831). The severity of a student's intellectual disability is related to their executive functioning skills with greater levels of severity yielding more significant deficits (Memisevic & Sinanovic, 2014). In the classroom, these deficits may appear in a student's difficulty in remembering and subsequently following directions (Alloway, 2010). Attention and behavior are also negatively impacted by executive functioning deficits. Response inhibition (like speaking without being called upon) is common in children with executive functioning issues, and problem-solving and shifting attention between tasks can be a particular challenge (Diamond, 2013). Dawson (2014) explains that as students' progress through their school grades and curricula, the demands on executive skills increase over time. Given these critical concerns, it is easy to comprehend the detrimental link between executive functioning deficits and lessened academic achievement as evidenced in the literature (Best et al., 2011; Bull et al., 2008).

Each student's executive functioning skills plays a vital role in their ability to acclimate and prosper in the classroom.

With regard to individual subject matter, reading is fundamental to classroom and academic progress as students must first learn to read in order to later read to learn. Extensive research has documented the struggle of reading for children and adolescents with intellectual disability. The intellectual disability often contributes to challenges across a variety of skills necessary for reading success, including auditory comprehension, phonological awareness, word decoding, perception skills, and comprehension (Afacan et al., 2018; Channell et al., 2013; Dessemontet & de Chambrier, 2015; Panopoulos & Drossinou-Korea, 2020; van Wingerden et al., 2017). These reading challenges are likely to present throughout the student's schooling and significantly impact other subject matter learning as well. Through their roles with advocacy and educational planning, school psychologists should know, explain, and assist in implementing teaching and intervention strategies that have been shown to be effective for readers and developing readers with intellectual disability. Some particularly effective strategies for reading instruction and intervention include systematic prompting on engagement, three-step decoding strategies, peer tutors, read-aloud techniques, sight-word instruction, and guided social interaction. More detail on this research and these strategies can be found in Alquraini and Rao (2020).

The difficulty with reading for students with intellectual disability leads to a corresponding challenge with writing. In school settings, writing is a common and expected way for students across the curriculum to demonstrate their understanding of subject matter content (Cannella-Malone et al., 2015). The ability to effectively communicate through writing includes subskills like planning, organizing, and revising (Hayes, 2012; Pennington & Delano, 2012). These subskills are similar in nature to the previously noted executive function deficits often experienced by children and adolescents with intellectual disability. School psychologists should be aware of and support the use of effective classroom practices for writing support with students with intellectual disability. The research highlights the following as productive approaches for increasing writing skills for children and adolescents with intellectual disability: incorporating word processing for early elementary students, using writing goals for late elementary and middle school students, explicit instruction, feedback from adults and/or peers, and self-assessment processes (Graham et al., 2016).

As with reading, the executive functioning deficits evidenced in students with intellectual disability impact mathematics skills in the classroom as well. Issues related to working memory, problem solving, and attention make math achievement a significant struggle for these students. Regardless of disability status, Spooner et al. (2019) highlight the importance of the student learning a progression of foundational skills through evidence-based teaching strategies that fit with the expected classroom content and are matched to the needs and skills of the child with intellectual disability. The most recent research regarding math instruction for students with intellectual disability supports the following classroom teaching strategies as effective: systematic instruction, in vivo instruction, system-of-least prompts strategy, constant time-delay strategy, and task-analytic instruction. For an explanation of these teaching techniques, the reader is encouraged to seek Hudson et al. (2018). The National Mathematics Advisory Panel (2008) also recommends teaching students to solve math problems with themes that are familiar to them in their current life activities.

IMPLICATIONS FOR SCHOOL PSYCHOLOGISTS

Assessment Role

Within the school setting, school psychologists are frontline workers in the evaluation process to determine whether a student has a disability that qualifies the student for special education eligibility under IDEA. This is particularly true in the case of intellectual disability, in which the school psychologist often plays a prominent role in the necessary cognitive, academic, and adaptive evaluations that are necessary to determine whether the child meets criteria for the disability and demonstrates a need for services. Depending on the severity of the child's deficits, the school psychologist will use a variety of formal and informal assessment tools, observations, and interviews to gather the data necessary for the team to make an eligibility decision. This assessment role must be undertaken with care, accuracy, and conscientiousness as the resulting decisions have significant life consequences for the child and family. These determinations not only impact current educational planning and delivery but also life-long academic and vocational opportunities.

Advocacy Role

One can argue that one of the most important roles that the school psychologist can play in the lives and well-being of students with intellectual disability is that of advocate. Due to the often compounded physical, social, emotional, behavioral, and academic challenges for children and adolescents with intellectual disability, many supports and services are necessary to advance their functioning. Thus, a multitude of agencies and professional personnel are needed for the child's progress. As such, the school psychologist is perfectly positioned (through training, ethics, and position) to serve as a liaison among the child, family, and service facilities. The school psychologist can direct the child and family to community-based opportunities to further development and care for the child and provide direction, attention, and resources for the family. The school psychologist can then serve a critical role in coordination and communication between community-based service providers and school-setting personnel.

Although school psychologists can offer critical collaboration efforts toward health and social–emotional planning with community partners, this advocacy role becomes even more essential when working toward a transition for students with disabilities. IDEA requires that transition planning from school life to adult life begin at the age of 16 and effective transition planning often leads to more positive outcomes for students with disabilities. Krieg et al. (2014) recommend that transition plans should be based in part on functional assessments, interest surveys, vocational evaluations, and interviews. The data from these evaluations and other relevant data points can be matched with community opportunities and resources to offer a realistic yet appropriately challenging transition plan to maximize the probability for the student with a disability to remain engaged in the community, develop positive self-esteem, and have a fulfilling role into adulthood. With their skills in data-based decision-making and collaboration, school psychologists are uniquely suited to enhance team efforts toward effective transition services for adolescents with intellectual disability.

Consultation Role

Beyond their role in consultation and collaboration for transition services, school psychologists can use their training and experience in these areas to provide other services and supports for students with intellectual disability. Through consultation, school psychologists can provide vital indirect services for improved behavioral, social–emotional, and academic functioning for students. Given that students with intellectual disability often experience challenges in all of these areas, the role of the school psychologist could be both relevant and impactful. School psychologists can and should support teachers through functional behavioral assessments, intervention planning, and intervention implementation to modify or replace maladaptive classroom behaviors. School psychologists may use their knowledge of social–emotional supports and services to advise intervention teams or other service providers regarding interventions directed at social skill development or emotion regulation for students with intellectual disability. Finally, school psychologists are positioned to apply their understanding of learning and cognition to better the group and individual academic interventions as delivered to the child or adolescent with intellectual disability.

Counseling and Therapy Role

When a student's needs go beyond what the school psychologist can provide through the indirect role of consultation, the psychologist may need to direct efforts toward direct service provision to support behavioral, social, and/or emotional needs of the student with intellectual disability. In those cases, the school psychologist may find it appropriate to engage in counseling or therapy services with the child or adolescent to assist with more socially appropriate behavior in the school, to help build a repertoire of prosocial skills, or to support students in understanding and regulating their emotions. As such, the school psychologist may choose to engage the student (with appropriate permission from the parent) in individual or group-based counseling or therapy services. The school psychologist would work with the child to develop goals and a treatment plan for working toward a level of adjustment that allows the child to improve functioning within their environment and create greater overall well-being. Also, given that children and adolescents with intellectual disability are at-risk in behavioral, social, and emotional areas in comparison to their typically developing peers, school psychologists may be called into crisis intervention roles in support of these students. Challenges with communication, emotion regulation, anxiety, and depression may lead to physical aggression, emotional excess, or even suicidal/homicidal ideation in the school setting. The school psychologist's training in crisis prevention and intervention would be vital in ensuring the safety of the student, their peers, and school staff members in the event of one of the aforementioned crisis situations. School psychologists should be confident in their training and prepared to respond when need arises to increase the probability of better outcomes for all.

EDUCATIONAL SUPPORTS

Educational planning and academic delivery for students with intellectual disability has changed dramatically since the enactment of IDEA and its requirements for a free and appropriate education within the least restrictive environment. Spooner and Browder (2015) explain that the implementation of IDEA as federal law represented the first time that many students with intellectual disability were allowed to attend public schools. Spooner and Browder (2015) have explored the important educational advancements for students with intellectual disability since that time. They posit that the use of operant conditioning strategies, the introduction of a functional skills curriculum, and the focus on standards-based instruction were critical developments in the education of children and adolescents with intellectual disability.

According to Project IDEAL (Informing and Designing Education for All Learners; an organization dedicated to helping teachers work with students with disabilities), functional skills should be an integral part of the curriculum for children and adolescents with intellectual disability in order to help them with future independent living. Functional skills focus on applied content like time, money, self-care, hygiene, and other concepts that help the individual progress toward the potential of living independently. However, they also note that as vital as these skills are, they should not be taught at the absolute expense of the academic curriculum as students with intellectual disability need literacy and quantitative skills. Project IDEAL specifically recommends the following teaching strategies for working with students with intellectual disability: breaking tasks or concepts into smaller parts, teaching concepts one step at a time, utilizing individual and small-group instruction, providing multiple opportunities to practice skills, using multimodal prompts, and positively reinforcing accuracy (Project IDEAL, n.d.). In addition, Spooner et al. (2012) conducted an extensive review of literature related to teaching students with severe disabilities and found that time-delay strategies and task-analytic instruction were effective evidence-based practices across reading, math, and science instruction. With respect to teaching written expression, Cannella-Malone et al. (2015) recommend that teachers approach the task using the ACCESS acronym. ACCESS represents accommodations and assistive technology, concrete topics, critical skills, explicit instruction, strategy instruction, and systematic evaluation in their processes.

> Functional skills focus on applied content like time, money, self-care, hygiene, and other concepts that help the individual progress toward the potential of living independently.

Finally, it is important to address the use of assistive technology in the classroom to support the education and development of students with intellectual disability. Although the term *technology* brings to mind some sophisticated electronic device, in actuality, assistive technology can be any physical object that is used for instructional purposes or functional purposes. Assistive technology for students with intellectual disability can fall along a continuum from something as low tech as a rubber pencil grip that allows a child to grasp a pencil more effectively to something as high tech as touch-screen technology for communication or response purposes. Assistive technology can be vital in academic, social, or functional life circumstances. Assistive technology allows the student with an intellectual disability to participate in the setting more fully and with their peers, thereby allowing a better quality of life. Some common examples of assistive technology include mobility devices, hearing and visual aids, voice-recognition and word-prediction software, and physical building modifications. It is in the best interest of the school psychologist to become familiar with the vast array of assistive technology tools and their uses to better support and advocate for children and adolescents with intellectual disability.

SCHOOL-BASED MENTAL HEALTH INTERVENTIONS AND SUPPORTS

Due to the nature of their disability, students with intellectual disability are at risk for a number of social, emotional, and behavioral challenges (Alimovic, 2013; Dekker et al., 2002; Emerson, 2003; Emerson & Einfield, 2010; Green et al., 2015; Maiano et al., 2018; Whitney et al., 2019). The social issues may include social exclusion and bullying (Jones et al., 2014), and the emotional concerns frequently manifest as anxiety and depression (Alimovic, 2013; Green et al., 2015; Maiano et al., 2018; Whitney et al., 2019). With regard to behavior, the executive functioning deficits of children and adolescents with intellectual disability may lead to issues related to following directions (Alloway, 2010), impulse control, and emotion regulation in the classroom (Diamond, 2013).

In order to address issues related to peer interactions (including social exclusion and bullying), social skills training has been found to be an effective intervention that can be delivered in the school setting to target the social concerns of children and adolescents with intellectual disability (Lappa & Mantzikos, 2019; Ledford et al., 2018; Plavnick et al., 2015). These interventions can be delivered in individual or small-group settings, and there is evidence to suggest that they demonstrate greater effectiveness when delivered in school or clinic settings (Ledford et al., 2018). Social skills include social-cognitive skills, communication skills, prosocial behavior, and emotional adjustment skills (Weiner, 2004). Social skills are rarely explicitly taught but learned through implicit interactions. Children and adolescents with intellectual disability struggle with intuiting the social cues that lead to prosocial interactions. In addition, due to the isolation that their disability often brings, children with intellectual disability also have fewer opportunities to practice what social skills they do acquire through their natural environmental interactions (Canney & Byrne, 2006). Beyond explicit social skill instruction, researchers have also found effectiveness in teaching social perception among adolescents with intellectual disability (Stauch et al., 2018). Given the plethora of evidenced-based social skills training interventions available, school psychologists are encouraged to research those specific to the social skill needs exhibited by the individual with whom they work. School psychologists are uniquely suited to understand the social skill challenges of students with intellectual disability, select an intervention with a high probability for success, implement that intervention with fidelity, and evaluate its effectiveness in the school setting with peers and other adults.

In their emotional functioning, children and adolescents with intellectual disability may need additional intervention to address issues related to anxiety and depression. It is particularly important to address the symptoms of anxiety as evidence suggests that children with both intellectual disability and anxiety are more likely to demonstrate problem behavior, and their higher rates of anxiety are long lasting (Green et al., 2015) Research has supported that the effectiveness of both positive behavior supports (Moskowitz et al., 2017) and cognitive behavioral therapy in assisting students with intellectual disability in the development of coping strategies (Hronis et al., 2019; Moskowitz et al., 2017; Reaven et al., 2011). Sadly, very little research has addressed the effectiveness of psychological interventions for children with intellectual disability and depression (Cameron et al., 2020). However, a few small studies have documented the effectiveness of cognitive behavioral therapy for targeting symptoms of depression in children with intellectual disability (Grieg & MacKay, 2005; Loades, 2015; Selvapandiyan, 2019). Thus, this seems to be the most promising course of action at this point. School psychologists who are trained to deliver cognitive behavioral therapy could provide this psychological intervention in the schools. Cognitive behavioral therapy focuses on maladaptive thought patterns and helps the individual learn coping skills and better understand their own behavior and others' motivations. There is an emphasis on current life circumstances to help the child or adolescent adapt to the present setting.

With regard to behavior, function-based interventions are found to be particularly effective with students with intellectual disability (Wong et al., 2015). School psychologists are trained and well versed in the functional behavioral assessment process and resulting positive behavioral supports. The assessment process includes conducting a series of systematic classroom observations of a target behavior for a student. The school psychologist uses information on the antecedent to the behavior and the consequences of the behavior to determine why the child is engaging in the behavior. In this context, the consequences are not necessarily punishments but anything that follows the behavior and increases the probability that it will occur again. The school psychologist determines whether the behavior is occurring due to a skill deficit that the child has or whether the child has the skill to be socially appropriate in the circumstance but is choosing not to use it. Then, the school psychologist identifies a socially appropriate replacement behavior that serves the same function for the child. That new behavior is taught, then reinforced for use in place of the previous, maladaptive behavior. School psychologists' skills in this process have long supported critical behavioral improvement for students with and without disabilities in the school setting.

CASE STUDY 3.1 ANTONELLA: CASE OF A BIRACIAL GIRL WITH INTELLECTUAL DISABILITY

Background

Antonella is a 7-year-old kindergarten student in a large urban district. Antonella's mother (Stacy) is White and originally from the Midwestern United States, and her father (Rodrigo) is an undocumented immigrant from Guatemala. Stacy was stationed in Guatemala with the U.S. Army and nearing the end of her military service when she became pregnant unexpectedly. She finished her service and moved to the metro-Chicago area. Shortly thereafter, Rodrigo moved the United States to be with Stacy. Stacy received early prenatal care and underwent testing at 15 weeks of pregnancy. The testing revealed an elevated risk of Down syndrome. Stacy's doctor recommended further testing with amniocentesis and suggested that she speak with the social worker affiliated with the medical practice to do some preplanning for services in case the baby was in fact born with Down syndrome. Stacy met with the social worker one time, but she and Rodrigo became fearful of the increased attention they were receiving due to Rodrigo's undocumented status. Stacy ceased seeking prenatal care at that point as well. At 38 weeks of pregnancy, Antonella was born in a Chicago hospital, and the Down syndrome diagnosis was confirmed through follow-up testing. Social workers again became involved and referred the family for early-intervention services. Throughout infancy and early toddlerhood, Antonella's maternal grandmother cared for her in her home while Stacy and Rodrigo worked full-time jobs. While in her home, Antonella received physical therapy, occupational therapy, and speech–language therapy as delays were evidenced in gross motor, fine motor, and speech skills. Antonella did not sit independently until after her first birthday and began walking at 2½ years old. She began feeding herself with her hands around 18 months but continues to struggle with using a spoon or fork. Her speech was very delayed with only a very small vocabulary available as she reached her third birthday. At the age of 3, it was recommended that Antonella enter an early-intervention preschool setting. The family again became fearful of that course of action due to Rodrigo's undocumented status. Rather than pursue the program, Rodrigo quit his job to stay home with Antonella. He continued to try to stimulate her progress through repeating the activities that he had seen

(continued)

3: INTELLECTUAL DISABILITIES

CASE STUDY 3.1 ANTONELLA: CASE OF A BIRACIAL GIRL WITH INTELLECTUAL DISABILITY (*continued*)

from the professionals and with some things that he had researched online, but professional services ceased. The family contemplated enrolling Antonella in kindergarten at the age of 5 but chose to continue the arrangement that they had developed instead. Over the course of the next 2 years, Antonella made little progress and even digressed behaviorally. At the age of 7, the family sought the services of a private pediatric psychologist, who diagnosed Antonella with intellectual disability based on her deficits in cognitive functioning and adaptive functioning, which had first appeared during the developmental period. At that point, the family decided to enroll Antonella in the local public school. Upon entry into a kindergarten class at the age of 7, Antonella has a vocabulary of 15 English words and two Spanish words. She cannot dress herself independently and struggles with frequent toileting accidents. In addition, Antonella frequently kicks, bites, and throws objects at peers and her teacher when she is frustrated. On the kindergarten admission screening, she could not answer any items correctly, including identification of shapes, colors, letters, and numbers to 10. School personnel sought and attained permission for a special education evaluation for Antonella.

Discussion

When the etiology of intellectual disability is identifiable, Down syndrome is a frequent cause. In fact, among the entire population of children and adolescents with intellectual disability, approximately 20% have Down syndrome. Down syndrome impacts brain development, and individuals with Down syndrome have a smaller brain volume and different brain shape than typically developing individuals. These differences are thought to cause the intellectual disability. In most cases of intellectual disability caused by Down syndrome, the level of severity is mild to moderate. In Antonella's case, the early onset of delays in gross motor, fine motor, and speech–language skills are hallmarks of intellectual disability. Those deficits continued throughout early childhood. Although her parents had justifiable fears regarding her father's undocumented immigrant status, Antonella's delays were likely exacerbated when her parents chose to remove her from the home-based early-intervention services as research supports that early intervention is critical to later developmental outcomes for children with intellectual disability. Likewise, her delayed school entry prevented Antonella from benefiting from the services available in that setting to address her cognitive and adaptive deficits. In addition to those concerns, her aggressive behavior puts her at risk for social exclusion among her kindergarten peers.

Given that Antonella's parents have granted permission for an evaluation, the school psychologist should begin the evaluation process. By law, the eligibility team (including the school psychologist) has 60 days to complete the evaluation and determine whether Antonella meets criteria as a student with an intellectual disability; however, since Antonella is not currently receiving any professional services for her deficits, it is imperative that the evaluation proceed immediately and with expediency. During the evaluation, the team will review records, complete classroom observations, and conduct interviews with the parents and teacher. The previous *DSM-5* diagnosis will represent a critical data point. The team will seek a release of information from the parents to receive those records from the private psychologist. Also, because Antonella has Down syndrome, they will also seek permission to obtain medical records from any providers involved in her care in that regard. The classroom observations may be completed by the school psychologist or another team member and will give the team valuable information about Antonella's functioning in the classroom relative to typically developing peers. The interviews with parents will focus on Antonella's early development and functioning within her home. This is a valuable data point to substantiate both early-delay information and adaptive behavior deficits. The interview with the teacher will give perspective on Antonella's academic, social, emotional, and behavioral performance at the present time. After these data points are compiled, the testing process is likely to begin. IDEA requires that Antonella be assessed in every area of suspected deficit. The school

(*continued*)

CASE STUDY 3.1 ANTONELLA: CASE OF A BIRACIAL GIRL WITH INTELLECTUAL DISABILITY (continued)

psychologist will be responsible for testing Antonella's cognitive ability with an individually administered IQ test. The psychologist will also assess Antonella's academic functioning with an individually administered academic achievement instrument. In addition, the school psychologist will likely be responsible for administering adaptive behavior assessments to Antonella's parents and her teacher to assess her adaptive skills. Finally, the school psychologist may be asked to complete a functional behavioral assessment as a part of the evaluation since Antonella is exhibiting behavioral concerns in the classroom and at home. As there are obvious issues with speech and language, the speech–language pathologist will evaluate Antonella's communication skills. If the eligibility team believes that Antonella continues to experience delays in gross and fine motor skills, then those testing processes will be conducted by a physical therapist and occupational therapist, respectively. Since Antonella is biracial and her family dynamics cross cultures, the team members will need to ensure that cultural considerations are taken into account in the evaluation process. They will also need to take the steps necessary to ensure that Antonella's father (who is not a native English speaker) can fully participate in the process. This may include such things as providing documents in Spanish or the use of a translator in interviews or meetings if appropriate. When all of the information necessary for the evaluation has been collected, then the eligibility team (professionals involved in the testing processes, general education teacher, special education teacher, LEA administrative representative, and parents) will meet for decision-making purposes. If the team determines that Antonella meets criteria for intellectual disability and displays a need for educational supports, then the team will determine that she is eligible for special education services under the IDEA eligibility of intellectual disability. The next task for the team will be to develop an IEP for Antonella. The IEP will discuss her present levels of performance based on the evaluation data, her education placement, yearly goals and objectives across all areas of need, and any related services (e.g., physical therapy, speech therapy, occupational therapy). The IEP team will meet yearly to discuss progress, review placement, and update Antonella's goals and objectives. Every 3 years, a re-evaluation will be conducted. Depending on the severity of her deficits and the team's decision, Antonella may be eligible for school-based services up to the age of 21.

Beyond the evaluation for special education services and when the needed educational supports are in place, the school psychologist will likely be involved in behavioral intervention for Antonella's aggressive actions in the classroom. The team will seek to have Antonella placed in the least restrictive environment (per IDEA) that will allow her to make progress toward her IEP goals. However, based on previous reports, some behavioral changes will be needed for Antonella to participate in the general education classroom. As such, the functional behavioral assessment conducted by the school psychologist during the evaluation will provide the basis for behavioral intervention. Research supports that function-based interventions are highly effective for modifying problematic behavior for students with intellectual disability. The school psychologist will use that information to determine the "why" behind Antonella's behavior. The school psychologist will decide what purpose the behavior is serving for Antonella and what is operating to maintain that behavior in the classroom. The school psychologist will determine whether Antonella is receiving something positive from her aggressive behavior, escaping something that she perceives as negative, or if it is stimulating to her. The school psychologist will then develop a behavior intervention plan that utilizes positive strategies to reinforce a new, socially acceptable replacement behavior that serves the same function for Antonella. The school psychologist will monitor the intervention plan as it is implemented and evaluate Antonella's progress over time. In addition, the school psychologist may also include Antonella in a social skills group. Many different forms of small-group social skill interventions have been shown to be effective for helping with cognitive, communication, and social problem-solving skills for children with intellectual disability.

SUMMARY POINTS

- In order to receive a *DSM-5* (APA, 2013) diagnosis of Intellectual Disability, the child must exhibit deficits in intellectual functioning and adaptive behavior with onset of symptoms during the developmental period.
- A child must meet the eligibility criteria for intellectual disability under IDEA and demonstrate a need for support in order to progress in the curriculum to qualify within the school setting for special education services.
- With regard to cultural considerations, the school psychologist should strive to understand the family's values, priorities, and expectations in order to engage them in the process and provide for better outcomes for the child.
- In practice, it is critically important for the school psychologist to understand and respect the family's position on discussing the child's disability status while also intervening and advocating in situations of social, emotional, or behavioral consequence for the child.
- For students with intellectual disability, their level of executive functioning plays a vital role in their ability to acclimate and prosper in the classroom.
- School psychologists can engage in many roles and functions to support the needs of students with intellectual disability.

TEST YOUR KNOWLEDGE

1. Which of the following is required for a *DSM-5* diagnosis of Intellectual Disability?
   a. Deficits in intellectual functioning
   b. Deficits in adaptive functioning
   c. Onset of symptoms in the developmental period
   d. All of the above

2. A *DSM-5* diagnosis of Intellectual Disability is required for a student to be eligible for school-based services under IDEA.
   a. True
   b. False

3. According to NASP's *Principles for Professional Ethics* (2020), a school psychologist may use a qualified translator during the assessment process when it is deemed appropriate based on cultural considerations.
   a. True
   b. False

4. Which of the following is a set of cognitive skills related to planning, organizing, and short-term memory?
   a. Metacognition
   b. Executive functioning
   c. Working memory
   d. Adaptive behavior

5. In vivo instruction and system-of-least-prompts strategy are evidenced-based practices for teaching writing skills to students with intellectual disability.
   a. True
   b. False

Answers: (1) d, (2) b, (3) a, (4) b, (5) b.

DISCUSSION QUESTIONS

1. Compare the *DSM-5* diagnostic criteria for Intellectual Disability with the IDEA eligibility criteria for intellectual disability.

2. Highlight some parental stressors for caring for a child with intellectual disability.

3. Discuss some ways of helping children with intellectual disability develop self-determination skills.

4. Explain how executive functioning deficits impact academic achievement for children with intellectual disability.

5. Detail one evidenced-based social–emotional intervention for students with intellectual disability.

CHAPTER RESOURCES

American Association on Intellectual and Developmental Disabilities—Promotes progressive practices for individuals with intellectual disability: www.aamr.org

Best Buddies—Nonprofit organization focused on promoting friendships and employment for individuals with intellectual disability: www.bestbuddies.org

Centers for Disease Control and Prevention *Facts About Intellectual Disability*: www.cdc.gov/ncbddd/childdevelopment/facts-about-intellectual-disability.html

National Association of Councils on Developmental Disabilities—Supports programs for self-determination and inclusion of individuals with disabilities: www.nacdd.org

National Center for Education Statistics *Students with Disabilities:* https://nces.ed.gov/programs/coe/indicator_cgg.asp#:~:text=In%202018%E2%80%9319%2C%20the%20number,percent%20had%20specific%20learning%20disabilities

Project IDEAL—Organization dedicated to help teachers support learners with disabilities: www.projectidealonline.org

Siskin Children's Institute—Dedicated to improving the lives of children with special needs: www.siskin.org

Special Olympics—Provides sports and competition opportunities for children and adults with intellectual disabilities: www.specialolympics.org

The Arc of the United States—Organization for promoting rights and opportunities for individuals with intellectual disabilities: www.thearc.org

U.S. Department of Education *IDEA:* https://sites.ed.gov/idea

KEY REFERENCES

Only key references appear in the print edition. The full reference list appears in the digital product on Springer Publishing Connect: connect.springerpub.com/content/book/978-0-8261-3587-2/part/part02/chapter/ch03

American Psychiatric Association. (2000). *Diagnostic and statistical manual of mental disorders* (4th ed., text rev.). American Psychiatric Press.

Carter, E. W., Lane, K. L., Cooney, M., Weir, K., Moss, C. K., & Machalicek, W. (2013). Self-determination among transition-age youth with autism or intellectual disability: Parent perspectives. *Research and Practice for Persons with Severe Disabilities, 38*(3), 129–138. https://doi.org/10.1177/154079691303800301

Emerson, E. (2003). Mothers of children and adolescents with intellectual disability: Social and economic situation, mental health status, and the self-assessed social and psychological impact of the child's difficulties. *Journal of Intellectual Disability Research, 47,* 385–399. https://doi.org/10.1046/j.1365-2788.2003.00498.x

Jones, L., Bellis, M. A., Wood, S., Hughes, K., McCoy, E., Eckley, L., Bates, G., Mikton, C., Shakespeare, T., & Officer, A. (2012). Prevalence and risk of violence against children with disabilities: A systematic review and meta-analysis of observational studies. *The Lancet, 380,* 899–907. https://doi.org/10.1016/S0140-6736(12)60692-8

Kimura, M., & Yamazaki, Y. (2016). Physical punishment, mental health, and sense of coherence among parents of children with intellectual disability in Japan. *Journal of Applied Research in Intellectual Disabilities, 29,* 455–467. https://doi.org/10.1111/jar.12198

Memisevic, H., & Sinanovic, O. (2014). Executive functioning in children with intellectual disability—The effects of sex, level, and aetiology of intellectual disability. *Journal of Intellectual Disability Research, 58*(9), 830–837. https://doi.org/10.1111/jir.12098

Patel, D. R., Cabral, M. D., Ho, A., & Merrick, J. (2020). A clinical primer on intellectual disability. *Translational Pediatrics, 9*(1), 23–35. https://doi.org/10.21037%2Ftp.2020.02.02

Saad, M. A. E., & ElAdl, A. M. (2019). Defining and determining intellectual disability (Intellectual Developmental Disorder): Insights from *DSM-5. International Journal of Psycho-Educational Sciences, 8*(1), 51–54.

Spooner, F., Knight, V. F., Browder, D. M., & Smith, B. R. (2012). Evidence-based practice for teaching academics to students with severe developmental disabilities. *Remedial and Special Education, 33*(6), 374–387. https://doi.org/10.1177/0741932511421634

Terhune, P. S. (2005). African-American developmental disability discourses: Implications for policy development. *Journal of Policy and Practice in Intellectual Disabilities, 2*(1), 18–28. https://doi.org/10.1111/j.1741-1130.2005.00004.x

U.S. Department of Education. (n.d.). *Individuals with Disabilities Education Improvement Act.* https://sites.ed.gov/idea

CHAPTER 4

Autism Spectrum Disorder

LEARNING OBJECTIVES

- Understand the *Diagnostic and Statistical Manual of Mental Disorders* (5th ed.; *DSM-5*; American Psychiatric Association [APA], 2013a) diagnostic criteria of Autism Spectrum Disorder (ASD).
- Describe the impact of ASD on a young child's social–emotional and behavioral functioning.
- Identify ways in which ASD may impact a young child's ability to learn in the classroom.
- Summarize the implications of how school psychologists can help to address the needs of children with ASD.
- Have knowledge of educational supports and school-based mental health interventions used to address the educational and mental health needs of children with ASD.

INTRODUCTION

Autism spectrum disorder (ASD) is a complex neurodevelopmental disorder that is characterized by deficits in two core areas: social communication and interaction and restricted repetitive patterns of behavior. According to the Centers for Disease Control and Prevention (CDC; 2021a), ASD occurs in approximately one in 44 children based on a study of eight-year-olds living in 11 communities. The CDC study also indicated that more children are being identified with ASD by age four. It is 4.2 times more likely to occur in boys than girls. It is important to also note that approximately one-third of eight-year-olds diagnosed with ASD also had an intellectual disability (CDC, 2021a). The *Diagnostic and Statistical Manual of Mental Disorders*, Fifth Edition (*DSM-5*; American Psychiatric Association [APA], 2013a), indicates that the worldwide prevalence of ASD is approximately 1% of the general population. Within the United States, it is reported that more than 3.5 million individuals have a diagnosis of ASD (Buescher et al., 2014).

DIAGNOSTIC ISSUES RELATED TO AUTISM SPECTRUM DISORDER

DSM-5 Diagnostic Criteria Related to Autism Spectrum Disorder

In the *DSM-5* (APA, 2013a), ASD is categorized as a Neurodevelopmental Disorder. This is a change from the *DSM-IV-TR* (APA, 2000), in which it was categorized as a subtype of Pervasive Developmental Disorders (PDD). The category of PDD had five subtypes: autistic disorder, Asperger's disorder, pervasive developmental disorder—not otherwise specified (PDD-NOS), Rett disorder, and childhood disintegrative disorder. According to APA (2013a), the decision to drop the individual subtypes was based on research studies that indicate that the subtypes were not consistently used across different medical and clinical professionals. However, it has been noted that individuals with a clear diagnosis of one of the four subtypes should still be given the diagnosis of ASD unless they only have marked deficits in social communication and do not meet other ASD diagnostic criteria for which an evaluation for social pragmatic disorder may be recommended (APA, 2013a). With regard to use of the term *spectrum*, the *DSM-5* (APA, 2013a) manual indicates that it is used to acknowledge the fact that symptom presentation of the disorder can differ substantially among individuals.

The *DSM-5* (APA, 2013a) manual indicates that the term *spectrum* is used to acknowledge that the symptom presentation of the disorder can differ substantially among individuals.

According to the *DSM-5* (APA, 2013a) diagnostic criteria, an individual must exhibit social communication and social interaction impairments that are continuous and evident across many contexts in order to apply the diagnosis. Information should be gathered from multiple sources, which might include interviewing the parent regarding the child's early history, conducting an observation of the child, and gathering information by interviewing the teacher and, if appropriate, the child (2013a). These deficits can be exhibited in various ways such as an impairment in social–emotional reciprocity that can range from an atypical social approach that is not characteristic of a typical back-and-forth conversation to a failure to either initiate or respond to others socially. Another way in which social communication and social interaction deficits can be manifested is in a demonstration of impairments in nonverbal communicative behaviors that are utilized for social interaction. A third example of how social communication and interaction deficits may be manifested is in establishing, maintaining, and comprehending interpersonal relationships that can range from difficulty in adjusting one's behavior to fit various social situations to a lack of interest in others (2013a).

The *DSM-5* also stipulates that restricted patterns of repetitive behaviors or interests are present for diagnostic purposes. These repetitive behaviors can be demonstrated in a variety of ways such as stereotyped or repetitive motor movements (hand flapping) or use of objects, for example, lining up small toys, or in repetitive speech as seen in echolalia. Another example of how restricted, repetitive behaviors may be evident is an insistence on sameness or inflexibility in regard to routine changes, which can lead to distress in the child. Or repetitive behaviors may be evident in restricted, fixated interests that are abnormally intense. Finally, another way in which a child may demonstrate restricted, repetitive behavior is in hyper- or hyporeactivity to sensory input or atypical interest in sensory aspects of the environment such as a negative response to particular sounds.

Unlike the *DSM-IV* (1994), which stipulated that autistic features had to be present before the age of 3, the *DSM-5*'s time frame for onset of symptoms is broader and now just has to be present in early development. The symptoms must have a significant adverse impact on the individual's functioning. It is important to note that the behaviors exhibited by the child must not be better explained by an ID or a global developmental delay. As part of the diagnostic criteria, the current level of severity for social communication and interaction as well as restricted, repetitive behaviors must be indicated. These levels of severity are based on the level of support needed (i.e., support needed, substantial support needed, and very substantial support needed; APA, 2013a).

Regarding differential diagnoses, there are several disorders that should be distinguished from ASD. Similar to ASD, Rett syndrome involves a disruption of social interaction, which typically occurs between 1 and 4 years of age, so its presentation is similar to ASD (APA, 2013a). However, social communication generally improves in children with Rett syndrome while autistic symptoms dissipate. The *DSM-5* manual notes that ASD should only be considered when all diagnostic criteria are evident (2013a). Unlike ASD and Rett syndrome, early development in a child with selective mutism follows a typical developmental course. Although the child may select not to speak in certain situations, there is evidence of developmentally appropriate communication skills in some settings as well as social reciprocity even during times when they are mute. In addition, children with selective mutism do not exhibit the restricted, repetitive behavior that is characteristic of ASD. In children with language disorders, communication difficulties may be evident, which could influence the child's social interactions if they are concerned that others will not understand them. However, the *DSM-5* (2013a) notes that atypical nonverbal communication is generally not linked to specific language disorder and that children with language disorder do not exhibit the repetitive behaviors that are present in ASD. Note also that social pragmatic communication disorder is distinct from ASD in that repetitive behaviors are not present. It is important to point out that, if the criteria for ASD are met, the child would be diagnosed with ASD rather than social pragmatic disorder (2013a).

In early childhood, differentiating ASD from ID can be challenging. A young child with ID may not yet have developed language skills or symbolic skills and may initially present as having ASD since repetitive behaviors are sometimes present in young children with ID (APA, 2013a). According to the *DSM-5* manual, the decision to give a diagnosis of ASD to a young child who has already been diagnosed with ID would be deemed appropriate if the child exhibits a significant impairment in social communication and interaction skills compared to the developmental level of nonverbal skills (APA, 2013a). However, it should be noted that ASD would not be diagnosed if the child's skills in social communication were developed similarly to their intellectual ability (APA, 2013a).

> According to the *DSM-5* manual, the decision to give a diagnosis of ASD to a young child who has already been diagnosed with ID would be deemed appropriate if the child exhibits a significant impairment in social communication and interaction skills compared to the developmental level of nonverbal skills (APA, 2013a).

As noted earlier, one of the diagnostic features of ASD is stereotypies, so stereotypic movement disorder would not be diagnosed if these symptoms are better explained by ASD (APA, 2013a). One thing to keep in mind, though, is that stereotypies can sometimes result in self-injury (APA, 2013a). In this case, a diagnosis of stereotypic movement disorder might be made. Another disorder to distinguish from ASD is attention deficit hyperactivity disorder (ADHD). Children with ASD exhibit attention abnormalities such as being easily distracted or overly focused. Consideration of a diagnosis of ADHD would be given if attentional problems or hyperactivity are more than what is typically seen in individuals of comparable developmental age (APA, 2013a). Schizophrenia in childhood may need to be distinguished from ASD when the symptoms of schizophrenia include odd interests or beliefs and social impairment, but other symptoms, such auditory hallucinations, are not present in ASD (2013a).

With regard to comorbidity, the *DSM-5* indicates that approximately 70% of people with ASD may be comorbid with a single mental health disorder, whereas 40% may have up to two or more disorders (APA, 2013a). Three disorders that ASD is often linked to in early development are ID, language disorder, and stereotypic motor movement. ASD and ADHD can coexist if criteria for both disorders are met. Some scholars report that ADHD is the most common disorder to coexist with ASD (Lord et al., 2018). As noted by Lord and colleagues (2018), it can have a considerable influence on the outcomes in youth with ASD who are of average intellectual ability or those who are intellectually disabled. Anxiety disorders have also been reported in children with ASD, as have behaviors of irritability and aggression, which can be manifested in mild physical aggression in youngsters and verbal aggression in adults (Lord et al., 2018).

School-Based Eligibility

Although use of the *DSM-5* criteria is required to make a medical diagnosis of ASD, a different classification system is used in the schools to determine whether a child with ASD is eligible for special education services. Federal legislation known as the *Individuals with Disabilities Education Improvement Act* (IDEA) ensures that students with disabilities are given a free public education in the least restrictive environment and provides special education services and related services (IDEA, 2004). Under Part B of this legislation, children between the ages of 3 and 21 may be determined to be eligible for one of 13 disability categories. A multidisciplinary team has 60 days to complete an evaluation of the child and then meets to review the data collected from the assessments conducted to determine whether a child is eligible for special education services. Before determining eligibility, the team must determine whether the child meets eligibility requirements of ASD and whether the child is in need of special education and related services (Salvia et al., 2016). If the child is found to be eligible for special education services, an Individual Education Program (IEP) will be established within 30 days following the eligibility determination. The IEP includes information about the child's current levels of achievement and functional performance, annual goals for the child, progress made toward the goals set for the child, special education and related services, and accommodations or modifications that may be needed (U.S. Department of Education, n.d.).

IDEA (2004) defines ASD as a developmental disability in which a child's verbal and nonverbal communication and social interaction are significantly affected. This federal definition indicates that signs of ASD are usually apparent before the age of 3. ASD can adversely impact a child's performance in school. This disability is characterized by the child's engagement in repetitive behaviors and stereotypic movement, resistance to change in daily routines or environmental change, and atypical responses to sensory experiences (IDEA, 2004). It should be noted that ASD would not be considered if it was determined that the child's adverse educational performance is mostly due to an emotional disturbance. In addition, a child who exhibits signs of autism after age 3 could be considered a child with autism (IDEA, 2004).

Although the child may have a medical diagnosis of ASD, the team may decide that the child is not eligible for special education services and may wish to consider the provision of accommodations through Section 504 of the Rehabilitation Act of 1973 (Office of Civil Rights, n.d.). This is civil rights legislation that was established to protect the civil rights of individuals with disabilities and to give them equal access to services at school. The multidisciplinary team will determine whether the child's disability inhibits a major life function which, in regard to ASD, includes learning. If the child is determined to be eligible under Section 504, a 504 plan will be developed that outlines ways in which the school will provide supports and remove any barriers in the school environment that hinder the child's access to services and ability to learn. The 504 plan outlines the specific supports and services the child will receive, who will provide the services and/or supports, and who will ensure that the plan is implemented as intended.

> If the child is determined to be eligible under Section 504, a 504 plan is developed that outlines ways in which the school will provide supports and remove any barriers in the school environment that hinder the child's access to services and ability to learn.

CULTURAL ISSUES RELATED TO AUTISM SPECTRUM DISORDER IN YOUTH

Risk Factors for Autism Spectrum Disorder

Environmental risk factors have been associated with ASD. Research studies have found an association between ASD and advanced maternal age (APA, 2013b; Lord et al., 2018) and advanced paternal age (Lord et al., 2018). Related to advanced maternal age, Lyall and colleagues (2014) found that a mild risk of ASD and developmental delay combined was associated with nonspecific factors during pregnancy, such as maternal metabolic conditions, increased weight, and hypertension along with more specific factors such as maternal hospital admissions due to infections or a family history of autoimmune disease. The use of valproate, a mood stabilizer intended to treat bipolar disorder and seizures, has also been found to be a risk factor (APA, 2013a; Lord et al., 2018). Studies have found an increased risk of ASD to be associated with preterm births, low birth weight, small-for-gestational-age status, and large-for-gestational-age status (Lampi et al., 2012; Moore et al., 2012).

Genetics have also been identified as a risk factor for ASD. According to the *DSM-5* (2013a), twin concordance rates have demonstrated heritability estimates of ASD ranging from 37% to more than 90% (APA, 2013a). Tick et al. (2016) conducted a meta-analysis and found heritability estimates of 74% to 93%. Other scholars conducting sibling research studies discovered that ASD seemed to occur in 7% to 20% of children born after an older child received a diagnosis of ASD and that prevalence increased in children who had two older siblings (Sandin et al., 2014).

Cultural Considerations

Research studies have indicated that ASD is not limited by culture or race (Dyches et al., 2004). According to the CDC (2021b), ASD exists in all racial, ethnic, and socioeconomic groups. A recent report by the CDC (2021b) indicated that the racial gap has decreased as evident in results that demonstrated "no overall differences in the percentage of Black, White, Hispanic, and Asian/Pacific Islander 8-year-old children identified with ASD" (p. 1). This is a change from earlier reports which indicated that ASD was more prevalent in White children than Black or Hispanic children (Autism Society of America, 2000 as cited in Dyches et al., 2004). The report, however, also indicated that, like previous findings, the number of Hispanic children with ASD remains lower in comparison to White or Black children (CDC, 2021b). Furthermore, recent CDC research also revealed that progress has been made in identifying ASD in children but more work is needed in identifying Hispanic children (CDC, 2021b).

ASD exists in all racial, ethnic, and socioeconomic groups.

Some studies have reported an increase in worldwide prevalence rates of ASD. Chiarotti and Venerosi (2020) provide a comprehensive summary of ASD prevalence estimates published since 2014. Overall, they reported a high variability in worldwide prevalence that is likely due to methodological differences in assessment methods and to the consistent increase of prevalence within each individual geographical area reviewed (Chiarotti & Venerosi, 2020). Similarly, Zaroff and Uhm (2012) conducted a review of worldwide studies on the prevalence of ASD and found differences in ASD prevalence across the studies reviewed and concluded that methodological factors most likely contributed to the differences observed. Chiarotti and Venerosi (2020) reviewed estimation data from countries across Europe, Asia, North America, the Middle East, Australia, and New Zealand. Based on the findings of these studies, it is clear that ASD extends across all cultures and races, and estimates of the prevalence of this disorder appear to be increasing. For a more thorough discussion, see Chiarotti and Venerosi (2020).

Relevant to school psychology and special education are ethnic differences in ASD eligibility determination for special education services. Researchers are examining the ethnic breakdown of ASD, which is one of the 13 disability categories considered under IDEA (2004). Morrier and Hess (2012) conducted a study that examined ethnic differences in over 295,000 school-aged students. Their findings revealed that 80% of states underrepresent the ASD population across ethnicities. The authors also found that "ethnic enrollment in special education under an autism eligibility proportionally in line with the general population percentages occurs in only 15 to 20% of states reporting data" (p. 60). They also found that Hispanic children were underrepresented in 95% of the 49 states whose data were reviewed, which, as the authors noted, reflects systemic problems in the identification of Hispanic school-aged children receiving special education services under the IDEA (2004) disability category of ASD. The authors point out that this is concerning given that Hispanics are "the fastest growing population in the United States" (Morrier & Hess, 2012, p. 60).

IMPACT OF AUTISM SPECTRUM DISORDER ON SOCIAL–EMOTIONAL AND BEHAVIORAL FUNCTIONING IN SCHOOL AND HOME ENVIRONMENTS

Social–Emotional and Behavioral Difficulties at School

Children with ASD may experience other mental health conditions. Because of the intensity of ASD behaviors, symptoms related to other conditions, such as anxiety, may go unnoticed. Within the literature, the most commonly reported mental health conditions observed in children with ASD include behavioral problems, ADHD, anxiety, and depression. Mental health conditions have been reported in approximately 45% of preschoolers with ASD and tend to become more prevalent as children with ASD get older (Kerns et al., 2020).

A review of the literature conducted by Vasa and colleagues (2020) revealed that children with ASD demonstrated higher levels of anxiety in comparison to children who did not have ASD. The authors noted that potential factors contributing to the anxiety experienced by children with ASD include sensory problems, sleep disturbance, and problematic behaviors. School psychologists working with children who have ASD should be sure to assess these problems in their work with children and their families.

To better understand the emotional and behavioral problems of children with ASD, Simonoff et al. (2008) conducted a study that examined comorbidity associated with ASD in a sample of children between the ages of 10 and 14. The study indicated that 70% of children in the sample had at least one comorbid disorder and approximately 41% had two or more disorders. The authors reported that the co-occurring disorders most often diagnosed included social anxiety disorder, ADHD, and ODD (Simonoff et al., 2008).

Behavioral problems may be related to difficulty regulating one's emotions. A child who has poor self-regulation may have a meltdown (as is seen with ASD) or an outburst, because they cannot control or manage their emotions, which manifest in their behavior. Scholars have also examined self-regulation and ASD in young children. A study by Ros and colleagues (2018) examined the role of ASD and ADHD behaviors in predicting self-regulation deficit in young children. The results of the study revealed higher ASD symptoms were linked with lower executive functioning for children demonstrating lower ADHD symptoms.

Social–Emotional and Behavioral Functioning at Home

One must look at the impact of emotional–behavioral problems not only on the individual child with ASD but on the family as well. The experience of trying to determine how best to respond to their child's problems can be stressful for parents. Scholars have found that the presence of emotional–behavioral problems in children with ASD are linked to parenting stress (Salomone et al., 2018). Not knowing how to respond to their child's behavioral problems may result in permissiveness in managing problematic behaviors. Such permissiveness and low levels of limit setting can be related to later behavior problems in children with ASD (Osborne et al., 2008). Similarly, some scholars have found lower levels of parenting efficacy and higher levels of stress among parents of children with ASD when compared to parents of typically developing children and even parents of children with other disabilities (Hayes & Watson, 2013). As seen earlier, ASD can also impact the child's family and home lives. Managing challenging behaviors, the high financial costs associated with various types of care that the child may need, loss of a caregiver's employment, and other such factors can contribute to stressful experiences for the family (Lopez & Magaña, 2020). Yet, caring for a child with ASD can be perceived as an experience that builds strength in the family (2020).

> Managing challenging behaviors, the high financial costs associated with various types of care the child may need, loss of a caregiver's employment, and other such factors can contribute to stressful experiences for the family (Lopez & Magaña, 2020).

Lopez and Magaña (2020) conducted a study to examine the impact of ASD on diverse families who had a child with ASD. The sample consisted of 46 Latina and 56 non-Latina White maternal caregivers with a child with ASD between the ages of 1 and 22. The researchers examined differences between these two groups in regards to their view on family difficulties that are associated with caring for a child with ASD and the level of pessimism they might have about their child's future. Lopez and Magaña (2020) examined the maternal caregivers' perceptions of problems within the family, optimism, and pessimism. The results of the study revealed that Latina maternal caregivers reported fewer perceived family problems and less pessimism about the child's future compared to their White counterparts.

IMPACT OF AUTISM SPECTRUM DISORDER ON LEARNING IN THE CLASSROOM

The cognitive abilities of children with ASD can range from a superior level of functioning to a level consistent with intellectual deficits. They may possess unique strengths and limitations that impact their success in the classroom (Williams et al., 2005). Spatial and nonverbal abilities have been found to be stronger than verbally mediated abilities for some children with ASD (Joseph et al., 2002). In addition, executive functioning deficits in children with ASD have been documented in the literature, and some studies have explored the link between executive functioning and language

(Joseph et al., 2005). A study by Joseph et al. (2005) found that children with ASD demonstrated lower language skills than a comparison group of typically developing peers. Within the group of children with ASD, no specific link was found between language ability and executive functioning. (Joseph et al., 2005). However, a positive association between executive performance and language ability was found in the comparison group. Joseph and colleagues (2005) indicated that the results suggested that "executive dysfunction in autism is not directly related to language impairment per se but rather involves an executive failure to use language for self-regulation" (Joseph et al., 2005, p. 361). In working with children with ASD, it is important to take into consideration executive dysfunction and language impairment as possible factors influencing the child's academic performance. According to Williams et al. (2005), there is no unique cognitive profile for ASD so it is important to remember that an individual child with ASD will have unique educational needs.

Barton and Harn (2012) recommend creating a structured classroom environment so that the child with ASD can "attend to important features in the classroom to promote learning and independence and minimize the likelihood of time to engage in nonfunctional stereotypical behavior" (p. 101). Given that ADHD can coexist with ASD, children with ASD may experience attentional problems. A highly structured classroom environment would help them to better attend to tasks and activities. In addition, children with ASD are often resistant to change and struggle with transitions. A highly structured classroom environment provides the predictability that is needed for children with ASD and helps the child know the routine and when transitions will occur. If a change in the routine is planned, it is helpful to give the child a 5-minute warning so that they can be prepared for the change.

Challenging behaviors in the classroom can impact learning. Self-regulation difficulties can result in outbursts that disrupt the classroom and stop instruction. Inflexibility in thinking and resistance to transitions can lead to disruptive behaviors. To address behavioral problems exhibited by the child, the teacher and school psychologist may do a behavioral assessment and develop a behavioral intervention plan (BIP) to help to increase prosocial and adaptive behaviors as well as reduce problematic behaviors that may interfere with the child's functioning in the classroom.

Given that children with ASD have an impairment in social communication and interaction, children with ASD may struggle in their interactions with peers. It is essential to promote positive peer interactions with the child who has ASD. With guidance from the school psychologist, the teacher of a young child with ASD can plan how to integrate skills such as initiating social contact with peers, taking turns, and sharing. Strategies, such as the use of scripts, modeling, and video modeling, may be useful tools to use to promote social interactions (Barton & Harn, 2012).

IMPLICATIONS FOR SCHOOL PSYCHOLOGISTS

Advocacy

In the role of advocate, school psychologists work with parents to learn their views on the needs of the child. The parents may have questions about ASD, so providing the parent with psychoeducational materials is an important way to help the parents better understand ASD and its impact on their child. The parent may have questions about services that the school can provide, so explain about the possible need for educational supports in the classroom. It is also important for the school psychologist to inform the parents about the Multi-Tiered Systems of Support that may be provided prior to a referral for a special education evaluation. If their child is referred for a special education evaluation, the school psychologist can explain the process, what types of assessment might be done (behavioral, intellectual, achievement, adaptive, communication, and developmental history), how long the process will take, and what will occur at the eligibility meeting. In addition, parents may have questions about what will happen if the child is found to be eligible for special education. An explanation of the purpose of an IEP and the type of information outlined on it will better help the parent understand the goals established on the IEP.

There may be times when the school psychologist may need to advocate for services outside the school. The parents may need assistance in finding community agencies that provide services such as mental health services, which children with ASD often need. By helping the parents maneuver through the school and outside agencies, the parents learn how to advocate for their child to ensure that the child receives the services that are needed.

Consultation

With inclusion, children with ASD are frequently placed in general education classrooms. Children with ASD frequently exhibit challenging behaviors that can interfere with learning by taking time away from instruction to manage the behavioral issues that are occurring in the classroom (Williams et al., 2005). Teachers may struggle with managing the special education child's behavior in the classroom because of a lack of knowledge about ASD and lack of prior training in behavioral management. General education teachers may not understand the unique social–emotional, behavioral, and learning needs of the child with ASD (Wilkinson, 2010). Results of a survey conducted by Wilkinson (2010) revealed that factual knowledge about ASD among educators was low. Eventually, the teacher may seek the help of the school psychologist. School psychologists are in a unique position to provide consultation services to general education teachers and can serve in a consultative supportive role to the teacher. As Williams et al. (2005) note, school psychologists can help establish a support network for children with ASD. School psychologists can draw on their knowledge of evidence-based interventions to help the teacher address a child's behavioral needs in the classroom.

Oftentimes, there are several interdisciplinary professionals, such as behavioral therapists, speech–language pathologists, clinical psychologists, occupational therapists, and so on, working with a child with ASD. School psychologists can also serve as a liaison between the school and any outside agencies that are providing services to a child with ASD. Issues may arise that hinder the collaboration process as evidenced in findings by Cheak-Zamora and Farmer (2015), which revealed that less than half (44%) of parents interviewed are pleased with the communication between the school and their primary care professional.

Shahidullah and colleagues (2020) contend this type of care coordination among interdisciplinary professionals involves effective communication and collaboration of the professionals involved in the provision of services for the child with ASD. Developing a partnership with outside professions in the community can be essential to the child's care. Shahidullah et al. (2020) note that school psychologists may encounter obstacles in the collaborative partnership such as a "mismatch in eligibility criteria for educational classifications versus medical diagnoses, lack of delineated roles and responsibility of other providers, and a limited infrastructure around information sharing" (p. 107). They recommend practices for school psychologists to consider in building effective partnerships. These practices include: (a) understanding and responding to the family's needs by focusing on the families' priorities and facilitating communication between the family and professionals; (b) improving communication with primary care and community-based partners by increasing communication frequency with the partners and streamlining the evaluation process as much as possible; (c) coordinating the use of evidence-based practices by being familiar with available research-based practices, incorporating collaboration in the delivery of tiered services, and using telehealth when possible; and (d) engaging in professional development and continuing education by pursuing professional development opportunities such as conferences and other continuing-education opportunities, and mentoring trainees and fellow school psychologists (Shahidullah et al., 2020). The authors emphasize the importance of building a strong partnership among interdisciplinary professionals and note that the responsibility of building future partnerships may fall on the school psychologist.

Assessment

School psychologists are engaged in the delivery of school psychological services for students identified as having ASD. One of these services is school-based assessments and evaluations. These evaluations may be related to special education eligibility determination, planning interventions, and progress monitoring (McClain et al., 2018). The type of evaluation used for the purposes of determining eligibility may be dependent on the requirements of the state where the school is located. For example, an initial evaluation for determination of ASD in the state of Georgia requires the following types of evaluations: (a) a complete psychological evaluation that includes an assessment of cognitive functioning and adaptive behavior; (b) an achievement evaluation to assess academic performance and present functioning levels; (c) a communication evaluation (by the speech–language pathologist) to assess the child's verbal and nonverbal communication, prosody, and pragmatic language using formal and informal measures; (d) a behavioral evaluation to assess behaviors that are typically associated with ASD such as social interactions with peers and adults, the ability to relate to others, stereotypic behaviors (e.g., hand flapping), abnormal responses to sensory stimuli, and resistance to change; (e) a developmental history that includes developmental delay and differences and the age of onset in early development of ASD behaviors (Georgia Rules and Regulations -160-4-7-.05-3 Eligibility Determination and Categories of Eligibility).

School psychologists need to be familiar with testing tools that are designed to assess autistic features. Screening instruments can be used to do a quick assessment of autistic behaviors to determine whether a more comprehensive assessment may be necessary. It is important to remember that screeners do not provide a diagnosis and do not provide a comprehensive assessment. An example of a screening tool used for young children is the Screening Tool for Autism in Toddlers and Young Children (STAT; Stone et al., 2000). This is an interactive tool that can be used if there is concern about the child's development. The STAT consists of 12 activities that assess the areas of play, communication, and imitation. The instrument can be administered in approximately 20 minutes. The Gilliam Rating Scale–Second Edition (GARS-2; Gilliam, 2005) is considered a diagnostic tool that assesses autistic behaviors. It is designed to be administered to individuals between the ages of 3 and 22. A comprehension assessment tool used to measure autistic behaviors is the Autism Diagnostic Observation Schedule–Second Edition (ADOS-2; Lord et al., 2012), which is designed for individuals between the ages of 12 months to adulthood. It assesses the areas of social interaction, communication, play, and imaginative use of materials and can be used if an individual is suspected of having ASD. It consists of an observational schedule of four 30-minute modules that are administered according to the person's expressive language level. It should be noted that administration of the ADOS-2 requires special training offered through training workshops hosted by professional organizations.

Behavioral assessments are another type of tool school psychologists often use in their work with a child who has ASD. To assess the child's behavior, the school psychologist conducts a functional behavioral assessment (Williams et al., 2005). A behavioral assessment involves observation during which the school psychologist looks for antecedents to the problem behavior and consequences of the behavior in order to determine the motivation (function) behind the behavior. As Williams et al. (2005) note, behavioral interventions should be developed on the information obtained from the functional assessment of the behavior.

EDUCATIONAL SUPPORTS

Many children with ASD are in general education classrooms with their typically developing peers. Research studies have found positive outcomes in children with ASD being placed in general education classrooms, including more frequent social interactions, less concern about disruptive behaviors, and improved academic/functional skills (National Autism Center, 2015). Given the unique needs of children with ASD and the increasing number of students being served in the general education classroom, educational supports for the child will need to be provided (Sansosti et al., 2018). Sansosti and colleagues (2018) emphasize the need for the school and family to work collaboratively so that there is consistency between the home and school in strategies used. According to Sansosti et al. (2018), supports that are provided for students with ASD should include the following components: (a) individualized supports that include choice-making, (b) functional programming, (c) evidence-based instruction, (d) home–school collaboration, and (e) person-centered planning. Regarding individualized supports that incorporate choice-making, Sansosti and colleagues (2018) recommend that the support should be designed so that the child with ASD is given a choice to select an activity from a group of options. Functional programming should utilize an approach that promotes prosocial skills while decreasing problematic behaviors. This prevent–teach–reinforce approach with students with ASD is designed to prevent problem behaviors, teaches replacement behavior, and provides contingent positive reinforcement (Sansosti et al., 2018). Another component of supports identified by Sansosti et al. (2018) includes evidence-based instruction within a structured environment. It is important to remember that the interventions are planned carefully and include frequent checks on success. With regard to home–school collaboration, it is vital that schools work collaboratively with families of children with ASD and involve them in educational planning and provision of supports and services so that students can utilize skills in both the school and home environments. According to Sansosti and colleagues (2018), this approach increases opportunities for learning and helps to maintain skills learned in the classroom and to be used across settings. The final component recommended by Sansosti et al. (2018) is person-centered planning, which focuses on the long-term goals of the student and ensures the provision of supports that help the child reach the identified academic, social, and behavioral goals (Sansosti et al., 2018).

In regard to specific educational supports used to address academic concerns, Sansosti and colleagues (2018) offer several supports that may be useful. One such educational support is to simplify instructions by using fewer words/steps and repeating multistep instructions. The teacher should remember to check in with the child to ensure that the instructions are understood. Another way of simplifying instructions includes using written lists of step-by-steps directions. Remember that the child may need time to process information so it is important to give the child time and to only ask a question a second time after several seconds have passed, so that the child's thinking is not disrupted. A third support offered by Sansosti and colleagues (2018) includes presenting materials in sections or including fewer items on a page or giving the child one page at a time. This technique helps the child to focus and stay on task as well as provides an opportunity for the child to receive feedback. Some children may find the use of color-coding enhances their organizations skills. Folders and other things could be color-coded so that a single color is used for a particular academic area. For supports related to specific academic areas, the reader is referred to Sansosti et al. (2018).

SCHOOL-BASED MENTAL HEALTH INTERVENTIONS AND SUPPORTS

A core feature of ASD is impairment in social communication and interaction. Children struggle to understand social situations and how to respond to others. Therefore, one of the most important interventions for children with ASD is social skills training (SST). They often need systematic teaching of social skills to be able to engage with others at school, home, and the community. SST is an evidence-based intervention that be effective in helping children with ASD build social skills (Bohlander et al., 2012; Tse et al., 2007). Through SST, a child with ASD could learn skills such as maintaining eye contact; how to greet someone; how to initiate a conversation; how to understand emotions and body language; how to have empathy; how to be assertive; and other similar skills (Bohlander et al., 2012). This intervention can be modified to an individual age and developmental level. Peer mentoring is a unique approach that incorporates children without ASD to serve as peer mentors. Peer mentors are given tasks to do with the child who has ASD. These tasks include how to facilitate interactions during social and play interactions. Another type of SST includes video modeling, which can be used to teach the child social concepts. For example, a child with ASD will watch a video demonstration of a skill and do that skill right after watching the video. Social stories involve using visual or written materials to describe a social skill concept. They can be adapted to incorporate the child's strengths and include techniques such as role playing (Bohlander et al., 2012). The fourth intervention is the University of California, Los Angeles (UCLA) Program for the Education and Enrichment of Relational Skills (PEERS; www.semel.ucla.edu/peers), which involves 90-minute sessions that are held on a weekly basis for approximately 3 to 4 months. This program can be used for children at the preschool age through adulthood. The sessions consist of lessons, group activities, and role playing that focus on promoting interactions. To encourage carry over of skills learned, a parent can attend the session and help the child practice the skills.

In addition to exhibiting a deficit in social communication and interaction, children with ASD exhibit challenging behaviors for which school-based services may be needed. As discussed earlier, school psychologists may consider conducting a behavioral assessment. The results of the behavioral assessment will guide the planning of a BIP (Williams et al., 2005). The purpose of the BIP is to eliminate problematic or inappropriate behavior and provide the child with an alternate behavior to replace the inappropriate behavior, known as the *replacement behavior*. The BIP provides a clear description of the behavior and possible explanation for why the behavior occurs. The plan includes strategies and supports that can be used to teach the child a replacement behavior. A functional behavioral assessment will determine what motivates the child to engage in the inappropriate behavior.

Techniques from applied behavioral analysis and cognitive behavioral therapy (CBT) could be integrated to address the child's problematic behaviors (Williams et al., 2005). Methods, such as the ones described here, which focus on enhancing social skills and reducing problematic behaviors, have been found to be effective when working with children with ASD.

CASE STUDY 4.1 JACK: A FIRST-GRADE STUDENT WITH AUTISM SPECTRUM DISORDER

Background

Jack is a 6-year-old boy who just started first grade. His parents report that he was born full term and that early developmental milestones occurred when expected with the exception of social interaction and communication. When he was approximately 18 months old, they noticed that he seemed "different" from other children in the play group they had joined. As a young child, Jack did not reciprocate when his parents played peek-a-boo with him, nor did he not attempt to smile back at them when they smiled at him. When they hugged him, he remained still instead of hugging them back. When he was around other children, Jack tended to play alone instead of interacting with them. He avoided eye contact with the parents and others and generally did not display facial expressions. When other children attempted to engage him, Jack just looked at them and did not respond. Other behaviors described by the parents included repetitive behaviors that he tended to exhibit when something occurred that overwhelmed him and confused him. The repetitive behaviors included hand flapping and flipping small objects. He also was resistant to changes in his routine, as noted by both the parents and teacher. According to the parents, Jack had an intense preoccupation with small cars, particularly the wheels of the car. These behaviors have impacted his ability to communicate in social situations and to interact with his peers. According to his teacher, Jack exhibits similar behaviors in the classroom and tends to keep to himself rather than initiate interactions with others. She also noted that he has difficulty paying attention in the classroom and gets easily distracted by stimuli in the room.

Once Jack's parents noticed the difference in his behavior compared to other children in the play group, they spoke to the pediatrician, who recommended an evaluation through the early-intervention program. The results revealed that Jack's cognitive and adaptive behaviors were in the average range. However, his social–emotional skills were in the deficit range. He received services through the early-intervention program until age 3. Although Jack was referred for an evaluation to determine preschool special education services, the parents moved to a different state and did not seek further help.

Discussion

Based on the description of Jack's behavior, he appears to be exhibiting signs of ASD. There are clear behaviors of a lack of social reciprocity such as his not smiling back to his parents. Other signs of an impairment in social communication and interaction include his lack of eye contact, lack of facial expressions, and a lack of interest in his peers. In addition, Jack exhibits repetitive behaviors of hand flapping and flipping objects. Restricted behaviors include his becoming upset when changes occur in his routine and a preoccupation with small cars. The parents first noted the onset of symptoms at 18 months, and the behaviors have had a significant impact on his ability to communicate and interact socially with others.

The school psychologist could have a pivotal role in helping Jack and his parents. Because Jack received early-intervention services, his parents may already have a good knowledge base about ASD. The school psychologist may still have a supportive role with the parents in helping them navigate the education system. The teacher may not have much experience working with children with ASD and, if that is the case, the school psychologist could provide psychoeducational materials to enhance the teacher's understanding of ASD. To address Jack's needs, educational supports may be provided. Those supports might

(continued)

> **CASE STUDY 4.1 JACK: A FIRST-GRADE STUDENT WITH AUTISM SPECTRUM DISORDER** (*continued*)
>
> include giving him a choice when possible and using the prevent–teach–reinforce approach to increase the likelihood of preventing problem behavior, replacing the behavior, and offering contingent positive reinforcement.
>
> If Jack does not respond to the supports that are provided, he may be referred for an evaluation by the school psychologist. It is important to obtain a developmental history to get a clear picture of when major developmental milestones were achieved. Areas that may be assessed include cognitive functioning, adaptive behavior, achievement, behavior, and communication. The two guiding questions that the multidisciplinary team will need to ask are whether Jack is a student who meets eligibility criteria for the IDEA category of ASD and whether he needs special education services to be successful in the general education classroom. If he is determined to be a student with a disability, an IEP will be established. Possible interventions for Jack include SST and perhaps behavior therapy if his behavior is problematic in the classroom.

SUMMARY POINTS

- ASD is a neurodevelopmental disorder that occurs in one out of 44 children.
- ASD is characterized by a deficit in social communication and interaction. Restricted, repetitive behaviors are also a feature of the disorder.
- ASD crosses all cultures and races and estimates of its prevalence indicate that it is increasing.
- SST is an effective tool in addressing social communication and interaction difficulties in children with ASD.

TEST YOUR KNOWLEDGE

1. What are the two core diagnostic areas of ASD?
   a. Social communication and interaction
   b. Inattentiveness
   c. Repetitive behaviors
   d. Both a and c

2. Approximately what percentage of people are comorbid with a single mental health disorder?
   a. 30%
   b. 50%
   c. 70%
   d. 90%

3. Research has found 80% of states report underrepresentation of ASD across ethnicities.
   a. True
   b. False

4. Which of the following are considered risk factors for ASD?
   a. Advanced maternal age
   b. Fetal exposure to valproate
   c. Low birth weight
   d. All of the above

5. One educational support that may be helpful to students with ASD is to simplify instructions.
   a. True
   b. False

Answers: (1) d, (2) c, (3) a, (4) d, (5) a.

DISCUSSION QUESTIONS

1. Summarize *DSM-5* criteria for ASD.
2. Highlight the IDEA criteria for eligibility under the category of ASD.
3. Identify components of educational supports that should be included when planning supportive educational services.
4. Describe how school psychologists can provide support for general education teachers of children with ASD.
5. List some effective classroom strategies for students with ASD.

CHAPTER RESOURCES

General Information Websites

American Psychiatric Association *What is Autism Spectrum Disorder?*: www.psychiatry.org/patients-families/autism/what-is-autism-spectrum-disorder

American Psychiatric Association *Expert Q&A: Autism*: www.psychiatry.org/patients-families/autism/expert-q-and-a

American Psychiatric Association *Adam's Story*: www.psychiatry.org/patients-families/autism/patient-story

American Psychological Association *Autism Spectrum Disorder*: www.apa.org/topics/autism-spectrum-disorder

Centers for Disease Control and Prevention *What Is Autism Spectrum Disorder?*: www.cdc.gov/ncbddd/autism/facts.html

Centers for Disease Control and Prevention *Real Stories from People Living with Autism Spectrum Disorder*: www.cdc.gov/ncbddd/autism/stories.html

Articles for School Psychologists

American Psychological Association *Diagnosing and Managing Autism Spectrum Disorder*: www.apa.org/topics/autism-spectrum-disorder/diagnosing

American Psychological Association *Helping People with Autism Reach Their Full Potential*: www.apa.org/monitor/2020/07/autism-potential

National Association of School Psychologists *Expanding the Role of School Psychologists for Children with Autism Spectrum Disorders*: www.nasponline.org/publications/periodicals/spf/volume-5/volume-5-issue-4-(winter-2011)

Books for School Psychologists

American Psychological Association *Autism Spectrum Disorder in Children and Adolescents: Evidence-Based Assessment and Intervention in Schools*: www.apa.org/pubs/books/4317328

American Psychological Association *Autism Spectrum Disorder: A Clinical Guide for General Practitioners*: www.apa.org/pubs/books/4317325

Books for Children

American Psychological Association *All My Stripes: A Story for Children with Autism*: www.apa.org/pubs/magination/441B163

American Psychological Association *Autism, The Invisible Cord: A Sibling's Diary*: www.apa.org/pubs/magination/441B101

American Psychological Association *Russell's World: A Story for Kids about Autism*: www.apa.org/pubs/magination/441B074

Factsheets for Families

Autism Society *Living with Autism: Going to Middle School*: www.autism-society.org/wp-content/uploads/2014/04/Transition_to_Middle_School.pdf

Autism Society *Living with Autism: Moving from Preschool to Kindergarten*: www.autism-society.org/wp-content/uploads/2014/04/Transition-Preschool_to_Kindergarten.pdf

Autism Society *Living with Autism: Planning for Successful Transitions Across Grade Levels*: www.autism-society.org/wp-content/uploads/2014/04/Transition_Across_Grade_Levels.pdf

Autism Society *Living with Autism: Preparing for a Lifetime*: www.autism-society.org/wp-content/uploads/2014/04/Transition-Preparing_for_a_Lifetime.pdf

Autism Society *Living with Autism: Preparing to Experience College Living*: www.autism-society.org/wp-content/uploads/2014/04/CollegeLiving.pdf

Autism Society *Living with Autism: Puberty and Children on the Autism Spectrum*: www.autism-society.org/wp-content/uploads/2014/04/LWA_Puberty.pdf

Autism Society *Living with Autism: Sibling Perspectives: Guidelines for Parents*: www.autism-society.org/wp-content/uploads/2014/04/LWA_Siblings.pdf

Autism Society *Next Steps: A Guide for Families New to Autism*: www.autism-society.org/wp-content/uploads/2017/02/nextsteps09.pdf

Autism Society *What Is Autism?*: www.autism-society.org/wp-content/uploads/2014/04/What_is_Autism_Final.pdf

Centers for Disease Control and Prevention *"Learn the Signs, Act Early" Program Factsheet*: www.cdc.gov/ncbddd/actearly/pdf/LTASE-program-one-pager-P.pdf

Books for Families

American Psychological Association *Autism and Your Teen: Tips and Strategies for the Journey to Adulthood*: www.apa.org/pubs/books/4441032

American Psychological Association *Parent Training for Autism Spectrum Disorder: Improving the Quality of Life for Children and Their Families*: www.apa.org/pubs/books/4317503

KEY REFERENCES

Only key references appear in the print edition. The full reference list appears in the digital product on Springer Publishing Connect: connect.springerpub.com/content/book/978-0-8261-3587-2/part/part02/chapter/ch04

American Psychiatric Association. (2013a). *Diagnostic and statistical manual of mental disorders* (5th ed.). https://doi.org/10.1176/appi.books.9780890425596

American Psychiatric Association. (2013b). *Autism spectrum disorder.* http://www.dsm5.org/Documents/Autism%20Spectrum%20Disorder%20Fact%20Sheet.pdf

Centers for Disease Control and Prevention. (2021a). *CDC's Autism and Developmental Disabilities Monitoring Network.* Author. https://www.cdc.gov/ncbddd/autism/pdf/ADDM_factsheet_2021-508.pdf

Dyches, T. T., Wilder, L. K., Sudweeks, R. R., Obiakor, F. E., & Algozzine, B. (2004). Multicultural issues in autism. *Journal of Autism and Developmental Disorders, 34*(2), 211–222. https://doi.org/10.1023/b:jadd.0000022611.80478.73

Lopez, K., & Magaña, S. (2020). Perceptions of family problems and pessimism among Latina and Non-Latina White mothers raising children with autism spectrum disorder. *Journal of Autism and Developmental Disorders, 50*(7), 2360–2374. https://doi.org/10.1007/s10803-018-3640-8

Sansosti, F. J., Harjusola-Webb, S., & Sansosti, J. M. (2018). *Autism spectrum disorder: Helping handout for school and home.* In G. G. Bear & K. M. Minke (Eds.), *Helping handouts: Supporting students at school and home* (S5H3). National Association of School Psychologists.

Shahidullah, J. D., McClain, M. B., Azad, G., Mezher, K. R., & McIntyre, L. L. (2020). Coordinating autism care across schools and medical settings: Considerations for school psychologists. *Intervention in School and Clinic, 56*(2), 107–114. https://doi.org/10.1177/1053451220914891

Williams, S. K., Johnson, C., & Sukhodolsky, D. G. (2005). The role of the school psychologist in the inclusive education of school-age children with autism spectrum disorders. *Journal of School Psychology, 43*(2), 117–136. https://doi.org/10.1016/j.jsp.2005.01.002

UNIT 3

MENTAL HEALTH DISORDERS IN CHILDREN AND ADOLESCENTS: DISRUPTIVE, IMPULSE-CONTROL, AND CONDUCT DISORDERS

CHAPTER 5

Conduct Disorder

LEARNING OBJECTIVES

- Summarize the diagnostic features for the *Diagnostic and Statistical Manual of Mental Disorders* (5th ed.; *DSM-5*; American Psychiatric Association [APA], 2013) diagnosis of Conduct Disorder.
- Highlight the cultural considerations for children and youth with conduct disorder.
- Describe common social–emotional and behavioral concerns for children with conduct disorder.
- Understand the classroom implications for a student with conduct disorder.
- Identify effective social, emotional, and behavioral interventions for students with conduct disorder.

INTRODUCTION

The *Diagnostic and Statistical Manual of Mental Disorders,* Fifth Edition (*DSM-5*; American Psychiatric Association [APA], 2013), classifies Conduct Disorder under the category of Disruptive, Impulse-Control, and Conduct Disorders. Conduct Disorder and the other disorders in this diagnostic area cover issues related to emotional and behavioral regulation. The behaviors in this category typically result in harm to others or significant conflict with rules, laws, and/or individuals in positions of authority. Some examples of other Disruptive, Impulse-Control, and Conduct Disorders include Oppositional Defiant Disorder (ODD; discussed in Chapter 6) and Intermittent Explosive Disorder (IED; addressed in Chapter 7).

In the *DSM-5* diagnosis of any of the Disruptive, Impulse-Control, and Conduct Disorders, context is particularly important. Some features of these disorders may be present in typically developing children and adolescents and even in functional adults; however, the consistency, severity, and intensity of the behaviors (as compared to individuals of similar age, gender, and culture) are the determinants of whether the behaviors represent common adjustment issues versus the clinical significance necessary for diagnosis of Conduct Disorder (APA, 2013).

DIAGNOSTIC ISSUES: *DSM-5* AND SCHOOL-BASED SERVICES

DSM-5 Diagnosis

Within the *DSM-5*, three criteria are required to be met in order to determine a diagnosis of conduct disorder. These criteria are as follows: (a) whether the individual exhibits multiple violations of the rights of other people, laws, and/or rules over a period of at least a year; (b) that the issues demonstrably impact the individual's functioning in school, work, or interpersonal interaction; and (c) a diagnosis of antisocial personality disorder has been ruled out (if an adult). The criterion related to the infringement on the rights of others and socially inappropriate violations is subdivided into 15 elements across four broad categories. Those categories are related to physical harm to other people or animals, damaging items that belong to others, stealing and theft by deception, and significant disregard of rules. In order to meet this criterion, the individual must display at least three of the elements over the prior year with at least one element having occurred within the most recent 6-month period (APA, 2013).

In addition to meeting the aforementioned criteria, upon diagnosis, the clinician must also specify diagnostic elements related to the age, emotionality, and severity of the symptoms of the individual with conduct disorder. A determination of *childhood-onset type* is given if at least one symptom was observed before the child turned 10 years old. It is important to note that individuals with childhood onset of conduct disorder often experience more significant and longer lasting symptomatology than those individuals with adolescent onset of conduct disorder (Dandreaux & Frick, 2009; Frick, 2016). If there were no symptoms present before the age of 10, then the type is determined to be adolescent onset. The median age of onset in the United States is 11.6 years (Nock et al., 2006). Research suggests that adolescent onset of conduct disorder appears to stem from exaggerated rebelliousness and a reaction against societal conventions (Dandreaux & Frick, 2009). Finally, if it is unclear whether symptoms began before or after 10 years of age, then a determination of *unspecified onset* is given. Dandreaux and Frick (2009) point out that it can be surprisingly difficult to determine the actual age of onset when assessing an older adolescent, but a triangulation of sources, such as self-report, parent report, and juvenile justice records, can be helpful in the process.

With regard to an emotionality specifier, a diagnosis of conduct disorder with limited prosocial emotions can be applied under certain circumstances. This specifier is based on the self-report of the individual under evaluation and corroborated with information from other knowledgeable sources like parents, school personnel, peers, or other service providers. If the individual and others note that the student has demonstrated at least two out of four characteristics (failure to experience remorse regarding harmful actions, failure to acknowledge the impact of their behaviors on others, lack of effort with school/employment, and muted or manipulative expression of emotions) across a variety of settings and over a period of at least 1 year, then the specifier can be added to the conduct disorder diagnosis. According to Scheepers et al. (2011), these callous and unemotional traits often delineate a subgroup of children and adolescents with a more significant form of conduct disorder. Frick et al. (2014) found that this group of children often exhibit more severe and calculated aggressive behavior even relative to other youth with significant behavioral concerns. However, Colins (2016) found that the specifier of limited prosocial emotions did not discriminate among the level of psychiatric symptoms in a group of incarcerated boys and argued against its clinical usefulness despite its inclusion in the *DSM-5*. Research supports that 25% to 30% of children with conduct disorder also demonstrate the characteristics consistent with limited prosocial emotions (Kahn et al., 2012). Although these children are by no means untreatable, researchers have found that they are more resistant to treatment than children who are not identified as having limited prosocial emotions (Frick, 2016; Frick et al., 2014).

Finally, a determination of the severity of the conduct disorder must be established. The severity indicators are mild (which represents few issues beyond meeting minimal diagnostic criteria), moderate (in a range between mild and severe), and severe (significant symptomatology that often causes significant harm to others). It is often necessary to solicit the input of multiple raters for accuracy in evaluating specifiers in the diagnosis of conduct disorder (APA, 2013).

> In addition to meeting the criteria for conduct disorder, upon diagnosis, the clinician must also specify diagnostic elements related to the age, emotionality, and severity of the individual with conduct disorder (APA, 2013).

PREVALENCE AND COMORBIDITY OF CONDUCT DISORDER

Although the *DSM-5* reports the overall prevalence of conduct disorder to be in a range from 2% to 10% of the population, other researchers have offered helpful statistics regarding children and adolescents with this diagnosis. Its worldwide prevalence among youth is estimated to be at 3.2% (Canino et al., 2010). According to the experts, there is a prevalence rate of 2% to 5% for children aged 5 to 12 and a 5% to 9% prevalence in youth from 13 to 18 years of age (INSERM Collective Expertise Centre, 2005). However, it is important to note that most studies regarding prevalence were conducted prior to the publication of the *DSM-5*. Although the changes in diagnostic criteria were minimal from prior editions of the *DSM* to the *DSM-5*, actual prevalence may change over time. Regarding age and conduct disorder, research supports that when diagnosed before the age of 11, children have a 5 times greater risk of being admitted to a psychiatric facility (Patel et al., 2018). In addition, children who first exhibit symptoms of conduct disorder in childhood (versus adolescent onset of symptoms) are more likely to engage in significant delinquent behavior and continue that behavior into criminal acts in adulthood (Gathright & Tyler, 2014; Institut national de la santé et de la recherche médicale (INSERM) Collective Expertise Centre, 2005; Odgers et al., 2008; Patel et al., 2018). The *DSM-5* also suggests that symptomology tends to become more significant over time with the presence of more severe behaviors that could result in lasting consequences (APA, 2013).

In relation to gender, at early ages boys are more likely to be diagnosed with conduct disorder than girls, but the gender-diagnosis gap narrows significantly during adolescence. During middle childhood (ages 5–12) boys are about 3 times as likely as girls to exhibit signs of conduct disorder (Moffitt et al., 2001). The estimated rates of conduct disorder diagnoses increase for both males and females in the teen years. Although the diagnosis among boys continues to be greater in frequency than that of girls, the actual ratio of diagnoses lowers to 2:1 (Loeber et al., 2000) during adolescence. Despite the increase in the proportion of females diagnosed with conduct disorder as teenagers, Patel el al. (2018) found that males are 3 times more likely to be admitted to a psychiatric facility for inpatient treatment of symptoms associated with conduct disorder as females. Because of these findings, some researchers have argued that the criteria for age of onset among girls should be marked by puberty as opposed to the 10-years-of-age criterion currently found in the *DSM-5*. They note that this is because adolescent onset of conduct disorder in girls is often associated with high-risk behaviors, such as sexual promiscuity and teen pregnancy. Also, as compared to boys with conduct disorder, girls with this diagnosis tend to engage in fewer acts of physical aggression but in more manipulative behaviors such as using indirect threats, spreading rumors, and gossiping about others (APA, 2013; INSERM Collective Expertise Centre, 2005).

With regard to comorbidity, research supports that children and adolescents with conduct disorder are highly likely to have symptoms associated with other clinical diagnoses as well (Gathright & Tyler, 2014; INSERM Collective Expertise Centre, 2005). Compared to a control group, children with conduct disorder are at 11 times greater risk for comorbid psychosis (Patel et al., 2018). Children and adolescents are commonly diagnosed with ODD prior to their symptoms rising to the intensity and severity needed for a diagnosis of conduct disorder, and children with conduct disorder frequently become adults with antisocial personality disorder. It is also common for children and adolescents with conduct disorder to have comorbid diagnoses of attention deficit hyperactivity disorder (ADHD), depression, and/or anxiety (INSERM Collective Expertise Centre, 2005). The *DSM-5* and other researchers specifically note the increased likelihood for particularly negative outcomes for children with conduct disorder who have also previously been diagnosed with ODD and ADHD (APA, 2013; INSERM Collective Expertise Centre, 2005). In addition, substance abuse issues and other high-risk behaviors are frequently seen in adolescents with conduct disorder. There is an especially elevated incidence of marijuana use among teen girls with conduct disorder (INSERM Collective Expertise Centre, 2005). Also, those high-risk behaviors may include suicidal ideation and suicide attempts (APA, 2013).

School-Based Eligibility

INDIVIDUALS WITH DISABILITIES EDUCATION IMPROVEMENT ACT REGULATIONS

For many years, teachers, administrators, parents, and other interested parties (including lawyers) have debated whether students with conduct disorder qualify for special education services under the Individuals with Disabilities Education Improvement Act (IDEA; Olympia et al., 2004; Sullivan & Sadeh, 2014; Theodore et al., 2004). In most circumstances, this debate has revolved around whether children and adolescents with conduct disorder can qualify under the category of Emotional Disturbance. In the federal law, the category of Emotional Disturbance is defined by the following: "(a) an inability to learn that cannot be explained by intellectual, sensory, or other health factors; (b) an inability to build or maintain satisfactory interpersonal relationships with peers and adults;

(c) inappropriate types of behavior or feelings under normal circumstances; (d) a general pervasive mood of unhappiness or depression; [and] (e) a tendency to develop physical symptoms or fears associated with personal or school problems" (U.S. Department of Education, n.d., Section 300.8 (c) (4) (i)). The law also notes that this does include children with schizophrenia. However, the law does not apply to students who are deemed to be socially maladjusted unless they additionally meet criteria for Emotional Disturbance (U.S. Department of Education, n.d.). This definition was originally derived from Bower's 1957 research of teachers who described their students as emotionally disturbed, although he later referred to these same children as *socially maladjusted* (Bower, 1982).

Although some people argue that the behaviors associated with conduct disorder do represent inappropriate types of behavior under normal circumstances as defined in IDEA (Olympia et al., 2004), the general consensus is that conduct disorder and its affiliated behaviors align with the concept of social maladjustment (Cloth et al., 2014). Perhaps contributing to the controversy is the fact that social maladjustment is not explicitly defined within the federal law but is left to interpretation by the states and its practitioners (Sullivan & Sadeh, 2014). For many years, scholars in this area have highlighted the problems associated with the lack of a definition of social maladjustment within IDEA. Those problems include inconsistent implementation across states, exclusion of many students, and a lack of reliable assessment tools for measuring social maladjustment (Olympia et al., 2004; Sullivan & Sadeh, 2014).

Despite the omission of a federal definition of social maladjustment, according to the American Psychological Association Dictionary of Psychology (n.d.), *social maladjustment* is defined as "1. An inability to develop relationships that satisfy affiliative needs. 2. A lack of social finesse or tact. 3. A breakdown in the process of maintaining constructive social relationships." In addition, Theodore et al. (2004) note that most attempts at distinguishing the concept of social maladjustment include a focus on antisocial types of behavior that are purposeful in nature. In other words, the socially maladjusted child understands their behavior and is in control of that behavior. This is in contrast to the child with emotional disturbance who exhibits primarily internalizing issues that are often not within the child's control. Further, it has been posited that despite not having an explicit definition for *social maladjustment*, the vastly different presentation of emotionally disturbed versus socially maladjusted children warrants very different treatments for the two groups of students (Theodore et al., 2004). The exclusion of students who exhibit behaviors solely associated with social maladjustment from the category of Emotional Disturbance has been supported through a number of court cases in the United States. These include *A.E. vs. Independent School District #25 of Adair County, Oklahoma, Springer v. Fairfax County School Board, N.C. v. Bedford Central School District, W.G. v. New York City Department of Education* to name a few. For a thorough treatment and discussion of these cases, the reader is encouraged to explore Sullivan and Sadeh (2014).

Beyond the IDEA disability category of Emotional Disturbance, others have argued that children and adolescents with conduct disorder could receive special education services under the designation of Other Health Impairment (OHI). According to the U.S. Department of Education (n.d.), "Other health impairment means having limited strength, vitality, or alertness, including a heightened alertness to environmental stimuli, that results in limited alertness with respect to the educational environment" (Section 300.8 (c) (9)). IDEA requires a determination as to whether the chronic health issue impacts the student's educational performance. The law specifies a variety of health conditions that should be considered under OHI. Those health conditions are inclusive of the following: ADHD, diabetes, epilepsy, heart conditions, hemophilia, lead poisoning, leukemia, nephritis, rheumatic fever, sickle cell anemia, and Tourette syndrome. However, the verbiage of the law makes it clear that this list of health conditions is not exhaustive and that other conditions can be considered if they meet the criteria (U.S. Department of Education, n.d.). Thus, the ability to include disorders beyond what is explicitly listed in IDEA is the basis for the contention that conduct disorder may apply and children with an OHI diagnosis may be eligible for special education services within the schools. Although most espouse that the spirit of the law was for the category of OHI to relate to medical care and medical concerns, such as missing school due to health appointments, poor attendance due to chronic health issues, or inability to fully participate in the curriculum due to a health-related issue, others (particularly parents' rights organizations and disability advocacy groups) insist that the terms "chronic health problems" that "adversely impact educational performance" are inclusive of the issues associated with conduct disorder.

Regardless of the intent of the law, special education eligibility for a student with conduct disorder would preserve some rights for the child that may be difficult for teachers and administrators to effectively navigate in practice. When a student is served in the schools under IDEA, the student must be able to receive services as they are outlined in the student's Individual Education Program (IEP). If the child is removed from school due to suspension or expulsion (which might be common disciplinary procedures for the behaviors often associated with conduct disorder; Frick, 2012), then the school must continue to provide those services (perhaps in the home or alternative setting). However, the legal protections under IDEA note that a child with a disability may not be removed for more than 10 days from their educational environment, and these 10 days do not have to be consecutive. If the child is to be removed for greater than 10 days, then this represents a change of placement. The school must initiate a manifestation determination hearing. At this hearing, the team must determine whether the child's IEP was being followed appropriately by school personnel and whether the child's inappropriate behavior was a result of the disability (U.S. Department of Education, n.d.). In the case of conduct disorder, failure to follow rules and adhere to societal norms is an inherent part of the disability (APA, 2013). Thus, the team may have no choice but to conclude that the conduct violation was a manifestation of the student's disability, and IDEA mandates that a child cannot be disciplined for an infraction that is a manifestation of their disability (U.S. Department of Education, n.d.). One can imagine that this might represent a significant challenge in the school system when trying to maintain safety and order in relation to a child or adolescent who is diagnosed with conduct disorder. However, it is critical to note that despite the long-standing reliance by schools on exclusionary practices for behavioral infractions, there is little evidence to suggest their efficacy in remediating current behaviors or preventing future behaviors. Further, significant data is indicative of its overuse with students from racial and ethnic minority backgrounds (Losen, 2015; Skiba et al., 2002, 2011).

> IDEA mandates that a child cannot be disciplined for an infraction that is a manifestation of the child's disability (U.S. Department of Education, n.d.).

SECTION 504

However, there is another (more common) pathway for providing school-based services to students with conduct disorder outside of IDEA. Section 504 of the Rehabilitation Act of 1973 represents landmark civil rights legislation that offers protections for and prevents discrimination of individuals with disabilities. All organizations and entities (including public schools) that receive federal funds are subject to the mandates of this federal law. Similar to IDEA, Section 504 requires that public schools provide a free and appropriate public education with any necessary related services and supports to students who have (or are suspected to have) a disability. Children and adolescents do not need to qualify under the eligibility criteria for IDEA in order to receive support under Section 504. It must merely be demonstrated through a school-based evaluation that the child has an impairment that "substantially limits one or more major life functions" (Office of Civil Rights, n.d., Section 104.3 (2) (iv)). According to Section 504, major life functions include caring for oneself, performing manual tasks, walking, hearing, seeing, speaking, breathing, learning, and working. However, it is noted that this list of major life functions is not exhaustive and other applicable life functions can and should be considered (Office of Civil Rights, n.d.).

Unlike IDEA, Section 504 does not list specific disabilities that may apply but focuses instead on types of impairment. The types of impairment are defined as follows: "and physiological disease or condition, cosmetic disfigurement, or anatomical loss affecting one or more of the following body systems: neurological; musculoskeletal, special sense organs, respiratory including speech organs; cardiovascular; reproductive; digestive; genito-urinary; hemic and lymphatic; skin; and endocrine; or any mental or psychological disorder, such as mental retardation, organic brain syndrome, emotional or mental illness, and specific learning disabilities" (Office of Civil Rights, n.d., Section 104.3 (2) (i)).

Although a diagnosis of conduct disorder certainly qualifies as a psychological disorder (per the impairment guidelines), the diagnosis alone is not sufficient for eligibility for services under Section 504. The law requires that a multidisciplinary team conduct an evaluation and collect enough information as is necessary to determine that the child or adolescent has a disability that does, in fact, impact a major life function (Office of Civil Rights, n.d.). In 2016, Zirkel and Weathers reported that 1.48% of public school students qualify for school-based services under Section 504. In cases in which a child or adolescent is found to qualify for those services, it is highly likely that the child's 504 plan for accommodations and modifications based on their disability will include a behavior intervention plan as well. Other common services that may be provided in the 504 plan for students with conduct disorder include counseling by a school counselor or school psychologist and medication distribution and management by a school nurse.

Given the range of options for the provision of school-based services for children and adolescents with conduct disorder, the school psychologist must be well versed regarding eligibility determinations, the resulting outcomes, and legal protections for these students. Due to their breadth and depth of knowledge related to special education law (IDEA) and other federal mandates (Section 504), school psychologists are often called upon to lead or participate in multidisciplinary teams that assess individuals, collect evaluation data, and make weighty educational decisions on behalf of students with conduct disorder. As such, it is critical that school psychologists are prepared for these roles, which may constitute life-altering decisions for these children and adolescents.

CULTURAL ISSUES RELATED TO CONDUCT DISORDER IN YOUTH

Risk Factors for Conduct Disorder

According to Frick (2016), a myriad of factors has been highlighted in the literature as risk factors for conduct disorder. Some of these issues include low serotonin (a mood stabilizing hormone) level, low resting heart rate, deficits in executive functioning, difficulties with social perception, challenges with emotion regulation, and personality factors. Also, these children (particularly those with limited prosocial emotions) may have temperamental issues that impede the normal development of a conscience (Frick, 2016). However, cultural issues have also been found to play a role in a child's predisposition to conduct disorder. For example, a number of factors related to poverty have also been associated with a greater probability of a diagnosis of conduct disorder in children (Gathright & Tyler, 2014; INSERM Collective Expertise Centre, 2005; Loeber et al., 2000; Patel et al., 2018). These factors include things such as poor-quality childcare, early exposure to violence in the home or community, and peers who engage in socially inappropriate behavior (Frick, 2016; Gathright & Tyler, 2014). Children with conduct disorder who come from impoverished homes are also 1.5 times more likely to be hospitalized for their symptoms than children from higher income households (Patel et al., 2018). In addition, family instability is a particular risk factor in the onset of conduct disorder in childhood (as opposed to adolescence). These children are often exposed to greater levels of family conflict and less effective parenting strategies than typically developing children (Frick, 2016).

> Children with conduct disorder who come from impoverished homes are 1.5 times more likely to be hospitalized for their symptoms than children from higher income households (Patel et al., 2018).

Gathright and Tyler (2014) also note the following environmental risk factors associated with conduct disorder: abuse, neglect, parental rejection, harsh discipline, inconsistent parenting, lack of supervision, single-parent status, parental criminality, and parental drug and alcohol abuse. However, it is important to note that environment alone does not create conduct disorder, rather it is believed to be an interaction between a child's disposition and their environment. In fact, research studies conducted with twins have found a combination of genetic and environmental factors contribute to the development of conduct disorder in children (APA, 2013; Gathright & Tyler, 2014; INSERM Collective Expertise Centre, 2005). As a caution, INSERM Collective Expertise Centre (2005) explains that, "It is clear that there is no single factor that, on its own, can either predict or explain why some children keep or adopt aggressive or antisocial behaviour patterns" (para. 6).

Despite these risk factors, Gathright and Tyler (2014) have highlighted a number of protective factors as well. Protective factors are those characteristics and actions that can inhibit the escalation of conduct disorder when it does occur in children and adolescents. Those protective characteristics are a family history free from other diagnoses of ODD or conduct disorder and when the child or adolescent does not exhibit symptoms associated with any comorbid condition. Protective actions that curtail the development of conduct disorder in children and adolescents include the provision of early assessment for conduct disorder and the implementation of effective treatments at a young age.

Cultural Considerations

According to Breslau and colleagues (2006), Hispanic people have the highest lifetime prevalence for conduct disorder at 6.9% of the population. This is followed closely by White individuals at 5% and Black people at 4.9%. However, even with similar symptomatology, African American children are more likely to be diagnosed with conduct disorder, and White children are more likely to be diagnosed with the less serious ODD (Proctor et al., 1992). In a very large research study, Patel et al. (2018) determined that White children represent the greatest frequency of children admitted to psychiatric hospitals for the treatment of conduct disorder; however, a larger proportion of African Americans and Hispanics with conduct disorder are hospitalized for care. Shockingly, African Americans are twice as likely to be admitted to the hospital for symptoms associated with conduct disorder as individuals from other races, and African American males under the age of 11 with conduct disorder are the most likely to be admitted to a psychiatric facility for treatment as compared to other children with conduct disorder. The researchers suggest that differences in parenting strategies may contribute to the differential rates of hospitalization among children. They note that African American parents are more likely to rely on physical forms of punishment and value obedience over families of other races. This combination may lead to more externalizing behaviors by teaching children to confront pain and challenges (like those associated with systemic racism) as opposed to comply in social situations (Patel et al., 2018). Research has also supported that African American boys are rated by teachers as significantly higher than their peers of other races on scales of externalizing behaviors, and African American boys from impoverished homes are rated significantly higher than their African American peers from other socioeconomic statuses on those same ratings of externalizing behavior (Schaeffer et al., 2003).

It is important to emphasize one other critical issue related to cultural context as highlighted by the *DSM-5*. The *DSM-5* notes that when conducting an evaluation for conduct disorder, a clinician must explore the cultural climate in which the behaviors of concern have occurred. They suggest that it would be inappropriate to give a diagnosis of conduct disorder when the child or adolescent is engaging in behaviors that are similar to what is occurring in their immediate surroundings. Some situations in which this might occur include areas with excessive violence as related to crime or war (APA, 2013). Finally, given the implicit racial bias documented throughout the health care system, it becomes even more critical for professionals to increase their awareness and guard against discrimination in the evaluation process (Merino et al., 2018). The clinician should be especially sensitive to judgments regarding which behaviors are considered aberrant since children and youth of racial and ethnic minority backgrounds are disproportionately labeled as such (Okonofua & Eberhardt, 2015; Okonofua et al., 2016).

IMPACT OF CONDUCT DISORDER ON SOCIAL–EMOTIONAL AND BEHAVIORAL FUNCTIONING IN SCHOOL AND HOME ENVIRONMENTS

Social–Emotional and Behavioral Functioning in School

Externalizing behavioral problems in the school setting is a defining feature for most children and adolescents diagnosed with conduct disorder. Their behaviors are frequent, intense, and highly disruptive. Students with conduct disorder consistently defy rules associated with behavioral expectations in that setting without remorse and engage in heated exchanges with teachers and administrators. Their behavior is characterized by lying, stealing, physical aggression, verbal aggression, and noncompliance with classroom academic expectations. In addition, children and adolescents with conduct disorder often perceive hostile intent even in neutral interactions with others and respond with greater hostility (Griffiths & Hart, 2016).

In response to the externalizing behavioral issues demonstrated by adolescents in the school setting, school administrators may be tempted to seek alternative placements for students with conduct disorder. These alternative settings frequently include rigid academic and disciplinary structures. Although it might seem that students with conduct disorder could benefit from the increased structure provided by these restrictive environments, research actually supports that they are counterproductive for students with conduct disorder at the secondary level. These environments often elevate the severity of conduct disorder symptomatology and lead to greater levels of school noncompliance. Also, these settings frequently exacerbate the social and academic issues already experienced by children and adolescents with behavioral challenges. Thus, it may not be surprising that these settings also increase the probability of the student with conduct disorder dropping out of high school (Powers et al., 2016).

Students with conduct disorder also frequently experience a negative social byproduct of their challenging behavior. Research consistently demonstrates that children and adolescents with conduct disorder often experience rejection from their peers due to their problematic behaviors, and this peer rejection pushes these students into even more deviant peer groups. In the deviant peer groups, the antisocial behavior is reinforced through peer attention, thus creating the likelihood that the behaviors will continue (Deater-Dekkard, 2001; Schaeffer et al., 2003). Children and adolescents with conduct disorder also frequently engage in bullying behaviors in the school setting, which may exacerbate their negative standing among peers (Kokkinos & Panayiotou, 2004).

Social–Emotional and Behavioral Functioning at Home

The earliest warning signs for conduct disorder are often first seen in the home environment. These include very early childhood issues with self-control and social interactions. The child or adolescent who is at risk for an eventual diagnosis of conduct disorder will frequently exhibit moodiness and impulsivity. They also tend to be aggressive and manipulative in interactions with both peers and adults. They exhibit a persistent pattern of defiance and often lack prerequisite skills associated with school readiness. At young ages, these children intentionally engage in socially maladaptive behaviors, including actions like lying, stealing, destroying property, and harming people or animals that are beyond what is considered developmentally appropriate (Gathright & Tyler, 2014).

Obviously, the home life for families with a child or adolescent with conduct disorder is uniquely challenging. This is likely compounded by the fact that some of the biological factors that contribute to the development of conduct disorder in children represent challenges in the parents themselves. According to Gathright and Tyler (2014), children with conduct disorder often also have parents with a greater probability of having alcohol dependence, antisocial personality disorder, ADHD, conduct disorder, and schizophrenia. There is also an increased incidence of having a sibling with either ODD or conduct disorder in the home. These compounded issues of psychopathology across multiple individuals in the home create complications with regard to financial stability, emotional well-being, communication, and familial relationships.

> According to Gathright and Tyler (2014), children with conduct disorder often also have parents with a greater probability of alcohol dependence, antisocial personality disorder, ADHD, conduct disorder, and schizophrenia.

In the most extreme circumstances, a child with conduct disorder requires placement in foster care. This can happen for a number of reasons. First, the behavior of a child or adolescent with conduct disorder may become so severe that it precludes them from remaining safely in the home (APA, 2013; INSERM Collective Expertise Centre, 2005). Second, given that there is a high co-occurrence of parental psychological problems and having a child with conduct disorder, the parent's own adjustment issues and concerns may inhibit their ability to effectively parent the child (APA, 2013). Third, there can be a mismatch between the child's intensive needs for structure, discipline, and boundaries, and the parenting style being employed in the home (INSERM Collective Expertise Centre, 2005). In these cases, out-of-home placement can occur. Social service providers would continue to monitor the child, the foster placement, and the home for progress toward meeting identified objectives with an ultimate goal of reintegrating the family at a point when the family can function safely and effectively.

In order to prevent these types of out-of-home placements, it is imperative that professionals involved with the family address parenting skills when needed and as early as possible as these types of interventions wane in their positive impact as children age into adolescence (Eyberg et al., 2008). Effective interventions for parenting often include assisting parents in developing and implementing a behavior plan in the home. Although the behavior plan should be focused on positive behavioral supports, the parents can also be taught more effective discipline strategies for when problematic behaviors do arise. Beyond the plan and its contingencies, parents should be encouraged to increase the quantity and quality of their interactions and communication with their child who has been diagnosed with conduct disorder (Frick, 2016). Since parent training interventions have consistently shown promise in the treatment of conduct disorder, it behooves professionals to advocate for these services for families in order to promote improved outcomes for all.

IMPACT OF CONDUCT DISORDER ON LEARNING IN THE CLASSROOM

Students with conduct disorder frequently struggle with deficits in executive functioning. Executive functioning is responsible for skills like attention, following directions, impulse control, and problem-solving. Research has found that challenges with executive functioning are particularly prevalent in children and adolescents with conduct disorder who also display physical aggression and violence (INSERM Collective Expertise Centre, 2005), and children who experience early difficulties with attention and concentration (as related to executive functioning deficits) have a higher probability of displaying antisocial behaviors later in life (Schaeffer et al., 2003). These deficits in executive functioning contribute to issues in the classroom for students with conduct disorder in meeting both academic and behavioral expectations. Schaeffer et al. (2003) describe the progression as follows: The child's struggle with attention and concentration yields more demands for compliance from teachers in the classroom. The child resists the demands, so the teacher's discipline becomes less consistent and harsher in response. These attempts at coercive types of discipline foster greater resistance from the child, and the pattern continues to escalate as both parties (child and teacher) struggle for control of the situation (Schaeffer et al., 2003). Thus, educational professionals should focus their efforts on helping children to build their repertoire of executive functioning skills while also disengaging from counterproductive power struggles in the classroom.

Although the behavioral impacts of conduct disorder in the classroom may be the most obvious area for intervention, academic issues must be addressed as well. It is well documented in the literature that students with conduct disorder often experience challenges with verbal ability and academic achievement (APA, 2013; Dery et al., 1999; INSERM Collective Expertise Centre, 2005). Their skills are often limited in vocabulary, comprehension, verbal fluency, oral expression, and written language, and these cognitive and academic deficits are associated with delinquency throughout adulthood as well (INSERM Collective Expertise Centre, 2005). In fact, these verbal deficits in students with conduct disorder are evident in research even when researchers control for socioeconomic status differences among the participants. This suggests that the verbal deficits are inherent with the conduct disorder as opposed to some other environmental variable that could contribute to challenges with verbal abilities and associated skills (Dery et al., 1999). Some researchers have even found that children and adolescents with conduct disorder have deficits in social pragmatic communication that is commensurate with those found in students with autism spectrum disorder. The struggle with verbal skills and associated communication issues may underlie much of their antisocial behavior (Gilmour et al., 2004). Recent research has also highlighted overall lower IQ scores among students with conduct disorder relative to comparable peers (Lazaratou et al., 2018).

It is well documented in the literature that students with conduct disorder often experience challenges with verbal ability and academic achievement (APA, 2013; Dery et al., 1999; INSERM Collective Expertise Centre, 2005).

Thus, teachers are charged with supporting students with conduct disorder through their academic challenges while also attempting to manage the students' emotional regulation and behavioral control issues. These intense and emotionally laden expectations for teachers of students with conduct disorder lead to burnout for the professionals in many situations (Brunsting et al., 2014). Despite the difficulties associated with students with conduct disorder within the classroom, teachers do have options for positive and productive engagement with these children and adolescents. With regard to effective practices for instruction, research supports that implementing a positive behavioral support plan in a classroom with a low student-to-teacher ratio and high-quality academic instruction is particularly effective. In addition, in order to address the impulse control issues in the context of the academic instruction, students with conduct disorder should be given multiple opportunities to respond and engage with instruction at a high frequency (Simpson et al., 2011). When these strategies are used and improvements in behavior and academic instruction are noted, the result is greater success opportunities for the student and higher teaching self-efficacy for the instructor (Brunsting et al., 2014).

IMPLICATIONS FOR SCHOOL PSYCHOLOGISTS

Assessment Role

In their assessment role, school psychologists are likely to be called upon to participate as a multidisciplinary team member in evaluations to determine eligibility for special services within the school setting. In many cases, this may take the form of an evaluation to determine eligibility for the categories of Emotional Disturbance or OHI under IDEA (see prior discussion in this chapter). Regardless of the category of disability under investigation in the evaluation, the functions of the school psychologist in the assessment process will vary little given the aspects explored through that evaluation for a student with conduct disorder.

After receiving parent permission for the evaluation, the team will have 60 days to complete the evaluation and determine whether the student is eligible under a disability category to receive special education services. This is a two-pronged eligibility decision. The team must decide whether the child or adolescent meets criteria as a student with a disability *and* whether the student demonstrates a need for services based on the educational impact of that disability. The team collects and uses a variety of data in making these decisions, and the work of the school psychologist is integral to the process.

In the case of a student with conduct disorder, the medical diagnosis of that condition and its associated features are critical for the team to explore. The team will pursue parental permission to access medical records related to the diagnosis. This may include pediatric, psychological, and/or psychiatric documentation of any prior evaluation and the resulting diagnosis. As noted previously in the chapter, the diagnosis is merely one piece of data and is not sufficient for any determination of school-based eligibility for services. Along with seeking these records, the team will heavily explore behavioral data available in the school setting. This is likely to include documentation regarding historical disciplinary infractions by the student as well as classroom observations of the student's current functioning.

These behavioral observations often constitute the first phase of the functional behavioral assessment portion of the evaluation, and the school psychologist may be the most qualified school-based professional to conduct the functional behavioral assessment. The aim of that assessment is to determine what setting events or occurrences precede problematic behavior, establish an operational definition of the target behavior, and pinpoint responses by others in the environment that closely follow the time of occurrence of the target behavior and serve to inadvertently reinforce the student's maladaptive behavior patterns. The functional behavioral assessment assists the team in determining why the behavior is happening in a particular setting and what psychological purpose it is serving for the student. If the team is trying to determine whether the student meets criteria under IDEA as a student with Emotional Disturbance, then the medical records and functional behavioral assessment are essential data in establishing whether or not the student's behavior constitutes social maladjustment. A student cannot be qualified to receive services under the category of Emotional Disturbance if their behaviors align with social maladjustment unless it can be determined that the student is exhibiting both emotionally disturbed and socially maladjusted behaviors. Finally, other components of a psychological evaluation (as conducted by the school psychologist) are likely to be considered in this determination as well. These should include behavioral assessments by other raters (like parents and teachers); interviews with parents, teachers, and the student; and measures of functioning in areas such as self-esteem, depression, and anxiety. Although these are team decisions, the school psychologist's knowledge and skills in this arena are invaluable to the process.

Beyond the aforementioned data, the team must also assess the student in any other area of suspected disability and detail their educational functioning. Again, the school psychologist plays a critical role in that the psychologist is often the only person on the team with competency to administer a cognitive assessment. Because research has established that students with conduct disorder often have concomitant issues with cognitive ability, then this line of inquiry should be pursued. As previously noted, adolescents with conduct disorder perform more poorly on verbal measures of intelligence and achievement (INSERM Collective Expertise Centre, 2005) than their peers, and this must be taken into account. Along with the cognitive assessment, academic achievement must also be measured to determine the individual's present levels of functioning and whether any disability has impacted the student's educational attainment and performance. This role, too, is often undertaken by the school psychologist. Throughout the process, it is imperative that the school psychologist engage in culturally competent assessment practices and guide the team in decision-making that is sensitive to diversity issues to mitigate the harmful effects of systemic bias.

When all relevant data have been collected, then the team will meet to make a determination of eligibility based on the IDEA disability category under consideration (e.g., Emotional Disturbance or OHI). If the child with a diagnosis of conduct disorder is found to meet the eligibility criteria for special education services, then the team would proceed to develop an IEP for that student. This plan would outline yearly goals and objectives, special education placement (location[s]) where services will be delivered, and necessary related services. As a part of this plan, the school psychologist may also be tapped to provide the related services. It may be determined that the psychologist will be a part of the student's needed behavioral supports, or the school psychologist may provide ongoing counseling or therapy in support of the student's academic and behavioral progress.

However, if the team determines that the student with a conduct disorder does not meet IDEA criteria as a child with a disability (as is often the case) or the student does not demonstrate a need for special education services, then a school-based team may consider the student's eligibility for services and supports under Section 504 of the Rehabilitation Act of 1973. The same data that was necessary for the special education evaluation is also critical in this evaluation. The key difference between the special education evaluation and the evaluation for a 504 plan is that Section 504 (see earlier discussion in this chapter) merely states that there is a disability (or suspected disability) that impacts a major life function. It is common for 504 eligibility teams to consider that a diagnosis of conduct disorder meets the established criteria as a psychological disorder and that the symptoms of the conduct disorder inhibit the child's ability to learn. When the team has made this determination of 504 eligibility, then a plan is developed to provide educational supports and services to increase the probability of the child's success and to give the child the opportunity to participate in the educational environment to the fullest extent possible despite the disability. As with the special education evaluation, in the 504 evaluation process, the school psychologist functions in critical roles related to assessment, data collection, interpretation, and decision-making.

Beyond their role in assessment for special education eligibility and services for students diagnosed with conduct disorder, school psychologists could also play a critical role in promoting universal social, emotional, and behavioral screenings in schools to promote early identification of students who are at risk for challenges like those associated with conduct disorder. School psychologists may develop and/or administer screening instruments across all grade levels. Given that early intervention is critical for successful outcomes for students with conduct disorder, it is imperative that these students be identified and provided with targeted interventions in areas of need. These interventions should support student skill development, adjustment within the school setting, and positively impact overall school climate issues.

Advocacy Role

Early assessment and intervention for children with conduct disorder has been found to lead to more positive outcomes in their present circumstances and into adulthood. Children and adolescents with conduct disorder frequently progress into adults engaged in criminality and who are diagnosed with antisocial personality disorder. However, early intervention can disrupt that negative progression. Experts suggest that public awareness is critical in this arena (INSERM Collective Expertise Centre, 2005). In that vein, school psychologists can play a critical role in educating school personnel and other stakeholders about typical versus atypical emotional and behavioral development in children as well as early warning signs of conduct disorder. This awareness could lead to better identification of and services for youth who are at risk for conduct disorder and its associated life complications.

In their advocacy role, school psychologists may also be called upon to play an indirect role in medication management for children and adolescents with conduct disorder. Although there is no specific U.S Food and Drug Administration (FDA)-approved medical treatment for addressing the needs of students with conduct disorder, a variety of medications are prescribed through community-based physicians to these children and adolescents (Gathright & Tyler, 2014; INSERM Collective Expertise Centre, 2005; Lillig, 2018). As such, within the school buildings, the school nurse is often tasked with dispensing any medications needed during the school day; however, the school psychologist may serve as a liaison between the school and any pediatrician or psychiatrist involved in outside care for the student. Specifically, the school psychologist may conduct behavioral observations in the school setting, report data back to medical providers, and provide feedback on behavioral progress associated with medicinal interventions. Given that the school psychologist has the opportunity to unobtrusively observe the student in a great variety of interactions across settings and times of day, the psychologist can offer invaluable insight into the child's school-based functioning to community-based partners for the child's care.

> Given that the school psychologist has the opportunity to unobtrusively observe the student in a great variety of interactions across settings and times of day, the psychologist can offer invaluable insight into the child's school-based functioning to community-based partners involved in the child's care.

Consultation Role

When consulting with parents of children and adolescents with conduct disorder, research can guide school psychologists in fulfilling an effective educational role. The literature suggests that professionals (like school psychologists) should help parents develop an understanding of what is normal versus abnormal behavior and conduct through the progressive developmental phases. In addition, school psychologists can also help parents with their parenting strategies. Since researchers have demonstrated that harsh, punishment-oriented discipline can exacerbate issues of conduct disorder, the school psychologist can help parents to develop more positive behavior supports for their homes, including recognizing and reinforcing appropriate behavior, ignoring minor behavioral infractions, and setting appropriate boundaries and limits. In addition, many of the effective treatments for children and adolescents with conduct disorders emphasize family involvement. Thus, the school psychologist should be aware of community-based options for parent training and family therapy. The psychologist can provide information and options for parents if they decide to seek this type of therapeutic assistance for their families.

Counseling and Therapy Role

Cognitive behavioral therapy has been shown to be effective with students with conduct disorder who are over the age of 10 (INSERM Collective Expertise Centre, 2005), and this is a role in which trained school psychologists can provide direct support to these students in the school setting. Cognitively based therapeutic treatments have been found to improve behavior among children and adolescents with conduct disorder across school, home, and community settings (Kazdin, 1997). This type of therapy is easily adapted to the school setting (Forman & Barakat, 2011), and it has been suggested that adding cognitive behavioral therapy to the repertoire of services provided by trained and experienced school personnel (like school psychologists) may be one of the most broadly effective psychosocial interventions available (Beidas et al., 2012).

Finally, considering the risky and often dangerous behaviors engaged in by students with conduct disorder, it is likely that school psychologists may be called into crisis work within the school setting. The necessary crisis management may be in response to threats of harm or violence, actual incidents of physical aggression against peers or teachers, or threats of self-harm. In this role, school psychologists must first take measures to ensure the safety of all involved in the present moment. Then, the psychologist must mitigate future risks of harm through the engagement of the appropriate familial, community, or law enforcement resources as necessary.

EDUCATIONAL SUPPORTS

Given their struggle with executive functions, students with conduct disorder may benefit from specific intervention in this area to assist with both academic and behavioral outcomes. Dawson (2014) suggests that executive function interventions can be effectively designed to target individual students, or they can be implemented at the classroom level. In cases in which a student with conduct disorder is demonstrating executive functioning deficits, educators should carefully consider whether those deficits are unique to the individual or whether there are systems or structures within the larger educational environment that are failing to promote the development of executive functions across larger groups of students (Dawson, 2014). This determination should guide the decision-making for the interventionist whether that individual is a school psychologist, building-based intervention specialist, or classroom teacher.

Students with conduct disorder and associated executive functioning deficits are often challenged with attentional issues, and classroom supports are necessary to enhance the students' probability of academic success. In her chapter on improving executive skills, Dawson (2014) offers a plethora of evidenced-based practices that could be applied when working with students with conduct disorder of all ages. Strategies, such as shortening assignments, are often helpful in building success in maintaining attentional focus and assignment completion. Modifying assignments to be more structured and less open-ended can also help to promote success and can be particularly beneficial for those students who have conduct disorder and also struggle with verbally loaded tasks and expectations. Beyond assignment modification, children and adolescents with conduct disorder benefit from classrooms that are designed for success. Structuring the furniture arrangement and classroom décor to minimize distractions and inhibit maladaptive and impulsive behavioral decisions can be helpful to these students with conduct disorder, their teachers who are charged with classroom management, and peers who are working in the environment. Providing a greater degree of explicit cognitive structure for the student with conduct disorder can be especially helpful. Giving directions in multiple modalities, modeling organizational tactics, rehearsing appropriate behavioral responses, and praising progress in executive functioning areas/skills promote successful classroom integration for the students with conduct disorder. Finally, Dawson (2014) promotes the overt practice of metacognitive strategies like planning, goal setting, and self-evaluation of task performance. She suggests that teachers or other educational personnel should use direct questions to the students with conduct disorder to prompt planning, problem-solving, and reflection (Dawson, 2014).

Students with conduct disorder and associated executive functioning deficits are often challenged with attentional issues, and classroom supports are necessary to enhance the students' probability of academic success.

Beyond those techniques that target issues with executive functioning, research has found that students with conduct disorder may benefit from other classroom-based strategies as well. Although not specific to students with conduct disorder, Harrison et al. (2013) offered an extensive review and analysis of the literature regarding empirically validated accommodations and modifications for a broader group of students with behavioral challenges. One such accommodation concerns choice-making. When children and adolescents are offered opportunities to make choices for themselves in the context of their classrooms, this simple technique serves to improve their on-task behavior, productivity, and accuracy in their academic work. Other practices that have also demonstrated some evidence of improving behavior and compliance in the classroom include provision of work around topics that students with behavioral challenges find of interest and increasing the pace of instruction to prevent opportunities for disruption (Harrison et al., 2013).

SCHOOL-BASED MENTAL HEALTH INTERVENTIONS AND SUPPORTS

Any school-based interventions to support students with conduct disorder should be focused on empirical factors that support success for these students, including the development of a support system for the family, the reinforcement of time spent with socially appropriate peers, the inhibition of interactions with peers who have their own challenging behaviors, and an increase in positive contacts with teachers and other school personnel (INSERM Collective Expertise Centre, 2005). Multitiered systems of intervention with intensive behavioral supports (rather than hierarchies of consequences) have been shown to have success with this population of students. As noted previously, exclusionary practices and restrictive educational placements are not only ineffective for adolescents with conduct disorder, but they have been found to have harmful outcomes. Adolescents who are placed in highly restrictive alternative placements frequently demonstrate an increase in maladaptive behavior and are at risk for dropping out of school (Powers et al., 2016).

One such program of multitiered support that has shown promise in positively impacting the behaviors of children and adolescents with conduct disorder is School-Wide Positive Behavior Support (SWPBS; Stewart et al., 2007). SWPBS is considered a primary prevention effort, and its positive impact on schools is well documented in the literature. Overall, schools implementing these programs have shown significant decreases in behavioral problems. Specific improvements include reductions in the percentages of behavioral referrals, decreased out-of-school suspensions, and reduced numbers of instructional days lost due to behavioral infractions among students (Curtis et al., 2010). In addition, research suggests that SWPBS is most effective when implementation begins at kindergarten. Along with reducing problem behaviors, SWPBS has even been shown to improve concentration, social–emotional functioning, and prosocial behavior in some examinations of its effectiveness (Bradshaw et al., 2012). Finally, longitudinal studies done in many schools even support long-term success off SWPBS when it is implemented with fidelity (Bradshaw et al., 2010).

The philosophy behind SWPBS is that behavioral issues are both predictable and preventable if the right support structures are in place. Research suggests that 10% to 20% of students in any school building are likely to exhibit some form of behavioral problem. The first step in preventing those problems is to accurately identify who those children may be and have staff members collaborate on a preliminary list of concerning behaviors along with when and where they occur. Once those foundational issues are highlighted, staff can then brainstorm simple solutions to prevent the issues from arising in the first place. The next step requires staff to come to consensus on the behavioral expectations that span the building, the classrooms, and its affiliated areas. Behavioral expectations are positively stated so that children are told what to do (instead of what not to do), and staff agree to a reinforcement structure. The students are reinforced for displaying the behavioral expectations and re-instructed when they fall short of the behavioral guidelines (Scott, 2001).

Social skills training in the schools has also been found to be effective for children and adolescents diagnosed with conduct disorder. These social skills interventions should focus on conflict resolution and teaching age-appropriate prosocial behaviors (INSERM Collective Expertise Centre, 2005). Role playing and modeling can be particularly effective techniques with these children who often struggle with abstract thinking and social problem-solving. Research has shown that social skills training specific to children with conduct disorder is related to reduction in externalizing behaviors overall, fewer incidents of aggression in the school setting, increased prosocial behavior with peers, and development of conflict management skills. These results are often maintained over time. However, one mitigating factor has been identified. Children with conduct disorder who have parents who are highly critical of the children and who rely on physical punishment do not show the same gains through social skills training as children who do not have those parental factors at play (Webster-Stratton et al., 2001).

A word of caution is warranted regarding small-group counseling settings for students with conduct disorder. Although small groups have shown effectiveness for a number of social issues, researchers argue that the small-group setting is not productive as a treatment modality for children and adolescents with conduct disorder. In fact, in the small-group setting, maladaptive behaviors can often be reinforced through peer attention. To be specific, the groups often devolve into deviant conversations that are counter to group and individual counseling goals. The laughter and shock of peers in response to the inappropriate verbalizations of the student with the conduct disorder will increase the probability that that student will engage in such speech and behaviors in other times and settings (Dishion et al., 1999; Theodore et al., 2004).

Although school personnel can and should offer interventions and supports within that setting for students with conduct disorder, the most effective interventions occur in multiple settings and are multidisciplinary in nature (Burns et al., 2003; Frick, 2016; Kazdin, 1997). The integration of services across all agencies involved in the lives and treatment of children and adolescents with conduct disorder is crucial. This often involves open communication, case management meetings, and shared documentation with regard to medical, social service, educational, and perhaps juvenile justice personnel. These coordinated efforts have the greatest probability of success through their elements of transparency and consistency (Burns et al., 2003).

> Although school personnel can and should offer interventions and supports within that setting for students with conduct disorder, the most effective interventions occur in multiple settings and are multidisciplinary in nature (Burns et al., 2003; Frick, 2016).

CASE STUDY 5.1 BRYCE: CASE OF AN AFRICAN AMERICAN BOY WITH CONDUCT DISORDER

Background

Bryce is an 11-year-old African American boy who lives in an impoverished area of New Orleans and attends a public school near his neighborhood. He was recently diagnosed with conduct disorder by his pediatrician. He is currently in the fifth grade; he was retained in the second grade due to academic and behavioral issues. Although the school year is only 2 months in, Bryce just finished serving his second out-of-school suspension after attempting to steal his teacher's wallet from her desk, throwing desks when confronted, and running from the building. Bryce had to be apprehended by the school resource officer on a nearby street corner. Bryce's academic history is replete with similar incidents.

Bryce was born into a two-parent home, but the family demonstrated dysfunction from the start. Bryce's father, Rick, dropped out of high school after a number of tumultuous years in the school system. Rick struggled academically throughout his schooling. He was served in special education under the disability category of specific learning disability due to his significant challenges in reading, but he demonstrated behavioral challenges as well. In early elementary school, Rick learned that he could escape difficult classroom tasks by engaging his teachers in arguments. Rick would intentionally taunt his teachers, be verbally abusive to peers, and run from the setting. The school personnel attempted increasingly restrictive placements, but by middle school, Rick was frequently truant and completely disengaged from academics when he was in the building. When he was not in school, Rick was active in gang culture and engaged in using and selling drugs. The school socially promoted Rick each

(continued)

CASE STUDY 5.1 BRYCE: CASE OF AN AFRICAN AMERICAN BOY WITH CONDUCT DISORDER (continued)

year through the grades. By the age of 16, Rick was expelled from school after threatening a classmate with a knife. He subsequently left school. Since that time, Rick has had a spotty employment history, rarely spending more than a few months at a time working in a variety of low-paying, manual-labor jobs. Rick is no longer involved with a gang, but he does use drugs recreationally and has taken antidepressants for about 3 years after a diagnosis of depression by a family physician. Bryce's mother, Shannon, had been married to Rick for almost 2 years when she discovered that she was expecting nearly 18 weeks into her pregnancy. She had been a casual marijuana user but stopped the use of all drugs and alcohol upon learning that she was pregnant. However, her relationship with her husband, Rick, has been volatile for the duration of their relationship. Shannon and Rick's arguments frequently escalated into shouting matches during which police were called by concerned neighbors, and Rick had physically assaulted Shannon on two occasions prior to her pregnancy and once during pregnancy. Bryce was born after a full-term pregnancy. He was an irritable baby from the start and introduced even greater stress into an already strained relationship. Rick lost his most recent job 8 weeks after Bryce's birth. His drug use increased, and he started bringing other unstable figures into the home. To support the family, Shannon went to work as an aide at a local nursing home. She worked 12-hour shifts, and Bryce was primarily home with Rick and Rick's friends. However, when Rick felt like going out, he would leave Bryce in the care of anyone who happened to be available within their apartment building. Oftentimes, these were people who Bryce had never met before and who had instability in their own homes. By the age of 3, Bryce began refusing to comply with many basic parental requests. He would often respond to a request by biting or kicking. By 4 years old, Bryce consistently used profanity (to the amusement of many of his dad's friends), had injured a neighbor's cat, and had been removed from a Mom's Day Out program that was run through a local church because of his challenging behaviors. When Bryce entered school at kindergarten, he had a well-established repertoire of maladaptive behaviors, including verbal and physical aggression, general noncompliance, and a tendency to elope from the classroom. The school had attempted some behavioral intervention and even suggested an alternative school at one point, but Bryce rarely made it through a few weeks' time without another out-of-school suspension due to a behavioral incident. Bryce was evaluated twice for special education services but found ineligible. Despite having overall low cognitive abilities and some deficits in reading, he did not meet criteria as a child with a specific learning disability and the team determined that his socially maladjusted behaviors disqualified him from services under the category of Emotional Disturbance. Throughout his early elementary years, Bryce's challenging behaviors continued in both the home and school settings. As he reached his 11th birthday, Shannon became concerned that Bryce might be beginning to affiliate with a local gang, and shortly after his birthday, Bryce was suspended yet again after the incident with his teacher's wallet and running from school. While on the suspension, Bryce's mother took him to the pediatrician who diagnosed him with early-onset conduct disorder, noted his severity as moderate, and started him on a mood-stabilizing drug. The pediatrician suggested that Shannon seek counseling services for Bryce. Because of the repeated incidents in the school, Shannon and Rick have decided to move in with Rick's aunt in another part of the city to give Bryce a fresh start in a new school.

Discussion

Bryce's background exhibits many of the factors associated with risk for conduct disorder. His father's history includes issues of learning problems and behavioral challenges as well. It is likely that he may have had undiagnosed conduct disorder himself. The family is living in poverty and within a high crime neighborhood. Rick has struggled with holding a job and has a diagnosis of depression. He has also been abusive with his wife. Bryce had early exposure to violence within his home and neighborhood and was often left with unstable caretakers during his early years. These issues are associated with an increased probability for developing a

(continued)

CASE STUDY 5.1 BRYCE: CASE OF AN AFRICAN AMERICAN BOY WITH CONDUCT DISORDER (continued)

conduct disorder, and that is precisely what has happened with Bryce. He has experienced early and continuing challenges with compliance in the school setting that appears to be escalating over time.

In the new school, a new team will attempt to better serve Bryce and his academic and behavioral needs. The school psychologist and other school personnel should review the previous evaluations along with any other academic and behavioral records available regarding Bryce's educational history. If the team finds that Bryce's prior evaluations were thorough and accurate, then the team should pursue the opportunity to provide more support for Bryce through Section 504 of the Rehabilitation Act of 1973. The team will seek parental permission to begin the evaluation process. All new data will be sought for classroom observations, parent and teacher interviews, and recent medical records. The school psychologist will be responsible for the educational and psychological portions of the evaluation. These include academic achievement testing; intellectual assessment; and use of behavior rating scales, depression inventories, and an anxiety scale to determine Bryce's current functioning in these areas. The school psychologist will also be primarily responsible for the functional behavioral assessment. Upon collection of the data, the team will meet to determine whether the cumulative data supports that Bryce's diagnosis of conduct disorder meets the Section 504 eligibility criteria of having a medical issue that impacts major life function. It is likely that it will be determined that Bryce's diagnosis of conduct disorder is a psychological disorder that impedes his ability to learn. The team will then proceed to determine the appropriate services and supports for Bryce. The team will use the functional behavioral assessment that was conducted as a part of the 504 evaluation as the basis for a positive behavior intervention plan to be implemented in the classroom, and they will use the academic data to define the educational supports necessary to address Bryce's difficulty with reading. Beyond those supports, the team will determine the related services that may help Bryce to function within the school and progress within the curriculum. Given that Bryce is now prescribed medicine for his conduct disorder, the school nurse will likely be included in the plan to support his medication management. In addition, related services with the school psychologist may be deemed necessary. Because Bryce has yet to receive any counseling related to his behavioral issues, he may benefit from school-based services with the school psychologist. Although the school psychologist will need to use an intake session to determine the direction of their work together, research suggests that students who exhibit behaviors like Bryce's can show improved outcomes through the use of cognitive behavioral therapy and social skills training. The school psychologist would need to develop goals, objectives, and evaluation procedures to assess the effectiveness of their counseling with Bryce. The school psychologist could initiate wraparound services to coordinate and collaborate with any outside service providers. Beyond the individual work with Bryce as outlined in the 504 plan, the school psychologist could serve him (and others) with additional services as well. The school psychologist could refer Bryce's family to community-based resources for culturally sensitive parent training and/or family therapy. Also, if the school does not currently have a program for SWPBS, the school psychologist could be instrumental in establishing and maintaining such a program for the betterment of the entire school population.

SUMMARY POINTS

- In order to receive a *DSM-5* diagnosis of Conduct Disorder, the child or adolescent exhibits multiple violations of the rights of other people, laws, and/or rules over a period of at least a year; that the issues demonstrably impact the individual's functioning in school, work, or interpersonal interaction; and that the individual (if an adult) does not meet criteria for antisocial personality disorder.
- With regard to etiology, the school psychologist should remember that environment alone does not create conduct disorder, rather it is believed to be an interaction between a child's disposition and the environment.
- The home life of families with a child or adolescent with conduct disorder is uniquely challenging.
- Students with conduct disorder often struggle with verbal ability and deficits in executive function.
- School psychologists can engage in many roles and functions to support the needs of students with conduct disorder.
- Any school-based interventions to support students with conduct disorder should be focused on empirical factors that support success for these students, including the development of a support system for the family, the reinforcement of time spent with socially appropriate peers, the inhibition of interaction with peers who have their own challenging behaviors, and increasing contacts with teachers and other school personnel.

TEST YOUR KNOWLEDGE

1. Which of the following is required for a *DSM-5* diagnosis of Conduct Disorder?
   a. Deficits in intellectual functioning
   b. Symptoms adversely impact the individual's function in school or work
   c. Onset of symptoms before age 5
   d. All of the above

2. Individuals who first exhibit symptoms of conduct disorder during adolescence have a greater incidence of criminality in adulthood than those individuals who experience childhood onset of conduct disorder.
   a. True
   b. False

3. Social maladjustment represents an exclusion for eligibility for Emotional Disturbance under IDEA.
   a. True
   b. False

4. Children with conduct disorder often struggle with which cognitive abilities?
   a. Verbal abilities
   b. Processing speed
   c. Working memory
   d. Visual-spatial skills

5. Social skills training in the schools has been found to be effective for children and adolescents diagnosed with conduct disorder.
   a. True
   b. False

Answers: (1) b, (2) b, (3) a, (4) a, (5) a.

DISCUSSION QUESTIONS

1. Describe the *DSM-5* diagnostic criteria for Conduct Disorder.
2. Discuss the possible ways that children and adolescents with conduct disorder may be eligible for school-based services.
3. Explain the environmental risk factors for conduct disorder.
4. Highlight the school psychologist's advocacy role in working with children with conduct disorder and their families.
5. Detail one evidenced-based social–emotional intervention for students with conduct disorder.

CHAPTER RESOURCES

American Academy of Child and Adolescent Psychiatry *Conduct Disorder*: www.aacap.org/AACAP/Families_and_Youth/Facts_for_Families/FFF-Guide/Conduct-Disorder-033.aspx

American Academy of Child and Adolescent Psychiatry *Conduct Disorder Resource Center:* www.aacap.org/AACAP/Families_and_Youth/Resource_Centers/Conduct_Disorder_Resource_Center/Home.aspx

American Academy of Child and Adolescent Psychiatry *Violent Behavior in Children and Adolescents:* www.aacap.org/AACAP/Families_and_Youth/Facts_for_Families/FFF-Guide/Understanding-Violent-Behavior-In-Children-and-Adolescents-055.aspx

American Psychiatric Association *Impulse Control and Conduct Disorder:* www.psychiatry.org/patients-families/disruptive-impulse-control-and-conduct-disorders/what-are-disruptive-impulse-control-and-conduct-disorders

Centers for Disease Control and Prevention *Behavior and Conduct Problems in Children*: www.cdc.gov/childrensmentalhealth/behavior.html

Johns Hopkins Medicine *Conduct Disorder*: www.hopkinsmedicine.org/health/conditions-and-diseases/conduct-disorder

Merck Manual *Conduct Disorder*: www.merckmanuals.com/professional/pediatrics/mental-disorders-in-children-and-adolescents/conduct-disorder

KEY REFERENCES

Only key references appear in the print edition. The full reference list appears in the digital product on Springer Publishing Connect: connect.springerpub.com/content/book/978-0-8261-3587-2/part/part03/chapter/ch05

American Psychiatric Association. (2013). *Diagnostic and statistical manual of mental disorders* (5th ed.). https://doi.org/10.1176/appi.books.9780890425596

Dandreaux, D. M., & Frick, P. J. (2009). Developmental pathways to conduct problems: A further test of the childhood and adolescent-onset distinction. *Journal of Abnormal Child Psychology, 37*, 375–385. https://doi.org/10.1007/s10802-008-9261-5

Dawson, P. (2014). Best practices in assessing and improving executive skills. In P. L. Harrison & A. Thomas (Eds.), *Best practices in school psychology: Student-level services*. National Association of School Psychologists.

Frick, P. J. (2016). Current research on conduct disorder in children and adolescents. *South African Journal of Psychology, 46*(2), 160–174. https://doi.org/10.1177/0081246316628455

Gathright, M. M., & Tyler, L. H. (2014). *Disruptive behavior in children and adolescents*. University of Arkansas for Medical Sciences Psychiatric Research Institute.

INSERM Collective Expertise Centre. (2005). *Conduct: Disorder in children and adolescents*. https://www.ncbi.nlm.nih.gov/pmc/articles/PMC6162794/#:~:text=Current%20data%20indicates%20that%20the,of%20conduct%20disorder%20than%20girls

Office of Civil Rights. (n.d.). *Protecting students with disabilities: Frequently asked questions about Section 504 and the education of children with disabilities*. https://www2.ed.gov/about/offices/list/ocr/504faq.html

Patel, R. S., Amaravadi, N., Bhullar, H., Lekireddy, J., & Win, H. (2018). Understanding the demographic predictors and associated comorbidities in children hospitalized with conduct disorder. *Behavioral Science, 8*(9), 80. https://doi.org/10.3390/bs8090080

Schaeffer, C. M., Petras, H., Ialongo, N., Poduska, J., & Kellam, S. (2003). Modeling growth in boys' aggressive behavior across elementary school: Links to later criminal involvement, conduct disorder, and antisocial personality disorder. *Developmental Psychology, 39*(6), 1020–1035. https://doi.org/10.1037/0012-1649.39.6.1020

U.S. Department of Education. (n.d.). *Individuals with Disabilities Education Improvement Act*. https://sites.ed.gov/idea/

CHAPTER 6

Oppositional Defiant Disorder

LEARNING OBJECTIVES

- Summarize the diagnostic features for the *Diagnostic and Statistical Manual of Mental Disorders* (5th ed.; *DSM-5*; American Psychiatric Association [APA], 2013) diagnosis of Oppositional Defiant Disorder (ODD).
- Highlight the risk factors for ODD in youth.
- Describe common social–emotional and behavioral concerns for children with ODD.
- Understand the classroom implications for students with ODD.
- Identify effective social, emotional, and behavioral interventions for students with ODD.

INTRODUCTION

The *Diagnostic and Statistical Manual of Mental Disorders,* Fifth Edition (*DSM-5*; American Psychiatric Association [APA], 2013), classifies Oppositional Defiant Disorder (ODD) under the category of Disruptive, Impulse-Control, and Conduct Disorders. ODD and the other disorders in this diagnostic area feature issues related to emotional and behavioral regulation. The nature of these concerns typically results in harm to others or significant conflict with rules, laws, and/or individuals in positions of authority. Some examples of other Disruptive, Impulse-Control, and Conduct Disorders include Conduct Disorder (discussed in Chapter 5) and Intermittent Explosive Disorder (IED; addressed in Chapter 7).

Many of the symptoms related to ODD may be found in typically functioning children, adolescents, and adults. However, the context for the behavior is critically important in diagnosis, in that those who would be manifesting the behaviors at a more clinical level would exhibit those symptoms more frequently and at greater levels of intensity (relative to others of similar age, gender, and culture) than more emotionally and behaviorally typical individuals. Thus, any clinician considering a *DSM-5* diagnosis of ODD for a child or adolescent must look beyond symptom expression and explore whether the behaviors are related to typical adjustment versus clinical significance (APA, 2013).

DIAGNOSTIC ISSUES: *DSM-5* AND SCHOOL-BASED SERVICES

DSM-5 Diagnosis

With regard to a *DSM-5* diagnosis of ODD, the first criterion denotes that the individual must exhibit at least four out of the eight defined symptoms in order to qualify for the diagnosis. The eight symptoms are clustered into three categories: Angry/Irritable Mood, Argumentative/Defiant Behavior, and "Vindictiveness." However, the identified symptoms for diagnosis may come from any of the three categories. The three angry/irritable mood symptoms include frequent demonstrations of losing one's temper, being easily annoyed, and appearing angry. The four argumentative/defiant behavior symptoms relate to conflict with individuals in authority, active noncompliance with rules or commands, intentionally annoying others, and failure to accept responsibility for actions. The vindictiveness category is only represented by the symptom of demonstrating vengeful actions at least two times in the prior 6-month period. Beyond simple alignment to the symptoms, the *DSM-5* further indicates that for very young children (less than 5 years of age), the symptoms must be expressed on a nearly daily basis for 6 months for diagnosis, whereas the symptom frequency for those individuals older than 5 years of age is at least weekly for the preceding 6-month period (APA, 2013). The frequency and intensity of the symptom expression should be beyond what is typical for an individual as compared to others of their gender, age, or culture.

The second and third criteria for diagnosis of ODD in the *DSM-5* both relate to context of the expression of the symptoms. The second criterion relates to the impact of the behaviors being expressed by the individual. In order to apply the diagnosis, the behavior must either lead to distress for the individual or their close relations or impair the individual's ability to function in social, academic, or employment settings. Impairment in these settings might include relationship issues, defiance of authority, and overall noncompliance that renders the individual unable to adapt and progress in the setting. The third criterion describes exclusions for the diagnosis. The behavioral incidents cannot result from issues related to drug/alcohol use, psychotic periods, depression, or bipolar disorder. The individual also cannot be diagnosed with ODD if they meet the criteria established for disruptive mood dysregulation disorder (APA, 2013).

Beyond the application of the diagnostic criteria, the clinician diagnosing a child, adolescent, or adult with ODD must also apply a specifier related to the extensiveness of the location(s) in the expression of the symptoms. The severity is determined to be mild if the person exhibits symptoms solely in a particular setting, but the severity is deemed moderate if the symptom expression occurs in at least two settings. Finally, the severe specifier is reserved for those individuals whose symptoms are present in three or more settings (APA, 2013).

The current criteria for ODD from the *DSM-5* represent a few changes from the prior version (the *DSM-IV-TR*). The grouping of the symptoms into the three categories represents a change from the diagnosis of ODD as described in the prior version of the *DSM*, and the previously-existing diagnostic exclusion related to conduct disorder has been removed. Additionally, the clinical guidance regarding symptom frequency by age level and the determination of severity are new considerations for the diagnosis of ODD (Gathright & Tyler, 2014).

The development of ODD is primarily found during the childhood period. According to the *DSM-5*, the earliest signs of ODD generally occur during the preschool years, and this disorder rarely manifests after adolescence (APA, 2013). The Centers for Disease Control and Prevention (CDC) notes that the onset of ODD is most often before a child reaches 8 years of age and rarely begins after the age of 12 (CDC, n.d.). Researchers have found the temperament and affective dimensions predictive of later diagnoses of ODD in children as young as 3 years old (Ezpeleta et al., 2012, 2019; Rowe et al., 2010; Stringaris, 2011). Even as infants, children who are later diagnosed with ODD are often described as fussy and reactive in nature (Gathright & Tyler, 2014). Although not specific to ODD, Gathright and Tyler (2014) note that some of the earliest warning signs for all disruptive behavior disorders include irritability, inattentiveness, impulsivity, and poor problem-solving skills.

According to the *DSM-5*, the earliest signs of ODD generally occur during the preschool years and this disorder rarely manifests after adolescence (APA, 2013).

According to the *DSM-5*, the overall prevalence of ODD across all populations (juvenile and adult) is approximately 3.3% (APA, 2013). In childhood, estimates of prevalence of ODD generally range from 1% to 3% (Boat & Wu, 2015), and in 2009, the National Research Council and Institute of Medicine noted the prevalence of childhood ODD at 2.8% in the overall population. Among samples of youth with other psychiatric disorders, the prevalence of ODD has been estimated as high as 4.6% in individuals aged 3 to 17 (Perou et al., 2013) and as high as 12.6% in adolescent clinical populations alone (Merikangas et al., 2010). When parsing out the prevalence in early childhood, Ezpeleta et al. (2019) found that among samples of children in the general population, the prevalence from ages 3 to 8 was 6% to 7%, but rose to 8.8% by age 9 in a 1-year incidence study. They report that the greatest risk for development of symptoms occurs in the preschool years, at 12.6%, and this risk declines to 9.3% in early childhood (Ezpeleta et al., 2019). Yet, Roberts et al. (2009) report that the 12-month incidence of new diagnoses of ODD among child and adolescent samples is 1.56%. Thus, these two studies further demonstrate the greater probability of the development of ODD symptoms in earlier childhood as opposed to adolescence. As with many psychiatric disorders early age of onset is associated with a greater probability for the development of comorbid psychiatric disorders (Ezpeleta et al., 2019; Kessler et al., 2007; Rutter et al., 1999), and Heflinger and Humphreys (2008) found that boys are more likely to be diagnosed at younger ages than girls. Once developed, symptoms show stability over time if left untreated (Hipwell et al., 2011; Loeber et al. 2009). With treatment, 67% of children and adolescents with ODD are symptom free within 3 years, but 30% will progress in their symptoms to a level consistent with a diagnosis of conduct disorder (Connor, 2002).

Although the *DSM-5* reports a prevalence 4 times greater in boys than girls prior to adolescence, other research is less definitive with regard to gender and frequency of diagnosis. In fact, some researchers even suggest that the criteria for diagnosis may be insufficient for girls in that the psychiatric research that forms the basis for those criteria are primarily focused on young males (Crick & Zahn-Waxler, 2003; Lahey et al., 1994; Munkvold et al., 2011). Nonetheless, in a large empirical study, Munkvold et al. (2011) found that among children aged 7 to 9, the prevalence of ODD for girls was 1.3% and boys was 4.0%, which is roughly equivalent to the estimate from the *DSM-5*. ODD symptoms may also appear as distinct between male and female children and adolescents as research has suggested that boys may experience a greater number of symptoms, be more physically aggressive, and demonstrate fewer prosocial behaviors than girls with the same diagnosis (McKinney & Renk, 2007).

ODD is highly comorbid with other mental health conditions in children and adolescents (APA, 2013). However, some data indicate that ODD is rarely the first diagnosis that a child or adolescent receives. Heflinger and Humphreys (2008) noted that children who enter the mental health system without pre-existing diagnoses are more likely to receive a first-time diagnosis of attention deficit hyperactivity disorder (ADHD) or depression than a diagnosis of ODD. Yet, children and adolescents who already have another diagnosis are 24% more likely to have an ODD diagnosis applied than those who do not have other diagnoses.

According to the *DSM-5* and other researchers, there is a particularly high co-occurrence of ODD and ADHD in youth (APA, 2013; Ezpeleta et al., 2019; van Lier et al., 2007). With regard to hyperactivity, research has found that teachers rate 73% of boys with ODD with elevated hyperactivity scores as compared to approximately 15% of boys without ODD. Rey and Walter (1999) found that children and adolescents with ODD are 4 times more likely to be diagnosed with ADHD than children without ODD. Beyond comorbid ADHD, ODD symptoms and diagnoses in children and adolescents often precede the development of conduct disorder in either childhood or adulthood (INSERM Collective Expertise Centre, 2005) though some research suggests that that developmental trajectory occurs with greater frequency in boys than in girls (Rowe et al., 2002; van Lier et al., 2007). Individuals with ODD are also more likely to develop issues related to anxiety, depression, and substance abuse (APA, 2013). Specifically, Ezpeleta et al. (2019) found that individuals who develop ODD symptoms in preschool have over a 5 times greater probability of experiencing symptoms of depression later in life than children who do not display ODD symptoms in preschool. Further research supports that girls with ODD are more susceptible to the development of depression than boys with ODD (Burke et al., 2010; Rowe et al., 2002). In addition, according to Munkvold et al. (2011), teachers rate over 46% of girls with ODD as displaying emotional concerns as compared to just over 10% of girls who do not have ODD diagnoses or symptoms. However, research by Burke (2012) found that affective symptoms, such as irritability in boys with ODD, is predictive of the development of depression.

Finally, Rey and Walters (1999) note that children and adolescents with ODD also often struggle with communication disorders and learning challenges, which frequently present issues for their functioning in the school setting. Research indicates that students with emotional and behavioral concerns exhibit academic issues resulting in achievement that is lower than their peers without these challenges, and this impaired educational progress crosses all core academic content (Kent et al., 2011; Lane, 2007).

School-Based Eligibility

INDIVIDUALS WITH DISABILITIES EDUCATION IMPROVEMENT ACT REGULATIONS

The Individuals with Disabilities Education Improvement Act (IDEA) is federal legislation that protects the rights of children and adolescents with disabilities served in public school settings. IDEA outlines 13 disability categories. The student under consideration must be evaluated in all areas of suspected disability, and, through a two-pronged process, eligibility teams determine whether (a) a student meets criteria for one of the disability categories, and (b) whether the child also demonstrates a need for special education services. If that multidisciplinary team decides that both conditions are met, then IDEA mandates that the child or adolescent must receive a free and appropriate public education in the least restrictive environment possible and any related services (e.g., counseling, speech therapy, occupational therapy) necessary for the student to progress in the curriculum (U.S. Department of Education, n.d.).

Although the evaluation and eligibility processes apply to all disability categories, these issues related to children and adolescents with ODD have been the source of decades of contentious debate (Olympia et al., 2004; Sullivan & Sedah, 2014; Theodore et al., 2004). Many school-based eligibility teams face the difficult decision of determining whether a child or adolescent with an outside diagnosis of ODD meets the federal criteria for the disability category of Emotional Disturbance. Within IDEA, *Emotional Disturbance* is defined as an inability to learn that cannot be explained by intellectual, sensory, or other health factors; an inability to build or maintain satisfactory interpersonal relationships with peers and adults; inappropriate types of behavior or feelings under normal circumstances; a general pervasive mood of anxiety, unhappiness, or depression; and a tendency to develop physical symptoms or fears associated with personal or school problems. Although the criteria specifically denote the inclusion of youth with schizophrenia under the category of Emotional Disturbance, the definition goes further to exclude from this category children and adolescents who are determined to be socially maladjusted from this category (U.S. Department of Education, n.d.).

Thus, the debate regarding whether children and adolescents with ODD meet criteria for Emotional Disturbance primarily centers on the concept of social maladjustment. Unfortunately, there is no definition of *social maladjustment* in the federal law, nor is there consensus in the literature of what those terms are meant to describe (Sullivan & Sedah, 2014). Many contend that the lack of a definition has led to challenges in consistency across assessment, application, and inclusion of students in the category of Emotional Disturbance (Becker et al., 2011; Olympia et al., 2004; Sullivan & Sadeh, 2014). Despite these issues, eligibility teams often distinguish between Emotional Disturbance and social maladjustment according to the purposefulness of the behavior. Although the determinant of inappropriate feelings or behaviors under normal circumstances may apply to both, decision makers often believe that students with Emotional Disturbance may be unable to control their actions and/or understand the resulting consequences of their actions and that the students with social maladjustment are typically intentional in their behavioral choices and fully cognizant of the potential outcomes. Because the behaviors of individuals with ODD are considered intentional in nature, they are often characterized as displaying social maladjustment. In fact, the *DSM-5* describes that individuals with ODD rarely see themselves as angry or defiant; rather, they believe their actions to be just and appropriate as a response to unreasonable demands being placed upon them (APA, 2013).

> Individuals with ODD rarely see themselves as angry or defiant; rather, they believe their actions to be just and appropriate as a response to unreasonable demands being placed upon them (APA, 2013).

Although the exclusion of children and adolescents with ODD is deemed controversial in educational and psychological communities, some support for making the distinction between children and adolescents with Emotional Disturbance versus those with social maladjustment has been noted. In particular, a number of court cases from varying judicial levels have upheld the exclusion of students with social maladjustment from special education eligibility under the Emotional Disturbance category. These cases include the following: *A.E. vs. Independent School District #25 of Adair County, Oklahoma*; *Springer v. Fairfax County School Board*; *N.C. v. Bedford Central School District*; and *W.G. v. New York City Department of Education* (Sullivan & Sedah, 2014). Beyond the court precedents, scholars have also described the importance of distinguishing between children and adolescents with Emotional Disturbance and those with social maladjustment based on their differing needs in treatment (Theodore et al., 2004).

A second IDEA disability category that may be considered by eligibility teams for students with ODD is that of Other Health Impairment (OHI). According to IDEA, OHI is intended to address chronic medical conditions that negatively impact a student's ability to function within the academic setting and progress within its associated curricula. Within the law, a number of health conditions are specified, including ADHD, diabetes, epilepsy, heart conditions, hemophilia, lead poisoning, leukemia, nephritis, rheumatic fever, sickle cell anemia, and Tourette syndrome. However, IDEA also explains that this list is not to be considered exhaustive and other conditions should be considered (U.S. Department of Education, n.d.). Although some may contend that ODD is a chronic mental health condition and its behavioral symptoms result in academic challenges for the student, other people believe that the spirit of OHI was intended for those who are exhibiting physical health challenges that result in frequent absences or sensory issues that inhibit their educational experiences.

The nature of the diagnosis of ODD may lead to frequent behavioral infractions for students within the school setting given its basis in rule-breaking and defiance toward authority figures (APA, 2013). In school settings, these types of behaviors often result in punishments that may include removal from the academic setting through placement in alternative settings and/or out-of-school suspensions, particularly for students with chronic emotional and behavioral challenges. Achilles et al. (2007) found that students with disabilities founded in emotional and behavioral concerns receive greater numbers of office referrals resulting in punishments involving removal from the classroom than students with other disabilities. These punishments continue with relative frequency in school settings despite evidence of racial disparity in their application and the lack of evidence supporting their effectiveness (Hess et al., 2014; Losen & Gillespie, 2012; Losen & Martinez, 2013; Skiba et al., 2002, 2011). Powers et al. (2016) found that students who are relegated to restrictive educational placements are more likely to be African American males from low socioeconomic backgrounds. Out-of-school suspensions result in a lack of access to learning experiences and greater educational gaps that often exacerbate conduct concerns, and alternative education placements increase the likelihood of continuing disruptive behavior, disengagement with school, and eventual school withdrawal. According to Hess et al. (2014), the risks associated with removal from the educational environment are even greater for students from diverse backgrounds whose exclusion may lead to "academic failure, social alienation, and future economic challenges" (p. 322).

When students are found to be eligible for special education services under IDEA, the federal legislation also offers some protections against the potential harmful effects of removing a child or adolescent with ODD from the school setting. IDEA mandates that students with disabilities must be able to access the services outlined in their Individual Education Program (IEP) and cannot be removed from those supports for more than 10 (consecutive or nonconsecutive) school days. If the school administration is seeking removal beyond the 10-day mark, then this represents a change of placement. The school must convene a manifestation determination meeting to examine whether the child's IEP was being implemented appropriately and whether the most recent behavioral infraction was a manifestation of the child's disability. If the behavior resulted from the symptoms of the disability (as may be probable in the case of a child or adolescent with ODD), then the student cannot be punished for that infraction (U.S. Department of Education, n.d.).

Section 504

Beyond the mandates of IDEA, another federal law offers the opportunity for students with ODD to access additional services and supports to accommodate their unique educational needs. Section 504 of the Rehabilitation Act of 1973 provides civil rights protections to individuals with disabilities in that they may not be discriminated against on the basis of their disability. Any institution that receives federal funding (including public schools) is subject to the application of Section 504. The criterion for Section 504 eligibility denotes that the individual has (or is suspected to have) a disability that inhibits performance of a major life function such as caring for oneself, performing manual tasks, walking, hearing, seeing, speaking, breathing, learning, and working (Office of Civil Rights, n.d.). However, it is crucial to note that the diagnosis alone is not sufficient for eligibility. A multidisciplinary team must conduct a comprehensive evaluation to determine whether the disability is, in fact, a detriment to a major life function for the child or adolescent in the school setting and with its associated expectations. In the case of students with ODD, it is possible that the symptoms of their disability (including rule noncompliance and defiance of authority figures) would disrupt their ability to learn and function in the academic classroom, thus making the case for Section 504 eligibility.

CULTURAL ISSUES RELATED TO OPPOSITIONAL DEFIANT DISORDER IN YOUTH

Risk Factors for Oppositional Defiant Disorder

Researchers have found that the development of ODD symptoms is also related to a number of familial variables. Early family experiences seem to be particularly related to future diagnoses of ODD in children and adolescents (Harvey et al., 2011). Specifically, children and adolescents who have experienced punitive parenting practices are more likely to develop ODD, as are children who have mothers with their own issues internalizing symptoms (Ezpeleta et al., 2019; Lavigne et al., 2013; Romano et al., 2005; Tung & Lee, 2014; Wakschlag & Keenan, 2001). Harvey et al. (2011) found that 3-year-old children with ODD symptoms were more likely to exhibit greater symptoms at 6 years old when their mothers had symptoms of depression and when they were parented with overly reactive responses from their parents.

These familial issues are often a result of and/or exacerbated by issues of poverty, and low socioeconomic status has also been related to the development of ODD and other behavioral concerns in children (Harvey et al., 2011). The issues connected to poverty may include exposure to domestic violence, looser parental supervision, and poor peer and adult models (Lahey et al., 2000). Wakschlag and Keenan (2001) also point to high parental stress, harsh discipline, maternal smoking during pregnancy, and viewing criminal acts as related to ODD. Research supports a link between the marital instability of parents and ODD in their offspring (Gathright & Tyler, 2014). Fathers with substance abuse issues are more likely to have children with ODD, but the link is merely through correlational research and causality has not been established. Finally, a relationship has been established between paternal antisocial behaviors and children with ODD (Frick et al., 1992).

With regard to familial issues, some researchers posit that boys are more likely to be exposed to adverse family situations than girls (Lahey et al., 2006; Moffitt & Caspi, 2001), but other empirical studies suggest that girls may be more influenced by challenging family circumstances when they are exposed (Sanson & Prior, 1999). Nonetheless, environmental variables related to the family along with certain genetic influences have been found to be powerful predictors in the development of ODD in children and adolescents. In fact, researchers have demonstrated that 67% of the variance in the development of symptoms (and eventual diagnosis) of ODD is accounted for by the combination of familial environment and biological factors (Burt et al., 2001; Cronk et al., 2002).

In relation to personality factors, Ezpeleta et al. (2019) found that children who exhibit early issues controlling their negative emotions and an overall struggle with emotional regulation are susceptible to the development of ODD. Sanson and Prior (1999) explain that negativism and issues with temperament can often be revealed as early as infancy, and other researchers theorize that children who are difficult to parent at the earliest stages may lead to the inconsistent and harsh parenting associated with ODD (Alvarez & Ollendick, 2003; Rey & Walter 1999). In addition, it is suggested that boys may be more prone to a temperament-based etiological pathway to ODD than girls (Sanson & Prior, 1999).

Although evidence indicates that there are relationships between a variety of factors and the development of ODD, a single clear pathway has not been established over time despite a multitude of research studies. However, McKinney and Renk (2007) attempted to consolidate the research into a theory for the development of ODD that provides for multiple pathways with regard to etiology. Their theory is referred to as an *interactional–developmental–etiological approach* whereby the associated genetic, environmental, and dispositional variables and their interaction through the developmental process may proceed along multiple pathways yielding disruptive behavior disorders.

Although the research has revealed risk factors that are associated with the development of ODD symptoms in children and adolescents, some encouraging protective factors have also been noted. Gathright and Tyler (2014) have explained that early identification, effective treatment strategies, the absence of a comorbid ADHD diagnosis, and a negative family history of disruptive behavior disorders may be associated with or promote better outcomes for youths with ODD. In addition, Lanza and Drabick (2011) found that families who maintain structured routines within their homes foster more positive adjustment for children with ODD. Structured routines may include things such as clear expectations, consistent rules and enforcement, and family schedules for meals and bedtime.

> Gathright and Tyler (2014) have explained that early identification, effective treatment strategies, the absence of a comorbid ADHD diagnosis, and a negative family history of disruptive behavior disorders may be associated with or promote better outcomes for youths with ODD.

Cultural Considerations

Although some research suggests ethnicity as a risk factor for the development of ODD among children and adolescents, a more culturally sensitive interpretation notes that it is a risk factor only as it relates to other complicating variables such as low socioeconomic status (McKinney & Renk, 2007). Communities with higher concentrations of ethnic minorities also tend to have higher levels of poverty and a greater concentration of children who exhibit physically aggressive behaviors (Romano et al., 2005). Thus, it is likely that the argument for the presence of challenging environmental conditions outweighs the correlation of ethnicity in the development of ODD symptomatology (McKinney & Renk, 2007).

In addition, clinicians should be aware of and sensitive to their own potential bias in the provision of any diagnosis, but research supports that they may need to be especially aware of cultural prejudice when considering ODD. In 2002, Day conducted a study to examine the impact of race on ODD diagnoses. He created vignettes of a child exhibiting symptoms of ODD; however, the child in the vignette was described as either Black, White, or the race was not specified. The vignettes were sent to clinicians who regularly perform diagnostic work. They were asked to provide a diagnosis for the hypothetical child and to rate their confidence in their own diagnosis. Day found that when the vignette indicated that a child was Black, the clinician applied more diagnoses and rated their confidence in their diagnoses as higher than when the hypothetical child was described as White or when the race was not noted (Day, 2002). Consistent with these results, Heflinger and Humphreys (2008) found that minority children were 38% more likely to receive an ODD diagnosis than their White peers, and they were also more likely to be diagnosed with ODD at younger ages than White children. Thus, it is imperative that clinicians examine their practices for signs of implicit bias and actively pursue improvement in their cultural competency.

IMPACT OF OPPOSITIONAL DEFIANT DISORDER ON SOCIAL–EMOTIONAL AND BEHAVIORAL FUNCTIONING IN SCHOOL AND HOME ENVIRONMENTS

Social–Emotional and Behavioral Functioning in School

Children and adolescents with ODD frequently engage in behaviors that are interpreted as challenging in the school setting. The nature of their disorder is such that defiance and rule breaking are common occurrences. According to Lahey et al. (2000), at younger ages, children with ODD exhibit higher levels of oppositional behavior, whereas in later childhood they tend to display more acts of aggression. Property destruction is more prevalent in adolescence. In the classroom, students with ODD may also present with low self-esteem and low frustration tolerance in comparison to typically developing peers (Cederna-Meko et al., 2014). The significance of the behaviors often strains the relationships between the student with ODD and their teachers and peers (Burke, Rowe, et al., 2014).

According to Lahey et al. (2000), at younger ages, children with ODD exhibit higher levels of oppositional behavior, whereas in later childhood they tend to display more acts of aggression.

Some have even suggested that the social skills deficits of children and adolescents with behavioral issues should be the primary concern within the school setting (Gresham, 2002). Mathys et al. (2012) posit that youth with ODD are frequently impaired in their social learning processes. To be specific, they note that neurobiological research supports that children and adolescents with ODD have difficulty learning appropriate behavior and inhibiting their own inappropriate behavior because of their inability to comprehend the relationship between their behaviors and potential positive or negative outcomes. These issues are then exacerbated by their struggles with attention, impulsivity, and overall problem-solving (Mathys et al., 2012). Difficulty with peer relationships and even rejection by peers are common social issues for children and adolescents with ODD (Burke, Rowe, et al., 2014; Munkvold et al., 2011; Pardini & Fite, 2010), and these concerns often result from the socially aggressive and bullying behaviors of the child or adolescent with ODD (Fite et al., 2014).

A solid body of research indicates that ODD may have two distinct symptom dimensions (Burke, Boylan, et al., 2014; Evans et al., 2016; Lavigne et al., 2015; Rowe et al., 2010). One dimension relates to those children and adolescents who express more irritability in their symptom expression, and the other dimension is indicative of youths who display greater levels of defiance. Whether displaying irritability or defiance, teacher ratings of children with ODD reflect more incidents of physical aggression, relational aggression, and peer rejection than their typically developing peers (Evans et al., 2016). Those children and adolescents with ODD whose symptoms include higher levels of irritability are the most likely to experience difficulty in their peer relationships (Stringaris & Goodman, 2009) and a tendency toward anxiety (Stringaris & Goodman, 2009; Whelan et al., 2013), depression, and reactive aggression (Evans et al., 2016). In contrast, those students with ODD who exhibit more defiance tend to also develop further conduct concerns, including proactive aggression (2016). Other findings also indicate that relationship difficulties with peers or teachers (as marked by defiance) are associated with subsequent ODD symptoms (de Moura & Burns, 2010; Li et al., 2018). Thus, both types of symptoms (irritability and defiance) may present significant challenges for the child, the teacher, and their peers with respect to school-based functioning, and Evans et al. (2016) proposes that the differing dimensions (irritable versus defiant) lend themselves to differing intervention pathways as well. They suggest that children and adolescents who primarily demonstrate irritability may benefit from interventions focused on emotional control and skill building, whereas those children whose symptom manifestation typically aligns with defiance would be better helped through teacher and parent training (Evans et al., 2016). Therefore, it is important for school psychologists to understand the two distinct dimensions of ODD and apply functional analysis skills to determine the most appropriate means for effecting positive change for children and adolescents with ODD.

Social–Emotional and Behavioral Functioning at Home

Empirical research has indicated a distinction exists between those children and adolescents with ODD who primarily exhibit antisocial types of behaviors toward adults (such as their parents), as opposed to those youths whose inappropriate behaviors are directed toward siblings or peers (Taylor et al., 2006). For example, children and adolescents with ODD who display temperament concerns as infants and who demonstrate more hyperactive behaviors are more likely to direct their oppositional behaviors toward parents (Frick & Morris, 2004). The following behaviors are common in the home in conjunction with this diagnosis: having tantrums, arguing, questioning/defying rules, intentionally annoying and being annoyed by others, failing to accept responsibility for actions, expressing anger or outbursts of rage, and seeking revenge for perceived slights (American Academy of Child and Adolescent Psychiatry [AACAP], 2009; Cederna-Meko et al., 2014). Girls are more likely to lie and be uncooperative, whereas boys tend to provoke family discord (AACAP, 2009).

Given the severity of these behaviors, parents may seek to regain control of the situation through stricter or more coercive discipline measures that have been demonstrated to be counterproductive in the parenting of children and adolescents with ODD (Ezpeleta et al., 2019). Sadly, these conditions may eventually lead to child maltreatment and/or placement outside of the home (Lewis et al., 2002). When child neglect, child abuse, or severe behaviors do warrant an out-of-home placement, it has been established that children and adolescents from ethnic minority and/or lower socioeconomic status backgrounds are disproportionality represented in foster-care settings (Pecora et al., 2009). In addition, youth with disruptive behaviors are 4 times more likely to be placed in highly restrictive placements such as residential care facilities (James et al., 2006).

Although adverse familial conditions and functioning may contribute to the development of ODD, research also demonstrates that positive family functioning may serve as a protective factor for some children with ODD. Lanza and Drabick (2011) found that structured family routines may create conditions that allow for children with ODD to experience better behavioral adjustment in the school setting. They discovered that families with greater structure in their routines and predictability in consequences led to lower teacher ratings of impulsivity and ODD symptoms in the school setting among their sample of low-income, urban, predominantly African American children. In addition, when mothers are taught the skills of emotion coaching and utilize them with children, this is also noted as a protective factor for ODD. Emotion coaching involves the direct instruction of expressing one's own emotions and awareness of emotions in others (Dunsmore et al., 2013; Katz & Windecker-Nelson, 2004). Thus, the research offers important implications for the conceptualization and treatment of ODD.

Lanza and Drabick (2011) found that family routines may create conditions that allow for children with ODD to experience better behavioral adjustment in the school setting.

IMPACT OF OPPOSITIONAL DEFIANT DISORDER ON LEARNING IN THE CLASSROOM

The research regarding the effects of ODD on education remains unclear at best, and conflicting at worst, with some empirical support for a direct role of ODD in impaired academic performance and other findings indicating the existence of an indirect role that is mediated by symptoms of ADHD (Liu et al., 2017; Serra-Pinheiro et al., 2008). At least one empirical study found ODD symptoms to be related to impaired academic function even when controlling for issues like attention, hyperactivity, and impulsivity (Burke, Rowe, et al., 2014). Likewise, Rhodes et al. (2012) found specific cognitive deficits in boys with ODD. The researchers noted that boys with ODD struggled with verbal memory, spatial memory, working memory, and long-term memory tasks. However, Mayes and Calhoun (2007) did not find differences between children with ODD and their typically developing peers in learning, attention, writing, and processing-speed tasks, and other research has noted that, in regard to school failure, oppositional symptoms do not play a role when symptoms of inattention are accounted for (Serra-Pinheiro et al., 2008). Regarding their results, Liu et al. (2017) state, "ODD did not show direct influence on academic achievement but contributed to social impairment and classroom behavioral problems" (p. 879).

Although not specific to ODD, and perhaps in support of the mediating effects of inattention, hyperactivity, and impulsivity, children and adolescents with behavioral challenges have been found to have deficits in executive functioning and verbal abilities (Alvarez & Ollendick, 2003; Loeber et al., 2000), and these deficits are commonly associated with symptoms of ADHD. Executive functioning skills include attention, following directions, impulse control, and problem-solving, and empirical research has demonstrated that early issues with attention and impulse control often develop into antisocial behaviors (including criminality) at later developmental stages (Schaeffer et al., 2003). Regardless, the presence of these deficits, along with the behavioral challenges inherent in ODD, frequently yield significant classroom and school setting challenges for children and adolescents with this mental health condition, and students with ODD have been found to have lower grades and a greater likelihood of receiving special education services than their typically developing peers (Greene et al., 2002).

Leadbeater and Ames (2017) note that the irritability and defiance that are hallmarks of ODD may limit children's and adolescents' compliance and perseverance with academic tasks, thereby impairing academic achievement in the present and educational outcomes in the future. They found that ODD symptoms in adolescence were related to lower levels of educational attainment in young, adult males (Leadbeater & Ames, 2017). Thus, their results emphasize the need for early academic supports to prevent the lingering and/or compounded impacts of ODD across the life span.

IMPLICATIONS FOR SCHOOL PSYCHOLOGISTS

Assessment Role

When the educational personnel or the parent of a child or adolescent with ODD requests a school-based evaluation for special services, the school psychologist will feature prominently in that process. Whether seeking services under IDEA or Section 504, a multidisciplinary team must convene to determine what data will be needed to make an eligibility determination. That team consists of the parent, a general education teacher, a special education teacher, an administrative representative, and someone qualified to interpret assessment results. The evaluation must be completed, an eligibility decision rendered, and services implemented (if the student is found eligible) within 60 school days of receiving parent permission for the process.

The team will collect data regarding the student's past and current functioning in all areas relevant to the concern. For a student who already has a diagnosis of ODD, record reviews are critically important. The school personnel will seek further permission from the parent to gather information from any outside service providers, including physical and mental health professionals. This may also include juvenile justice records if the child or adolescent has had law enforcement involvement. Records will be evaluated from within the school setting to investigate both academic and behavioral histories. This data may relate to grades, standardized test scores, discipline referrals, and prior academic or behavioral interventions. Beyond the existing files for the child or adolescent, these data points will also be explored through interviews with the parent, teacher, and student. The school psychologist is frequently responsible for gathering some (if not all) of the aforementioned information for the evaluation.

Beyond the collection of existing data, new information is required for the assessment as well. Because a student with ODD is likely exhibiting behavior issues in the school setting, the school psychologist will conduct behavioral observations as a first step in their functional behavioral assessment to analyze the target behavior, its associated settings, and the likely cause of the behavior. If the team is considering whether the child or adolescent meets IDEA eligibility criteria for Emotional Disturbance, then these observations and analyses will represent important indicators regarding the exclusionary criteria related to social maladjustment. The school psychologist is also likely to evaluate the child's emotional and behavioral status with other measures as well. When assessing a student with ODD, it would be common to use tools that assess behavior, anxiety, depression, and self-esteem.

Educational data that measures present levels of functioning will be collected to determine the need for services and supports. The school psychologist may administer an individual cognitive assessment and also an academic achievement battery. With IDEA evaluations, the team is required to determine whether the child meets criteria as having a disability and whether the child demonstrates a need for services in order to function within the curriculum. See the "School-Based Eligibility" section for more detailed information on IDEA (Emotional Disturbance and OHI) and Section 504 criteria. If a child is found to qualify for support under the criteria of either federal law, then a plan is developed and enacted to provide any and all necessary educational services to assist the child or adolescent with their school-based progress.

Outside of the individual assessment process, the school psychologist should promote other screening/assessment processes as well. The school psychologist should be a leader in assisting with universal screenings to identify students who are at risk for social, emotional, and behavioral challenges like those children and adolescents with ODD. Once identified, students should be provided with targeted interventions for the prevention or remediation of issues that impair their overall school adjustment. See the section "School-Based Mental Health Interventions and Supports" for more information on Multi-Tiered Systems of Support.

Advocacy Role

Given that many of the behavioral manifestations of ODD in children and adolescents may occur in the school setting, school psychologists' combined experience in both psychological and educational realms makes them uniquely suited to advocate for the student with ODD and their professional providers outside of the school system. School psychologists may provide important observations and monitor progress related to medication management for pediatricians or psychiatrists who are working with children and adolescents with ODD. It is important to note that medication alone has not been shown to be effective in the treatment of ODD (AACAP, 2009; Woolgar & Scott, 2005). Thus, school psychologists should advocate for the provision of additional psychoeducational and therapeutic interventions (either inside the school environment or external to that setting) to improve the outcomes for students with ODD.

> School psychologists may provide important observations and monitor progress related to medication management for pediatricians or psychiatrists who are working with children and adolescents with ODD.

Consultation Role

Parent-Management Training has been identified by the AACAP and others as one of the most effective treatments for children and adolescents with ODD (AACAP, 2009; MacKenzie, 2007). Although it would likely be most beneficial for families to seek this intervention through trained, community-based practitioners, some may be hesitant to do so due to resource constraints, including limits to both time and money. Thus, school psychologists may be in a position to provide consultation regarding parenting strategies to help with familial adjustment and more positive functioning for the child or adolescent with ODD. School psychologists can help parents to understand the importance of relying on positive parenting practices and the ineffective/counterproductive results caused by harsh and punitive discipline. Parents can also be trained to be consistent in their expectations and responses with regard to their child's behavior. The implementation of these simple strategies may improve parenting effectiveness, familial stability, and child compliance. In addition, Markward and Bride (2001) indicate that it is appropriate for this type of family-centered practice to originate in the school setting.

Aside from parent consultation, school psychologists are uniquely suited through their training and experience to offer consultation services for teachers regarding students with ODD in their classrooms. These students likely display behavioral concerns in the academic setting, and those issues may coexist with and/or create challenges with educational progress as well. School psychologists are trained to offer objective guidance, analysis, and assistance with the development, implementation, and measurement of behavioral and academic interventions. They apply their psychological background to the school environment in order to effect positive change for students (and their teachers) through the use of targeted, evidenced-based interventions. This may also include consultation with administrators to determine appropriate natural consequences rather than exclusionary practices in the event of disciplinary infractions.

Counseling/Therapy Role

School psychologists are experienced providers of counseling and therapy for students in the educational environment. Children and adolescents who are diagnosed with ODD often need these services to develop more appropriate coping strategies to adjust across many domains of functioning. Cognitive behavioral therapy and social skills training are easily adapted to the school setting and have been shown to be effective therapeutic interventions for children and adolescents with ODD (Battagliese et al., 2015). The provision of these services by school psychologists expands needed mental health treatments while also easing financial and logistical burdens for families. Although the hope is that interventions such as these build skills to prevent escalation of behaviors, school psychologists may also be called upon to provide crisis-intervention services if the behaviors or statements of children and adolescents with ODD create (or imply) safety threats for themselves or others. School psychologists are frequently the most experienced professionals within schools to navigate the crisis and the critical follow-up procedures.

EDUCATIONAL SUPPORTS

According to Harrison et al. (2013), both IDEA and the empirical literature have failed to provide sufficient guidance on the accommodations needed for children and adolescents whose behavioral challenges serve as an impediment to their academic attainment in the classroom. Therefore, they conducted an extensive review of classroom accommodations for students with behavioral concerns to determine effectiveness across methodologies and samples. Although not specific to ODD, their review established that a number of educational supports show promise for improving the classroom adjustment for children and adolescents whose ODD symptoms of noncompliance and defiance are manifested in classroom settings.

One accommodation that demonstrates promise for targeting oppositional types of behavior was providing choices in the classroom setting. With this simple strategy, teachers provide the student with a list of task options on which to work. The student chooses the option that they are willing to complete, thereby producing compliance, engagement, and, potentially, academic progress. Harrison et al. (2013) found that offering choices not only reduced problematic behaviors (with often large effect sizes) but subsequently increased work completion and academic accuracy on classroom assignments beyond conditions where choices were not provided. Thus, providing choices for academic or nonacademic classroom tasks is a simple strategy that allows the educator to control the parameters of acceptable choices while also promoting desirable outcomes for the student.

A second classroom strategy explored across empirical studies by Harrison et al. (2013) involved adding elements of interest to the student to the academic practice assignments like worksheets. Including simple drawings, cartoons, or pictures to the sheets that piqued student interest produced beneficial effects when working with children who frequently create classroom disruption. Providing elements of interest to the assignment yielded both decreases in noncompliant behavior and increases in compliant behavior across multiple empirical studies. Therefore, the classroom experiences for both students and teachers may be enhanced through the use of this strategy.

Although evidence of their effectiveness may be less clear than with the aforementioned strategies, other accommodations were also examined and show promise as educational supports for students demonstrating disruptive behaviors like those often exhibited by children and adolescents with ODD. Some basic supportive conditions for positive student engagement in the classroom include shortening assignment length to facilitate on-task behavior and providing greater opportunities to respond during instruction (Harrison et al., 2013). Finally, given the variety of memory deficits associated with ODD in their findings, Rhoades et al. (2012) recommend the use of written notes and reminders to facilitate the performance of classroom tasks and expectations. These effective classroom strategies are likely already familiar to teachers, are simple to implement, and result in more positive outcomes.

> Some basic supportive conditions for positive student engagement in the classroom include shortening assignment length to facilitate on-task behavior and providing greater opportunities to respond during instruction (Harrison et al., 2013).

Beyond these classroom practices, the interactional style of the teacher can be important in working with students with ODD. Danforth (2016) highlights the importance of tone of voice. It is particularly important for educators to avoid yelling or using sarcasm, which often serve to exacerbate tense situations and may even reinforce the defiance of children and adolescents with ODD. Rather, teachers and other authority figures in the school should use a neutral tone of voice when providing instructions and rely on firm but steady tones when issuing necessary reprimands. In times of praise or encouragement, light and cheerful tones of voice are more likely to elicit the desired response from the student (Danforth, 2016).

SCHOOL-BASED MENTAL HEALTH INTERVENTIONS AND SUPPORTS

The AACAP (2009) has described its perspective on the most effective treatments for ODD by age. It indicates that treatment for preschoolers should focus primarily on parent-management training and education regarding the diagnosis. For children, school-based interventions combined with parent training and individual therapy have the greatest potential for positive change, and for adolescents, AACAP advocates a combination of individual therapy and parent-management training (AACAP, 2009). With regard to parent training, research indicates that children are more amenable to treatment during the ages of 3 to 8 than later in childhood or adolescence (Dishion & Patterson, 1992). Thus, to yield more successful outcomes, early intervention is critical.

The individual therapeutic approach often touted as the most successful option for children and adolescents with disruptive behavior disorders is cognitive behavioral therapy, which may focus on problem-solving and anger management (Battagliese et al., 2015). The research even supports its adapted use with very young children with ODD (Calub et al., 2021). Cognitive behavioral therapy techniques include techniques like relaxation, role playing, journaling, and cognitive restructuring to assist the child in reformulating unhelpful thoughts. School psychologists are commonly trained in these therapeutic interventions and can positively impact the lives of students with ODD through the provision of services in the school setting while also minimizing the strain on familial resources that may be experienced with external treatment for children and adolescents whose symptoms of ODD necessitate intervention.

Although cognitive behavioral therapy has shown benefits for children and adolescents with ODD, those treatments are based on social learning theory. Mathys et al. (2012) suggest that these treatments may be limited in their effectiveness with students with ODD for this reason. Their theory suggests that neurobiological impairments in youths with ODD cause challenges in social information processing related to potential positive and negative outcomes resulting from their behaviors. They believe that the outcomes from cognitive behavioral interventions could be improved through individualized assessment of each child's or adolescent's social learning capabilities. To be specific, therapists (like school psychologists) should conduct standardized behavioral observations of the youth's response to reward and punishment, evaluate their executive functions, and interview parents and teachers about these skills in order to tailor any interventions for the strengths and weaknesses of that particular student. Standard elements of cognitive behavioral therapy can be easily adapted to maximize the probability of positive outcomes (Mathys et al., 2012).

Perhaps due to issues with social learning, another intervention with an established base for realistic success for children and adolescents with behavioral concerns in the school setting is social skills training. Given that students with ODD struggle with social learning and often also experience challenges with peer relations, social skills training may be effective in building a repertoire of skills that promote more successful interactions and relationships. Empirical research supports that children with ODD may experience improved social competence, feelings of well-being, and ability to identify their own emotions after social skills training interventions (Behan & Carr, 2000; Goertz-Dorten et al., 2019; Gresham et al., 2004; Zabihi Hesari et al., 2019). Gresham et al. (2004) conducted a grand meta-analysis of five other meta-analyses of social skills training interventions and found that across all of the included empirical studies, 65% of intervention participants showed improvement in their social skills after treatment. Social skills training often uses a behavioral approach to attempt to build, maintain, and generalize social skills across settings in a way that also inhibits problematic behaviors from occurring. According to Frey et al. (2014), social skills instruction is most effective when it involves modeling of the necessary skills, practice of the skills, feedback and reinforcement of the skills, and review. School psychologists who implement these interventions in the school setting may do so through the use of any of a number of published programs or by simply following the aforementioned steps in an individualized and goal-directed manner for the child or adolescent with ODD.

> According to Frey et al. (2014), social skills instruction is most effective when it involves modeling of the necessary skills, practice of the skills, feedback and reinforcement of the skills, and review.

Beyond individually based counseling and therapy interventions, Multi-Tiered Systems of Support (MTSS) in schools have shown promise in promoting positive behaviors for children and adolescents (similar to students with ODD) who engage in frequent disruptions and rule infractions in that setting. MTSS deliver an array of interventions of increasing intensity and specificity to students based on their level of need. Hess et al. (2014) also notes that the use of these supports may also help to address the disproportionality of racial and ethnic minority students receiving punishments that involve exclusion from the classroom while simultaneously improving behavioral outcomes for many students. Hess et al. (2014) specifically recommends the implementation of three steps to ensure cultural sensitivity in the process. These steps include parsing relevant behavioral data across various student groups, intentionally addressing cultural variables in problem-identification and problem-analysis phases of intervention development, and choosing interventions and supports with demonstrated effectiveness for diverse populations.

According to Stoiber (2014), MTSS have a goal of "optimizing schooling outcomes for all students" (p. 45). The MTSS tenets are especially beneficial for the subset of students in need of specialized attention to progress in a similar manner as their typically developing peers. MTSS generally focus on three levels (though can range from two to four) for prevention and intervention when applied to behavioral concerns. Tier 1 encompasses the general population of students (80%–90% of the student body) who have not been identified as in need of special support to participate in the school environment and to progress in the curriculum as expected. Behavioral expectations are established and implemented consistently across the school setting, including universal programming to facilitate positive behavioral outcomes like social–emotional learning programs and/or school-wide positive behavioral intervention systems that provide reinforcement for the display of appropriate behaviors. Tier 2 features targeted interventions and supports for smaller groups of students who need more focused attention. The interventions supplement or enhance those basic structures in place for Tier 1. Tier 2 must also incorporate progress monitoring to determine the effectiveness of interventions over time for students who are receiving supports at this level. Implementation at this level of intervention normally requires 6 to 12 weeks of effort prior to decision-making regarding effectiveness. If students continue to struggle with meeting expectations after Tier 2 interventions, then school-based teams may move the child or adolescent to Tier 3 for an even more intensive level of intervention and supports that are normally delivered in very small group or individual formats. Approximately 1% to 5% of students will need this level of intervention. In addition to the increasing intensity of intervention offered at Tier 3, these supports tend to be longer in duration and require even more focused progress monitoring (Stoiber, 2014). For a more detailed discussion of MTSS implementation, see Stoiber (2014).

CASE STUDY 6.1 CALLIOPE: CASE OF A WHITE GIRL WITH OPPOSITIONAL DEFIANT DISORDER

Background

Calliope is 8 years old and lives with a foster family in a rural Midwestern state. Calliope was born to a single teen mother. At the time of her birth, Calliope's mother, Tressa, was living at home with her biological parents. Tressa's father was unemployed, and her mother worked a low-wage job as a convenience store clerk. The mother's wages were just enough to pay rent and utilities. The family relied on government assistance and local charities for food, but this often ran short at the end of the month. Prior to Calliope's birth, Tressa ate free daily breakfast and lunch at her public high school but would frequently leave school after she had eaten lunch. She would go home to go back to bed. Tressa had been treated for depression as a young child, and her symptoms of depression were managed through community-based counseling and antidepressants prescribed through a psychiatrist working at that facility. However, the clinic was 30 miles from her small community, and Tressa's family had to stop her treatment when they could no longer afford the travel to and from appointments. When Tressa's father complained about her being at home during the day, she started going to a friend's home instead of her own when she would leave school. Tressa and her friend's older brother started a relationship, and she became pregnant just as he was moving to Arkansas to live with an elderly aunt.

(continued)

CASE STUDY 6.1 CALLIOPE: CASE OF A WHITE GIRL WITH OPPOSITIONAL DEFIANT DISORDER (continued)

Originally, Tressa's family had planned for Calliope to stay in the home with her biological grandfather while Tressa finished her last 2 years of high school. When Calliope was born, she was an extremely fussy baby. She was irritable and difficult to soothe even as an infant. Calliope's needs were too demanding for her grandfather, and Tressa withdrew from school to stay home with her. However, it was difficult for Tressa's mother's income to meet the needs of the family. Tressa decided to move into a low-rent, weekly motel room with two friends and try to find a job. She worked a series of minimum-wage jobs and left Calliope in the care of a variety of others living in the motel. However, by toddlerhood, it became difficult for Tressa to find a babysitter for Calliope due to her challenging behavior. She exhibited extreme tantrums that would include hours of screaming and physically aggressive acts when she was corrected or disciplined in any form. Caregivers attempted to avoid confrontations by giving in to her, but she would continue to engage in more extreme behaviors until they had to respond due to safety issues, then she would often leave bruises and marks on their bodies from hitting, biting, and scratching in response. When she had exhausted all of her childcare resources, Tressa enrolled Calliope into a free daycare program operated by a local cooperative of charitable and religious organizations. In that setting, Calliope demonstrated noncompliance with virtually all expectations, was defiant with the volunteer caregivers, and injured two staff members and two children in her first week of the program. When Tressa was called to pick Calliope up early on each of her first 5 days, she decided to quit her job and stay home with Calliope until she could start prekindergarten in 8 months' time. The new arrangement would cause even greater strain on her lean finances, but Tressa believed that a firmer hand in discipline would help to correct Calliope's problematic behaviors. Tressa started spanking Calliope when she would engage in physical aggression. This only served to escalate Calliope's behaviors. Tressa then resorted to physical punishment for smaller transgressions, but (not surprising), Calliope's behaviors continued. By the time that Calliope entered school, she was exhibiting significant behaviors on a near-daily basis at home and at school. In addition to her defiance and physical aggression, Calliope would engage in vengeful behavior in response to perceived slights. For example, when her teacher removed her from the library center for throwing books at peers, Calliope smashed the family portrait on the teacher's desk. And, when a peer took the yellow marker that Calliope wanted, she shoved him down and put glue in his hair. After these incidents, Tressa sought help from her pediatrician, who diagnosed Calliope with ODD. He recommended counseling for her, but Tressa was unable to manage the drive to the out-of-town clinic. Calliope's behavior continued despite school personnel attempting to manage her behavior through a hierarchy of consequences. Tressa's frustrations with Calliope's behavior and her own stress grew to the point that she resorted to even harsher physical punishments. By the time Calliope reached her eighth birthday, social services had become involved after school personnel reported significant bruising on Calliope's body from severe physical punishment. Calliope was placed in a therapeutic foster-care home, and Tressa started taking steps toward family reintegration after a misdemeanor child abuse conviction.

Discussion

Calliope's early history demonstrates a number of risk factors for ODD. She was born to a mother with a history of depression. She was also difficult to soothe as an infant and demonstrated behavioral challenges like defiance and physical aggression as a very young child. The frequency and intensity of her behaviors are consistent with ODD. In response to the behavioral issues, her mother attempted harsher forms of discipline, which are often counterproductive to management of ODD symptoms.

Within the school setting, rather than resorting to punishment-oriented strategies, the school should seek the input and services of the school psychologist. The school psychologist would first begin the functional behavioral assessment process to determine the antecedents and/or setting events that precipitate Calliope's behaviors and the consequences that follow the behavior and serve to maintain it. The process is undertaken to determine the function

(continued)

CASE STUDY 6.1 CALLIOPE: CASE OF A WHITE GIRL WITH OPPOSITIONAL DEFIANT DISORDER (continued)

of the behavior and answer the question of why it is occurring. This knowledge of the function will be the basis for a behavioral intervention plan that positively reinforces Calliope for socially appropriate behaviors that are inconsistent with the display of the problematic behavior. When the behavior plan is in place, the school psychologist may also find it helpful to begin individual counseling with Calliope as well. Both cognitive behavioral therapy and social skills training have been found to be effective with students with ODD. Calliope may benefit from these interventions geared toward the development of better adjustment and prosocial behaviors. Given Tressa's legal situation, it is likely that her reintegration plan includes parent-training components, but the school psychologist could be available for future support with the development of parenting strategies or advocacy for the family. Finally, in light of the school's initial, reactive approach with Calliope, the school psychologist should help the staff with the development of a more proactive approach for the prevention and remediation of behavioral issues beyond Calliope's situation. The school psychologist should lay the groundwork for MTSS at the building level. The school psychologist can consult with the personnel to enact universal screening procedures and a system of tiered interventions to support students in the development of and engagement in prosocial behaviors in the school setting. These systems of support have demonstrated effectiveness across the spectrum of students within educational environments.

SUMMARY POINTS

- In order to apply a *DSM-5* diagnosis of ODD, a child or adolescent must exhibit at least four symptoms from the first criterion.
- With regard to etiology, the school psychologist should remember that familial and biological factors contribute significantly to the development of ODD.
- Structured family routines and emotional coaching may serve as protective factors in the home for children and adolescents with ODD.
- Parent-management training is one of the most effective intervention strategies for children and adolescents with ODD.
- School psychologists can engage in many roles and functions to support the needs of students with ODD, including assessment, advocacy, consultation, and counseling and/or therapy.
- Social skills training has demonstrated effectiveness in the treatment of children and adolescents with ODD.

TEST YOUR KNOWLEDGE

1. What is the severity specifier for a *DSM-5* diagnosis of ODD based on?
   a. Number of symptoms
   b. Number of settings for symptoms
   c. Age of onset
   d. Etiology

2. A student with ODD automatically meets criteria for Emotional Disturbance under IDEA.
   a. True
   b. False

3. Research does not support a genetic component for ODD.
   a. True
   b. False

4. Which of the following is an empirically supported treatment for ODD?
   a. Parent-management training
   b. Out-of-school suspension
   c. Special education services
   d. Alternative education placements

5. ODD symptoms most often begin in adolescence.
   a. True
   b. False

Answers: (1) b, (2) b, (3) b, (4) a, (5) b.

DISCUSSION QUESTIONS

1. Describe the *DSM-5* diagnostic criteria for ODD.
2. Explain why children and adolescents with ODD may not meet IDEA criteria for Emotional Disturbance.
3. List the familial factors that may contribute to the development of ODD.
4. Explain the school psychologist's advocacy role in working with children with ODD.
5. Detail one evidenced-based social–emotional intervention for students with ODD.

CHAPTER RESOURCES

American Academy of Child and Adolescent Psychiatry *ODD: A Guide for Families*: www.aacap.org/App_Themes/AACAP/docs/resource_centers/odd/odd_resource_center_odd_guide.pdf

American Academy of Child and Adolescent Psychiatry *Oppositional Defiant Disorder*: www.aacap.org/AACAP/Families_and_Youth/Facts_for_Families/FFF-Guide/Children-With-Oppositional-Defiant-Disorder-072.aspx

American Academy of Child and Adolescent Psychiatry *Oppositional Defiant Disorder Resource Center*: www.aacap.org/AACAP/Families_and_Youth/Resource_Centers/Oppositional_Defiant_Disorder_Resource_Center/Home.aspx

Cedars-Sinai *Oppositional Defiant Disorder in Children*: www.cedars-sinai.org/health-library/diseases-and-conditions---pediatrics/o/oppositional-defiant-disorder-odd-in-children.html

Centers for Disease Control and Prevention *Behavior or Conduct Problems in Children*: www.cdc.gov/childrensmentalhealth/behavior.html

Intervention Central *School-Wide Strategies for Managing Defiance/Non-Compliance*: www.interventioncentral.org/behavioral-interventions/challenging-students/school-wide-strategies-managing-defiance-non-complianc

Mayo Clinic *Oppositional Defiant Disorder*: www.mayoclinic.org/diseases-conditions/oppositional-defiant-disorder/diagnosis-treatment/drc-20375837

National Federation of Families *Oppositional Defiant Disorder Resources:* www.ffcmh.org/resources-odd

KEY REFERENCES

Only key references appear in the print edition. The full reference list appears in the digital product on Springer Publishing Connect: connect.springerpub.com/content/book/978-0-8261-3587-2/part/part03/chapter/ch06

American Psychiatric Association. (2013). *Diagnostic and statistical manual of mental disorders* (5th ed.). https://doi.org/10.1176/appi.books.9780890425596

Burke, J. D., Rowe, R., & Boylan, K. (2014). Functional outcomes of child and adolescent oppositional defiant disorder symptoms in young adult men. *Journal of Child Psychology and Psychiatry, 55*, 264–272. https://doi.org/10.1111/jcpp.12150

Evans, S. C., Pederson, C. A., Fite, P. J., Blossom, J. B., & Cooley, J. L. (2016). Teacher-reported irritable and defiant dimensions of oppositional defiant disorder: Social, behavioral, and academic correlates. *School Mental Health, 8*, 292–304. https://doi.org/10.1007/s12310-015-9163-y

Ezpeleta, L., Granero, R., de la Osa, N., Penelo, E., & Domenech, J. M. (2012). Dimensions of oppositional defiant disorder in 3-year-old preschoolers. *Journal of Child Psychology and Psychiatry, 53*(11), 1128–1138. https://doi.org/10.1111/j.1469-7610.2012.02545.x

Gathright, M. M., & Tyler, L. H. (2014). *Disruptive behavior in children and adolescents.* University of Arkansas for Medical Sciences Psychiatric Research Institute.

Harrison, J. R., Bunford, N., Evans, S. W., & Sarno Owens, J. (2013). Educational accommodations for students with behavioral challenges: A systematic review of the literature. *Review of Educational Research, 83*(4), 551–597. https://doi.org/10.3102/0034654313497517

Stoiber, K. C. (2014). A comprehensive framework for multitiered systems of support in school psychology. In P. L. Harrison & A. Thomas (Eds.), *Best practices in school psychology: Student-level services.* National Association of School Psychologists.

Sullivan, A. L., & Sadeh, S. S. (2014). Differentiating social maladjustment from emotional disturbance: An analysis of case law. *School Psychology Review, 43*(4), 450–471. https://doi.org/10.1080/02796015.2014.12087415

U.S. Department of Education. (n.d.). *Individuals with Disabilities Education Improvement Act.* https://sites.ed.gov/idea

CHAPTER 7

Intermittent Explosive Disorder

LEARNING OBJECTIVES

- Summarize the diagnostic features for the *Diagnostic and Statistical Manual of Mental Disorders* (5th ed.; *DSM-5*; American Psychiatric Association [APA], 2013) diagnosis of Intermittent Explosive Disorder (IED).
- Highlight the risk factors for IED in children and adolescents.
- Describe common challenges within the school and home for children and adolescents with IED.
- Understand the educational supports needed for students with IED to progress in the classroom.
- Identify effective interventions for the adjustment and mental health of students with IED.

INTRODUCTION

Intermittent Explosive Disorder (IED) is classified along with similar mental health conditions under the category of Disruptive, Impulse-Control, and Conduct Disorders by the *Diagnostic and Statistical Manual of Mental Disorders*, Fifth Edition (*DSM-5*; American Psychiatric Association [APA], 2013). These disorders share features related to controlling one's emotions and behaviors as they relate to others. Individuals with these disorders frequently infringe upon the rights, authority, and/or property of others. Examples of other Disruptive, Impulse-Control, and Conduct Disorders include Conduct Disorder and Oppositional Defiant Disorder (ODD).

As with any of the Disruptive, Impulse-Control, and Conduct Disorders, a clinician considering a *DSM-5* diagnosis of IED for a child or adolescent must consider that the associated symptoms may also occur in typically developing youth. Thus, symptom expression alone is not indicative of a clinical need for diagnosis. The context of the behaviors and emotional control issues is of utmost importance as to whether the nature, severity, and frequency of those challenges is of sufficient intensity to warrant diagnosis. In order to apply the diagnosis, children and adolescents should exhibit symptoms at clinical levels relative to others of similar age, gender, and cultural contexts (APA, 2013). For example, a typically developing child may ask for a new toy in the store, whine when denied repeatedly, and escalate into a crying and screaming episode in the checkout line. In contrast, a child with IED in the same circumstance may indicate that they want a new toy, and when denied initially, they might stomp on the toy, throw it at the parent, and scream profanities without apparent escalation.

DIAGNOSTIC ISSUES: *DSM-5* AND SCHOOL-BASED SERVICES

DSM-5 Diagnosis

The *DSM-5* outlines six criteria for the diagnosis of IED. The first criterion describes failure of the individual to inhibit socially inappropriate and significant aggressive behaviors. This criterion also includes two subcriteria that further define the frequency and intensity of behavioral incidents. The subcriteria are as follows: (a) the problematic behaviors may be either verbal or physical (yet nondestructive/damaging/injurious) in nature and occur at a frequency of about twice per week over a 3-month time frame, or (b) there may be three incidents of physically injurious behaviors directed toward others over a 1-year time span. The second, third, and fourth criteria elaborate upon the first criterion. The second criterion notes that the explosive behavioral outbursts are excessive or extreme as compared to the events or conditions that led to them, and the third asserts that they are neither planned nor intended for the aggressor's gain. The fourth criterion explains that the outbursts yield significant negative consequences for the individual. Those consequences could be emotional, relational, monetary, or legal. The fifth criterion for consideration in the application of the diagnosis of IED is more objective in that it states that the individual must be at least 6 years old. Finally, the sixth criterion excludes the individual from diagnosis if their behaviors are the result of another mental, physical, or substance-induced condition. This criterion further states that the behaviors under observation cannot be related to another adjustment-related condition in children and adolescents. The behavioral outbursts of the child or adolescent are obviously a key determinant in the diagnosis of IED. The *DSM-5* explains that these violent episodes typically last less than 30 minutes in duration and may seem drastically out of proportion to an observer in regard to the precipitating situation. The aggressive incidents are impulsive and often begin with few warning signs prior to initiation of the outburst (APA, 2013).

Children must be at least 6 years of age to be considered for a diagnosis of IED (APA, 2013).

Although the criteria and features for what is currently termed *IED* has roots back in the original *DSM* from 1952, the *DSM-5* criteria for IED underwent some changes from prior versions (Coccaro et al., 2014). One key change in the most current version relates to the subcriteria of the first criterion. According to Coccaro et al. (2014), the differing frequencies and time spans for the aggressive incidents are meant to distinguish between individuals whose outbursts are of high frequency and low intensity versus those that are of low frequency but high intensity. Coccaro et al. (2014) conducted the research that formed the basis for the subcriteria of IED for the *DSM-5*. The concept of significant behavioral incidents as high frequency and low intensity was previously included as an associated feature of IED in the *DSM-IV-TR* (APA, 2000). Based on empirical research, an individual with IED may display only high-frequency and low-intensity outbursts. Conversely, they may demonstrate solely low-frequency and high-intensity incidents. However, Coccaro et al. (2014) found that approximately 70% of participants with IED symptoms in a large, clinical research study engaged in both high-frequency/low-intensity and low-frequency/high-intensity episodes of aggression. Individuals with only high-frequency and low-intensity behaviors accounted for an additional 20% of their sample, and 10% of the participants only engaged in low-frequency and high-intensity behaviors. Despite the differing behavioral manifestations across their study, the authors explain that there were no other meaningful differences between these subsets of individuals with IED, and therefore, they should be considered as one under the IED diagnosis and offered similar treatments (Coccaro et al., 2014). Finally, it is important to note that the research for these subcriteria included only adult participants within their clinical sample. Thus, application to children and adolescents is an extrapolation beyond these findings despite the criterion stating that children 6 years of age and older can be diagnosed with IED.

Although IED may manifest during adulthood, it is most commonly developed within the childhood or adolescent period (APA, 2013). In the early 2000s, the National Comorbidity Survey Replication Adolescent Supplement found the average age of onset of IED to be 12 years across a sample of over 6,000 adolescents (McLaughlin et al., 2012). Despite these findings, Coccaro (2012) reports a range of average onset across multiple studies to be from 13 to 21 years of age, and Oliver et al. (2016) found an average age of onset of 10 years in their sample of Black adolescents. The average duration of symptoms associated with IED is 12 years' time (Kessler et al., 2006).

According to Coccaro (2012), a disorder consisting of impulsive aggression was included in the original *DSM* in 1952, but IED was originally believed to be rare relative to other mental health conditions. However, research studies that emerged in the mid-2000s suggested greater prevalence than had been suspected for the preceding 5 decades. This research found a weighted lifetime prevalence of 5.4% or approximately 16 million people in the United States. That figure is consistent with research by McLaughlin et al. (2012), which found lifetime prevalence to be 5.3% among adolescents. Yet, Oliver et al. (2016) indicated that prevalence among Black and Caribbean Black adolescents may be as high as 9.0% and 12.4%, respectively. Data from the World Mental Health surveys indicated that the United States has the highest lifetime prevalence among all measured nations at 7.4% (Kessler et al., 2011). Kessler et al. (2011) explained that data from the vast majority of countries notes prevalence rates at less than half of what is found in the United States. Beyond lifetime prevalence statistics, the *DSM-5* reports a 1-year prevalence of 2.7% across all age groups (APA, 2013), and McLaughlin et al. (2012) found a 1-year prevalence rate of 1.7% in a large, adolescent-only sample. Twelve-month prevalence among a sample of Black adolescents was measured at 6.7%, and a 1-year prevalence for Caribbean Black adolescents was 11.5% (Oliver et al., 2016). Prevalence data varies broadly across geographic regions with the lowest reported rates in Asia and the Middle East. It is unclear whether these differing prevalence rates represent a true difference in frequency of IED across cultures or whether the difference may be due to a measurement or reporting issue (Coccaro, 2012).

Likewise, the prevalence of IED across genders lacks clarity in the literature as well. Although some studies suggest that males outpace females in the diagnosis of IED by 2:1 (APA, 2013; Coccaro et al., 1998; Kessler et al., 2011; McElroy et al., 1998), other empirical studies supported a range from 1.4 to 2.3 males for every female diagnosed in the overall population (APA, 2013; Kessler et al., 2006; Yoshimasu & Kawakami, 2011). Among Black adolescents, Oliver et al. (2016) found males significantly more likely to be diagnosed with IED than females. However, McLaughlin et al. (2012) explained that although boys are more likely than girls to display extreme anger episodes (among juvenile samples), IED appears to occur in equal frequency among male and female children and adolescents (McLaughlin et al., 2012). Galbraith et al. (2018) suggested that boys and girls may engage in differing forms of aggression associated with their IED as well. They noted that boys are more prone to proactive aggression associated with callous and unemotional traits, whereas girls generally display reactive aggression that is linked to emotion regulation issues.

Regarding comorbidity, the *DSM-5* indicates that a number of other issues may co-occur for individuals diagnosed with IED. These include concerns with depression, anxiety, and diagnoses associated with disruptive behavior such as attention deficit hyperactivity disorder (ADHD), ODD, and conduct disorder. Research conducted with adolescents found that youths with IED were 3.5 times more likely to be diagnosed with an anxiety disorder as adolescents without IED (Galbraith et al. 2018). The *DSM-5* further notes that individuals with antisocial personality disorder and borderline personality disorder are susceptible to the development of IED symptoms and/or diagnoses (APA, 2013). Finally, clinical research supports that individuals with IED frequently have comorbid substance abuse issues as well (Coccaro et al., 1998, 2005). In fact, substance abuse and depression are 3 and 4 times more likely, respectively, to be present in individuals with IED as compared to people without IED diagnoses (Coccaro, 2012; Coccaro et al., 2005; Kessler et al., 2006; Yoshimasu & Kawakami, 2011).

> Research conducted with adolescents found that youths with IED were 3.5 times more likely to be diagnosed with an anxiety disorder as adolescents without IED (Galbraith et al., 2018).

According to Kessler et al. (2006, 2011) even when individuals eventually exhibit symptoms of multiple mental health conditions, the IED is frequently the first to manifest. McLaughlin et al. (2012) report consistent results with IED originating prior to comorbid disorders like generalized anxiety disorder (GAD), major depression, posttraumatic stress disorder, comorbid panic disorder, and substance abuse. Evidence from research by Medeiros et al. (2018) is indicative of IED development prior to comorbid major depressive disorder. Likewise, Radwan and Coccaro (2020) noted that IED diagnoses are generally applied prior to diagnoses of ODD or CD in cases in which the individual demonstrates symptoms of more than one disorder. In contrast, McLaughlin et al. (2012) found that IED is often diagnosed after phobias and separation anxiety disorder, and Radwan and Coccaro (2020) report that when IED is comorbid with ADHD, the age of onset and diagnosis of ADHD typically precedes that of IED. Despite its comorbidity with a variety of other mental health conditions, it is surmised that IED symptomatology represents a distinct disorder that is not better described by other diagnoses (Radwan & Coccaro, 2020).

When IED is comorbid with other disorders, research has supported that IED symptoms are often expressed with greater severity. Medeiros et al. (2019) found that individuals who have comorbid IED and GAD report higher levels of hostility than those individuals with IED alone. The authors contend that the combination of IED and GAD may increase the severity of aggression directed toward others. Similarly, research by Galbraith et al. (2018) on comorbid IED and anxiety disorders (including social phobia, specific phobia, panic disorder, and GAD) discovered that adolescents with both diagnoses are more likely to have issues with academic, social, and overall functioning due to their explosive outbursts than adolescents with a singular diagnosis of IED. Those adolescents with both IED and an anxiety disorder are also more likely to experience substance abuse and receive additional psychiatric diagnoses as well. Finally, in research on comorbid IED and major depressive disorder, evidence suggests that people with both diagnoses fare worse with regard to assaultive behavior, hostility, and social adjustment (Medeiros et al., 2018). Thus, the already significant symptomatology of IED appears intensified with certain comorbid diagnoses.

School-Based Eligibility

INDIVIDUALS WITH DISABILITIES EDUCATION IMPROVEMENT ACT REGULATIONS

The Individuals with Disabilities Education Improvement Act (IDEA) is a federal law that requires school systems that receive any form of government funding to provide a free and appropriate public education to students who meet criteria as having any one of the 13 disabilities outlined by the legislation. As such, some children and adolescents who are diagnosed with psychological disorders may be eligible for services under IDEA that include specialized supports designed to assist the child or adolescent in progressing in the curriculum despite their disability (U.S. Department of Education, n.d.). One disability category in which students with mental health issues are often served is that of Emotional Disturbance.

According to IDEA, the eligibility criteria for Emotional Disturbance are as follows: an inability to learn that cannot be explained by intellectual, sensory, or health factors; an inability to build or maintain satisfactory relationships with peers and teachers; inappropriate types of behavior or feelings under normal circumstances; a general pervasive mood of unhappiness or depression; and a tendency to develop physical symptoms or fears associated with personal or school problems. The child or adolescent must exhibit one or more of those criteria "over a long period of time and to a marked degree that adversely affects a child's educational performance" (U.S. Department of Education, n.d., Section 300.8 (c) (4)). Although the criteria that reference difficulty with interpersonal relationships and inappropriate behaviors would certainly be characteristic of children and adolescents with IED, IDEA further denotes that children with schizophrenia are included under its tenets, but children who exhibit social maladjustment are not considered to meet criteria under the Emotional Disturbance category. Therein lies the complication for children and adolescents with IED.

The federal law does not include an operational definition of *social maladjustment*, and many scholars in this area contend that this has led to significant inconsistency in its interpretation and application (Olympia et al., 2004; Sullivan & Sadeh, 2014). In addition to the variability in implementation, the lack of a federally based definition of *social maladjustment* has created considerable debate among parents, school personnel, legal representatives, and academicians over the past few decades. Nonetheless, the general consensus (which has typically been upheld through court cases) is that behaviors associated with social maladjustment are intentional in nature and under the control of the child or adolescent. Further, the individual engaging in the behaviors chooses the problematic behaviors despite understanding the likely consequences. In contrast, the concerns for a child or adolescent who is eligible under the category of Emotional Disturbance are primarily driven by internalizing issues that are not under the individual's conscious control (Theodore et al., 2004). Therefore, in most cases, youth with IED are not found eligible for special education services under the IDEA disability category of Emotional Disturbance unless they are exhibiting separate issues that would be associated with Emotional Disturbance.

When school personnel or parents initiate a referral for a special education evaluation under IDEA for a child or adolescent with IED, another disability category for consideration might be that of Other Health Impairment (OHI). According to the U.S. Department of Education, OHI is intended to serve students with chronic health issues that impact their ability to function and progress within the standard curriculum due to their disability (U.S. Department of Education, n.d.). Although the IDEA definition for OHI lists a number of eligible health conditions that meet criteria if determined to adversely impact the child's school performance (and IED is not one of the listed conditions), it further notes that other chronic issues may be considered as well if the condition is directly related to an impairment in functioning that impedes the student's progress. Although one could certainly argue that the aggressive outbursts associated with IED would likely inhibit progress in the school setting for the child or adolescent with this diagnosis, most educational personnel believe that the category of OHI was designed for students who struggle with physical ailments whereby the symptoms of those disorders or needs associated with those disorders create the impediment to progress in the school setting commensurate with typically developing peers. Thus, it may be rare for a school-based eligibility team to find a child or adolescent with IED who qualifies for services under this category.

SECTION 504

Although it seems rare for students with IED to be provided with special education and support services under IDEA, another piece of federal legislation may be more suited to children and adolescents who are diagnosed with this condition: Section 504 of the Rehabilitation Act of 1973. This federal civil rights legislation for individuals with disabilities applies to any entity or organization (including public schools) that receives any form of government funding. Section 504 has been commonly invoked for children and adolescents with IED, and its use in this manner has been supported through the court system.

Section 504 establishes that schools must provide the services and supports needed for a child or adolescent to appropriately function and progress in the curriculum if they have a disability or are suspected of having a disability. This determination is based on impairment in any major life function. Although the list is not exhaustive, the following activities are considered major life functions under Section 504: caring for oneself, performing manual tasks, walking, hearing, seeing, speaking, breathing, learning, and working. With regard to the types of impairments, Section 504 offers the following guidance "any physiological disease or condition, cosmetic disfigurement, or anatomical loss affecting one or more of the following body systems: neurological; musculoskeletal, special sense organs, respiratory including speech organs; cardiovascular; reproductive; digestive; genito-urinary; hemic and lymphatic; skin; and endocrine; or any mental or psychological disorder, such as mental retardation, organic brain syndrome, emotional or mental illness, and specific learning disabilities" (Office of Civil Rights, n.d., Section 104.3 (2) (i)).

A diagnosis of IED would certainly meet the impairment guidelines related to a mental or psychological disorder; however, a school-based eligibility team is charged with determining whether the disability impacts a major life function. In this case, that major life function is likely to be learning as the behavioral disruption caused by the verbal or physical aggressive outbursts would create interruptions to the teaching processes and curricular sequences. This may be especially true if the school relies on a reactive approach to discipline that uses removal from the classroom as punishment for rule infractions. If a multidisciplinary team of professionals and the child's parent deem the child to be eligible for services, then a 504 plan of accommodations and modifications will be developed to support the student's progress. For a child or adolescent with IED, this plan includes a behavioral intervention plan produced from a functional behavioral assessment process that established positive behavioral supports aligned with the variable or variables that are maintaining the socially inappropriate behavior in the school setting. Additional support services may be included in the plan to provide school-based counseling or therapeutic intervention by the school psychologist or school counselor, and if applicable, school nursing services for medication management.

CULTURAL ISSUES RELATED TO INTERMITTENT EXPLOSIVE DISORDER IN YOUTH

Risk Factors for Intermittent Explosive Disorder

A substantial body of research supports familial and genetic impact on the development of IED. One study found that 32% of individuals with IED also have a first-degree relative with the disorder (McElroy et al., 1998), and another study found increased risk for IED among families even when other mental health conditions and behavioral variables were accounted for (Coccaro, 2010). Further, two studies support that aggressive tendencies are often genetic in origin (Yeh et al., 2010). However, according to Lee et al. (2014), parenting style is also highly correlated with the development of IED. They found that aversive parenting (low in parental care and high in parental control) is found substantially more frequently in families in which a member develops IED versus families with members with other forms of psychopathology or no clinical diagnoses at all. The authors explain that, based on their results, IED may be particularly related to low parental warmth (especially from the mother). Similarly, Smeijers et al. (2018) found parental rejection (as defined by high hostility, undifferentiated rejection, and low warmth) to be associated with aggression in adult psychiatric patients. Finally, according to McLaughlin et al. (2012), the size and structure of a child's or adolescent's family is related to their probability of developing IED. Specifically, the demographic variable most closely associated with IED concerns parents residing in the home. Children and adolescents who live in homes without two parents are more likely to be diagnosed with IED. Also related to family composition, children and adolescents who have no siblings have increased duration of IED symptoms (McLaughlin et al., 2012).

Another emerging risk factor related to the development of IED is trauma. Individuals who have been victims of crime, experienced the trauma of a death of a close friend or relative, and/or contended with multiple traumatic events are at greater risk for the development of IED (Fincham et al., 2009). Nickerson et al. (2012) found that early exposure to trauma is particularly problematic with regard to IED. Childhood exposure to trauma is more highly associated with diagnoses of IED than even repeated traumatic events that occur during adulthood.

> Individuals who have been victims of crime, experienced the trauma of a death of a close friend or relative, and/or contended with multiple traumatic events are at greater risk for the development of IED (Fincham et al., 2009).

In addition, other researchers have found that one form of trauma experienced during the developmental period is uniquely predictive of IED diagnosis—that of child abuse (Fanning et al., 2014; Puhalla et al., 2020). Both Fanning et al. (2014) and Puhalla et al. (2020) have noted significantly higher incidence of child abuse in their samples among participants with IED as compared to control group respondents, and empirical research by Puhalla et al. (2020) found that the participants with IED who had experienced child abuse also reported higher levels of aggression than their control group counterparts. The history of child abuse not only predicted overall aggression, but it further differentiated participants with IED from participants with other forms of psychopathology (Puhalla et al., 2020). Among all forms of child abuse, Fanning et al. (2014) discovered physical abuse (as opposed to emotional or sexual abuse) to specifically predict IED; however, Nickerson et al. (2012) found that sexual trauma in childhood (rather than adulthood) is associated with the development of IED. Researchers in this area posit that the early abuse experiences may lead to social information processing deficits in which the child believes that the world is hostile and uses aggressive behaviors as a means of protecting themselves in situations that they perceive as threatening (Coccaro et al., 2016; Fanning et al., 2014; Puhalla et al., 2020). It has also been proposed that early traumatic experiences impede children's development of emotion regulation. This lack of emotion regulation yields explosive anger (consistent with IED), which then further serves as a detriment to interpersonal relationships throughout the life span (Cloitre et al., 2009; Coccaro et al., 2016; Zlotnick et al., 2008).

Beyond the aforementioned environmental variables, other research points to neurological distinctions that are associated with IED and the social–emotional information processing deficits. Some theorists purport that IED is primarily a disorder of emotion regulation, and research by McCloskey et al. (2016) provides some support for this notion. They found that when presented with images of angry faces, individuals with IED experienced an increased response in the amygdala of the brain. The amygdala is responsible for fight-or-flight responses. In contrast to the amygdala hyperactivity in IED participants, subjects in the McCloskey et al. (2016) study without IED displayed arousal in other brain structures that suggest distinct differences in the way individuals with

IED process emotions versus people who do not have IED symptoms. In addition, other research has discovered white matter abnormalities in the superior longitudinal fasciculus regions of the brains of adults with IED (Lee et al., 2016). White matter is brain tissue that is composed of nerve fibers and plays a role in relaying information between brain structures. The abnormalities would result in decreased connectivity to structures related to executive functions like problem-solving and impulse control that would be consistent with the behavioral patterns of expression by children and adolescents with IED. Neurological research also supports the distinction between IED and other impulse-control disorders (Dell'Osso et al., 2006).

Cultural Considerations

Beyond the prevalence rates reported for IED among various ethnic subgroups, a few researchers have sought to explore the relationship between IED and other cultural variables. For example, Ortega et al. (2008) compared IED diagnosis across Latino subgroups living in the mainland United States and explored the relationship between IED and acculturation. They found that Puerto Ricans have the greatest probability of IED diagnoses as compared to Cubans, Mexicans, and other Latinos. The authors note that this finding is consistent with other research that suggests that Puerto Ricans have higher rates of diagnosed psychopathology as compared to other groups with similar sociodemographics and that this may be due to a greater cultural acceptance of mental health issues in the Puerto Rican population (Ortega et al., 2008). Researchers suggest that although Puerto Ricans are bestowed U.S. citizenship at birth, they may actually feel higher levels of discrimination than other Latino groups (Alegria et al., 2007). With regard to acculturation, Ortega et al. (2008) noted that Latino individuals with higher levels of English proficiency and who are born within the United States have a greater likelihood of IED diagnosis. The researchers suggest that cultural issues related to social investments and religious practices may provide coping pathways for immigrants less acculturated to the United States as compared to immigrants who experience greater acculturation within the United States.

As previously noted, Oliver et al. (2016) engaged in a large research project focused on IED among Black adolescent populations. They found that Caribbean Black adolescents were significantly more likely to be diagnosed with IED than African American teens. They explain that these findings mirror other research that reports higher rates of mood and anxiety disorders among Caribbean Black males as compared to African American males. The researchers contend that more empirical work is needed in this area to determine whether Caribbean Black adolescents express their psychological distress with greater aggressive tendencies (consistent with IED diagnosis) than African American adolescents. However, despite the finding of greater prevalence of IED across the Caribbean Black youth participants, Oliver et al. (2016) found that when they do exhibit IED symptoms, African American adolescents experience more severe impairment in their functioning as compared to Caribbean Black youth. Again, more research is warranted to investigate the nature of these ethic group differences in the prevalence and expression of IED.

IMPACT OF INTERMITTENT EXPLOSIVE DISORDER ON SOCIAL–EMOTIONAL AND BEHAVIORAL FUNCTIONING IN SCHOOL AND HOME ENVIRONMENTS

Social–Emotional and Behavioral Functioning in School

In relation to the impact of IED on school functioning and the academic environment, McLaughlin et al. (2012) suggest that the earliest warning signs of IED may be most likely detected in the school setting (as opposed to home or community settings) due to the young average age of onset as compared to other mental health conditions. A number of research studies report that individuals with IED may exhibit behaviors (beyond the episodes of physical and verbal aggression) that impair the development and maintenance of interpersonal relationships with adults and peers. These ancillary behaviors are likely to be of concern within the school setting as they create discord and potentially disrupt the environment.

One behavior of concern for relationship building and peaceful social interactions is that of relational aggression. *Relational aggression* refers to tactics that are undertaken to harm another person's image or social status. Some examples may include bullying, gossiping, insults, and social exclusion. Compared to typically developing individuals, people with IED exhibit higher levels of relational aggression (Murray-Close et al., 2010). Although the research on relational aggression comes from adult samples with IED, given that relational aggression is common during the childhood and adolescent periods, it stands to reason that youths with IED would likely engage in these socially harmful behaviors as well.

Another issue likely to cause strife in peer and adult relationships within the school setting relates to the manner in which individuals with IED perceive social interactions. Even when interactional events are neutral in tone, people with IED are more likely to interpret those interactions as negative than their typically developing peers (Coccaro et al., 2009, 2016) and to respond with hostility to those events with hostility. In fact, Coccaro et al. (2016) utilized neutral vignettes to assess social attributions of adults with IED. They found that the individuals with IED attributed higher levels of hostile intent and lower levels of benign intent to the scenarios as compared to both typically developing control subjects and participants with other psychiatric diagnoses. In addition, when presented with socially appropriate responses to the vignettes, individuals with IED indicated that they were unlikely to pursue those choices and predicted less probability of a successful outcome from those responses (Coccaro et al., 2016). These issues with negative attribution can lead to conflicts with others and may trigger an aggressive outburst consistent with the individual's IED symptomatology. Kessler et al. (2011) explain that disproportionate responses to perceived provocation are central to the expression of IED. Those responses are frequently explosive in nature, in that they are extremely rapid in onset, exhibit rage, and are short in duration. The outbursts often serve to exacerbate strained social and interpersonal relationships. Specific to boys' adolescent peer relationships, research has demonstrated that young males who engage in reactive aggression have fewer friends and lower quality friendships than adolescents who are proactively aggressive (Poulin & Bouvin, 1999). Lope et al. (2018) also found evidence for strained peer and adult relationships among aggressive adolescents in the school setting. Their research indicated that these youths have fewer friends in the classroom, perceive themselves as receiving lesser support from teachers, and rate their attitudes more negatively toward school in general than their peers.

> Even when interactional events are neutral in tone, people with IED are more likely to interpret those interactions as negative than their typically developing peers (Coccaro et al., 2009, 2016) and to respond with hostility to those events with hostility.

An additional concern in the school setting for children and adolescents with IED is the aggressive outbursts that are central to the diagnosis. McLaughlin et al. (2012) found adolescents with IED to engage in an average of 18.3 such incidents per year, and Fanning et al. (2019) revealed that individuals with IED conduct aggressive acts impulsively at a significantly higher rate than both typically developing people and individuals with other psychiatric disorders. Given the amount of time spent in the school environment, it is highly likely that many of those outbursts would occur during the school day. Although the aggressive outbursts of a child or adolescent with IED may represent a challenge for the school setting, the outbursts may yield psychological and emotional consequences for the student as well. Kulper et al. (2015) found that before and during an incident of aggression, the aggressor experiences negative emotions and physical distress. These students also often feel a lack of control over their own behaviors. The intensity of the psychological consequences of an aggressive incident are significant for the child or adolescent with IED. Thus, it is imperative for schools to have both proactive, positive behavioral supports and also crisis response protocols in place to support the adjustment and safety for all students in the school setting.

Social–Emotional and Behavioral Functioning at Home

Dodge (2006) theorized that the hostile attribution bias (as seen in children and adolescents with IED) may be the result of parental rejection and lack of warmth in the home. Hostile attributions cause an individual to perceive neutral events and interactions as negative and/or threatening. Dodge (2006) explained that hostile attributions are a universal default, but most children learn the skills to make benign attributions. However, lack of warmth from caregivers in early life experiences may impair the development of the skills that support prosocial interactions. This hostile attribution bias is a type of cognitive distortion that causes the child or adolescent to engage in aggressive behaviors. The aggressive behavior then reinforces the cognitive distortion, leading to a cycle of increasingly violent behavior (Barriga et al., 2000, 2008).

These faulty attributions and cognitive distortions may lead to further discord, dysfunction, or even violence within the home environment, which may already be strained by parenting issues. According to Barriga et al. (2008) and Smeijers et al. (2018), self-serving cognitive distortions (like those of children and adolescents with IED) yield physical aggression because the person believes that others are deserving of their assaultive behavior. Although verbal aggression is also the result of cognitive distortions, the impetus is more oppositional in nature. The individual experiencing the cognitive distortions believes that rules and structures should not apply to them and justifies their actions and choices without remorse. In support of these propositions by Barriga et al. (2008), de Vries et al. (2016) conducted research that highlighted that the link between parental rejection and aggressive behavior is mediated by cognitive distortions, and Smeijers et al. (2018) also noted a direct link between parental rejection and aggressive behavior. When adolescents display aggressive behavior in the home, Lope et al. (2018) noted a link between those behaviors and negative associations with family relationships. To be specific, adolescents who display aggressive tendencies rate their levels of offensive communication and family conflict as high and give low ratings to measures of open communication in the home and family cohesion.

According to Barriga et al. (2008) and Smeijers et al. (2018), self-serving cognitive distortions (like those of children and adolescents with IED) yield physical aggression because the person believes that others are deserving of their assaultive behavior.

In addition to issues of parenting, some family relationships and home lives may be further strained due to the heritability of IED. As previously noted, research supports that many children and adolescents with IED also have a close relation (perhaps in the home) who has a diagnosis of IED as well (Coccaro, 2010; McElroy et al., 1998). The challenges in the home represented by any individual displaying unpredictable rage-like behaviors would introduce heightened alertness, anxiety, apprehension, and even fear throughout the family unit; however, if more than one individual in the home displays IED symptoms, the distress within the home may be exponentially increased as the two people with IED interact with each other and with other family members through a lens of hostile attribution bias and cognitive distortion. It is probable that the presence of more than one individual with IED in the home significantly increases the likelihood of verbal and physical assaults across all members within the home.

IMPACT OF INTERMITTENT EXPLOSIVE DISORDER ON LEARNING IN THE CLASSROOM

It stands to reason that the significant behavioral issues and explosive outbursts inherent with IED are likely to cause disruptions to the learning environment for both students with IED and their peers. These acts of rage would necessitate that the instruction would cease in order to address behavior management and safety needs associated with the outburst. Depending on the school and/or district's approach to discipline, this interruption to the learning process may also lead to exclusion for the student, including means such as suspension, restrictive alternative placements, or expulsion. Although these methods have been used extensively in American educational practice, research indicates that their application often results in further harm to the student, including exacerbation of behavioral issues and increased probability of dropping out of school (Hess et al., 2014; Powers et al., 2016).

In addition to these concerns, Boxmeyer et al. (2018) indicate that the psychosocial impairment related to anger in students often persists beyond those classroom incidents. They note that students who struggle to contain their anger often experience concerns with academic performance, other behavioral infractions within the school, and issues of criminality outside the educational environment. Thus, it is imperative to offer both prevention and intervention strategies to disrupt the negative cycle of anger for children and adolescents with IED or those who exhibit symptomatology similar to that of IED.

IMPLICATIONS FOR SCHOOL PSYCHOLOGISTS

Assessment Role

In the event that a school-based support team determines that evaluation for special services is appropriate for a student with IED, it is likely that the school psychologist will feature prominently in the evaluation and eligibility decision-making processes. Whether the team is pursuing qualification for the student as an individual with a disability under IDEA or Section 504, the process is quite similar. Either process requires initiation of the referral and signed parent permission in order to proceed. Then, the evaluation team has 60 days to determine eligibility and offer services from the point of receiving the signed consent to evaluate. The team makes a plan to assess the child or adolescent in any area of suspected disability.

In the case of a child or adolescent with IED, critical components of the evaluation are likely to include record reviews, observations, interviews, functional behavioral assessment, and psychometric testing. The school psychologist may or may not be charged with reviewing the relevant extant data from records. Those records should include any school-based files, including attendance, grades, standardized test scores, and behavioral/discipline referrals. For students with IED, it is also probable that records will need to be collected and reviewed from outside the school as well. If the child is receiving outside psychological, psychiatric, and/or medical services, then the team will seek additional permission from the parent to access reports and records from community mental health providers, psychologists, psychiatrists, and/or pediatricians who are involved in the student's care. In some instances, a child or adolescent with IED may also have had law enforcement involvement due to their extreme aggressive incidents. If that is, in fact, applicable, then juvenile justice or probation records may be sought by the team to help establish the extent and severity of the behavior.

Beyond file review of historical data, observations of the child or adolescent will also be conducted as a component related to present levels of performance. The observations should take place across a variety of structured and unstructured settings/situations with both formal and informal observation techniques. Interviews are another piece of data that provide context regarding the student's current functioning in both school and home environments as information is explored with the student, parent, and teacher(s) about these critical factors in evaluating overall functioning. In addition, these observations and interviews also provide critical data for the functional behavioral assessment. The intent of the functional behavioral assessment is to examine the target behavior of concern (likely verbal and/or physical outbursts for a student with IED) to analyze the setting events that precipitate that behavior and the consequences that follow and help to maintain the behavior. The goal of functional behavioral assessment is to understand why the behavior is occurring and create and reinforce socially appropriate replacement behaviors that serve the same need for the student as the target behavior. The school psychologist is trained and experienced in the collection of all of the aforementioned data.

The school psychologist is uniquely suited to conduct the psychometric testing that may be needed for evaluation purposes. Given the frequently comorbid concerns for children and adolescents with IED, it will be necessary to examine additional behavioral, emotional, and social factors through the use of behavioral rating scales and personality instruments. Depending on the circumstances, it might be prudent to assess issues like depression, anxiety, and self-esteem.

Aside from these pieces of the psychological assessment, the school psychologist is likely to evaluate the child's or adolescent's academic and cognitive functioning as well. This is especially important if the team is evaluating for eligibility under IDEA. IDEA mandates a two-pronged eligibility determination. First, the team must decide whether the data support that the student meets the criteria under one of the 13 disability categories, then they must also determine whether the youth exhibits a need for special education services. This need is evaluated based on the student's academic performance and ability to progress in the curriculum without specialized service provision. Thus, the academic and cognitive testing (along with record review and work sample data) establish the basis for that decision. Overall, the data collection and determinations are guided by a team of professionals and the child's parent, but the school psychologist is integral to the process.

Advocacy Role

Early diagnosis and treatment are imperative for children and adolescents with IED as the aggressive behavior that is a hallmark of IED is associated with a plethora of adverse life outcomes, including academic challenges, criminality, and substance abuse (Fergusson et al., 2005; Radwan & Coccaro, 2020). In fact, studies from the United States found that youths with IED were significantly more likely to be arrested for theft, burglary, and violent crime than children and adolescents without an IED diagnosis (McLaughlin et al., 2012). Similar research among adolescents with IED in China reported that these subjects are more likely to engage in violent crime (such as rape and assault) and also represent repeat offenders in the juvenile justice system (Shao et al., 2019). If they are not providing the services themselves, school psychologists can advocate for the family to access community-based supports to decrease the probability of adverse, life-altering outcomes for the child or adolescent with IED. Fergusson et al. (2005) suggest that a programmed approach to therapeutic intervention for children and adolescents with aggression issues should incorporate social, familial, and individual factors, and school psychologists are uniquely positioned to offer support and advocacy across these domains.

> Studies from the United States found that youth with IED were significantly more likely to be arrested for theft, burglary, and violent crime than children and adolescents without an IED diagnosis (McLaughlin et al., 2012).

School psychologists may also play a vital role in advocacy related to medication management for those children and adolescents with IED who have prescriptions from pediatric or psychiatric medical providers. Psychiatric treatment studies have found that prescription drug intervention is effective in reducing impulsive aggression in individuals with IED (Coccaro, 2012). The pharmacological options may include mood stabilizers, antipsychotics, and selective serotonin reuptake inhibitors, although the drug treatment studies often include individuals with aggressive tendencies who do not necessarily meet diagnostic criteria for IED (Dell'Osso et al., 2006). The role of the school psychologist may include observations and progress monitoring in the school setting related to efficacy of prescriptions and dosing as medical providers work toward finding the most appropriate pharmacological intervention for the child or adolescent with IED. School psychologists can offer objective data for decision-making regarding the student's academic, behavioral, and social functioning in a setting that would otherwise be off limits to the physician.

Consultation Role

Through their function as consultants, school psychologists can offer their psychological expertise to the academic environment regarding academic, behavioral, social, and emotional concerns. Given the behavioral manifestations of IED, it is likely that a student with IED may occasionally experience aggressive outbursts of a verbal or physical nature in the classroom with peers or the teacher. This type of situation could be volatile given that the outbursts are frequently disproportionate to the triggering event and often arise without warning. Thus, school psychologists should work within their school buildings to create, implement, and support proactive strategies that promote prosocial behavior with the hope of preventing problematic behaviors from occurring. Multi-Tiered Systems of Support, positive behavioral intervention support, social–emotional learning programs, and violence prevention programs are within the expertise of the school psychologist, and they can provide invaluable guidance to school personnel regarding their design and program evaluation. However, school psychologists should also prepare staff members for crisis response when dangerous situations surface.

School psychologists should be involved in drafting the school's crisis plan to include best practice response to a variety of situations (including aggressive assaults like those often exhibited by children and adolescents with IED). The crisis response protocols should include planning for incidents at either the building, classroom, or individual level. When proper safety precautions have been conceptualized, documented, and rehearsed with thoughtful student-centered approaches, then communities reap the rewards of a more secure environment for teachers and school personnel. Given the two subtypes of IED (high frequency/low intensity behavioral incidents versus low frequency/high intensity behavioral incidents), school psychologists should prepare schools to work with students with IED through both behavioral intervention and safety plans.

Counseling/Therapy Role

The importance of early intervention and treatment for people with IED has been highlighted in the literature. Rynar and Coccaro (2018) noted that addressing IED symptoms at earlier stages may help to prevent some of the negative outcomes associated with IED in adulthood, including impaired quality of life, poorer life satisfaction, employment instability, and marital discord. In addition, a study with adults with IED has noted associations between IED and negative physical health conditions. Though not causal in nature, IED is significantly correlated with increased risks in adulthood for coronary heart disease, hypertension, stroke, diabetes, arthritis, back/neck pain, ulcers, headaches, and other chronic pain (McCloskey et al., 2010). Thus, treatment for IED is imperative in an effort to address both current and future functioning for the child or adolescent with IED. Despite the need for intervention services, McLaughlin et al. (2012) suggest that a significant proportion of children and adolescents with IED do not receive treatment, and among those who do, few treatments address their emotional needs and concerns. In their research, only 6.5% of adolescents with IED had received treatment for their anger in the preceding 12 months (McLaughlin et al., 2012). Oliver et al. (2016) found treatment rates to be especially low among Black adolescents with IED. According to Galbraith et al. (2018), the youths with comorbid IED and anxiety disorders are more likely to have treatment opportunities than adolescents with IED alone. However, when treatment is sought for IED, research supports the effectiveness of cognitive behavioral therapy in reducing both impulsive aggression and negative attributions (McCloskey et al., 2008). Counseling and therapeutic interventions are well within the purview of the school psychologist's training, experience, and competency. Thus, school psychologists should ensure that their roles and functions within their practice settings fully utilize their potential to positively impact both the current and future functioning of students with IED within their buildings.

EDUCATIONAL SUPPORTS

Although the literature base is scant regarding the academic support needs for students with IED, there are more plentiful resources associated with children and adolescents who exhibit aggression outside of an IED diagnosis. In addition, it is clear that students who engage in aggressive behaviors in the school setting demonstrate greater academic need. In a very large and recent European study, it was found that across a variety of ages, instruments, and raters, those students who demonstrate greater levels of aggressive behaviors also have poorer academic performance as measured by grades and standardized test results (Vuoksimaa et al., 2021). These findings are consistent with other researchers who have noted causal evidence between childhood and adolescent aggression and lower school performance and educational attainment (Fergusson et al., 2005; Hinshaw, 1992).

Savage et al. (2017) noted that the relationship between increased aggression and decreased academic achievement is present in a meta-analysis of empirical studies even when controlling for other variables like parent levels of education and the family's socioeconomic status. Studies indicate that the causes for the link between aggression and impaired academic performance are both genetic and environmental (Hinshaw, 1992; Lewis et al., 2017; Porsch et al., 2016). Despite the overwhelming evidence establishing the connection between violent behavior and poor academic achievement, Savage et al. (2017) argue that schools are virtually ignoring academic intervention as a pathway for lowering violence and improving the levels of aggressive behavior among children and adolescents who exhibit assaultive outbursts in the educational environment. Consistent with this recommendation, Lekwa et al. (2019) found that teachers' instructional practices predicted academic engagement (which is associated with academic achievement) in ways that classroom behavior management practices did not. Therefore, educational supports and intervention may be necessary to address academic achievement gaps among students with IED and may subsequently reduce aggressive behaviors in the classroom as well.

Studies indicate that the causes for the link between aggression and impaired academic performance are both genetic and environmental (Hinshaw, 1992; Lewis et al., 2017; Porsch et al., 2016).

Increasing academic engagement in the classroom may be one way to improve the academic achievement (and thereby improve behavioral performance) for children and adolescents with IED. In their chapter focused on best practices for increasing academic engagement, Gettinger and Miller (2014) recommend a number of classroom strategies to promote progress in this area of instruction. They group the strategies into three areas as follows: managerial strategies, instructional strategies, and student-regulated strategies. The managerial strategies include organizational and leadership qualities that promote student engagement in the day-to-day activities of the educational environment. They include such recommendations as designing the classroom layout to allow for student management, reducing transition time, and building and maintaining positive teacher-student relationships. Instructional strategies relate to teacher and task variables. A few best practice techniques in this area include facilitating active participation by students, allotting teacher attention appropriately, and designing adequate scaffolding for learning. The final category of academic engagement, student-regulated strategies, are those aspects of the classroom that promote independence of the learners. Gettinger and Miller's (2014) recommendations include the following: promoting metacognition among pupils, teaching self-monitoring skills, and encouraging goal setting. The authors further suggest that school psychologists should have a working knowledge of the principles and techniques of academic engagement in order to effectively consult with teachers for the betterment of the classroom environment and the students' academic and behavioral outcomes.

SCHOOL-BASED MENTAL HEALTH INTERVENTIONS AND SUPPORTS

McLaughlin et al. (2012) recommend the use of school violence prevention programs to address issues associated with IED, and Lester et al. (2017) conducted a systematic review of systematic reviews to investigate the most effective approaches to preventing violence in the school environment. The authors found that cognitive behavioral interventions may be effective at preventing peer victimization, especially when delivered at the whole-school level. Further, when investigating the reduction of verbal and physical aggression among peers, social–emotional learning and peer mediation demonstrate consistent effectiveness across a variety of programs (Lester et al., 2017). In general, social–emotional learning programs teach children and adolescents to recognize and understand their own emotions, demonstrate empathy toward others, and foster positive relationships, whereas peer mediation programs train select students to work as impartial negotiators to help their peers solve conflicts.

When investigating the reduction of verbal and physical aggression among peers, social–emotional learning and peer mediation demonstrate consistent effectiveness across a variety of programs (Lester et al., 2017).

At the individual level, cognitive behavioral therapy has been found to be particularly effective for individuals with IED when it includes relaxation components along with cognitive restructuring and instruction on using coping skills (McCloskey et al., 2008). Research studies note the effectiveness of this therapeutic approach in both individual and group formats (Costa et al., 2018; McCloskey et al., 2008). It has also been found to be effectively delivered in hybrid formats that include face-to-face and online components (Lochman et al., 2017). The use of cognitive behavioral therapy with individuals with IED has been associated with improvements in aggression, anger, hostility, and depression. The empirical work by Smeijers et al. (2018) regarding cognitive distortions supports that "Cognitive therapeutic interventions should be more focused on specifically targeting the cognitive distortions . . . instead of employing a general approach during cognitive therapy" (p. 502). Their belief is that this targeted approach to therapy will produce greater reductions in aggressive behaviors. Coccaro et al. (2016) also promote targeting social information processing deficits with therapeutic intervention for individuals who exhibit aggressive behaviors.

It may be particularly important to address social cues and emotional awareness through therapeutic intervention as well. Even adults with IED have been shown to struggle with appropriately identifying emotions in vignettes. While they were adept at identifying scenarios related to anger, they also often attributed anger to vignettes that were not related to anger. Additionally, individuals with IED demonstrated a particular struggle identifying the emotion of sadness in the research vignettes (Patoilo et al., 2021). Recognizing and identifying the emotions of oneself and others are concepts that fall under the category of *emotional intelligence*. Coccaro et al. (2015) found that individuals with IED are indeed impaired in emotional intelligence compared to peers even after controlling for demographic and cognitive variables, and they assert that direct intervention in this area may be beneficial in reducing the aggressive tendencies of people with IED. Specifically, they note that individuals with IED struggle with understanding emotions and managing emotions. They further explain that these difficulties are likely related to their hostile attributions in neutral interactions (Coccaro et al., 2015). For the school psychologist delivering the therapeutic intervention, the approaches may mirror those of social–emotional learning programs delivered at the whole-school level but with a more intensive, individual-delivery focus. These efforts could help to address some of the relationship issues that complicate interactions with adults and peers for the student with IED.

Finally, though more research is needed to explore its effectiveness, preliminary case study research has found child-centered play therapy to be promising as a treatment for IED with younger children (Paone & Douma, 2009). The authors found significant symptom reduction in a 7-year-old boy (who was not receiving pharmacological treatment) through the use of play therapy. They believe that the play therapy helps children to develop self-awareness and problem-solving skills that are beneficial to individuals with IED. Until a more solid empirical base is established for the use of play therapy for students with IED, it would behoove school psychologists to continue to monitor the research literature for efficacy studies in this regard.

CASE STUDY 7.1 DENVER: CASE OF A WHITE BOY WITH INTERMITTENT EXPLOSIVE DISORDER

Background

Denver is a 14-year-old boy who lives in a large metropolitan area. He was born to a single mother and has no siblings. Denver's father has never been involved in his life. Prior to his birth, Denver's mother, Emily, struggled with depression and had a significant bout of postpartum depression after his birth. Due to the severity of her symptoms, she was unable to care for Denver, and a friend moved into their small apartment to help with him. The friend was Denver's primary caregiver for the first 7 months of his life before she joined the navy and moved out. When Emily took over Denver's care at that time, she was relatively unfamiliar with his routines and disinterested in building their relationship. Emily's parenting was detached with little affection for her young son. As Denver grew, Emily's expectations for him were inconsistent. She frequently disengaged from his daily life but would occasionally exhibit rageful behaviors when he did not behave as she anticipated. By the time Denver was 4, Emily's boyfriend had moved into the home. Emily continued to have verbally aggressive outbursts directed toward Denver, and her boyfriend began physically abusing Denver

(continued)

CASE STUDY 7.1 DENVER: CASE OF A WHITE BOY WITH INTERMITTENT EXPLOSIVE DISORDER (continued)

in an effort to correct even minor misbehavior. Their parenting style became increasingly controlling, and Denver started to respond with sudden, explosive tantrums in response to changes in routine or perceived criticism. Those behavioral incidents included screaming, breaking items, hitting others, and cursing. In his preschool setting, when Denver's teacher corrected a response or attempted to show him a new way of doing a task, he displayed similar verbal aggression. These behavioral patterns persisted throughout Denver's early school experiences and resulted in frequent calls to his home. The disciplinary calls home further increased the strain and frustration in that environment to the point where Emily's boyfriend left the home. Although Denver no longer suffered from the physical abuse from the boyfriend, Emily became even more critical of Denver and his behavior. After a particularly frightening outburst at the age of 11, Emily took Denver to a pediatrician to inquire about his behavior. The pediatrician referred them to a local psychiatrist. The psychiatrist diagnosed Denver with IED. She recommended a combination of cognitive behavioral therapy, family therapy, and prescription medication. Emily chose to fill the prescription but did not pursue any form of therapy for Denver or herself. Denver has continued on the medication since that time. For nearly 3 years, his behavioral outbursts decreased in intensity but not in frequency; however, they have recently returned to pretreatment levels, and school personnel and peers have been frightened by threatening posture and rage-like verbalizations. Denver is also failing three of his six eighth-grade courses. The school principal has requested the school psychologist's assistance in working with Denver.

Discussion

First, the school psychologist requested a meeting with Emily to gather information and discuss Denver's current status in school. Emily agreed to meet due to her frustration with the situation. At the meeting, Denver's mother shared that she has become fearful of Denver's outbursts since his recent growth spurt. He is now physically larger than Emily and uses his size to intimidate her during his outbursts though he has never attempted bodily harm with her. Emily also indicated that Denver's prescription medication has remained the same for the past 2 years despite his significant change in weight and size. Given that the medication appears no longer effective, the school psychologist seeks and receives written permission from Emily to contact Denver's psychiatrist. The school psychologist also sought permission to begin cognitive behavioral therapy with Denver after Emily expressed that she believed Denver needed intervention but did not have the time or money to pursue it through community-based services.

After the meeting, the school psychologist reached out to the psychiatrist to discuss Denver's challenging behavior, the recent changes in behavior, and his increase in size. Through their discussion, they devised a plan for the school psychologist to provide observational data and teacher interview information to the psychiatrist. When this was concluded, the psychiatrist decided to keep Denver's current medication but include an additional dose midmorning. The school psychologist then coordinated with the school nurse and Emily to establish procedures for the nurse to administer this dose of medication during the school day in hopes of better managing the outbursts for Denver.

While working through the medication management issues, the school psychologist also began initial treatment sessions with Denver. During the intake, the school psychologist realized that Denver struggled to identify emotions in others and demonstrated the hostile attribution bias that is common in adolescents with IED. The school psychologist designed a treatment plan using cognitive behavioral therapy to address these deficits and worked with school personnel to design a positive behavioral intervention plan for the prevention of behaviors and a safety plan to mediate risks when incidents do arise.

With regard to learning, the school psychologist hoped to improve Denver's academic progress. Through a series of interviews with his teachers and observations in the classroom, the school psychologist found that Denver was rarely engaged in the classroom, and his

(continued)

CASE STUDY 7.1 DENVER: CASE OF A WHITE BOY WITH INTERMITTENT EXPLOSIVE DISORDER (continued)

aggressive outbursts occurred primarily when he was disengaged. The school psychologist decided that many teachers could benefit from new information and strategies for academic engagement for the betterment of all students. The school psychologist arranged with the school principal to provide a training session on academic engagement at the upcoming inservice day. Further, the school psychologist will follow up with Denver's teachers to discuss the strategies that might be particularly effective for him, including new classroom arrangements, reduction in transition time, and instruction in metacognitive techniques. Finally, the school psychologist arranged for a meeting with the principal, teachers, Emily, the psychiatrist, and the school nurse in 6 weeks to discuss new data regarding Denver's school-based academic and behavioral progress.

SUMMARY POINTS

- In order to apply a *DSM-5* diagnosis of IED, a child or adolescent must meet a criterion related to the frequency and intensity of their aggressive outbursts.
- With regard to etiology, the school psychologist should remember that familial issues may be risk factors for the development of IED.
- Children and adolescents with IED apply hostile attributions to neutral interactions or events.
- Hostile attributions and cognitive distortions may lead to aggressive incidents for children and adolescents with IED.
- School psychologists can engage in many roles and functions to support the needs of students with IED, including assessment, advocacy, consultation, and counseling and/or therapy.
- Mental health interventions should target cognitive distortions and emotional awareness.

TEST YOUR KNOWLEDGE

1. A child cannot be diagnosed with IED if younger than what age?
   a. 3
   b. 6
   c. 13
   d. 18

2. The United States has a lower prevalence of IED than most countries.
   a. True
   b. False

3. Cognitive distortions are not common in children and adolescents with IED.
   a. True
   b. False

4. Which type of aggression is undertaken to harm another person's reputation or social status?
   a. Reactive aggression
   b. Relational aggression
   c. Regimented aggression
   d. Residual aggression

5. Trauma is a risk factor for developing IED.
   a. True
   b. False

Answers: (1) b, (2) b, (3) b, (4) b, (5) a.

DISCUSSION QUESTIONS

1. Describe the *DSM-5* diagnostic criteria for IED.
2. Explain why children and adolescents with IED may be considered socially maladjusted under IDEA.
3. List the familial factors that may contribute to the development of IED.
4. Discuss how hostile attributions may impair interpersonal relationships for children and adolescents with IED.
5. Detail one evidenced-based social–emotional intervention for students with IED.

CHAPTER RESOURCES

American Psychiatric Association *What Are Disruptive, Impulse Control, and Conduct Disorders?*: www.psychiatry.org/patients-families/disruptive-impulse-control-and-conduct-disorders/what-are-disruptive-impulse-control-and-conduct-disorders

Mayo Clinic *Intermittent Explosive Disorder*: www.mayoclinic.org/diseases-conditions/intermittent-explosive-disorder/symptoms-causes/syc-20373921

National Institutes of Health *Intermittent Explosive Disorder Affects Up to 16 Million Americans*: www.nih.gov/news-events/news-releases/intermittent-explosive-disorder-affects-16-million-americans

KEY REFERENCES

Only key references appear in the print edition. The full reference list appears in the digital product on Springer Publishing Connect: connect.springerpub.com/content/book/978-0-8261-3587-2/part/part03/chapter/ch07

American Psychiatric Association. (2013). *Diagnostic and statistical manual of mental disorders* (5th ed.). https://doi.org/10.1176/appi.books.9780890425596

Coccaro, E. F., Fanning, J., Keedy, S. K., & Lee, R. J. (2016). Social cognition in intermittent explosive disorder and aggression. *Journal of Psychiatric Research, 83*, 140–150. http://doi.org/10.1016/j.jpsychires.2016.07.010

Coccaro, E. F., Lee, R., & McCloskey, M. S. (2014). Validity of the new A1 and A2 criteria for *DSM-5* intermittent explosive disorder. *Comprehensive Psychiatry, 55*, 260–267. https://doi.org/10.1016/j.comppsych.2013.09.007

Galbraith, T., Carliner, H., Keyes, K. M., McLaughlin, K. A., McCloskey, M. S., & Heimberg, R. G. (2018). The co-occurrence and correlates of anxiety disorders among adolescents with intermittent explosive disorder. *Aggressive Behavior, 44*, 581–590. https://doi.org/10.1002/ab.21783

Gettinger, M., & Miller, K. (2014). Best practices in increasing academic engaged time. In P. L. Harrison & A. Thomas (Eds.), *Best practices in school psychology: Student-level services*. National Association of School Psychologists.

Lester, S., Lawrence, C., & Ward, C. L. (2017). What do we know about preventing school violence? A systematic review of systematic reviews. *Psychology, Health, & Medicine, 22*(51), 187–223. http://doi.org/10.1080/13548506.2017.1282616

McLaughlin, K. A., Green, J. G., Hwang, I., Sampson, N. A., Zaslavsky, A. M., & Kessler, R. C. (2012). Intermittent explosive disorder in the National Comorbidity Survey Replication Adolescent Supplement. *Archives of General Psychiatry, 69*(11), 1131–1139. https://doi.org/10.1001/archgenpsychiatry.2012.592

Oliver, D. G., Caldwell, C. H., Faison, N., Sweetman, J. A., Abelson, J. M., & Jackson, J. S. (2016). Prevalence of *DSM-IV* intermittent explosive disorder in Black adolescents: Findings from the National Survey of American Life, Adolescent Supplement. *American Journal of Orthopsychiatry, 86*(5), 552–563. https://doi.apa.org/doiLanding?doi=10.1037%2Fort0000170

Puhalla, A. A., Berman, M. E., Coccaro, E. F., Fahlgren, M. K., & McCloskey, M. S. (2020). History of childhood abuse and alcohol use disorder: Relationship with intermittent explosive disorder and intoxicated aggression frequency. *Journal of Psychiatric Research, 125*, 38–44. https://doi.org/10.1016/j.jpschires.2020.02.025

U.S. Department of Education. (n.d.). *Individuals with Disabilities Education Improvement Act*. https://sites.ed.gov/idea

UNIT 4
MENTAL HEALTH DISORDERS IN CHILDREN AND ADOLESCENTS: ANXIETY DISORDERS

CHAPTER 8

Generalized Anxiety Disorder

LEARNING OBJECTIVES

- Summarize the diagnostic features of the *Diagnostic and Statistical Manual of Mental Disorders* (5th ed.; *DSM-5*; American Psychiatric Association [APA], 2013) diagnosis of Generalized Anxiety Disorder (GAD).
- Highlight the risk factors for GAD in children and adolescents.
- Describe common social–emotional and behavioral concerns for children with GAD.
- Understand the classroom implications for students with GAD.
- Identify effective social, emotional, and behavioral interventions for students with GAD.

INTRODUCTION

Imagine suffering alone with generalized anxiety disorder (GAD). The weight of anxiety is pushing down on your chest every moment. You try to fight it, and it tightens its grip. When it is happening to you, you are isolated and live within the constraints of your own mind. It is difficult to see any way out of this prison of your mind. You might withdraw from the people closest to you, frightened of hurting them by behaviors that seem out of your control. You see yourself as different from other people. You are angry and emotionally exhausted. Each day is painful, and you just endure it. It is a daily battle, and you are not sure anyone will understand you. It is exhausting. For children and adolescents, this can be compounded by having no other point of reference. Some may not know that there is any other way to feel, may not have words to describe what they are feeling, and may be concerned about how they will be judged. GAD can be a debilitating disorder.

DIAGNOSTIC ISSUES: *DSM-5* AND SCHOOL-BASED SERVICES

DSM-5 Diagnosis

The first criterion from the *Diagnostic and Statistical Manual of Mental Disorders*, Fifth Edition (*DSM-5*; American Psychiatric Association [APA], 2013), classifies Generalized Anxiety Disorder 300.02 as extreme levels of anxiety or anticipation of aversive circumstances that are prominent on most days for minimum of a half year. The second criterion denotes the individual's struggle to contend with the worry. The third criterion states that for an adult to be diagnosed with GAD, the person must exhibit an additional three symptoms. For children, only one additional symptom is required for diagnosis. These symptoms include restlessness or feeling on edge, fatigue, difficulty concentrating, irritability, muscle tension, and/or sleep disturbance (APA, 2013). These symptoms are consistent with previous editions of the *DSM*; however, prior to the publication of the *DSM-5*, some scholars called for the removal of fatigue, difficulty concentrating, irritability, and sleep disturbance as symptoms due to their relative infrequency with GAD in children and adolescents and their overlap with depression. It was further suggested that the inclusion of these symptoms might lead to an underdiagnosis of GAD in youth. In fact, empirical research found that up to 11% of children and adolescents who would otherwise meet criteria for GAD would likely be excluded based on the associated symptoms criteria (Comer et al., 2012). Despite the concerns expressed by scholars, the symptoms remain part of the diagnosis, but this accounts for the difference between the number of symptoms required for diagnosis in adults versus only requiring the presence of one for children and adolescents. The fourth criterion indicates that the excessive anxiety and worry must cause inhibitory distress or impairment in typically occurring settings and situations. The fifth and sixth criteria explain that the anxiety may not be the result of another chemical substance or mental health condition, respectively (APA, 2013). It is interesting to note that children and adolescents were not even eligible for a diagnosis of GAD prior to the *DSM-IV* (APA, 1994; Keeton et al., 2009).

The key element for the diagnosis of GAD is the idea of excessive or extreme levels of anxiety, worry, and/or fear. Most of us experience anxiety throughout life. When does the worry and anxiety cross the line into excessive worry and anxiety? The *DSM-5* discusses three elements that note the difference between nonpathological anxiety and GAD. First, these worries should "interfere significantly with psychosocial functioning" (APA, 2013, p. 222). Psychosocial functioning can be described as typical daily activities, relationships, and meeting the demands of one's existence (APA, 2013). Second, the worry and anxiety are not proportional to the anticipated event. Likewise, the intensity, duration, and frequency of the worry and anxiety are also disproportionate to the focus of these thoughts (APA, 2013). In children, this often manifests as anxiety related to performance (e.g., worries over school, sports, social skills). Third, it is more likely that the worry and anxiety are accompanied by physical symptoms (ranging from pain to restlessness; APA, 2013). In nonpathological anxiety, one can typically quell worry. In GAD, this is very difficult if not impossible.

Within the *DSM-5*, GAD is classified under the category of Anxiety Disorders. Examples of other disorders in this subsection include Separation Anxiety Disorder (SAD), Social Anxiety Disorder, and Selective Mutism (APA, 2013). These additional anxiety disorders are covered in Chapters 9, 10, and 11, respectively, in this text. These mental health conditions are similar in their significant association with anxieties and fears beyond what would be considered typical. It is also important to note that the diagnoses within the classification of Anxiety Disorders frequently overlap and co-occur, and thus, it is recommended that clinicians look carefully at all related disorders in making a diagnostic determination (APA, 2013). Further complicating the matter, researchers warn that instruments designed for the assessment of anxiety often cannot distinguish between children with GAD and children with symptoms of other anxiety disorders (Keeton et al., 2009).

> Researchers warn that instruments designed for the assessment of anxiety often cannot distinguish between children with GAD and children with symptoms of other anxiety disorders (Keeton et al., 2009).

The *DSM-5* indicates that the average age of onset of GAD is well into adulthood and later than the age of onset of other related anxiety disorders (APA, 2013). However, among pediatric samples, researchers have determined that the onset of GAD generally ranges from 10 to 13 years of age (Beidel & Turner, 2005; Costello et al., 2003; Weems, 2008), although at least one large study found a much younger onset: 8.5 years (Keeton et al., 2009). Regarding age, the literature indicates that the focus of children's worries changes throughout childhood and into adolescence. As reported in Jarrett et al. (2015), children from 6 to 9 years of age commonly report fears of animals, children 10 to 13 have recurring fears associated with personal danger and death, and adolescents from 14 to 17 often express worry related to social situations and/or performance. Unlike the consensus regarding the developmental progression in types of worries, studies within the literature are conflicting about the level of GAD symptoms seen across age ranges. Some studies have found no differences in the number of symptoms reported at younger versus older ages in childhood and adolescence (Masi et al., 1999), but other researchers have found that children self-report more symptoms at older ages than they do at younger stages (Kendall & Pimentel, 2003). Finally, Jarrett et al. (2015) discovered equivalent levels of symptomatology between younger and older students but differing foci. Younger students reported higher levels of harm avoidance, and older adolescents indicated experiencing more issues with attention, emotion regulation, and school-related worry.

With regard to prevalence of GAD, it is estimated that 2.2% to 3.6% of children globally have met or could meet criteria for a diagnosis of GAD (Costello et al., 2005). The prevalence of GAD among children and adolescents within the United States is near the higher end of that range at 3% (Burnstein et al., 2014), and the *DSM-5* reports the 12-month prevalence among adolescents to be at 0.9% (APA, 2013). *Twelve-month prevalence* refers to the percentage of adolescents who reported experiencing symptoms of GAD in the 12 months preceding their participation in research. The risk for the development of GAD appears to rise as children age into adolescence (Mohammadi et al., 2020), but overall, the Centers for Disease Control and Prevention (CDC) reports that approximately 4.4 million children and adolescents ages 3 to 17 in the United States have a diagnosis of anxiety (though that diagnosis is not specific to GAD and could refer to any of the anxiety disorders within the *DSM-5*). The CDC also indicates that anxiety among children and adolescents in the United States is growing. When asked whether a child had ever been diagnosed with anxiety, the percentage of respondents answering affirmatively rose from 5.5% in 2007 to 6.4% in 2011 (CDC, n.d.). Research on prevalence further demonstrates that girls are at significantly higher risk for a GAD diagnosis than boys (Beesdo et al., 2009; Lewinsohn et al., 1998; Mohammadi et al., 2020), but the number of GAD symptoms and their levels of severity across genders appears to be roughly equal (Masi et al., 2004).

School-Based Eligibility

INDIVIDUALS WITH DISABILITIES EDUCATION IMPROVEMENT ACT REGULATIONS

The Individuals with Disabilities Education Improvement Act (IDEA) applies to all public schools and defines a number of disabilities that qualify a child as a student with a disability under the Act (see 34 C.F.R. § 300.8(c)(1)–(13)). If a child qualifies as a student with a disability, then that child must be provided with a free and appropriate public education in the least restrictive environment. The category most relevant to children with GAD or other mental health issues is that of Emotional Disturbance, which is codified at 34 C.F.R. 300.8(c)(4). According to the U.S. Department of Education (n.d.), "(i) Emotional Disturbance means a condition exhibiting one or more of the following characteristics over a long period of time and to a marked degree that adversely affects a child's educational performance" (Section 300.8 (c) (4)). The five characteristics include challenges with educational achievement not due to other cognitive or medical conditions, difficulty in establishing and keeping social relationships, atypical emotional and behavioral responses under normal circumstances, frequently depressed mood, and somatic symptoms associated with individual problems. The criteria also specify that a child with schizophrenia can be identified as having a disability under the category of Emotional Disturbance, but a child who exhibits socially maladjusted behaviors is excluded from this category.

The criterion of Emotional Disturbance related to physical symptoms associated with personal or school problems offers a parallel to the criteria and symptoms of GAD as described in the *DSM-5*. However, this element is more global in nature and could encompass several other anxiety disorders, such as SAD, selective mutism, specific phobia, social anxiety disorder, panic disorder, and agoraphobia. As previously noted, these disorders are all affiliated in the *DSM-5* in the category of Anxiety Disorders and may all have physical symptoms and/or fear associated with personal or school problems. If a school-based eligibility team determines that a student with GAD does, in fact, meet the criteria for Emotional Disturbance, then they must also satisfy the second question of the two-pronged eligibility requirement. This means that the evaluation must demonstrate that the GAD and its symptoms are directly and negatively impacting the child's ability to learn in the school setting, and he/she needs additional services (i.e., special education) and supports in order to progress in the academic curriculum to his/her potential. The symptoms of GAD may impair the student's ability to function in the academic setting due to issues related to attendance, attention, and/or behavior. Although the category of Emotional Disturbance has been one of significant debate over decades, many agree that the spirit of the law is intended to provide support for students with internalizing problems like GAD. However, it is critical to note that diagnosis of GAD alone is neither necessary nor sufficient for a child to qualify for special education services under IDEA.

As an alternative eligibility category to Emotional Disturbance, some school-based teams have used the IDEA category of Other Health Impairment (OHI), coded at 300.8(c)(9) to qualify children and adolescents with GAD for special education services to meet their needs. OHI is defined by three criteria. The first is that the child or adolescent is experiencing "limited strength, vitality, or alertness, including a heightened alertness to environmental stimuli" that impairs focus in the school setting

(U.S. Department of Education, n.d., Section 300.8 (c) (9)). The second is that that condition of impaired alertness is related to a chronic or acute medical condition, and the third is that that condition subsequently hinders school performance. Although the definition of OHI specifies a number of medical concerns that apply here (and GAD is not one of those specified), it further states that the list is not exhaustive and other conditions should be considered eligible if the criteria are met otherwise (U.S. Department of Education, n.d.). As such, one can certainly surmise that an educational evaluation team could determine (with appropriate evaluations and data) that a student with GAD meets the criteria as having a disability under the category of OHI, and the student's symptomatology could demonstrate a need for special support, services, accommodations, and modifications in order to fully access the academic curriculum.

Beyond the special education eligibility offered through IDEA, a child or adolescent with GAD could also presumably qualify for additional supports within the school setting under Section 504 of the Rehabilitation Act of 1973. This federal legislation applies to all entities, organizations, and offices that receive any form of federal financial support. It is considered a form of civil rights legislation for individuals with disabilities, and public schools are mandated to apply its tenets. Section 504 is designed to provide equal access and to eliminate discrimination based on disability status. Like IDEA, Section 504 requires that students with disabilities be provided with a free and appropriate public education with necessary supports consistent with the person's disability. However, unlike IDEA, Section 504 merely requires that the student have a disability (or be suspected of having a disability); it does not dictate that the disability must have direct impact on educational attainment (Office of Civil Rights, n.d.). Thus, a student with GAD who could not qualify for services under IDEA due to the adverse educational impact requirement, may be found eligible for similar supports under Section 504 if the school-based eligibility team determines that the child or adolescent does have a disability that inhibits the individual in one or more major life functions. Learning is considered to be a major life function within Section 504 (Office of Civil Rights, n.d.). Thus, there are multiple pathways for the student with GAD to access needed educational services with regard to their mental health needs.

CULTURAL ISSUES RELATED TO GENERALIZED ANXIETY DISORDER IN YOUTH

Risk Factors for Generalized Anxiety Disorder

Recent research has revealed a number of risk factors associated with the development of GAD. One such risk factor is genetics (Beesdo et al., 2009; Eley et al., 2003; Kendler et al., 2002). One large study of preschoolers found particularly high genetic influences related to general distress and noted that genetic factors likely account for 30% to 40% of variance in anxiety symptoms, whereas environmental factors account for only 10% to 20% (Eley et al., 2003). The *DSM-5* offers a similar estimate by indicating that genetic factors are responsible for approximately one third of the risk for GAD (APA, 2013). One model suggests a relationship between familial history of anxiety, maternal internalizing symptoms, and the development of clinical levels of anxiety (Kendler et al., 2002). Finally, research has also shown a relationship with the amygdala (Biederman et al., 2001; DeBellis et al., 2000). The amygdala is the part of the brain where fight-or-flight responses originate. It plays a role in memory, decision-making, and stress responses (i.e., anxiety), and scholars have found that the amygdala in the brains of children with GAD were significantly larger than in children without GAD; however, it is unclear whether this size difference is due to genetic factors or the environmental conditions of the child (DeBellis et al., 2000).

Although research suggests a significant genetic component to the development of GAD, some environmental factors are also related to the anxiety that may precede its presence in children and adolescents (APA, 2013; Keeton et. al., 2009). Parents may unwittingly contribute to increased anxiety in their children through their parenting approaches. To be specific, overprotective parenting often leads to higher levels of fear in children and fewer coping skills for managing those fears (Keeton et al., 2009; Wood et al., 2003). In addition, theorists have suggested that both parental rejection of the child (i.e., withdrawal and lack of warmth) and parental control (i.e., overinvolvement and encouragement of dependence) are related to anxiety in children and adolescents, but McLeod et al.

(2000) found that parental control is more highly related to childhood anxiety than parental rejection. Pella et al. (2018) found that parenting style is also related to treatment barriers for children with anxiety. Children with anxiety who have parents with an anxious childrearing style report a greater number of barriers to seeking treatment for anxiety within the school setting.

Beyond parenting style, other familial factors have also been associated with GAD in children and adolescents, including lower socioeconomic levels (Kendler et al., 2002; Kessler et al., 2012), parental anxiety disorders (Kawakami et al., 2012), lower levels of maternal education, maternal illiteracy, and maternal history of psychiatric hospitalization (Mohammadi et al., 2020). A final environmental variable that may play a role in the development of GAD among children and adolescents relates to traumatic life experiences (Kendler et al., 2002). In their review of GAD in youth, Imran et al. (2017) found evidence to support that experiences of trauma, exposure to violence, and living in a congested urban area were all related to this mental health condition.

Parents may unwittingly contribute to increased anxiety in their children through their parenting approaches.

Personality variables may also be considered risk factors for the development of GAD in children and adolescents. Kendler et al. (2002) has described the following early-childhood dispositions as associated with a diagnosis of GAD: inhibited temperament, anxiety, depression, and withdrawal. In later childhood and adolescence, they note that conduct problems, low self-esteem, and high negative emotionality are related to the development of GAD. Along with these issues, children and adolescents with GAD may struggle with perfectionism (APA, 2013; Jarrett et al., 2015) and may need more feedback and reassurance regarding their efforts across a variety of domains (APA, 2013).

Finally, children and adolescents with GAD experience high comorbidity with other psychiatric diagnoses as well. As mentioned previously, GAD frequently co-occurs with other anxiety disorders (APA, 2013). In fact, Masi et al. (2004) note that up to 75% of children with GAD also meet criteria for another anxiety disorder. The most common comorbid diagnoses (in order of likelihood) are social phobia, SAD, and specific phobias (SP). Keeton et al. (2009) state, "Co-occurrence of GAD, SP, and SAD is the rule rather than the exception; up to 60% of anxious children meet the criteria for two of the three disorders, and 30% meet the criteria for all three disorders" (p. 172). Beyond the affiliated anxiety disorders that exhibit significant symptom overlap, GAD in youth is also highly comorbid with major depressive disorder (Moffitt et al., 2007), where rates of comorbidity are approximately 15% (Costello et al., 2003). In addition, children and adolescents with GAD are commonly diagnosed with attention deficit hyperactivity disorder (ADHD) and oppositional defiant disorder (Masi et al., 2004) as well as concerns with substance abuse (Kaplow et al., 2001; Sartor et al., 2007). Finally, those with anxiety disorders are more likely than typically developing children and adolescents to develop psychiatric conditions in adulthood (Costello et al., 2003; Imran et al., 2017).

Cultural Considerations

With regard to cultural considerations for GAD, the *DSM-5* highlights a distinction in the presentation of its features across cultures. Specifically, it explains that individuals from some cultures are more likely to experience physical symptoms associated with their diagnoses, whereas people from other cultures are at greater risk for cognitive symptomatology (APA, 2013). However, this symptom expression is noted within adult populations with GAD and has not been studied in the young. Thus, it is not known whether this pattern holds for children and adolescents.

Additional cultural considerations are related to the race of people manifesting GAD. In their study, which compared U.S. immigrants of a variety of racial and ethnic backgrounds to American-born White people, Budhwani et al. (2015) found the highest prevalence of GAD among the American-born White sample. When comparing foreign-born subjects (i.e., Asian, Hispanic, and Afro-Caribbean) to their American-born counterparts of similar racial background, they discovered that the American-born participants had a greater frequency of GAD diagnosis across all comparisons. Foreign-born individuals of Afro-Caribbean ethnicity exhibited the lowest prevalence of GAD overall. It is suggested that this mental health advantage for immigrants may be due to the fact that people who choose to immigrate likely have greater health than their peers who do not immigrate, and their health advantage persists despite often having lower incomes than their American-born counterparts (Budhwani et al., 2015). The Budhwani et al. (2015) findings are consistent with the work of Asnaani et al. (2010), who found that White people are diagnosed with GAD at higher rates than African Americans, Hispanic Americans, and Asian Americans. Finally, Breslau et al. (2007) also report lower rates of GAD diagnoses among racial and ethnic minority individuals.

One additional cultural consideration relates to treatment for anxiety issues in the school setting. Research has revealed some relationships between family demographics and children's perceived barriers to accessing mental health services within their schools. To be specific, Pella et al. (2018) found that children of parents with lower levels of education were likely to identify a greater number of barriers to seeking treatment. In addition, children from African American homes perceive more barriers to treatment than children of White descent.

IMPACT OF GENERALIZED ANXIETY DISORDER ON SOCIAL–EMOTIONAL AND BEHAVIORAL FUNCTIONING IN SCHOOL AND HOME ENVIRONMENTS

Social–Emotional and Behavioral Functioning in School

The school setting is replete with pressures that are likely to trigger anxiety among children and adolescents with GAD. These include the academic work itself along with peer and teacher relationships (Barrett & Heubeck, 2000). Socially, children and adolescents with anxiety symptoms and GAD struggle with their peer relationships. Huberty (2014) explains that children with anxiety experience a plethora of social issues including social entry, conversation entry, and group participation. According to research, same age peers tend to rate students with anxiety as more withdrawn (Coplan et al., 2007) and less likable than other typically developing peers (Nelson et al., 2005). According to Strauss et al. (1998), children with anxiety disorders may even be more socially neglected by peers than children who exhibit conduct disorder. Students with GAD also report that they perceive themselves as lower in social competence and expect to be rejected by peers in social situations (Chansky & Kendall, 1997).

However, Alfano et al. (2011) differs in their perspective of the social relationships of children and adolescents with GAD. They offer that those social relationships may not be as problematic as those of students with other types of anxiety disorders. In their research, they found that (as compared to typically developing peers), children with GAD had fewer friends overall but reported equivalent ratings with regard to having a best friend and participating in social activities. Parents of children with GAD also rate them as comparable to peers in their social competence. The researchers posit that the nature of GAD may actually facilitate some social relationships and friendship dimensions. Because children and adolescents with GAD are both conscientious and rule-abiding, this may support their peer relationships over those experienced by children with other anxiety disorders. Their relatively fewer number of friends may be the result of their own selectivity in friendships in that they would likely seek to avoid peers who engage in behaviors that they deem as too dangerous.

According to Alfano et al. (2011), children with GAD have fewer friends overall but report equivalent ratings with regard to having a best friend and participating in social activities.

Social–Emotional and Behavioral Functioning at Home

In addition to their expression of anxiety, children and adolescents with GAD may also experience problems with sleep in the home (Shanahan et al., 2014). In their research on sleep and childhood psychiatric issues, Shanahan et al. (2014) found that just over 26% of participants reported at least one concern with sleep in the preceding 2 months. The most commonly reported sleep concerns for children with anxiety were difficulty falling asleep and restlessness in sleep. In addition, girls with anxiety were 3 times more likely to report consistent feelings of fatigue than boys with anxiety. With regard to age differences and sleep problems, children with anxiety between the ages of 9 and 12 were more likely to report insomnia and nightmares, but participants from 13 to 16 were more likely to report fatigue after sleep. Hypersomnia was also found to be associated specifically with children and adolescents with GAD. These sleep issues are especially concerning since sleep is critical in emotion regulation and school performance (Shanahan et al., 2014). Thus, parents should monitor both the sleep habits and sleep quality in their children with GAD.

Another complication for the families of children and adolescents with GAD arises if the student's anxiety becomes so pervasive that they begin to refuse school attendance. According to Suldo and Ogg (2014), the disruption to families caused by school refusal crosses multiple domains of concern. Because most states have truancy laws that mandate attendance by minors, parents may quickly run afoul of the law when absences due to school refusal surpass any legislated absence cutoffs. However, these absences do not merely impact the parents' legal standing, they can also negatively affect their occupational status as well. Depending on the age of the child, the school refusal might also force workplace tardiness and/or absences for the parent. This, in turn, may yield subsequent employment and financial instability for the family.

Even if these dire consequences do not manifest, the family is still likely subject to significant emotional strain and conflict due to the child's or adolescent's school-refusal behavior during which children or adolescents engage in significant behavioral outbursts and emotional dysregulation related to school attendance (Suldo & Ogg, 2014). Unfortunately, for children with anxiety, school refusal and the resulting absences may be automatically reinforcing for the child. The student experiences anxiety related to school. Then, they miss school, thereby reducing the anxiety. That reduction in anxiety increases the probability that the child will refuse school again. Interventions directed at school refusal must be function based and should likely incorporate a gradual return to school with positive reinforcements in place (Suldo & Ogg, 2014).

IMPACT OF GENERALIZED ANXIETY DISORDER ON LEARNING IN THE CLASSROOM

Despite the prevalence of GAD among children and adolescents, Mychailyszyn et al. (2010) lamented the sparsity of research regarding anxiety and school performance among students. However, Langley et al. (2004) found that anxiety in children is also associated with inhibited performance in the classroom and issues with school competence (particularly in older children; Ialongo et al., 1994; Jarrett et al., 2015; Kessler et al., 1995). Jarrett et al. (2015) found that younger children with GAD have fewer learning problems and appear happier based on teacher report and as compared to older children with GAD. This might suggest the importance of early intervention as school-related problems may increase for children and adolescents with GAD as they age and progress in the academic curriculum. These results are consistent with research by Mychailyszyn et al. (2010) in which teachers endorsed more negative scores for children with anxiety disorders on work ethic, learning, academic achievement, and happiness as compared to children who are not experiencing symptoms of anxiety. From a parent perspective, parents of younger children with GAD also rate their children's school competence higher than parents of older children with GAD (Jarrett et al., 2015). Mothers also indicate that their children with anxiety disorders perform more poorly in school-related tasks than mothers of children without anxiety disorders (Mychailyszyn et al., 2010).

> Jarrett et al. (2015) found that younger children with GAD have fewer learning problems and appear happier based on teacher report and as compared to older children with GAD.

According to Wood (2006), the academic performance deficits and struggles experienced by children and adolescents with anxiety may be due to other perceived threats rather than the academic work itself. When a student is feeling anxious, a physiological arousal results. This arousal serves to focus the child's or adolescent's attention on the target of that anxiety. As their focus narrows to the threat, it minimizes the child's ability to provide attentional resources to other stimuli (i.e., schoolwork) that is not considered threatening in that circumstance. Correlational research supports the inverse relationship between anxiety symptoms and academic achievement in both reading and math (Ialongo et al., 1994). A related point: although it has already been noted that girls have an overall higher prevalence of anxiety, some research suggests that boys may be more susceptible to academic anxiety (Carey et al., 2017).

One target for anxiety specific to the school setting is that of test anxiety. The presence of test anxiety has been denoted as a possible early-warning sign for the development of more pervasive anxiety and anxiety disorders (Beidel & Turner, 1998). The anxiety associated with classroom assessments for children and adolescents with anxiety has been related to poorer academic performance overall (Call et al., 1994; Dusek et al., 1975; Pintrich & DeGroot, 1990). These results of students without anxiety outperforming their peers with test anxiety were also replicated in a sample composed solely of African American children (Turner et al., 1993). Thus, this area may warrant particular intervention emphasis to improve overall classroom functioning for students with GAD.

Beyond these findings, a research study conducted in Canada also offers important insight into some negative outcomes associated with learning and students with anxiety disorders. Though this work was not specific to GAD, the authors found that adults with anxiety disorders report significant distress associated with general nervousness in the classroom and difficulty speaking in front of their peers as children and adolescents (Van Ameringen et al., 2003). This type of school-based anxiety often precedes school-refusal behaviors. The first indicators of budding school refusal include frequent visits to the nurse's office with somatic complaints and appeals to call home to be released early from school (Suldo & Ogg, 2014). According to Van Ameringen et al. (2003), over 34% of their participants reported that their anxiety and affiliated symptomatology caused them to avoid school and have long-term absences (Van Ameringen et al., 2003). This is consistent with the literature, which supports that students who chronically refuse to attend school likely have diagnosed or undiagnosed anxiety disorders (Berg, 1992; Last & Strauss, 1990). In fact, Heyne and King (2004) found that 5% to 7% of students with anxiety will also exhibit school refusal behaviors.

School absences (particularly when they are chronic or extended) serve to tremendously impact the delivery of the curriculum in ways that likely create gaps in learning and significant struggle in progressive academic skills (Suldo & Ogg, 2014). Absences also negatively impact the ability of a student to access special education supports. During IDEA eligibility evaluations, the team must rule out access to education as the variable (as opposed to disability) that is causing deficits. When absences are extensive, it is challenging for the evaluation team to determine that the student has in fact had adequate opportunity to learn and advance in the curriculum. Also, the Van Ameringen et al. (2003) study revealed that approximately 49% of their adult anxiety disorder participants had dropped out of school prior to completing their high school education, and 24% of those who withdrew early explained that their anxiety was the primary reason for doing so. Dropping out of high school often has severe implications for an individual's lifetime educational attainment, occupational pursuits, and financial well-being.

IMPLICATIONS FOR SCHOOL PSYCHOLOGISTS

Assessment Role

As previously noted, the child or adolescent with GAD could potentially qualify for special services and supports under two different forms of federal legislation—IDEA and Section 504 of the Rehabilitation Act of 1973. Regardless of the path used for the provision of services, the role of the school psychologist features heavily in the evaluation. The school psychologist would likely be responsible for the assessment of the child's or adolescent's cognitive, academic, and psychological functioning, along with observations, file reviews, interviews, and record reviews. The resulting assessment data would be used by the multidisciplinary team to make eligibility determinations and any subsequent decisions regarding the necessary services and supports for the child or adolescent with GAD to be able to function and progress in the academic curriculum to their fullest potential.

Advocacy Role

Given their diagnosis of GAD, it is highly probable that students with this mental health condition are involved with community-based providers. These providers may include pediatricians, psychologists, and/or psychiatrists, depending on their engagement with therapy-based or medication protocols. As such, the school psychologist is perfectly positioned through their training, background, and experiences to serve as a liaison between those professionals and the school setting. Because a child or adolescent with GAD spends a great deal of their waking hours in the school, their adjustment within that environment is likely to be of interest to external providers. The school psychologist may offer insights (with appropriate parental permission) into attendance, classroom behavior, academic achievement, and peer relationships to those responsible for treatment outside of the school. These observations can serve as a critical progress-monitoring component for the maintenance or adjustment of therapy and/or prescriptions used in the management of GAD and its affiliated symptoms for children and adolescents. If, however, the child is not involved with external providers for the treatment of their symptomatology associated with GAD, the school psychologist may steer the family toward appropriate community resources and services. The school psychologist may even facilitate communication between the family and those professionals.

Consultation Role

Although consultation for behavioral intervention in the classroom is normally thought to target the elimination or minimization of a challenging behavior, a more helpful and beneficial perspective is to direct these same strategies toward building a repertoire of positive, adaptive, and prosocial behaviors. The school psychologist can collaborate with the teacher to design positive behavioral support plans to increase school functioning with skills like classroom participation, assignment participation, or even attendance issues. When the child or adolescent with GAD has been taught to recognize their anxiety triggers, then they can be prompted to utilize adaptive coping skills and appropriately reinforced for using these skills in the classroom setting. This will serve to increase the probability of the use of those strategies in future anxiety-provoking situations.

> The school psychologist can collaborate with the teacher to design positive behavioral support plans to increase school functioning with skills like classroom participation, assignment participation, or even attendance issues for students with GAD.

Beyond the school setting, school psychologists may be called upon to consult with parents of children and adolescents with GAD as well. Given that parents often unintentionally enable or reinforce their children's anxiety through their own parenting approach, school psychologists may offer parent training or psychoeducation directed at modifying parenting techniques or broadening their skill set. In order to minimize adverse reactions in the child with anxiety, parents should be taught the importance of consistency in their responses, positivity in their interactions, and clarity in their expectations with their child (Huberty, 2014). These simple strategies may promote a stronger parent–child bond and security and stability for the child or adolescent with GAD.

Counseling/Therapy Role

In any intervention undertaken because of anxiety experienced in the school system, Huberty (2014) indicates that a goal of complete elimination of symptoms would be unhelpful and unrealistic. Rather, school psychologists should aim to assist students in managing their symptoms in a way that facilitates the child's or adolescent's overall adjustment. In support of the idea that improvement of symptoms produces multiplicative positive effects, Wood (2006) found that parents reported perceived improvement in their child's school performance as their symptoms of anxiety reduced due to therapeutic intervention. This may be due to greater levels of engagement by the children or to increased attentional resources for the schoolwork.

One of the most consistently effective interventions used to address children's and adolescent's symptoms of GAD is cognitive behavioral therapy, which focuses on the interactions of the student's thoughts, feelings, and behaviors. (See the section in this chapter titled "School-Based Mental Health Interventions and Supports" for a more thorough treatment of this topic.) Mychailyszyn et al. (2011) has also highlighted the school environment as an appropriate venue for delivery. Yet, despite the promise of cognitive behavioral therapy as an effective intervention for children with GAD and its amenability to school-based delivery, Creed et al. (2015) suggest that its actual practice within the school setting has been insufficient to the need and effectiveness of this evidenced-based practice. As such, school psychologists should look to expand their offering of cognitive behavioral therapy to address the prevalent anxiety issues of children and adolescents in that setting. Creed et al. (2015) specifically promote the use of cognitive behavioral therapy in schools due to the unique opportunities that it offers for students to practice their new skills in a setting where they may be experiencing significant anxiety. However, in order to promote this expanded practice, school psychologists should also be aware of the barriers to its use and success. In their research, Pella et al. (2018) found that over 45% of their child participants reported worrying about missing academic content while attending school-based therapy, over 37% expressed fears related to the taboo of mental health services, and nearly 37% feared questions from their classmates about leaving class for therapy. Yet, children and adolescents still maintain higher rates for therapy attendance in schools than in community-based facilities (Atkins et al., 2006).

EDUCATIONAL SUPPORTS

Given that issues with anxiety may specifically inhibit focused attention to classroom work, students with GAD may benefit from any of a number of teaching strategies to focus their efforts on the task at hand and manage their associated symptoms. Huberty (2014) offers a myriad of simple strategies to address the needs of children and adolescents with anxiety in the classroom. These include structuring classroom routines for consistency so that students know what is to be expected in the sequence of classroom activities at any given time, thereby reducing the anxiety associated with the unknown. With regard to classroom performance, both expectations for academic output and their affiliated evaluation should be clear. Assignments can be modified for presentation in smaller components to minimize their intimidation for students, and students can be taught to subdivide assignments themselves to increase their coping skills toward potentially overwhelming academic stimuli. Finally, using peer models to practice social skills and prompting the child to use relaxation strategies can help with overall classroom adjustment (Huberty, 2014).

SCHOOL-BASED MENTAL HEALTH INTERVENTIONS AND SUPPORTS

Research consistently indicates that children and adolescents with GAD are highly amenable to treatment. Imran et al. (2017) notes that therapy should be the first-line approach. Specifically, cognitive behavioral therapy has documented success across a number of research studies of children with GAD (Imran et al., 2017; Ishikawa et al., 2007; Keeton et al., 2009; McLoone et al., 2006; Rapee, 2000; Wood, 2006). Clinical research in this area has demonstrated that up to 80% of children with anxiety may exhibit long-lasting improvements in their symptomatology after treatment with cognitive behavioral therapy (Barrett et al., 2001; Rapee, 2000). In children and adolescents with GAD, cognitive behavioral therapy combined with prescription medications (i.e., selective serotonin reuptake inhibitors [SSRIs]) has been shown to have positive impacts beyond either cognitive behavioral therapy or medication use alone (Creswell et al., 2014; Imran et al., 2017; Piacentini et al., 2014). However, parents have reported a preference and greater acceptability for cognitive behavioral therapy as an intervention for their children's anxiety over the use of pharmacological-based treatment (Brown et al., 2007; Chavira et al., 2003). They also note a belief that cognitive behavioral therapy is more credible than prescription drugs in the treatment of children's anxiety (Brown et al., 2007).

Parents have reported a preference and greater acceptability for cognitive behavioral therapy as an intervention for their children's anxiety over the use of pharmacological-based treatment (Brown et al., 2007; Chavira et al., 2003).

Cognitive behavioral therapy uses techniques like relaxation, role playing, journaling, graduated exposure to anxiety producing stimuli, and cognitive restructuring to assist the child in reformulating unhelpful thoughts. School psychologists commonly have training and experience in conducting cognitive behavioral therapy, and research suggests that it may be effectively delivered in the school setting. Delivery by trained therapists during the standard school day minimizes academic time lost due to outside appointments and reduces the financial and logistical strain for families in seeking treatment for children with mental health conditions (Creed et al., 2013, 2015).

McLoone et al. (2006) specifically highlight the use of two cognitive behavioral therapy programs for the treatment of anxiety within the school setting. The first program is called *Cool Kids* and is delivered in small-group format (Misfud & Rapee, 2005). The *Cool Kids* program features 10 1-hour sessions. It is recommended that groups be composed of approximately six students. The program is appropriate for use with children and adolescents aged 7 to 16, but it is important for the group members to be relatively homogeneous in age. In addition to the student sessions that are led by a trained therapist (like a school psychologist), there are also two meetings between the facilitator and a parent of each participant. These sessions take place prior to the start of the group and at the midpoint. They serve to educate parents on the expectations for the group and to promote their engagement in the process. The aims of the group are to reduce children's and adolescent's overall anxious symptomatology but also to advance their skills in confronting and managing situations that trigger their fears. The *Cool Kids* program has demonstrated significant success in the reduction of anxiety based on child, parent, and teacher report of symptoms (Misfud & Rapee, 2005).

The second program described by McLoone et al. (2006) for use in the schools is the FRIENDS program developed by Lowry-Webster et al. (2001). This program is implemented at the classroom level (primary or secondary) by a trained teacher who serves as facilitator and is considered a prevention strategy. Lowry-Webster et al. (2001) note that a particular advantage of the FRIENDS program is that it eliminates the stigma associated with intervention since it is delivered to all children in the classroom rather than a pull-out group of selected students. The FRIENDS program uses exposure and relaxation techniques to reduce anxiety and fears over 10 sessions lasting an hour each. The program builds skills to allow the child to increase their social circle through activities with peer group members. There are also three parent sessions to educate parents on the group goals and process and to teach some behavioral reinforcement strategies. In clinical studies, over 75% of children and adolescents in the FRIENDS program are able to reduce their symptoms of anxiety to subclinical levels upon completion of the group (Shortt et al., 2001).

A final program for treatment of GAD in children and adolescents worth noting for the treatment of GAD in children and adolescents is perhaps the most popular, well-researched, and widely adapted cognitive behavioral therapy. It is the Coping Cat program. The Coping Cat offers manualized treatment for children ages 7 to 17 across its childhood and adolescent curricula. The program includes the following four components: comprehending physical and emotional responses to anxiety, identifying thoughts in anxious situations, creating plans to cope with anxiety, and self-assessment of performance. The 16-week program features 50- minute sessions and a parent component. The program is available in English, Chinese, Hungarian, Spanish, Japanese, and Norwegian. Its effectiveness in reducing anxiety in short- and long-term research has been established (Kendall, 1994; Kendall & Southam-Gerow, 1996; Lenz, 2015; McNally Keehn et al., 2013; Norris & Kendall, 2020; Oldham-Cooper & Loades, 2017; Santesteban-Echarri et al., 2018). Thus, school psychologists have a variety of evidenced-based treatment protocols to choose from to assist children and adolescents with improvement of their GAD within the school setting.

CASE STUDY 8.1 MIA: CASE OF A WHITE FEMALE WITH GENERALIZED ANXIETY DISORDER

Background

Mia is a 13-year-old girl from a middle-class family in the Midwest. Mia is described as a child who has worried about everything from birth. She is shy, quiet, and very compliant. Mia's family consists of herself, her mother (Susan), her father (John), and her older brother (Sam, 16 years old). Their extended family lives out of town, but the maternal and paternal grandparents play an important role in the family's lives. Susan has her bachelor's degree and is currently working as an office manager in a local chiropractic office. John has a bachelor's degree and is currently employed as an insurance agent, working from home and occasionally traveling for work. Susan and John expect their children to further their education and life goals by either going to a technical school, going into the military, or pursuing a 4-year degree. Susan mentioned that she wants to make sure that she has prepared her daughter to support herself before she enters into any relationship. Primary caregiving is split between Susan and John. According to Susan, Mia has five close female friends that she has made at school and while in the school band. These friends are around Mia's same age. When interacting with her friends, Mia has mostly verbal interactions, video chatting to discuss schoolwork, and playing video games while video chatting to communicate on the game they are playing together. However, over the past year she has played less and less with her friends. If she continues in this direction, Susan believes she will have no friends.

Mia is described by her teachers as being a decent student for the most part. However, her attendance is spotty, and her math grade has been dropping. She has missed several days due to a stomachache. Her pediatrician can find no reason for her stomach problems and refers to it as her *nervous stomach*. Her teacher has indicated that her concentration varies at times. She stated that Mia "zones out" frequently in class. Mia's grades are all Bs except for in mathematics, where she has a low C (72). Susan mentioned that Mia has usually had lower grades in mathematics compared to her other courses, but this was the first year that she has been this low. Mia's favorite subjects this year are English and history. Her least favorite subject is mathematics. Susan has mentioned that Mia seems to be showing more frustration with mathematics homework than in her previous grades. She seems to "short circuit" and just stop functioning. Before and after working on homework, Mia seems to get incredibly anxious. Her insecurity, need for constant reassurance, and school absenteeism are frustrating and upsetting for her parents.

Mia states that when she was younger, she worried about dying. She doesn't recall any specific cause of death. She just worried about it. Mia is currently worried she will not be able to get into college and that she is a failure. No matter how she does on a test, she believes it is not good enough. She stated that she cannot even discuss homework or tests with her friends or she "shuts down." Mia does not think her friends "get" her and has been withdrawing from them. She states she is unable to control her worrying and cannot discuss it with her parents. It is overwhelming and occurs all the time. Accompanying this excessive and uncontrollable worry are difficulty falling asleep, impatience with others, and difficulty focusing at school.

Discussion

The intensity, frequency, and duration of anxiety is out of proportion to anything occurring in Mia's life. She is worried about her school performance and being able to get into college, but her worry is extremely excessive. Her worry is not controllable and has been going on for quite some time. She has difficulty falling asleep, is impatient, and has trouble focusing. Her relationships and academics are suffering due to the anxiety.

Mia is struggling with her peer relationships. Most of her contact is electronic, and she continues to withdraw from those contacts. She is less likely to enter social situations, initiate social contact, feel comfortable with strangers, and participate in group activities. Her academics continue to decline, specifically her math grade. Math can be challenging, because there is a clear right and wrong. Math is self-reinforcing. An individual struggling is aware of the struggle, and this can add to the anxiety.

(continued)

CASE STUDY 8.1 MIA: CASE OF A WHITE FEMALE WITH GENERALIZED ANXIETY DISORDER (continued)

A comprehensive assessment of Mia and her academic performance would be helpful. With this information, the team could decide how to intervene with her math issues. It should also help in developing a clear plan to deal with the absenteeism. It would also guide the team in the best approach to use to deal with her anxiety and social interactions. The academic intervention would occur in the school and may occur at home. The anxiety and social interaction would most likely need to be addressed with counseling or therapy. This may occur at school with the school psychologist or outside the school with a private practitioner. Cognitive behavioral therapy would be a good method to deal with her issues. It utilizes techniques like relaxation, role playing, journaling, graduated exposure to anxiety-producing stimuli, and cognitive restructuring to assist the child in reformulating unhelpful thoughts. It can also develop Mia's skills in confronting and managing situations that trigger her fears of failure. It can also help her understand the physical and emotional responses to anxiety. From all of these, she can begin to work with the therapist to develop a plan to cope with anxiety. If a private practitioner is used, the school psychologist may then work in a consultative role with the practitioner. He or she can gather data or conduct some check-ins with Mia. The school psychologist may also work with teachers to share some simple strategies they can use in the classroom to address the needs of children and adolescents with anxiety in the classroom. For example, structuring classroom routines for consistency to help Mia reduce her anxiety associated with the unknown. Give her clear expectations for academic performance and how she will be evaluated. Assignments can be modified for presentation in smaller components to minimize her intimidation, especially in math assignments. Mia's symptoms are intense, but with a comprehensive assessment and data-driven interventions, Mia's anxiety can be managed.

SUMMARY POINTS

- In order to apply a *DSM-5* diagnosis of GAD, a clinician must distinguish between the anxiety that most of us experience throughout life and the extreme levels of anxiety associated with GAD.
- With regard to etiology, the school psychologist should remember that both genetic and environmental factors play a role in the development of GAD.
- Homes that include a child with GAD may face serious consequences if the student exhibits school-refusal behaviors.
- The anxiety symptoms may inhibit a student's ability to focus on academic content in the classroom.
- School psychologists can engage in many roles and functions to support the needs of students with GAD, including assessment, advocacy, consultation, and counseling and/or therapy.
- Cognitive behavioral therapy has demonstrated effectiveness in the treatment of children and adolescents with GAD.

TEST YOUR KNOWLEDGE

1. A student with GAD may qualify for special education services under which IDEA category?
   a. Anxiety Disorders
   b. Emotional Disturbance
   c. Specific Learning Disability
   d. Intellectual Disability

2. A student with GAD automatically meets criteria for Emotional Disturbance under IDEA.
   a. True
   b. False

3. Research does not support a genetic component to GAD.
   a. True
   b. False

4. Which of the following is often an early-warning sign for school refusal?
   a. Lack of participation in extracurricular activities
   b. Peer relationship concerns
   c. Test anxiety
   d. Frequent visits to the nurse's office

5. Cognitive behavioral therapy and SSRIs are more effective together than cognitive behavioral therapy alone in the treatment of children and adolescents with GAD.
   a. True
   b. False

Answers: (1) b, (2) b, (3) b, (4) d, (5) a.

DISCUSSION QUESTIONS

1. Describe the *DSM-5* diagnostic criteria for GAD.
2. Highlight the IDEA criteria for eligibility under the category of Emotional Disturbance.
3. List the genetic factors that may contribute to the development of GAD.
4. Explain the school psychologist's consultation role in working with children with GAD.
5. Detail one evidenced-based social–emotional intervention for students with GAD.

CHAPTER RESOURCES

American Academy of Child and Adolescent Psychiatry *Anxiety Disorders Resource Center*: www.aacap.org/AACAP/Families_and_Youth/Resource_Centers/Anxiety_Disorder_Resource_Center/Home.aspx

American Academy of Child and Adolescent Psychiatry *Anxiety Disorders: Parents' Medication Guide*: www.aacap.org/App_Themes/AACAP/docs/resource_centers/resources/med_guides/anxiety-parents-medication-guide.pdf

Anxiety and Depression Association of America *Childhood Anxiety Disorders*: https://adaa.org/find-help/by-demographics/children/childhood-anxiety-disorders

Centers for Disease Control and Prevention *Anxiety and Depression in Children*: www.cdc.gov/childrensmentalhealth/depression.html

Mayo Clinic *Antidepressants for Children and Teens*: www.mayoclinic.org/diseases-conditions/teen-depression/in-depth/antidepressants/art-20047502

Merck Manual *Overview of Anxiety Disorders in Children and Adolescents*: www.merckmanuals.com/professional/pediatrics/mental-disorders-in-children-and-adolescents/overview-of-anxiety-disorders-in-children-and-adolescents

National Association of School Psychologists *Anxiety and Anxiety Disorders in Children: Information for Parents*: www.nasponline.org/resources-and-publications/resources-and-podcasts/mental-health/mental-health-disorders/anxiety-and-anxiety-disorders-in-children-information-for-parents

Stanford Children's Health *Generalized Anxiety Disorder in Children and Teens*: www.stanfordchildrens.org/en/topic/default?id=generalized-anxiety-disorder-in-children-and-adolescents-90-P02565

KEY REFERENCES

Only key references appear in the print edition. The full reference list appears in the digital product on Springer Publishing Connect: connect.springerpub.com/content/book/978-0-8261-3587-2/part/part04/chapter/ch08

Alfano, C., Beidel, D., & Wong, N. (2011). Children with generalized anxiety disorder do not have peer problems, just fewer friends. *Child Psychiatry and Human Development, 42*(6), 712–723. https://doi.org/10.1007/s10578-011-0245-2

American Psychiatric Association. (2013). *Diagnostic and statistical manual of mental disorders* (5th ed.). https://doi.org/10.1176/appi.books.9780890425596

Costello, E. J., Mustillo, S., Erkanli, A., Keeler, G., & Angold, A. (2003). Prevalence and development of psychiatric disorders in childhood and adolescence. *Archives of General Psychiatry, 60*, 837–844. https://doi.org/10.1001/archpsyc.60.8.837

Eley, T. C., Bolton, D., O'Connor, T. G., Perrin, S., Smith, P., & Plomin, R. (2003). A twin study of anxiety-related behaviours in pre-school children. *Journal of Child Psychology and Psychiatry, 44*(7), 945–960. https://doi.org/10.1111/1469-7610.00179

Imran, N., Haider, I. I., & Azeem, M. W. (2017). Generalized anxiety disorder in children and adolescents: An update. *Psychiatric Annals, 47*(10), 497–501. https://doi.org/10.3928/00485713-20170913-01

Jarrett, M. A., Black, A. K., Rapport, H. F., Grills-Taquechel, A. E., & Ollendick, T. H. (2015). Generalized anxiety disorder in younger and older children: Implications for learning and school functioning. *Journal of Child and Family Studies, 24*, 992–1003. https://doi.org/10.1007/s10826-014-9910-y

Keeton, C. P., Kolos, A. C., & Walkup, J. T. (2009). Pediatric generalized anxiety disorder: Epidemiology, diagnosis, and management. *Pediatric Drugs, 11*(3), 171–183. https://doi.org/10.2165/00148581-200911030-00003

Kendler, K. S., Gardner, C. O., & Prescott, C. A. (2002). Toward a comprehensive developmental model for major depression in women. *American Journal of Psychiatry, 159*, 1133–1145. https://doi.org/10.1176/appi.ajp.159.7.1133

Kessler, R. C., McLaughlin, K. A., Koenen, K. C., Petukhova, M., & Hill, E. D. (2012). The importance of secondary trauma exposure for post-disaster mental disorder. *Epidemiology and Psychiatric Sciences, 21*(1), 35–45. https://doi.org/10.1017/s2045796011000758

Van Ameringen, M., Mancini, C., & Farvolden, P. (2003). The impact of anxiety disorders on educational achievement. *Anxiety Disorders, 17*, 561–571. https://doi.org/10.1016/s0887-6185(02)00228-1

CHAPTER 9

Separation Anxiety Disorder

LEARNING OBJECTIVES

- Differentiate the revised *Diagnostic and Statistical Manual of Mental Disorders* (5th ed.; *DSM-5*; American Psychiatric Association [APA], 2013) criteria for Separation Anxiety Disorder (SAD) from the *DSM-IV* (APA, 1994) and earlier *DSM* versions.
- Understand how federal protections for education (e.g., Individuals with Disabilities Education Improvement Act [IDEA] and Section 504) may apply to students who have a *DSM-5* diagnosis of SAD.
- Gain knowledge about prevalence, comorbidity, risk factors, and correlates of SAD from a culturally sensitive perspective.
- Identify well-validated assessments and interventions for SAD.

INTRODUCTION

Separation Anxiety Disorder (SAD) is listed in the *Diagnostic and Statistical Manual of Mental Disorders* (5th ed.; *DSM-5*) under the category of Anxiety Disorders (American Psychiatric Association [APA], 2013). Based on revisions made in the *DSM-5*, adults can now receive this diagnosis. Children and adolescents with a *DSM-5* diagnosis of SAD experience extreme debilitating fear and anxiety when anticipating or actually separating from key attachment figures, such as parents and caregivers. SAD symptoms have a potentially profound negative impact on all aspects of life functioning, including academics, behavior, social–emotional/mental health functioning, as well as peer and adult relationships.

Evidence-supported treatments for SAD exist, particularly cognitive behavioral therapy (CBT). School psychologists are in a unique position to support children/adolescents and their families who have a *DSM-5* SAD diagnosis through provision of a wide range of direct (i.e., cognitive behavioral interventions) and indirect (i.e., consultation, psychoeducation, data monitoring) roles.

DIAGNOSTIC ISSUES: *DSM-5* AND SCHOOL-BASED SERVICES

DSM-5 Diagnostic Criteria

According to the APA's (2013) *DSM-5*, SAD falls under the category of Anxiety Disorders (coded as 309.21; APA, 2013). According to the APA, "separation anxiety disorder [SAD] is excessive fear or anxiety concerning separation from home or attachment figures" (APA, 2016, p. 4). Under the *DSM-5*, clinicians must consider four main criteria for a diagnosis of SAD (APA, 2013). The first major inclusionary criterion has to do with extreme fear or anxiety with regard to being separated from major attachment figures (APA, 2013, p. 190). For this category to be met, the individual must meet *three of eight specific criteria*. The first two criteria are as follows: (a) the individual is very worried or distressed when expecting and/or actually encountering separation from an attachment figure; (b) the individual is highly fearful that other close persons (i.e., parent, caregiver) or they themselves will be seriously hurt. As one example, the individual may fear being struck with a dreaded disease that would cause separation from a loved one. A third criteria, which has a clear impact on school and academic functioning, is that the individual is very reluctant to leave the attachment figure because of anxiety caused by separation. This criteria, if present among children and adolescents who have SAD, may be particularly debilitating for school and academic performance because it could result in refusal to attend school. Additional *DSM-5* criteria include anxiety over being on one's own without the attachment person, concerns about sleeping without the attachment figure being visible, somatic symptoms when thinking about or actually separating from the attachment figure, and nightmares about separation.

To make a *DSM-5* diagnosis of SAD, a clinician must also consider how long the fear or anxiety about separation from attachment figures has been present. The length of time required for the diagnosis is minimally 4 weeks for children and adolescents, whereas it is 6 months or more in adults.

An additional component that must be present for a diagnosis of SAD is that there must be a clinically significant impact on major areas of functioning, such as social, academic, occupational, or other critical areas. Academic and social development are critical development areas for school-aged children and adolescents. Therefore, school psychologists should be mindful of academic performance and how symptoms of SAD may be impacting the willingness of children and adolescents to attend school due to excessive anxiety over being separated from key attachment figures. Relatedly, children and adolescents with SAD may be misunderstood by school personnel as having chronic truancy, which could lead to discipline referrals and punitive school responses rather than social–emotional support and mental health treatment. The final category that must be met for a diagnosis of SAD is that another *DSM-5* diagnosis is not a better fit for what is being observed. For example, the *DSM-5* offers different diagnoses to consider, such as autism, psychoses, agoraphobia (fear of going outside), or another type of anxiety disorder, such as generalized anxiety disorder (GAD)/illness anxiety disorder (APA, 2013).

Changes in Separation Anxiety Disorder Diagnostic Criteria: *DSM-IV* to *DSM-5*

The most notable change in the SAD diagnostic criteria in *DSM-5* (APA, 2013), compared with the *DSM-IV* (APA, 1994), is that SAD was moved from the category of disorders "Usually Diagnosed in Infancy, Childhood and Adolescence" to fall under "Anxiety Disorders" (APA, 2013; Center for Behavioral Health Statistics and Quality, 2016). As a result, adults can now be diagnosed with SAD (Center for Behavioral Health Statistics and Quality, 2016). Related changes made to the updated *DSM-5* (APA, 2013) concern the duration of SAD symptoms for adults as 6 months or longer, dropping the required onset before 18 years of age, an additional functional impact of SAD is now work, as well as some changes to the diagnoses that clinicians must rule out (i.e., autism, symptoms of illness identity disorder, and generalized identity disorder (Center for Behavioral Health Statistics and Quality, 2016). The specifier of early onset before age 6 years was also dropped. Practically speaking, the changes specific to adult onset will not likely impact the daily work of school psychologists working primarily with children and adolescents. However, the early-onset specifier may impact professionals working with young children in early-childhood settings.

The main changes to the *DSM-5* criteria for making a diagnosis of separation anxiety is that it now falls under the Anxiety Disorder category and adults can receive this diagnosis (APA, 2013).

Applications to the Individuals With Disabilities Education Improvement Act

A student with a *DSM-5* (APA, 2013) diagnosis of SAD needs to have symptoms and behaviors that meet the criterion for one of 13 special education categories defined under the Individuals with Disabilities Education Improvement Act (IDEA; 2004) to receive special education and related services (i.e., counseling/psychological services) through an Individual Education Program (IEP). School psychologists play a large role in conducting special education evaluations as part of a multidisciplinary team and contribute to the development and execution of IEPs with students who qualify. Although no research was found that provided data about the percentage of students diagnosed with SAD who also meet the special education criteria, the category of "emotional disturbance" (IDEA, 2004) has several potential overlapping symptoms and behaviors with SAD. The criteria for Emotional Disturbance are as follows:

(i) Emotional disturbance means a condition exhibiting one or more of the following characteristics over a long period of time and to a marked degree that adversely affects a child's educational performance:
(A) An inability to learn that cannot be explained by intellectual, sensory, or health factors.
(B) An inability to build or maintain satisfactory interpersonal relationships with peers and teachers.
(C) Inappropriate types of behavior or feelings under normal circumstances.
(D) A general pervasive mood of unhappiness or depression.
(E) A tendency to develop physical symptoms or fears associated with personal or school problems.
(ii) Emotional disturbance includes schizophrenia. The term does not apply to children who are socially maladjusted, unless it is determined that they have an emotional disturbance under paragraph (c) (4) (i) of this section. (IDEA, 2004, Section 300.8 (c) (4))

For a student to qualify under the Emotional Disturbance category, one might argue that children with SAD are not able to have satisfactory interpersonal relationships with those in school due to anxiety and distress about being away from key attachment figures. One could also argue that children with SAD show somatic (physical) symptoms or fears associated with SAD-related anxiety. In order to become eligible for any special education category, an adverse effect on educational performance must also be present. In other words, children with SAD may have significant anxiety and interpersonal challenges but if they are performing adequately in school, they would not typically qualify under IDEA (2004). Although each individual case is different, many children with SAD would most likely be excluded from receiving special education services through eligibility for the Emotional Disturbance category. School psychologists are key players who make such judgments as part of a multidisciplinary team and are looked upon for their expertise in disentangling the origins and impact of social–emotional and behavioral concerns in the educational context. Recent data provided by the U.S. Department of Education Office of Special Education Programs (OSEP; 2020) indicate that the percentage of students with disabilities (special education eligibility and IEPs) who qualify under the category of Emotional Disturbance is only 5.45%, with a wide range reported by states (from 1.65% to 17.36%). These data reflect that in most cases, a relatively low percentage of children qualify for special education under the category of Emotional Disturbance. These findings are in contrast with the national data showing that children show much higher rates of mental health issues and disorders, including anxiety-related disorders like SAD. For example, one national study shows that the prevalence of children with at least one mental health disorder is estimated at 16.5%, with nearly half (49.4%) of those meeting this criteria not having access to mental health treatment (Whitney & Peterson, 2019).

Applications to Section 504 of the Rehabilitation Act of 1973

It is arguably more likely that students who have a *DSM-5* (APA, 2013) diagnosis of SAD would qualify for educational protections under Section 504 of the Rehabilitation Act of 1973 rather than for special education services under IDEA (2004). Under Section 504 "individuals with disabilities are defined as persons with a physical or mental impairment which substantially limits one or more major life activities" (U.S. Department of Education Office for Civil Rights [OCR], 2006, para. 3). Mental and psychological disorders are included in this definition, but a designated list is not offered through the statute due to concerns over not being inclusive (OCR, 2016). Although learning is included in the description of the major life activities impacted by one's disability, along with others (i.e., seeing, hearing, thinking, etc.), OCR cautions that school districts should not only consider how learning is impacted, but if and how the disability may impact the student's participation in any of the school's programs and offerings (2016). Essentially, Section 504 (1973) ensures that students are not discriminated against due to their disability status under Section 504 and should be provided the same access that students without disabilities would have. In order to comply with Section 504, school districts must ensure, similar to IDEA, that students with disabilities have access to a free and appropriate public education (FAPE; 2016). To meet the FAPE standard, it is incumbent upon the school district to show how it is meeting the needs of students with disabilities just as it does for children without disabilities through the "provision of regular or special education and related aids and services" (2016, p. 11). Therefore, in practice there are many processes and procedures that are similar in both IDEA and Section 504, which include appropriate evaluation and placement activities, as well as reevaluation and due-process rights of families (i.e., right to receive notice, right to a hearing; 2016). Although not technically required under the Section 504 mandates, most school districts outline how they are in compliance through a formal written 504 plan, which contains the educational services being provided. Unlike IDEA (2004), which requires that the disability has an adverse effect on educational performance, this is not the case for Section 504 (2016). School psychologists have an important role as part of a team charged with conducting Section 504 evaluations and determining appropriate educational supports. Examples of Section 504 accommodations and supports that might be provided to a student who has SAD could be a behavior plan/anxiety reduction intervention (practicing coping skills when separated from loved ones; Kendall & Hedtke, 2006), collaboration with parents, consultation with teachers, and providing social skills training.

> Children with SAD may qualify for special education services under IDEA (2004), with the most likely category being Emotional Dsturbance. It is more likely that students with SAD will qualify for a Section 504 plan.

Prevalence and Onset of Separation Anxiety Disorder

Time will tell how the changes made to the *DSM-5* (APA, 2013) will impact estimated prevalence rates of SAD, as studies are completed relatively infrequently due to the large-scale nature of most of the studies published. The prevalence data that are available have varied outcomes, which depend on a range of factors, including how the data are collected (Vaughan et al., 2017). Further, most of the available studies are not based on the *DSM-5* but early versions of the *DSM*.

U.S. Studies

The available epidemiological studies paint a picture of how common SAD is among children, adolescents and adults, with adult-onset being relatively common (Shear et al., 2006). As one example, Shear et al. (2006) reported prevalence of common *DSM-IV* (APA, 1994) disorders using data gathered through the National Comorbidity Survey Replication (NCS-R) study (Kessler & Merikangas, 2004) with a U.S. national community sample. These data were collected by nonclinical lay persons. The NCS-R findings were that the estimated lifetime prevalence of SAD among children was 4.1%, whereas it was 6.6% in adults. Lifetime prevalence means that a case is counted if it happens at least once in a person's life (National Institute of Mental Health, 2017). The authors also reported that most individuals who met their criteria for adult SAD cases experienced an initial onset as adults (77.5%), showing evidence in support of adding an adult-age onset for SAD to the *DSM-5* (APA, 2013) criteria. In addition, their findings were that a high percentage of children who have SAD continue to meet the criteria as adults (36.1%), showing evidence that SAD is often a long-term struggle. School psychologists have a critical role in identifying children at risk for SAD and advocating for treatment to prevent lifelong distress that is prevalent based on these findings.

In a similar study focused on adolescents (ages 13–17) and adults (18–64), Kessler et al. (2012) reported the prevalence of SAD using the NCS-R (Kessler & Merikangas, 2004) survey and a supplement to it used for adolescents (NCS-A; Merikangas et al., 2009). For the entire sample of all anxiety disorders (not including specific and social phobias), SAD had the highest lifetime prevalence at 6.7% (followed by posttraumatic stress disorder [PTSD] at 5.7%). Further, adolescents had higher estimated rates of SAD compared with adults. Among adolescents, lifetime prevalence rates were significantly higher for females (9.5%) compared with males (5.9%). Among adults, females also had significantly higher rates of SAD (8.2%) compared with males (4.7%). Kessler et al. (2012) also reported 12-month prevalence rates (meeting criteria for SAD in the year prior to the survey completion) as 1.5% for adolescents and 1% for adults. The authors compared the ratios of 12-month prevalence to lifetime prevalence estimates (12 months/lifetime prevalence), finding a very low ratio for SAD, meaning that only roughly 20% of the identified lifetime cases were presented in the 12 months before the study was conducted. Kessler et al. (2012) interpreted this finding as due to the more common resolution of SAD as children transition to adolescents relative to other *DSM* disorders. Kessler et al. (2012) also reported the lifetime morbid risk (LMR) ratio, which is another metric used to understand prevalence. These authors describe how the LMR ratio includes both a prediction of how many people are expected to get a particular disorder and who already meets criteria for it at the time of a study. Kessler et al. (2012) note that this is a less frequently reported metric (Oakley-Browne et al., 2006, as cited in Kessler et al., 2012) but one that is important for policy and treatment planning. SAD had the highest ratios (along with phobias) of lifetime prevalence compared with LMR projections, indicating that most of the adolescent and adult participants who would ever be likely to meet the SAD study criteria at any time in their lives would already have done so by the time they participated in the study. Further, the age of onset was the earliest for both SAD and phobias compared with the other *DSM-IV* (APA, 1994) disorders.

Lewinsohn et al. (2008) provide additional information about the prevalence of SAD as well as age-of-onset data, based on a community sample from Oregon that participated in a longitudinal study. The average age of onset was among the youngest in their sample, at roughly 7 years of age with an estimated duration of 3 years. In addition, only roughly 6% of adolescents who met the SAD criteria prior to age 16 years (the first point of contact) continued to do so when they were assessed again at age 17 (the second point of contact).

There are many different metrics used to determine the prevalence rates of SAD and other mental health disorders. In one U.S. study, Shear et al. (2006) estimated the lifetime prevalence of SAD in children at 4.1%, and 6.6% in adults.

Worldwide and International Studies

As part of the World Health Organization (WHO) World Mental Health Survey Initiative, surveys were conducted through in-person interviews across 17 countries located throughout Africa, the Americas (e.g., the United States, Mexico and Columbia), the Middle East, Europe, and Asia (Kessler et al., 2007). Kessler et al. (2007) conducted one of the largest worldwide epidemiological studies to date, with over 85,000 study participants. Lay interviewers conducted these assessments, which resulted in *DSM-IV* and *International Classification of Diseases, Tenth Revision* (ICD-10; WHO, 1991), diagnoses. The findings specific to anxiety disorders are the most relevant to SAD. Kessler and colleagues found that among anxiety disorders, SAD and phobias had an early age of onset, with medians that ranged from 7 to 14. Kessler et al. also reported interquartile ranges (IQR) from a low of 25th percentile (8 years old) to the 75th percentile (age of 11). One can see the earlier age of onset among those diagnosed with SAD in contrast with other anxiety disorders, such as GAD, panic disorder (PD) and PTSD. For these three disorders, the median age of diagnosis ranged from 24 to 50, with the lower (25th IQR) age of 31 and the higher (75th IQR) of 41. These findings are consistent with the Kessler et al. (2012) study, which showed a relatively early age of onset for SAD compared to other disorders, particularly anxiety disorders.

Mohammadi et al. (2020) conducted a more recent prevalence study of SAD using a national community sample of Iranian children and adolescents (ages 6–18), resulting in 29,699 participants. Clinical psychologists trained researchers to use a semi-structured interview, the Persian version of the Kiddie Schedule for Affective Disorders and Schizophrenia Present and Lifetime (K-SADS-PL; Ghanizadeh et al., 2006) to evaluate the percentage of the sample that met criteria for a wide range of mental health disorders. The SAD prevalence rates for the total sample were 5.3%, with no significant difference found by gender, unlike Kessler et al. (2012) reported previously. Mohammadi et al.

(2020) also found that SAD prevalence rates were highest among the younger children in the sample (ages 6–9) at 7.2%. These researchers also found higher rates of SAD prevalence in urban (5.6%) participants compared with those living in rural settings (3.5%).

> Compared with other anxiety disorders, SAD and phobias have an earlier age of onset (Kessler et al., 2007).

Comorbidity and Stability of Separation Anxiety Disorder With Other *DSM-5* Disorders

There have been several studies that have looked at the comorbidity and long-term predictability of SAD with other disorders. For example, Kearney et al. (2003) evaluated a sample of 60 Nevada preschool children using *DSM-IV* criteria (APA, 1994), finding that most of the children who met the criteria for SAD when they were, on the average, three-and-one-half years old did not continue to do so at a three-and-a-half-year follow-up assessment. The sample size was fairly small, particularly when comparing the nine who met full SAD criteria initially with the three who continued to do so at the second touch point. However, these data do point to the lack of stability of SAD diagnoses in young children. School psychologists should be mindful when working in early-childhood settings about the developmental nature and expectations for separation and attachment of young children with their caregivers, as well as the importance of early intervention and support of families in navigating separation issues. Kearney et al. (2003) also found that children who met the SAD diagnostic criteria at age 6 were more likely to have comorbid diagnoses, based on parent ratings on the Parental Investment in Children (PICH) Separation Anxiety subscale, as well as more anxiety, somatic complaints, and internalizing concerns (at age 3 and 6) compared with children who did not have SAD symptomatology. These findings support the need for school psychologists to work with others on their team to monitor SAD symptoms in young children and to support them over time, as necessary, given the findings of this study.

In a study focused on a population of adults (average age of 34.8), deMathis et al. (2013) examined the comorbidity of obsessive-compulsive disorder (OCD) with other psychiatric diagnoses. Their sample of 1,001 participants was drawn from six cities in Brazil. Clinicians arrived at the current and lifetime *DSM-IV* (APA, 1994) psychiatric diagnosis based on interviews with the adult participants. The results were that SAD was the most common psychiatric comorbid disorder found, as well as the diagnosis with the earliest average age of onset (5.9 years of age). Further, individuals whose first psychiatric diagnosis was SAD were more likely to have PTSD when experiencing a trauma, scored significantly higher on the sexual/religious dimension of the Dimensional Yale-Brown Obsessive Compulsive Scale (DY-BOCS) and showed higher scores on the Beck Depression Inventory (Beck et al., 1961) and Beck Anxiety Inventory (Beck et al., 1988). Based on these findings, deMathias and colleagues (2013) concluded that those with a current OCD diagnosis and a history of SAD are particularly at risk for acquiring a host of anxiety-related disorders. This comorbidity study is important for school psychologists because screening for, monitoring, and treating students who either fully meet or have symptoms of SAD appears critical for mitigating student risk for acquiring additional anxiety disorders later in life. The findings with respect to PTSD are also important because school psychologists who work with students who have SAD should be mindful and aware of how exposure to trauma and related stressors may be particularly triggering for them.

Lewinsohn et al. (2008) contributed to the knowledge about comorbidity of SAD with other psychiatric disorders in their longitudinal study with a community sample in western Oregon, drawn from a larger project about adolescent depression. There were four data collection times, with the first and second times occurring when the participants were adolescents (roughly 16 and 17 years old) followed by the next two times, when they had reached adulthood (at approximately ages 24 and 30). Diagnostic interviews were conducted to determine the existence of *DSM-III-R* (APA, 1987) psychiatric diagnoses. The participants were asked to provide both current and retrospective information (i.e., lifetime prevalence) about psychiatric concerns at each data collection time period. The researchers created four separate groups of participants to test whether meeting different types of psychiatric diagnoses at 18 made any difference in predicted meeting future diagnostic psychiatric criteria as a young adult (19–30). The four groups were as follows: (a) a control group deemed to not have any psychiatric disorder besides anxiety; (b) participants who met the SAD criteria at all four data collection points; (c) a group who had been categorized as having any type of anxiety disorder besides SAD; and (d) those who had not met the criteria for any psychiatric disorder before the age of 19. The authors controlled for differing demographics in each group and comorbid disorders before the age of 19, and then calculated odds ratios through multiple hierarchical logistic regression. Based on these statistical analyses, Lewinson et al. (2008) found that those with an SAD diagnosis at age 18 had a higher chance of subsequently meeting the criteria for PD (in the age range of 19–30) compared with the other three groups. In addition, those in the study with SAD at 18 were more likely to meet the *DSM* depression criteria as young adults when compared with those who never evidenced a psychiatric disorder prior to the age of 19 and those who met the criteria for other disorder(s) except for anxiety.

Kossowsky et al. (2013) conducted a meta-analysis of 25 studies that included nearly 15,000 participants. Based on odds ratios, children with SAD were more likely to develop any type of anxiety disorder and PD at a later point, yet were not more likely to develop depression at a later point. The authors found that SAD did not predict later substance disorders, but this was based on a limited number of five studies in the meta-analysis. Kossowsky et al. (2013) argue that a developmental psychopathology approach is needed in the study of anxiety disorders, including SAD.

Aschenbrand et al. (2003) found somewhat contradictory findings to Lewinsohn et al. (2008) and Kossowsky et al. (2013) with respect to earlier SAD diagnoses predicting PD in adulthood. Their follow-up study of participants who had been treated for anxiety in a clinic the previous 5 to 9 years was a clinical sample in contrast to that of Lewinsohn et al (2008). Participants all had an earlier diagnosis of a principal anxiety disorder (based on either *DSM-III-R* [APA, 1987] or *DSM-IV* [APA, 1994] diagnoses) when they were referred for treatment between 9 and 13 years of age. At follow-up, the participants (90% agreed to be part of the follow-up) were assessed by a clinical psychologist and two advanced doctoral candidates using age-based variations of the Anxiety Disorders Interview Schedule for Children completed by the young persons and their parents (ADIS-C/ADIS-P; Silverman & Albano, 1997) and the Anxiety Disorder Interview Schedule for *DSM-IV* Lifetime (ADIS-IV-L; DiNardo et al., 1994). At the time of the follow-up study, the average age of participants was approximately 19 (with a range from 15.5 to 22.75 roughly). Aschenbrand and colleagues created groups based on a principal diagnosis, which was the primary diagnosis viewed as interfering with one's life. These groups were as follows: (a) those with a principal SAD childhood diagnosis, (b) those with a GAD diagnosis (no SAD diagnosis), and (c) those with a principal diagnosis of social phobia (no SAD diagnosis). Similar to Lewinsohn et al. study, odds ratios were calculated to determine the degree to which having a primary diagnosis of SAD as a child predicted a later mental health diagnosis as a late adolescent/young adult. Unlike the findings of Lewinsohn et al. (2008), having a diagnosis of SAD as a child did not increase the chances of meeting the diagnostic criteria for PD or agoraphobia at follow-up compared with those in the study who had other types of anxiety disorders as children (e.g., GAD and social phobia). The same findings held for major depressive disorder. However, at follow-up, those with a childhood diagnosis of SAD were more likely than their counterparts with other childhood anxiety disorders to meet the diagnostic criteria for the following types of anxiety disorders: OCD, specific types of phobias, PTSD, and acute stress disorder.

Although the findings across the two studies just reviewed differ, specifically related to the role of SAD in predicting PD, these differences could be attributed to differences in the samples. As Aschenbrand et al. (2003) point out, differing findings in their study could be due to their sample having been previously treated for anxiety. The Aschenbrand et al. (2003) sample would be considered a clinical sample, whereas the Lewinsohn et al. (2008) study was based on a community sample.

When facing trauma, children and adolescents with a history of SAD are at risk for future psychiatric disorders, such as PD (Kossowsky et al., 2013; Lewinsohn et al., 2008) and PTSD (deMathis et al., 2013).

Predictors of Separation Anxiety Disorder: Risk Factors and Correlates

There is literature that guides our understanding of risk factors and correlates of SAD. As noted by Milrod et al. (2014), "Separation anxiety has both heritable (genetic) and social (experiential/epigenetic) origins" (p. 35). Biological factors have been identified among those who are at risk for (SAD). As a neurological explanation for the origins of SAD and related anxiety disorders, researchers point to those with SAD and PD showing heightened reactions to CO_2 exposure (Esquivel et al., 2010 as cited in Battaglia, 2015; Magnotta et al., 2012 as cited in Battaglia, 2015). Lebowitz et al. (2016) found that a clinical sample of children and adolescents (between the ages of 7 and 16 years) with a *DSM-5* (APA, 2013) diagnosis of SAD had lower levels of oxytocin (OT) compared with those who had other anxiety disorders. Further, the researchers found that youths with lower OT levels were more likely to have mothers who helped them to avoid anxiety-related distress, referred to as *family accommodation* (Lebowitz et al., 2016, p. 39). Similarly, youths with lower OT levels also reported more distress at not being accommodated in their anxiety. The findings for family accommodation were based on the entire sample of participants, who had a wide range of anxiety disorders. Milrod et al. (2014) point to the potential of neural drivers of SAD being highly involved in fear circuitry when one is separated from attachment figures, with overarousal of reward mechanisms upon reunification. At the same time, Milrod and colleagues caution against concluding that these neural systems are causal, but likely related to other underlying systems in persons who have SAD, such as social and cognitive thought processes (Paquette et al., 2003, as cited in Milrod et al., 2014).

Further research should specifically examine how family accommodation plays out in SAD, which has clear implications for the role of school psychologists in understanding and facilitating the treatment of children who suffer from SAD. The Lebowitz et al. (2016) study illustrates the importance of school psychologists working with families to help their children manage their anxiety rather than entirely avoid it. Families that make accommodations for their children to avoid anxiety-related stress associated with SAD inadvertently reinforce and maintain SAD symptoms by not exposing children to anxiety triggers (i.e., parents leaving) and therefore SAD cannot be effectively treated (Philipps et al., 2020). Philipps et al. (2020) found that parents of children who had interfering symptoms (i.e., engaging in anything to keep their parent home, crying, not being able to go to sleepovers) were the most likely to engage in accommodating behaviors relative to families with low levels of SAD symptoms or moderate SAD symptoms without interfering behaviors.

> Children with SAD tend to have lower levels of oxytocin compared with children who have other types of anxiety (Lebowitz et al., 2016).

Familial and environmental risk factors have also been explored in SAD. Battaglia (2015) notes that although it is difficult to tease out the potential parental hereditary role in the development of SAD, there is evidence that children who experience adverse early life events, particularly losing or being separated from a parental through divorce or death, are at heightened risk for developing SAD, along with PD. A link between SAD and comorbidity/subsequent PD diagnosis has been found in other research described previously (Kossowski et al., 2013; Lewinsohn et al., 2008). Others have explored the role of early parental attachments in the development of SAD. For example, Sirin (2019) conducted a retrospective study in Turkey with over 1,500 college-age students who were asked to report whether they experienced acceptance or rejection by their parents as children and if they described their current romantic relationships as secure or insecure (e.g., anxious or avoidant). The participants also completed a tool to determine whether they met diagnostic criteria for adult SAD. Based on structural equation modeling, the connection between perceptions of parental rejection in childhood and having adult SAD was mediated by insecure attachment, with reports of anxious attachment being stronger than avoidant attachment. The findings show the complexities of these relationships and how close intimate relationships in adulthood are impacted by beliefs about early parental rejection and the likelihood of developing SAD as an adult. As the authors point out, the study is limited by the sample not having been diagnosed with a mental health disorder. However, it is possible that diagnostic criteria were met for one or more mental health diagnoses, but the information was not collected in this study.

CULTURAL ISSUES RELATED TO SEPARATION ANXIETY DISORDER IN YOUTH

A discussion of cultural issues in SAD and mental health disorders needs to occur in the larger context of racism found in all systems like healthcare settings and schools and related inequities in access to culturally responsive and effective mental health treatment among minoritized persons (Alegria et al., 2010; American Psychological Association, 2017). The American Academy of Pediatrics (AAP) published a position statement articulating the contributing role of racism in all forms (individual, structural and systemic) on the disparate health outcomes experienced by minority youth (Trent et al., 2019). The AAP position statement contained recommendations that included prioritizing implicit bias training for healthcare providers (i.e., pediatricians) and educators as well as conducting mental health evaluations with patients/clients who experience racism.

The U.S. Department of Health and Human Services, Office of Minority Health, established in 1986 to promote health policies that mitigate racial and ethnic bias and disparities in healthcare, publishes profiles of specific racial/ethnic minorities groups, which include disparate healthcare access and outcomes. Each profile clearly documents consistent health disparities among racial/ethnic minority youth and families, which are connected with a broader range of social health determinants (i.e., unemployment, housing discrimination, living in under-resourced areas, not having insurance, lack of qualified diverse healthcare providers (U.S. Department of Health and Human Services, 2019a). As one of many statistics documenting health outcomes, African American females in grades 9 to 12 are 60% more likely to attempt suicide compared with non-Hispanic peers (U.S. Department of Health and Human Services, 2019b). School psychologists are encouraged to access the information and resources available on the U.S. Department of Health and Human Services website, which includes important information about healthcare access and outcomes, including mental health treatment among racial/ethnic minority groups.

When working with students suspected of or diagnosed with SAD, cultural issues should be considered beyond individual student-perceived deficits, but within the larger context of biased systems. For example, French et al. (2020) offer a new framework for psychology, called *radical healing* (p. 14) in relation to trauma that shifts from focusing on individuals in psychological treatment to focusing on healing. The radical healing framework is contextualized within historical systems of racial oppression but also recognition is given to the enormous resiliency and strong cultural heritage and contributions that persons of color have made to our society.

Such a model could be applied to cultural considerations with respect to SAD. For example, when considering cultural issues specific to children and adolescents who have SAD, school psychologists should consider the daily lived experience of racism, bias, discrimination, and microaggressions that persons of color experience and how child and adult responses to separation from loved ones may be impacted by this reality. As described at the start of the chapter, one of the inclusionary criteria for a *DSM-5* diagnosis of SAD is being extremely fearful and distressed when not around a loved one (APA, 2013). Given the larger historical context of racism and recent tragic events, which include the killing of George Floyd, and many other persons of color throughout U.S. history, clinicians must consider the potentially real fear of leaving the house and everyday racism that Black and Brown persons experience (Nir, 2020). It is important not to pathologize individual behavior that may be connected to the realities of racism that Black and Brown individuals experience every day when leaving home. School psychologists must work to understand these realities while working alongside families in assessing and treating SAD-related symptoms.

Research specific to race, culture, and ethnicity with respect to SAD in children and adolescents is scant. Sood et al. (2012) studied whether acculturation to American culture, religious beliefs, and ethnicity predicted how mothers of Puerto Rican, Indian American (South Asian), and European backgrounds would interpret childhood SAD symptoms as presented in four vignettes. The participants were asked whether they would seek help from a religious leader, a mental health professional, or a physician. Mothers who were more acculturated to American culture were more likely to attribute the causes of SAD symptoms to psychological issues and to seek help from a mental health professional. Another important finding was that the mothers' identification with their own cultural heritage did not impact how they responded to SAD causes or who they would get help from. Mothers who endorsed being more religious were more likely to seek help from a religious leader. However, there were some variations within ethnic groups, as mothers who identified as Sikh were less likely than those who identified as Catholic to seek help from a religious leader (after controlling for the strength of their religion). Sood et al. (2012) note that these findings underscore the importance of not generalizing findings from one religious group to another. Further, the authors stress how limited the psychology and mental health work is to date with respect to the study of South Asians. The recent rise in hate crimes, violence, and racism with Asian American Pacific Islanders (AAPIs), connected with centuries long anti-AAPI racism and violence and racist trauma, underscores the need for more work and understanding (Truong et al., 2021).

Sood et al. (2012) also found that mothers who identified as Puerto Rican, compared with mothers who identified as European American, were more likely to attribute medical causes to SAD symptoms. The authors interpreted their findings as important for treatment goals to be co-constructed with the children and families of Puerto Rican backgrounds who may be more likely to stress how the mind and body are connected. They also draw on prior research in their conclusions, which supports that Latinx children may experience mental health concerns as physical (somatic) complaints (Pina & Silverman, 2004, as cited in Sood et al., 2012). Latinx newcomers and recent immigrants may be particularly prone to mental health concerns due to trauma, including racist and xenophobic trauma they may have experienced, which may particularly be the case in recent years among Latinx immigrant populations, who may have realistic fears of being separated from loved ones. These fears may impact the expression of SAD symptoms, as well as the likelihood that Latinx families seek mental health treatment (Diaz & Fenning, 2017).

The consideration of cultural, racial/ethnic, and broader systems of racism and oppression are necessary in the diagnosis and treatment of SAD, anxiety disorders, and broader mental health concerns. There is not a one-size-fits all approach and each child and family should be considered within a larger historical context, which would involve considerations of the potential role of their personal racial/ethnic identities as well as additional intersected, and possibly oppressed identities they may hold (i.e., class, gender, gender identity, sexual orientation, immigration status, language, etc.; Crenshaw, 2016). It should not be assumed that children, adolescents, and families who identify as racial/ethnic minorities and/or hold additional oppressed identities should be treated in a uniform manner on the basis of these identities. It is important for school psychologists, educators, and clinicians who work with children of color who have and/or are suspected of having SAD to consider the larger social context of racism, bias, and discrimination and to seek support and training to become more culturally responsive in assessment and treatment.

The diagnosis and treatment of SAD must be considered within the larger cultural context in which children and families live, particularly racial/ethnic minority children and families with inequitable access to healthcare systems tied to broader systems of racism, bias, and discrimination (U.S. Department of Health and Human Services, 2019a).

IMPACT OF SEPARATION ANXIETY DISORDER ON SOCIAL–EMOTIONAL AND BEHAVIORAL FUNCTIONING IN SCHOOL AND HOME ENVIRONMENTS

Social–Emotional/Behavioral Needs

SAD, by definition, is marked by fear and extreme distress at the prospect of being separated from key attachment figures or being away from home (APA, 2013). As described throughout this chapter, the prospect of being separated from primary attachment figures/caregivers (i.e., parents) results in anxious and distressed behavior that may involve throwing temper tantrums as well as crying to avoid the separation (Pincus et al., 2008). Pincus et al. (2008) also describe key times when such externalizing behaviors may be present, which include evenings when the child is asked to sleep alone and wants to remain with the parent(s). Another key time when behaviors escalate is when the child must separate from parents to attend school (Pincus et al., 2008). The behavioral avoidance of school, which will be described in the text that follows in the "Functioning at School" section, is a key issue that needs to be considered and addressed by school psychologists. Relatedly, social aspects of SAD include the limited opportunity for developmentally appropriate interactions with peers due to missing out on social interchanges, like being involved in sports, sleepovers, and spending time with peers, because of distress over separation (Pincus et al., 2003; Vaughan et al., 2017).

Impact on Child Development

As described throughout this chapter, children with SAD are at great risk for not meeting a broad range of developmental milestones, particularly because they avoid the opportunity to engage in expected tasks, such as attending school and having social opportunities with peers (Vaughan et al., 2017). Erikson's psychosocial stage of development (Erikson, 1963) helps to explain why separation from parents/key attachment figures is necessary for children and adolescents to progress through the psychosocial stages of development. For example, Erikson's stage 4 of "industry versus inferiority," typically happens between the ages of 5.5 and 12, during the school years, when children achieve more independence from attachment figures so they are able to perform activities viewed as critical in a society. In the United States and Western cultures, separation from attachment figures is needed so that children can learn in school and form friendships on their own, which are not managed by their parents/caregivers.

Functioning at School

Children and adolescents with SAD who engage in avoidant behaviors and miss school are at risk for school failure and the opportunities to interact and form relationships with teachers and peers as part of typical school experiences. Close to 75% of children and adolescents who have SAD have at least one incident of school refusal (Hella & Bernstein, 2012, as cited in Elliott & Place, 2019). Another estimate is that roughly 30% to 38% of children who meet the diagnostic criteria for SAD engage in school-refusal behaviors (Heyne et al., 2004, as cited in Doobay, 2008). Elliott and Place (2019), in an updated literature review about school refusal, note how there isn't consensus about the definition of *school refusal* and although broadly resolved, a debate continues as to how it differs from truancy (see Elliott, 1999). Broadly speaking, school refusal is experienced by children who suffer from SAD and anxiety-related disorders, but also those who would simply be considered truant (Elliott & Place, 2019). School refusal also differs from SAD in that it is not considered a *DSM-5* (APA, 2013) diagnosis (Elliott & Place, 2019). School psychologists are well positioned to examine attendance data so they can work with school teams to determine root-cause drivers of why attendance/school avoidance issues are occurring.

Another area of school functioning that may be impacted is social relationships and the social–emotional learning that happens in school (Mahoney et al., 2018). Given that schools are primary environments where problem-solving, conflict resolution, cooperation, and making friends happens, when children and adolescents avoid school entirely or their time in the classroom is disrupted with frequently wanting to check in with caregivers or they are unavailable because of anxiety even though present in class (APA, 2016), then opportunities to meet social developmental milestones are limited.

Functioning at Home

Families with children and adolescents who suffer from SAD can have very disruptive home lives as a result. By definition, SAD symptoms include distress at the prospect or actual separation from key attachment figures (APA, 2016). To avoid separation, children and adolescents engage in highly combative and disruptive behaviors at home (Philipps et al., 2020). These interactions may cause significant stress in the family that can challenge the relationship that parents have with their children (Cunningham & Renk, 2017). Cunningham and Renk note the importance of integrating attachment theory (i.e., Bowlby, 1982) and the parent–child relationship in treating SAD. In their treatment of a young child who met criteria for both SAD and Tourette's disorder, Cunningham and Renk (2017) integrated parts of a parenting intervention (called *Circle of Security–Parenting*), along with traditional cognitive behavioral intervention with positive results. School psychologists can collaborate with outside therapists in supporting their treatment of children and families to facilitate more positive interactions in the home and to reinforce cognitive behavioral interventions that focus on treating the anxiety associated with SAD that results in children and adolescents refusing to leave home to attend school (Doobay, 2008).

> Children with SAD and their parents benefit from interventions that include work on how they interact and relate to one another (Cunningham & Renk, 2017).

IMPACT OF SEPARATION ANXIETY DISORDER ON LEARNING IN THE CLASSROOM

One of the key learning factors among children and adolescents who have SAD is the risk of missing many days of school due to separation issues and therefore, instructional time is lost. Although the empirical literature about the role of SAD in academic functioning is limited, there has been some research that has looked at how well reading performance, based on fluency and decoding measures, predicts separation anxiety symptoms (Grills-Taquechel et al., 2012). Grills-Tacquechel et al. (2012) explored two models looking at whether anxiety predicts academic achievement or whether it is the other way around. Their findings were based on a sample of first graders who completed self-report anxiety measures and reading assessments at the middle and last part of the school year. The findings differed according to the type of reading assessment, as children with reading decoding skills in the middle of the year were more likely to have higher self-reported anxiety-related harm avoidance in the final days of school (i.e., wanting to do things exactly correctly, being obedient with adults), whereas children with reading fluency challenges at the middle of the year reported higher anxiety-related separation symptoms at the end of the year. The authors interpreted the findings as being related to the type of task presented, as those with decoding problems may be less worried about doing things precisely because they are self-aware about their decoding concerns. In contrast, the authors hypothesized that those with fluency concerns are more likely to want to avoid school because they are anxious about academic failure, particularly when presented with time-pressure tasks like reading fluency measures. These findings have implications for school psychologists who have an opportunity to collect data related to anxiety when conducting standard reading assessments, and who can also analyze the findings to determine those who may be at risk for or have SAD. More research is certainly needed, as well as clinical observation in practice to determine how academic performance and outcomes are related to SAD. Clearly, those with SAD are at risk for their learning to be impacted if they are not in school due to avoidance because of separation anxiety. It should also be noted that children with SAD often want to contact their parents/key attachment figures frequently even when they are at school, furthering the potential for their instruction to be disrupted even when they are at school (APA, 2000, as cited in Doobay, 2008).

> One of the most challenging aspects of SAD is that children avoid school due to anxiety about separating from loved ones, putting them at risk for academic challenges and further anxiety when approached with academic tasks (APA, 2000, as cited in Doobay, 2008).

IMPLICATIONS FOR SCHOOL PSYCHOLOGISTS

Assessment

There are many different types of assessment tools, including structured/semi-structured interviews and rating scales, which have been developed and used to screen/diagnose the full range of anxiety disorders that children and adolescents face, including SAD (see Silverman & Ollendick, 2005). As noted by Orenes et al. (2017), a common tool used by clinicians to evaluate SAD is the Anxiety Disorders Interview Schedule for Children for *DSM-IV* Child/Parent Version (ADIS-IV-C/P; Silverman & Albano, 1997). The ADIS-IV-C/P is a semi-structured interview used with both parents and children that contains dichotomous (yes or no) questions about anxiety symptoms that align with *DSM-IV* anxiety-related classifications and impact on life functioning (APA, 1994; Silverman & Albano, 1997; Silverman et al., 2001). The ADIS-IV-C/P is a well-researched measure showing excellent test–retest reliability for a SAD diagnosis using only parent and child interview information, as well as data from both (Silverman et al., 2001).

Rating scales have also been developed specifically for the assessment of SAD. For example, the Separation Anxiety Assessment Scale Children and Adolescent Version (SAAS-C; Eisen & Schaefer, 2005) and the Separation Anxiety Assessment Scale Parent Version (SAAS-P; Eisen & Schaefer, 2005) are rating scales that have specific domains that align with SAD symptoms in children and adolescents. Although there has been relatively limited research done about the reliability and validity of the SAAS-C and SAAS-P scales, available findings are that the internal consistency for both versions of the tool is adequate (on the order of 0.68; Hahn et al., 2003, as cited in Chessa et al., 2012). Further, validity studies comparing the SAAS-C to similar anxiety tools show adequate to strong relationships (Chessa et al., 2012).

In international research, Chessa et al. (2012) translated the SAAS-C into Italian and administered it to a sample of nonclinical elementary-age Italian students (between 6 and 10 years of age), finding adequate internal consistency and convergent validity with two related anxiety measures. In another study, Orenes and colleagues (2017) administered a Spanish translation of the SAAS to a sample of school-aged children enrolled in grades 3 to 6 in southern Spain. Their findings showed good to strong psychometrics of the translated tool with respect to internal consistency, temporal stability, and convergent validity with another measure of separation anxiety and two others evaluating similar symptoms.

In addition to measures that focus only on the diagnosis of SAD, there are also tools that focus on multiple forms of anxiety and contain subscales that measure SAD. The Screen for Child Anxiety Related Emotional Disorders (SCARED; Birmaher et al., 1997) is one such tool, which in its earlier version was an 85-item parent and child rating scale, and was subsequently reduced to a 35-item version. Birmaher et al. reported strong internal consistency (ranging from 0.74 to 0.93) for the SCARED, and evidence for the discriminative validity of the tool in differentiating anxiety from other mental health disorders and among specific subtypes of anxiety. Runyon et al. (2018) conducted a meta-analysis of 65 studies evaluating the psychometrics of the SCARED, based on studies published from 1997 to 2017, not including those that could not be translated into English. Their findings also showed support for the psychometrics of the SCARED, including strong internal consistency of the total score, as well as for the SAD subscale and others that are part of the SCARED. Further, Runyon and colleagues found evidence of test–retest reliability and parent–child agreement that ranged from moderate to large. The findings of these studies document that the SCARED (Birmaher et al., 1997) is a psychometrically sound tool that can be used by both researchers and clinicians in the assessment of anxiety, and for specific subtypes of anxiety like SAD (Runyon et al., 2018).

Another commonly used parent and child rating scale of anxiety is the Multidimensional Anxiety Scale for Children (MASC), which is now in its second edition (March, 2013). The MASC has both a self- and parent-report variation, and measures anxiety and a number of subtypes, including a subscale in the second edition called *separation anxiety/phobias* (March, 2013). Wei et al. (2014) conducted a study examining the psychometric properties and validity of the earlier edition of the MASC (March et al., 1997) with a sample of children between 7 and 17 years of age, all of whom met criteria for having an anxiety disorder. They found that the separation/panic subscale, which is the scale that was developed to measure separation anxiety, had reasonably high internal reliability and was predictive of both childhood and adolescent SAD diagnoses, based on both parent and self-ratings, with the stronger predictive validity among adolescents.

There are a number of rating scales, direct-observation tools, and interviews now available to school psychologists and clinicians to assess the presence of SAD and related anxiety disorders, reflecting advances in the research validation of both the measures and processes involved with arriving at a diagnosis of anxiety and its subtypes (Silverman & Ollendick, 2005). We have highlighted a few examples and direct the reader to comprehensive reviews of the multitude of tools that assess SAD and related anxiety disorders. For example, see Silverman and Ollendick (2005) and Spence (2018) for a more recent detailed overview of the available anxiety assessment tools, along with information about age ranges included in the measures, along with coverage of reliability and validity data.

Consulting With Parents, Outside Agencies and Teachers, and Discipline Deans

School psychologists have a critical role to play as consultants with parents and key family members who support the family's efforts in the delivery of mental and educational interventions with their children (described in more detail in the text that follows). School psychologists can serve as supportive professionals for families who are often facing significant distress and disruptions in their own lives due to the challenges related to SAD symptoms. School psychologists are also particularly suited to consult with teachers in developing behavior and academic intervention plans to support classroom functioning. School psychologists are trained to deliver consultation and engage in data-based decision-making consistent with National Association of School Psychologists Standards (National Association of School Psychologists [NASP], 2020). Further, school psychologists can play a key role in providing psychoeducation with discipline deans, attendance coordinators, and others who may interact with children and adolescents who have SAD and not be aware of the importance of treating the underlying SAD symptoms through mental health supports rather than invoking punitive discipline, which would not work and inadvertently reinforces students with SAD to avoid school through measures such as school suspensions (Allen et al., 2018).

Advocacy Efforts on Behalf of the Child

As some of the best trained school-based mental health professionals working in schools, school psychologists are important advocates on behalf of children and adolescents with SAD. They are trained to understand how SAD symptoms, and the related anxiety and distress, impacts behavior, mental health, and school functioning. In addition to their consulting roles with school personnel and families, as well as being involved in mental health, behavioral, and academic supports, they are instrumental in determining the needs children and adolescents may have for Multi-Tiered Systems of Support (MTSS; Jimerson et al., 2016). Further, school psychologists are instrumental in decisions as to whether children with SAD should be considered for either a Section 504 (1973) plan or be evaluated for special education services and related supports under IDEA (2004). School psychologists have an ethical obligation to ensure that students with SAD receive the necessary educational, behavioral, and mental health support in schools (NASP, 2020). They also have the expertise to communicate with outside service providers, such as therapists, who they can collaborate with and consult once proper parental consent has been secured, to determine ways that any outside treatment can be supported in the school building.

EDUCATIONAL SUPPORTS

School psychologists have a key role in delivering educational and mental health support with children and adolescents who experience SAD. Their role can be either as direct treatment agents or in taking a more supportive role in which they support treatment that is happening elsewhere.

For example, school psychologists can work with school team members to develop behavior intervention plans that support students successfully entering and remaining in school, possibly in conjunction with cognitive behavioral therapeutic interventions. Further, school psychologists can also be essential in collecting data on an ongoing basis to determine whether interventions and supports are working and to collaborate with professionals internal and external to the school as needed. Another educational support that may be useful would be social skills training because of the likely detrimental impact of SAD symptoms on social development (Doobay, 2008). School psychologists can implement individual and group-level social skills interventions with children who have SAD and can also work with families to support their children in having more social exchanges with peers in the community.

SCHOOL-BASED MENTAL HEALTH INTERVENTIONS AND SUPPORTS

With respect to the mental health treatment of SAD and anxiety disorders more broadly, CBT that includes exposure as part of the intervention has consistently emerged as the treatment of choice for those who have SAD (Friedl et al., 2017). Suveg et al. (2009) point out that CBT focuses specifically on thinking errors (i.e., cognitive distortions) and avoidant behaviors that are common in SAD and other forms of anxiety. As one example of the efficacy of CBT in treating children with anxiety and related disorders, Suveg and colleagues evaluated CBT with a sample of children (ages 7–15) using both a randomized control trial and treatment in a clinic. The children were diagnosed with a range of anxiety disorders, including SAD. The results were that the children who received CBT had several positive outcomes, which included self-reported reductions in anxiety, based on the MASC, improved self-efficacy, better coping skills and emotional regulation shown through being less worried. However, the CBT did not result in changes in how children modulated emotions in areas not directly targeted through the CBT, like angry or sad feelings. The authors explained their findings as positive for emotions targeted as part of CBT, but also showed a lack of treatment generalizability to nontargeted feelings/emotions.

A common evidence-supported manualized CBT intervention used to treat anxiety in children and perhaps familiar to many school psychologists due to its use in schools is Coping Cat (Kendall & Hedtke, 2006; The California Evidence-Based Clearinghouse for Child Welfare, 2018). A version of Coping Cat, referred to as the *CAT program*, is available for adolescents up to age 17 (Walkup et al., 2008). The original Coping Cat developed by Kendall and Hedtke is 16 sessions long and contains both a therapist treatment manual and a client workbook. The program has both instructional and applied practice pieces, which include helping the client to identify anxiety-related feelings, somatic responses, and thought patterns as well as opportunities to practice newly learned coping skills in actual real-world anxiety-provoking situations (Kendall & Hedtke, 2006). There are also two parent sessions as part of the treatment. With the support of the therapist, the client evaluates how well the skills are applied (The California Evidence-Based Clearinghouse for Child Welfare, 2018). Crawley et al. (2013) developed, implemented, and evaluated a less-time intensive eight-session version of a manualized cognitive behavioral therapy to treat anxious youth modeled from Coping Cat. The most essential components were retained, specifically the exposure piece and those deemed important by expert clinicians. Once the revised materials were developed, Crawley et al. implemented them with a group of children between the ages of 6 to 13, all of whom met the criteria for one of several anxiety disorders, including SAD. The findings were promising in that over 42% of the children receiving the treatment were no longer diagnosed with the anxiety disorder they had prior to the intervention. These findings held up for 33% of children in the treatment condition at a 2-month follow-up. A computer-based variation of Coping Cat, called *Camp Cope-A-Lot (CCAL)* has also been developed (Kendall & Khanna, 2008). It was implemented with a group of 7- to 13-year-old children, all of whom had a *DSM-IV* Anxiety Disorder diagnosis, some of whom had SAD (APA, 1994; Khanna & Kendall, 2010). Variations for CCAL (Kendall & Khanna, 2008) were that the intervention was reduced to 12 computer-based sessions. In the first half, the child developed skills in a self-paced fashion using the manual. Following this, the therapist supported the child in exposure to stressors and practice of coping skills in actual individualized anxiety-producing events. Khanna and Kendall (2010) showed positive results when comparing CCAL to two other randomly assigned treatments, which were one of the following: (a) individual CBT based on 12 sessions of Coping Cat (Kendall & Hedtke, 2006) or (b) Computer-Assisted Education, Support, and Attention (CESA), a control condition, in which children spent time with a therapist, were taught about anxiety, and had computer game time. The lessons used to teach about anxiety in this condition were drawn from prior anxiety intervention work (Kendall et al., 2008). The findings were positive for the use of CCAL and the other CBT intervention, as they resulted in better anxiety-related outcomes compared with CESA following treatment and at 3-month follow-up. Community clinicians, including five school psychologists, implemented treatment. The studies reviewed here, along with long-standing decades-long well-controlled studies support the use of CBT in the treatment of a range of anxiety disorders in children and adolescents, including those who have SAD (Kendall & Hedtke, 2006; Labellarte et al., 1999).

There is more controversy and less information about the use of medications in the treatment of SAD, either as the sole intervention or in combination with CBT (Labellarte et al., 1999; Walkup et al., 2008). Walkup et al. (2008) conducted a well-designed randomized control trial comparing treatment outcomes with children between the ages of 7 and 17, all with an anxiety disorder diagnosis of either GAD, SAD or social phobia. The participants were placed in one of four varied conditions: (a) provided with only 14 sessions of CBT (Coping Cat; Kendall & Hedtke, 2006);

(b) received just the psychopharmacologic (medication) sertraline, which is a selective serotonin uptake inhibitor (SSRI); (c) received both the medication and the CBT in combination; or (d) received the medication as a placebo. The findings were that the combination of medication and CBT produced the best outcome compared to either CBT or medication alone, based on levels of anxiety evaluated prior to the treatment (i.e., baseline) and then at three follow-up points 1, 2, and 3 months out from the treatment. Walkup et al. (2008) pointed out the importance of considering the family's comfort level in treatment selection, including medication. School psychologists can play a key role in the delivery and evaluation of mental health interventions. They can also support and consult with other school personnel, such as the school nurse and physician, in helping to collect school-based outcome data if medication is deemed appropriate. With respect to cognitive behavioral interventions, school psychologists have the knowledge and expertise to implement interventions such as Coping Cat, which come with training opportunities (see The California Evidence-Based Clearinghouse for Child Welfare, 2018). Further, they can support therapists providing outside CBT, particularly in supporting the exposure component of CBT when children must leave home and attend school. School psychologists can reinforce the coping techniques that children are taught in therapy, either as part of school-based implementation or through supporting outside therapy by prompting and reinforcing children and adolescents with SAD when they apply such techniques at school.

CASE STUDY 9.1 HILARY: CASE OF A LATINX FEMALE WITH SEPARATION ANXIETY DISORDER

Background

Hilary is 8 and lives with her parents, Caroline and Jim, as well as her older sister, Mira, who is 16. The family identifies as Latinx. Caroline's parents immigrated from Mexico, and Caroline was born in the United States. Hilary is in the third grade at the local public elementary school. Jim's parents have been in the United States for two generations. Jim's dad was a career military person, and Jim moved frequently with his own family. Jim is a surgeon on active duty in the military and has been deployed three times since Hilary was born, the most recent deployment being the longest at 9 months. The family has also had one military move, from the Tacoma, Washington, area to a military installation near Huntsville, Alabama. Caroline is an elementary school teacher who has primary responsibility for the family when Jim is deployed and engaged in required military training activities. Caroline takes short-term teaching appointments and substitute teaches. Caroline's parents and Jim's dad are now retired and are strong supports for the family, frequently coming to help Caroline when Jim is deployed or busy with military activities. Jim's mother passed away about 5 years ago. Hilary has always been extremely close with her parents and grandparents. At about age 4, she started to have extreme temper tantrums when her dad would leave for a deployment or her grandparents would leave after an extended visit. The tantrums involve physically clinging to her dad and grandparents when they announce they are leaving. She also clings to Caroline during any type of separation, such as when she left Hilary in the care of grandparents, a babysitter, or her older sister when running errands or leaving for work. These tantrums escalate when Jim is gone because of a deployment or when he is in military training. Hilary doesn't cling to her sister but does seek her attention. Mira thinks of her sister as a pest.

Hilary had a difficult transition to kindergarten and Caroline decided to home school her, particularly since the family was moving to Huntsville, Alabama, at the time. The family's decision to re-enroll Hilary in the public school starting in third grade has resulted in an escalation in Hilary's temper tantrums and extreme distress when Caroline asks her to get ready for school and leave home. At times, Caroline reports that Hilary is aggressive toward her and her sister when it is time to go to school because she wants to stay home. Hilary also has extreme bouts of crying when getting ready for school in the morning. Often, Caroline gives in and lets Hilary stay home to avoid escalation of her behaviors and anxiety.

From about the age of 5, Hilary has refused to sleep alone, resulting in her sleeping with her parents or only Caroline when Jim is gone. She also sleeps with her sister at times. Hilary is more willing to leave the house to visit her grandparents, but still shows distress when she is separated

(continued)

CASE STUDY 9.1 HILARY: CASE OF A LATINX FEMALE WITH SEPARATION ANXIETY DISORDER (continued)

from her parents. However, Hilary asks to call Caroline multiple times throughout the day when with her grandparents. When she can be coaxed to go to school, Hilary will also frequently ask her teacher to call home and make sure everyone in her family is all right. Hilary reports being worried that her dad is going to get hurt when gone due to his military service. She is also worried that her mom, sister, and grandparents will get in a car accident and she won't be there to help them. Caroline and Jim are "ready to give up" and revert back to home schooling. With the aid of a 504 plan, they have been able to get the support of an instructional assistant and behavioral plan, which is helping somewhat with getting Hilary to school, but her attendance is very inconsistent, as she has missed over 20 days of school at the midpoint of the year. When Hilary is in school, she frequently goes to the office, reporting that she has a stomachache. The family, especially Caroline, are exhausted and want some relief. They haven't had solid sleep in years. Caroline and Jim are also worried that Hilary is not only suffering from constant distress and anxiety about being separated from her family, and worries about harm coming to them, but she is lacking social skills, the opportunity for making friends, and doing things other children her age do. Hilary is at grade level in reading, but is somewhat behind in math. Caroline and Jim are also concerned that as schoolwork gets harder, Hilary will get further behind.

Discussion

Hilary shows classic symptoms of SAD, which include her extreme distress and anxiety when separated from her parents, which results in tantrums and crying. Hilary is also worried that harm will befall her family—specifically, that her dad will be hurt during his military service and that her other family members will get in a car accident. To ease the anxiety and related tantrums/crying, Hilary's family engages in accommodating behaviors (Philipps et al., 2020), which likely reinforce her anxiety and related behaviors. There are multiple ways that school psychologists can support Hilary and her family. First of all, it would be helpful for the school psychologist to convene the Section 504 team to review the plan and make adjustments. If there is no behavioral plan or an insufficient one, then it should be revised particularly around transition time and staying at school, including a data-collection plan to evaluate outcomes. The school psychologist and team may want to consider whether a special education evaluation is warranted. With respect to assessment, the school psychologist could administer the SCARED (Birmaher et al., 1997) as a screening tool.

Hilary would likely benefit from CBT, such as the manualized Coping Cat intervention (Kendall & Hedtke, 2006), which could be implemented by the school psychologist if trained in its use and/or by an outside therapist with the school psychologist's support. Hilary and her family could benefit from a parent support group with children who have anxiety-related disorders. The school psychologist and team members can also work with Hilary's parents and grandparents to provide support and devise a plan to support Hilary in school as well as involve all family members in the plan, including extended family (i.e., grandparents). The school psychologist would also be an important consultant with the classroom teaching staff and could help with a plan for when Hilary asks the teacher to leave the classroom to call home or reports somatic complaints. Further, the school psychologist could provide psychoeducation to all school staff about the characteristics of SAD and ways to address it in school. The school psychologist will want to consult with all team members in the school, including the school nurse, administrators, and others engaged in discipline and attendance, so there is coordination and a consistent plan is implemented at school. Further, the school psychologist should closely monitor how Hilary is performing academically and help to determine whether secondary (Tier 2) and/or tertiary (Tier 3) interventions are warranted. Finally, due to Jim's military service, the school psychologist should be mindful of potential military moves and consult with any new school that the family transitions to, aligned with the Military Interstate Compact, which has been adopted by all 50 states to provide military youth with flexibility and support during military moves and transitions to new schools (Department of Defense Education Activity, 2020). It is particularly important to consult with a receiving school about any special education supports, Section 504 plans, and supports/interventions provided in the school (Department of Defense Education Activity, 2020).

SUMMARY POINTS

- SAD in children and adolescents is characterized by excessive fear and worry over being separated from loved ones (APA, 2013), often with serious implications for school due to fear of leaving home.
- Under the revised *DSM-5* criteria (APA, 2013), SAD is now placed under the broad category of Anxiety Disorders and adults can receive a SAD diagnosis.
- Children and adolescents with SAD are at risk of developing other mental health disorders later in life, including PD. Therefore, it is important for psychologists to pick up on early signs of SAD so that is can be treated.
- There are a host of empirically and psychometrically sound tools available to assess and diagnose SAD, including parent and child rating forms and interviews.
- Cultural factors are important when considering whether a SAD diagnosis is appropriate and treatment should be handled in a culturally responsive manner.
- CBT is a well-researched and empirically supported mental health treatment for SAD.
- School psychologists play a key role in helping families and other school professionals understand that SAD should not be equated with truancy.

TEST YOUR KNOWLEDGE

1. SAD can be diagnosed in adults.
   a. True
   b. False

2. Children and adolescents with SAD may show the following symptoms:
   a. Extreme distress when being separated from attachment figures
   b. Crying and tantrums
   c. Irrational fear of harm befalling themselves or loved ones
   d. All of the above

3. The mental health intervention that has the most empirical support in treating SAD is:
   a. Psychodynamic therapy
   b. Cognitive behavioral therapy
   c. Humanistic therapy
   d. Dialectical behavior therapy

4. The most likely mental health disorder that children and adolescents are likely to face later in life is:
   a. Schizophrenia
   b. Panic disorder
   c. Bipolar disorder
   d. Conduct disorder

5. Children and adolescents with SAD may require the following educational supports:
   a. Social skills development
   b. A behavior intervention plan
   c. Academic intervention
   d. All of the above

Answers: (1) a, (2) d, (3) b, (4) b, (5) d.

DISCUSSION QUESTIONS

1. Describe how the *DSM-5* (APA, 2013) diagnostic criteria for SAD have changed from the prior *DSM* editions.

2. Discuss biological and familial factors that may contribute to a diagnosis of SAD and/or the severity of its expression.

3. Articulate how you would implement and/or consult with an outside provider in delivering CBT with a child or adolescent who has SAD.

4. Specify how school psychologists can use their consultation and collaboration skills with families and school personnel (i.e., teachers, discipline deans, administrators).

5. Summarize how a school psychologist could be helpful in addressing academic, behavioral, or social–emotional challenges that a child or adolescent with SAD may have.

CHAPTER RESOURCES

American Counseling Association *Anxiety Resources:* www.counseling.org/knowledge-center/mental-health-resources/anxiety

American Psychiatric Association *What Are Anxiety Disorders?:* www.psychiatry.org/patients-families/anxiety-disorders/what-are-anxiety-disorders

American Academy of Child and Adolescent Psychiatry *Anxiety Disorders Resource Center:* www.aacap.org/aacap/Families_and_Youth/Resource_Centers/Anxiety_Disorder_Resource_Center/Home.aspx

Center for Disease Control and Prevention *Anxiety and Depression in Children*: www.cdc.gov/childrens mentalhealth/depression.html

Anxiety and Depression Association of American (ADAA) *What Is Anxiety?*: https://whatisanxiety.adaa.org/?gclid=CjwKCAjwieuGBhAsEiwA1Ly_nfNRqXgaLybhP3QhzeqEZ88l1jJU-Dum3v774cf7Hmz7UJiInWVPLxoC0z8QAvD_BwE

KEY REFERENCES

Only key references appear in the print edition. The full reference list appears in the digital product on Springer Publishing Connect: connect.springerpub.com/content/book/978-0-8261-3587-2/part/part04/chapter/ch09

Birmaher, B., Khetarpal, S., Brent, D., Cully, M., Balach, L., Kaufman, J., & Neer, S. M. (1997). The Screen for Child Anxiety Related Emotional Disorders (SCARED): Scale construction and psychometric characteristics. *Journal of the American Academy of Child Adolescent Psychiatry, 36*, 543–553. https://doi.org/10.1097/00004583-199704000-00018

Crawley, S. A., Kendall, P. C., Benjamin, C. L., Brodman, D. M., Wei, C., Beidas, R. S., & Podell, J. L. (2013). Brief cognitive-behavioral therapy for anxious youth: Feasibility and initial outcomes. *Cognitive Behavior Practice, 20*(2), 1–9. https://doi.org/10.1016/J.cbpra.2012.07.003

Doobay, A. F. (2008). School refusal behavior associated with separation anxiety disorder: A cognitive-behavioral approach to treatment. *Psychology in the Schools, 45*(4), 261–272. https://doi.org/10.1002/pits.20299

Grills-Taquechel, A. E., Fletcher, J. M., Vaughn, S., & Stuebing, K. K. (2012). Anxiety and reading difficulties in early elementary school: Evidence for unidirectional or Bi-Directional relations? *Child Psychiatry Human Development, 43*, 35–47. https://doi.org/10.1007/s 10578-0110246-1

Hella, B., & Bernstein, G. A. (2012). Panic disorder and school refusal. *Child and Adolescent Psychiatric Clinics of North America, 21*, 593–606. https://doi.org/10.1016/j.chc.2012.05.012

Kearney, C. A., Sims, K. E., Pursell, C. R., & Tillotson, C. A. (2003). Separation anxiety disorder in young children: a longitudinal and family analysis. *Journal of Clinical Child and Adolescent Psychology, 32*(4), 593–598. https://doi.org/10.1207/S15374424JCCP3204_12

Kendall, P. C., & Hedtke, K. (2006). *Coping Cat workbook* (2nd ed.). Workbook Publishing.

Kendall, P. C., & Khanna, M. S. (2008). *Camp Cope-A-Lot: The Coping Cat DVD* [DVD]. Workbook. http://workbookpublishing.com

Kessler, R. C., & Merikangas, K. R. (2004). The National Comorbidity Survey Replication (NCS-R): Background and aims. *International Journal of Methods in Psychiatric Research, 13*(2), 60–68. https://doi.org/10.1002/mpr.166

Kessler, R. C., Petukhova, M., Sampson, N. A., Zaslavsky, A. M., & Wittchen, H. U. (2012). Twelve month and lifetime prevalence and lifetime morbidity risk of anxiety and mood disorders in the United States. *International Journal of Methods in Psychiatric Research, 21*(3), 169–184. https://doi.org/10.1002/mpr.1359

Khanna, M. S., & Kendall, P. C. (2010). Computer-assisted cognitive behavioral therapy for child anxiety: Results of a randomized clinical trial. *Journal of Consulting and Clinical Psychology, 78*(5), 737–745. https://doi.org/10.1037/a0019739

CHAPTER 10

Social Anxiety Disorder

LEARNING OBJECTIVES

- Describe the *Diagnostic and Statistical Manual of Mental Disorders* (5th ed.; *DSM-5*; American Psychiatric Association [APA], 2013) criteria for Social Anxiety Disorder (SOC*), highlighting key changes in the *DSM-5* SOC specifier.
- Highlight relevant educational federal protections (e.g., Individuals with Disabilities Education Improvement Act [IDEA; 2004a] and Section 504 of the Rehabilitation Act of 1973 [U.S. Department of Education, Office for Civil Rights, 2016]) that may apply with students who have SOC.
- Gain knowledge about prevalence, comorbidity, risk factors, and correlates of SOC from a culturally sensitive perspective.
- Understand the social–emotional, social, academic, and behavioral implications of SOC in educational settings.
- Identify evidence-supported social, behavioral, and mental health interventions that are used to treat children and adolescents who have SOC and how they could be adapted for use in schools.

INTRODUCTION

According to the American Psychiatric Association's (APA's; 2013) *Diagnostic and Statistical Manual of Mental Disorders* (5th ed.; *DSM-5*) social anxiety disorder (SOC*; also known as *social phobia*) falls under the category of Anxiety Disorders (coded as 300.23; APA, 2013). Children and adolescents with a *DSM-5* diagnosis of SOC have extreme anxiety when presented with social situations. Another characteristic of SOC is extreme fear of being evaluated by others in a critical manner. The majority of children and adolescents who have SOC do not receive treatment, despite empirically-validated treatments being available (Chavira et al., 2004a). Children with SOC are at risk of not meeting important social developmental milestones.

This chapter covers diagnostic issues in SOC that are important for school psychologists, including an overview of the *DSM-5* criteria and potentially applicable legal protections in schools, such as the Individuals with Disabilities Education Improvement Act (IDEA; 2004a) and Section 504 of the Rehabilitation Act of 1973 (U.S. Department of Education, Office for Civil Rights, 2016). Comorbid conditions that are commonly found among children and adolescents who have SOC are also covered, along with their potential impact on social–emotional, behavioral, and academic functioning. Implications for the role of school psychologists are organized into their assessment, consultation, and advocacy roles. Evidence-based interventions that could be implemented in schools or in community settings are offered. To be specific, research supporting the use of cognitive behavioral therapy (CBT), along with social skills training and parent/family involvement, are emphasized (Herbert et al., 2009; Warner et al., 2007). The role of school psychologists is weaved throughout the chapter, particularly how they can contribute to the implementation of Multi-Tiered Systems of Support (MTSS) to help children and adolescents who have SOC (Doll, 2019), along with their engagement in consultation and collaboration with families, teachers, and community-service providers.

---

*In Chapter 10, social anxiety disorder is abbreviated as *SOC* so as not to confuse it with separation anxiety disorder (SAD). SOC is an accepted acronym for *social anxiety disorder* in the psychiatric and mental health fields.

DIAGNOSTIC ISSUES: *DSM-5* AND SCHOOL-BASED SERVICES

DSM-5 Diagnostic Criteria

According to the *DSM-5*, there are 10 diagnostic criteria that are considered when making an SOC *DSM-5* diagnosis (APA, 2013). Persons with SOC have debilitating anxiety or fearfulness about being in social settings, which is a key symptom of this condition (APA, 2013). Further, those who have SOC are also highly anxious about being judged by others in a negative manner (APA, 2013). Of particular importance to school psychologists is the fact that in order for an SOC diagnosis to be made with children, extreme anxiety must occur with peers, not only with adults (APA, 2013). In children, SOC symptoms can look like what may be perceived as disruptive/acting-out and challenging behaviors like throwing tantrums, being very clingy with others, crying, or not talking in social contexts (APA, 2013). Another area to consider is that for an SOC diagnosis to be made, the anxiety or fearfulness in social encounters must happen almost all the time, and the individual actively avoids or is very fearful/anxious in social contexts (APA, 2013). In addition, in order for an SOC diagnosis to be made, the level of anxiousness/fearfulness shown when exposed to a particular situation is totally out of proportion to any real threat to the person (APA, 2013). One must also look at how long the symptoms last before arriving at an SOC diagnosis, which requires a duration of symptoms of approximately 6 months or more. Further, there must be a detrimental impact on major life spheres (i.e., social, career/job, etc.; APA, 2013). There are other diagnoses that must be ruled out, particularly those with symptomatology similar to SOC, such as other anxiety disorders and autism (2013). Finally, if the person has a medical diagnosis, the level of anxiety or fear must not be related to it and SOC characteristics can't be the result of drugs, alcohol, or a medical substance (APA, 2013).

CHANGES IN SEPARATION ANXIETY DISORDER DIAGNOSTIC CRITERIA—*DSM-IV-TR* TO *DSM-5*

The one substantial change made to the diagnostic criteria for SOC under the *DSM-5* is that a "performance-only specifier" has replaced a generalized specifier (Chou et al., 2015). According to the *DSM-5*, a "specifier" is noted when making a diagnosis of SOC if the anxiety/fear being shown in a social situation is *exclusive* to speaking or performing in front of others (i.e., athletics, dance, etc.)—this is called a *performance-only specifier* (APA, 2013). In contrast, the *DSM-IV-TR* had a "generalized" specifier under SOC (APA, 2000), which was dropped in the *DSM-5* (Center for Behavioral Health Statistics and Quality, 2016). As the name implies, the "generalized specifier" was a demarcation of severe anxiety and fear in response to many different social scenarios and not simply in response to performing in some way (Chou et al., 2015). The clinical utility of the *DSM-5* new SOC specifier focused only on anxiety in performance situations has been questioned due to a lack of evidence for it in the literature (Chou et al., 2015; Kerns et al., 2013). Research to date suggests that a very low percentage of children and adolescents who meet the criteria for an SOC diagnosis show only performance-based anxiety (Burstein et al., 2011; Kerns et al., 2013). Burstein et al. (2011) used a portion of the National Comorbidity Survey Replication Adolescent Supplement (NCS-A; Merikangas et al., 2009) to determine, in part, the percentage of the nationally representative nonclinical sample of adolescents who met criteria for what ultimately became the SOC performance specifier. They found that less than 1% (0.8%) of adolescents who met the SOC criteria met the performance SOC subtype. In contrast, Burstein et al. (2011) found that over 55% of adolescents with SOC also met the *DSM* generalized SOC subtype in place when the study was done. Kerns et al. (2013) conducted a study with children and adolescents who had SOC, based on *DSM-IV-TR* criteria, finding that none of them showed just performance-based anxiety, but just over 64% showed generalized forms of anxiety. The authors also found that the study participants with the generalized subtype showed more serious SOC symptoms, and were more likely to be depressed compared with those who did not have this subtype. These findings have important implications for school psychologists, who may be among the first to see SOC symptoms in children and adolescents in schools. For example, children and adolescents with SOC may avoid situations in class when they are to be evaluated in a public way or avoid informal social environments where peers will be present, like the playground, lunch room, and hallways.

The main changes to the *DSM-5* criteria for a diagnosis of SOC compared with the prior *DSM-IV-TR* version is that the generalized specifier was replaced by a performance-only specifier when making the SOC diagnosis (APA, 2013; Center for Behavioral Health Statistics and Quality, 2016).

Applications to the Individuals With Disabilities Education Improvement Act

Children who have a *DSM-5* diagnosis of SOC may be served under IDEA (2004a) if they meet one or more of 13 possible special education categories and there is a documented adverse impact on educational performance. A *DSM-5* diagnosis of SOC does not necessarily qualify one for special education and related services (i.e., psychological, social work, speech) under IDEA. One IDEA category that children with SOC could arguably meet the criteria for is Emotional Disturbance (ED; Sulkowski et al., 2012):

(i) Emotional disturbance means a condition exhibiting one or more of the following characteristics over a long period of time and to a marked degree that adversely affects a child's educational performance:
  (A) An inability to learn that cannot be explained by intellectual, sensory, or health factors.
  (B) An inability to build or maintain satisfactory interpersonal relationships with peers and teachers.
  (C) Inappropriate types of behavior or feelings under normal circumstances.
  (D) A general pervasive mood of unhappiness or depression.
  (E) A tendency to develop physical symptoms or fears associated with personal or school problems.
(ii) Emotional disturbance includes schizophrenia. The term does not apply to children who are socially maladjusted, unless it is determined that they have an emotional disturbance under paragraph (c)(4)(i) of this section. (IDEA, 2004b, Section 300.8 (c) (4))

The ED criteria related to forming and maintaining satisfactory interpersonal relationships with peers would be particularly relevant for children and adolescents who have SOC. Given that, by *DSM-5* definition, children and adolescents experience high anxiety in social situations, specifically with peers, it is conceivable that this criterion would be met. The anxiety symptoms in social situations that are part of SOC could definitely prohibit the establishment and maintenance of social relationships that are part of healthy development. Further, educational functioning could be impacted given that classroom activities and assignments frequently require students to interact with one another to complete them. If students have high anxiety in social situations, including peer learning experiences, then evidence of this could show the ways in which SOC symptoms inhibit educational success.

In addition to possibly meeting the IDEA category for ED, students who have SOC could alternatively meet the criteria for "other health impaired (OHI)" (Sulkowski et al., 2012). The criteria for OHI (IDEA, 2004c) follows:

9. Other health impairment means having limited strength, vitality, or alertness, including a heightened alertness to environmental stimuli, that results in limited alertness with respect to the educational environment, that—
   (i) Is due to chronic or acute health problems such as asthma, attention deficit disorder or attention deficit hyperactivity disorder, diabetes, epilepsy, a heart condition, hemophilia, lead poisoning, leukemia, nephritis, rheumatic fever, sickle cell anemia, and Tourette syndrome; and
   (ii) Adversely affects a child's educational performance. (IDEA, 2004c, Section 300.8 (c) (9))

Similar to the required criteria for ED, students who could potentially qualify under OHI would need to show that the observed impairments have a negative impact on the student's functioning in school. Sulkowski et al. (2012) make the important point that some state statutes contain added language beyond what is in IDEA (2004) requiring a medical doctor to confirm an anxiety diagnosis for students to qualify for special education under OHI criteria. Further, they note that although anxiety disorders are not explicitly listed in federal IDEA (2004) language, some states do make reference to anxiety under their regulations. Therefore, it is really important for school psychologists to become proficient in understanding not only federal regulations, but also what is in place in the state they practice in. School psychologists are commonly looked to as the experts in the building and as the professionals who ensure compliance with educational laws and guidance, in addition to best practices in providing equitable mental health support as part of their daily practice (National Association of School Psychologists [NASP], 2020a).

It is the case that many students who have social anxiety, and other forms of anxiety as well, may not have symptoms that meet the criteria for a formal *DSM-5* diagnosis and/or special education services. However, school psychologists can be instrumental in implementing MTSS in schools (i.e., Response to Intervention [RtI]) by preventing and responding to the earliest signs of anxiety through Tier 1 supports (Sulkowski et al., 2012). Although not responding specifically to SOC, Sulkowski et al. offer recommendations for school psychologists to use to address anxiety that is focused on Tier 1 supports for all students, Tier 2 supports for groups of students and more intensive individualized supports for students who do not respond sufficiently to less intensive forms of intervention. At the Tier 1 level, Sulkowski recommends practices such as universal screening for anxiety and other mental health concerns, as well as group and individualized interventions that fall along the MTSS/RtI continuum. Please see Sulkowski et al. (2012) for more detailed recommendations regarding the types of services they recommend in the treatment of anxiety in general. School psychologists can be integral to implementing MTSS for children with all forms of anxiety as school-based mental health professionals. Prevention, early intervention, and treatment with children who have a formal SOC *DSM-5* diagnosis or the precursor to it would benefit from use of tiered supports aligned with MTSS/RtI, which is increasingly being focused on in schools as an efficient and prevention-oriented way of supporting students with internalizing disorders (Collins et al., 2019; Doll, 2019). MTSS systems are supportive of students who fall along a continuum of needed supports and it is important to note that children who have mental health concerns and issues like SOC—whether or not they qualify for special education—benefit from school supports that match their need along a continuum of support. As noted by Munson (n.d.), a common misunderstanding is that what is often referred to interchangeably as RtI in federal IDEA statute and MTSS in the field is synonymous with special education, under which students must qualify for under IDEA to receive services. However, this is not the case, as RtI/MTSS supports should incorporate general and special education supports (Munson, n.d.). Therefore, children with SOC could receive tiered support to help them overcome anxiety in a variety of social situations and contexts through use of a tiered system.

Children with SOC may meet the criteria for special education services and support under ED or OHI (APA, 2013; Center for Behavioral Health Statistics and Quality, 2016; IDEA, 2014b; IDEA, 2014c).

Applications to Section 504 of the Rehabilitation Act of 1973

Children with SOC may be eligible for services under Section 504 of the Rehabilitation Act of 1973. Section 504 specifically defines individuals (students) with disabilities "as a person who: (1) has a physical or mental impairment that substantially limits a major life activity; (2) has a record of such an impairment; or (3) is regarded as having such an impairment. (Section 504 of 1973)" (U.S. Department of Education, Office for Civil Rights, 2016, p. 3). Mental and psychological disorders are included in this definition, but a designated list is not offered through the statute due to concerns over lack of inclusivity (U.S. Department of Education, Office for Civil Rights, 2016). Under Section 504, a plan could be written to support students with SOC through practice of anxiety-reduction techniques in the classroom and planning for peer exposure as part of cognitive behavioral interventions implemented during peer group learning activities or during unstructured recess time, at lunch, and when making class presentations in front of an audience.

Prevalence and Onset of Social Anxiety Disorder

As noted by Khalid-Khan et al. (2007), SOC is a fairly prevalent mental health disorder seen in children and adolescents and has an early age of onset. Unfortunately, SOC is underdiagnosed, which results in a lack of mental health treatment for children and adolescents who need it, calling on primary care physicians to address this issue (Khalid-Khan et al., 2007). School psychologists can also play a pivotal role in identification of students who have SOC, as they work in communities and neighborhoods just like pediatricians and other physicians who see children and adolescents on a routine basis. School psychologists work in schools where children and adolescents are and therefore are in an excellent position to screen for anxiety using the universal procedures aligned with many MTSS systems, which are emerging or already in place in many schools across the country (Sulkowski et al., 2012). Further, school psychologists can work hand-in-hand with healthcare providers in the community, such as mental health providers and those working in community counseling centers, to diagnose and subsequently provide the treatment that children and adolescents with SOC desperately need and are not getting.

U.S. Studies

Epidemiological studies can help school psychologists and other clinicians know how frequently a particular mental health disorder occurs so they can get a better understanding of how to look out for students who may show such symptoms individually and see challenges that a larger population in the local school context may have (Doll & Cummings, 2008). Kessler, Avenevoli, Green, et al. (2009) examined prevalence rates of *DSM-IV* (APA, 1994) disorders among a sample of adolescents (ages 13–17) who participated in the large NCS-A study (Kessler, Avenevoli, Costello, et al., 2009). Kessler, Avenevoli, Green, et al. (2009) evaluated the percentage of adolescents who met criteria for SOC using the following two assessments: (a) the Composite International Diagnostic Interview (CIDI; Merikangas et al., 2009), which was completed by nonclinicians; and (b) the Kiddie Schedule for Affective Disorders and Schizophrenia for School-Age Children (K-SADS) interview (Kaufman et al., 1997) done by mental health clinicians who completed an assessment with both the adolescent and their parent as part of a follow-up about 77 days later. *Lifetime prevalence* is defined as the mental health condition occurring at least one time in one's life (National Institute of Mental Health, 2017). The findings were that the lifetime prevalence rates for social phobia were 9.8% using the CIDI and 9.2% using the K-SADS. The authors found that social phobia was the second most common anxiety disorder in the study. Kessler, Avenevoli, Green, et al. (2009) also found strong consistency for the types of assessments used in evaluating the presence of SOC in adolescents. These findings are important not only to gain a better understanding of how relatively common SOC is among adolescents, but also to understand the consistency of evaluation instruments used in large-scale research studies with more intensive clinical interviews used to measure a range of *DSM* diagnoses.

Chavira et al. (2004a) studied both the prevalence of several types of anxiety disorders among a community-based sample of children (ages 8–17) randomly selected from a larger list of those who had visited their pediatrician in the last year, and their parents completed a number of tools and an interview. The parent and child questionnaires specific to rating SOS symptoms were the Social Anxiety Scale-Children Revised (SAS-C; LaGreca et al., 1988) and Social Anxiety Scale-Adolescents (SAS-A; LaGreca & Lopez, 1998). In addition, the Anxiety Disorders Interview Schedule for Children (Silverman & Albano, 1996) was given to parents and children to assess a range of anxiety-related disorders, including SOC. The results of the questionnaires were that 18% of children in the sample were above the clinically significant level on the scale on the SAS-C, whereas 12% of adolescents fell in this range on the SAS-A. Further, close to 7% (6.8%) of the sample met the criteria for SOC, based on the Anxiety Disorders Interview Schedule for Children and based on prevalence rates of 1 year. Of all anxiety disorders (including SOC), only 31% of those diagnosed received medication or counseling at some point in their lives. Being a White adolescent predicted receiving psychotherapy. These findings have important implications for school psychologists, as they reinforce that children and adolescents with SOC are not identified and are missed by mental health professionals and therefore students do not receive intervention. The findings of Chavira et al. (2004a) about White adolescents being the most likely to receive intervention underscores broader concerns about the lack of available equitable mental health services for historically minoritized students (U.S. Department of Health and Human Services, Office of Minority Health, 2019). The findings also suggest that younger children may not be identified for services. School psychologists should be particularly mindful of the importance of individual, systemic, and structural biases and racism in both the identification and treatment of children suspected of having SOC when working with students who are historically minoritized by race/ethnicity and may hold additional intersected oppressed identities, such as being identified as having a disability, by gender, gender identity, and/or sexual orientation (Annamma et al., 2020; Staats, 2015–2016; Sullivan et al., 2020).

WORLDWIDE AND INTERNATIONAL STUDIES

Stein et al. (2017) conducted a large worldwide epidemiological study that was based on a community sample of households drawn from Africa, North/South America, Eastern Europe, Western Europe, Western Pacific, and the Eastern Mediterranean. Their findings were that SOC was estimated to have a 30-day prevalence of 1.3%, a 12-month prevalence of 2.4%, and a lifetime prevalence of 4% respectively across all the countries. In addition, there were differences in SOC prevalence across the globe and by country income. For example, SOC prevalence was lowest in low/lower middle-income countries and identified less frequently in African and Eastern Mediterranean nations. In contrast, SOC was determined to have the highest prevalence in high-income countries as well as North/South America and in the Western Pacific. SOC was most long-lasting in the highest economic strata (highest and upper middle-income countries), the Eastern Mediterranean, and Africa. These worldwide findings are important to consider as they demonstrate that SOC occurs across the globe, yet there are differences in the numbers of individuals identified, with higher rates, broadly, in countries in the highest income bracket and in particular regions, including the Americas. Future research is needed to better understand what may be driving the differing prevalence rates in affluent versus less affluent countries and more broadly, the difference in prevalence rates of SOC across the world.

Mohammadi et al. (2020) conducted a study in Iran to assess prevalence rates of SOC. The children in the sample were between the ages of 6 and 18. Epidemiological rates were based on a *DSM-IV* (APA, 1994) diagnosis made by clinical psychologists who interviewed parents and children (for young children a parent was present) using a Farsi language version of the Kiddie Schedule for Affective Disorders and Schizophrenia for School-Aged Children/Present and Lifetime Versions (K-SADS-PL; Kaufman et al., 1997). Please see Ghanizadeh et al. (2006) for reliability and validity information about the Farsi version of the K-SADS-PL used by Mohammadi et al. in their study. The lifetime prevalence of SOC in the sample (which was weighted) was 1.8%. Older children between the ages of 15 and 18 were more likely than younger children to meet the SOC criteria. It is unclear why these age differences were found, but one might hypothesize that there were potential differences in the developmental expectations for children compared with adolescents.

> Similar to other *DSM* disorders, there is variability in the estimated SOC prevalence rates among children and adolescents based on the type of sample and the methods used. SOC prevalence rates in a community-based sample were found to be 7% and more commonly found in adolescents (Chavira et al., 2004a). SOC is a common form of anxiety, yet it is frequently left untreated (Chavira et al., 2004a).

Comorbidity of Social Anxiety Disorder With Other *DSM-5* Disorders

Children and adolescents who have SOC frequently have comorbid mental health disorders. Chavira et al. (2004b) studied comorbidity of a range of *DSM* disorders in a sample of children and adolescents (ages 8–17) who visited a pediatric community health setting. They used the Anxiety Disorders Interview Schedule for Children-Parent Version (Silverman & Albano, 1996), which includes a module that measures social anxiety, among other *DSM* disorders. Their findings were that SOC was found to be comorbid with major depression, attention deficit hyperactivity disorder (ADHD), and two types of anxiety disorders: generalized anxiety disorders (GAD) and specific phobias. This comorbidity was for the general subtype of SOC and not the nongeneralized type. These findings are consistent with the Kerns et al. (2013) study described earlier, which supports that children with the generalized subtype of SOC are more likely to be depressed and to present with more serious symptoms in general.

Garber and Wearsing (2010), based on their review of the research, offer potential reasons why anxiety and depression are comorbid in children and adolescents. First, they offer that the rating forms used to evaluate both conditions (Cole et al., 1997, as cited in Garber & Wearsing, 2010), as well as how similar the symptoms look to us, despite being based on different underlying factors, play a role. Second, Garber and Wearsing (2010) point to the literature suggesting that expression of anxiety and depression is marked by negative affectivity in both disorders, which has to do with expression of distressed emotions (Clark & Watson, 1991, as cited in Garber & Wearsing, 2010). Finally, Garber and Wearsing (2010) point to research documenting that children with anxiety disorders are more likely to have parents with anxiety or depression (Weissman et al., 1997). These findings are important for school psychologists, who engage in psychological evaluations as well as review reports from outside clinicians, as they underscore the overlap in symptoms of depression and anxiety. A comprehensive evaluation of social–emotional and mental health functioning is critical to ensuring the school-based team has a clear understanding of the student. In addition, Garber and Wearsing (2010) also stress the need to prioritize prevention and potentially treating children who are anxious with the goal of avoiding the onset of depression later. Their recommendations also have implications for the role of school psychologists, who can engage in prevention-oriented Tier 1 screening and supports to identify children who are at risk for anxiety. These findings show that a potential positive outcome would be to ameliorate not only anxiety but the risk for depression.

Grant et al. (2005) conducted a U.S. epidemiological study of SOC using a national sample of persons ages 18 and over. Based on findings from the National Epidemiological Survey on Alcohol and Related Conditions (Grant et al., 2004), they found that those who met the *DSM-IV* (APA, 1994) criteria for SOC were statistically more likely to have GAD, bipolar 1 disorders, as well as avoidant and dependent personality disorders. These findings held whether they looked at the 12-month prevalence of 2.8% or the lifetime prevalence of 5.0%. They also found that the mean age of onset was in adolescence (15.1 years), whereas the median onset was 12.5 years. Consistent with Chavira et al. (2004a), most persons with SOC were not provided with any treatment (more than 80%) and those who did had a mean age of approximately 27 years of age before accessing any. These findings are compelling for school psychologists, who are in positions in schools to identify and support the mental health treatment of persons who have SOC, so these individuals have access to the support they need and not living with SOC well into early adulthood and beyond. Further, Grant et al. (2005) found racial/ethnic differences, which are not commonly reported. Indigenous persons were more likely to have SOC compared with White persons, whereas individuals who identified as Black, Asian, and Hispanic were less likely to have SOC compared with White persons. Finally, another important demographic is that persons in rural communities compared with those in urban/more populated areas were less at risk for acquiring SOC. It is critical for school psychologists to be aware of these findings. Given the shortage of school psychologists, particularly in rural areas, collaboration with mental health practitioners in the community and finding creative ways to train more school psychologists to work in rural areas is critical to support persons with SOC and mental health concerns more broadly (Lahman et al., 2006). Further, school psychologists should engage in culturally responsive treatment by affirming the identities and world views of children, adolescents, and families who identify as Indigenous, including how traditional White-centered mental health treatment may be perceived, and by working to dismantle personal biases and larger systems of racism and oppression (NASP, 2020b).

Schneier et al. (2010) conducted a study looking, in part, at the comorbidity of SOC with alcohol abuse and dependence. A national sample of adults were interviewed using the Alcohol Use Disorder and Associated Disabilities Interview Schedule-*DSM-IV* Version (Hasin et al., 2007). They found that persons who met the SOC criteria had higher odds of also having alcohol-related disorders—both alcohol dependence and abuse. Further, women who had alcohol dependence had higher chances of also having SOC, but this comorbidity was less likely for individuals who identified as African American and Hispanic compared with those who identified as White. Although this study is focused on adults, there are implications for school psychologists as prevention and early intervention with children and adolescents who have SOC is critical. In addition, tiered interventions in schools could be developed that focus on healthy coping techniques and not alcohol and drug abuse, which could be embedded into the health curriculum as components of universal/Tier 1 supports. Therefore, this effort could support children who not only meet the criteria for SOC, but those who have other mental health issues and also act as a prevention strategy as part of population-based supports (Doll & Cummings, 2008).

Asher and Aderka (2018) used National Comorbidity Survey Replication (NCS-R) epidemiological data (Kessler & Üstün, 2004) to determine whether there were gender differences in the prevalence rate of SOC. Their sample met the *DSM-IV* (APA, 1994) criteria for 12-month prevalence of SOC. Women were statistically more likely to suffer from SOC than men for both 12-month and lifetime prevalence estimates. There were also gender differences in the comorbidity of SOC with other mental health conditions. When considering the 12-month prevalence rates, men were more likely to also have drug and alcohol dependence and use, as well as conduct disorder as a comorbid condition. Women, on the other hand, were more likely to have anxiety-related comorbid conditions (e.g., specific phobia, GAD, and posttraumatic stress disorder). Women also had a higher probability of having had a prior panic attack. Although these findings are based on adults, it is likely that precursors to these conditions were seen during the school-aged years. Boys with conduct problems may be viewed as having disciplinary issues and not receive mental health and supports for social concerns. Girls may have internalized mental health issues through anxiety and their issues may not have risen to school personnels' attention if they were not disruptive. Clearly, it is not possible to conclusively draw these conclusions. Having an understanding of how SOC may be expressed, in conjunction with additional diagnoses, is helpful for school psychologists as they engage in prevention-oriented efforts to address and treat social and peer-related issues in schools, of which a *DSM-5* (APA, 2013) diagnosis of SOC may be a component.

Children and adolescents with SOC are at risk for having a number of comorbid *DSM* disorders, such as depression, anxiety, ADHD, GAD, specific phobias (Chavira et al., 2004b), as well as bipolar I, and personality disorders (Grant et al., 2005). Adult epidemiological studies have found comorbidity of SOC with alcohol dependence and abuse (Schneier et al., 2010). Females may have higher rates of SOC compared with males (Asher & Aderka, 2018).

Predictors of Social Anxiety Disorder: Risk/Protective Factors and Correlates

Festa and Ginsburg (2011) completed a number of child and parent report measures to look at predictors of social anxiety in a sample of children between the ages of 7 and 12 years. A range of child and parent measures were completed that measured social support, social acceptance, and parenting behaviors. Levels of child social anxiety were determined through interviews with parents and children using Anxiety Disorders Interview Schedule for *DSM-IV* Child Version (ADIS-C; Silverman & Albano, 1996) and through child ratings on the Screen for Child Anxiety Related Emotional Disorders-Child Version (SCARED-C; Birmaher et al., 1999). Independent observers also evaluated how parents interacted with their children as an external assessment of parental overcontrol. There were a number of significant findings reported in the study. Children with higher levels of perceived social support and social acceptance and validation from peers were more likely to have lower levels of social anxiety. The degree to which certain factors predicted social anxiety in children depended on who was doing the rating and type of measure used. The strongest predictors of child social anxiety were the anxiety levels of parents as determined by an outside evaluator, and the quality of children's friendships. When children rated their own anxiety, controlling behaviors of parents and perceptions of social acceptance were the strongest predictors. The authors point to their findings as showing the importance of addressing anxiety in parents and also considering peer relations in both assessment and interventions. These findings are important for school psychologists who can observe peer interactions in a wide range of settings and help children and adolescents with SOC form friendships and engage in positive social interactions with peers in the natural setting of schools.

Weissman et al. (1997) added to the knowledge base about the role of parental mental health in children's anxiety and other mental health challenges. They studied the children of parents who did and did not meet *DSM-III* (APA, 1980) and *DSM-III-R* (APA, 1987) criteria for major depressive disorder.

Both *DSM-III* (APA, 1980) and *DSM III-R* (APA, 1987) versions were used at different points in the study. They found that children with one or more parents facing depression were more likely to have depression, phobias, panic disorder, and greater social difficulties. They also found that anxiety disorders were much more likely to happen earlier in children whose parents were diagnosed with depression.

CULTURAL ISSUES RELATED TO SOCIAL ANXIETY DISORDER IN YOUTH

The cultural norms and beliefs of children and their families influence the students' social and peer interchanges (Chen & French, 2008). The ways in which children approach and value peer relations and whether they are perceived as shy or withdrawn is culturally and contextually specific (2008). Applied to a diagnosis of SOC, one could argue that the *DSM-5* (APA, 2013) criteria are defined through Western eyes. Children's identities based on race/ethnicity, gender, social class, language, immigration status, gender identity, sexual orientation, and additional intersected status influence social expression, social interactions, and meaning-making in relationships with peers. Cultural and individual identities of children and families contribute to potential biases in the ways in which minoritized students are assessed for SOC and the types of interventions and supports that are recommended. School psychologists need to be mindful of the individual identities and cultures of students who are referred for/suspected of having SOC. Evaluations and treatment should be considered in a culturally responsive manner. It is also important to remember that individuals do not fall into a particular social stereotype based on their cultural and racial identity. School psychologists need to consider the totality of the student within the contexts where they function, including school, home, and community. They must consider when and if social issues are deemed problems and by whom. School psychologists should be astute in listening and honoring the voices of children and their families, as well as other key individuals in their lives, such as teachers and other educators as well as other individuals who are important to the child and family.

Hofmann et al. (2010) described several cultural considerations in diagnosing and treating SOC. They presented epidemiological data about SOC showing racial/ethnic differences in prevalence rates, some of which was described earlier in this chapter. They pointed specifically to one culturally based expression of SOC that appears to happen more frequently among those from Japanese and Korean cultures, but this version of SOC is also seen among individuals who identify from additional cultures as well. Termed *Taijin kyofusho* (*TKS*; Hofmann et al., 2010, p. 1119), symptoms include being concerned about doing something that will bring embarrassment or offend another person, so this is an outerdirected form of SOC. A phonetic pronunciation of TKS is found in *How to Pronounce* (n.d.). As some examples of this fear, the individual worries that their physique or something they do will result in this effect on another person. This version of SOC is found in the Japanese psychiatric classification system. It is important for school psychologists to be aware of TKS when working with youths, but be cautious not to stereotype behaviors of children and adolescents who may identify as Korean or Japanese and make assumptions on the basis of students' cultural identity.

More broadly, Hofmann et al. (2010) describe a number of cultural considerations that must be considered when making an SOC diagnosis or providing an intervention. Culturally, students and their families may adhere to a more collective culture, in which there is a focus on community and adherence to group social norms. A collective culture differs, broadly, from those that take more of an individualist approach, consistent with Western European thinking. Further, there may be cultural differences in the level of independence and autonomy present in one's self-identity versus being more dependent on others, which may also intersect with gender norms and expectations in a particular culture. Once again, it is important not to generalize these broad constructs to a particular subgroup or individual student. However, at the same time, it is important to think about cultural expectations students may have and ensure that children and adolescents are not pathologized on this basis.

> School psychologists should consider the cultural norms and beliefs of students and their families (Chen & French, 2008). Although it is important not to stereotype or generalize cultural factors to any one student, school psychologists must be mindful that they do not pathologize students from minoritized communities on the basis of their culture and their individual identities.

IMPACT OF SOCIAL ANXIETY DISORDER ON SOCIAL–EMOTIONAL AND BEHAVIORAL FUNCTIONING IN SCHOOL AND HOME ENVIRONMENTS

Social–Emotional/Behavioral Needs

Children with SOC, by definition, struggle in social situations due to the anxiety they experience (APA, 2013). The expression of SOC symptoms can impact social–emotional functioning in many ways because children and adolescents will avoid social situations and interchanges that promote healthy social–emotional development. The symptoms of SOC may also impact behavior through outbursts that may materialize through tantrums, crying, and so on (APA, 2013). Given that one of the *DSM-5* criteria (APA, 2013) is that social anxiety with peers is present, a key social–emotional/behavioral area to address would be helping students to manage their anxiety when they are around peers. In addition, a primary point of intervention would likely be helping students to develop social coping skills during peer interactions. Schools are places where being around peers and working with them happens throughout the entire day. Students with SOC will need social–emotional supports that could be delivered along a continuum of tiered supports consistent with MTSS, as referenced throughout this chapter (Doll, 2019). These supports could begin with the delivery of social–emotional learning on a school-wide or classroom basis, using an evidence-based curriculum. Collaboration for Academic, Social, and Emotional Learning (CASEL) is an organization which offers substantial evidence-based social–emotional learning resources on its website to help teams plan, deliver, and evaluate social–emotional support in classrooms and schools (CASEL, 2021). Further, there is substantial evidence to support the implementation of cognitive behavioral interventions in children and adolescents with SOC. Such interventions could be offered to supplement the social–emotional learning of all students in the building (CASEL, 2021; Mohatt et al., 2014). As with other tiered interventions, cognitive behavioral interventions could be offered along a continuum of supports at the group and/or individual level (Doll, 2019).

Children and adolescents with SOC may also have behavioral needs. For example, a functional analysis of behavior (FBA)/behavior intervention plan (BIP) could be developed to individually support students who show acting-out behavior in response to the debilitating anxiety felt in social situations. School psychologists are key professionals in the building who have the behavioral expertise to complete FBAs/BIPs. When conducting an FBA, one gathers data about the "function" the behavior serves, which is an understanding of the purpose behind the behavior (Loman et al., 2019). For example, students may engage in undesirable behavior to get something they want (i.e., adult attention) or escape/avoid something they don't want (i.e., difficult work, social interactions). Once the function of the behavior is determined, a behavior plan is built to help the student meet the same function but by learning or performing a desired behavior (Loman et al., 2019). The Center on Positive Behavioral Interventions and Supports (PBIS; www.pbis.org) has a wealth of resources on FBA/BIPs (www.pbis.org/resource/basic-fba-to-bsp-trainers-manual) as well as school-wide behavior supports that are very useful in designing and implementing behavioral practices at all tiers of support.

Impact on Child Social Development

The development of children and adolescents who have SOC may be disrupted, particularly in the social realm. According to Erikson's theory of psychosocial development (Erikson, 1963), children, adolescents, and adults must navigate social worlds in order to master healthy social development. While one could see the impact of SOC symptoms across all stages of Erikson's theory, including among young children who must navigate social interactions through cooperative play, the middle childhood years (stage 4; children roughly 5.5–12 years), "industry vs. inferiority" (stage 5; adolescence), "identity versus isolation" and young adulthood (stage 6; 1963) may be particularly impacted. According to Erikson, in stage 4, children focus on learning the activities that are important for their particular culture. During middle childhood, a great deal of social development occurs and children are focused on peer acceptance and engage in social comparison (Eccles, 1999). Therefore, children who have extreme anxiety and avoid social interaction are at great risk for not meeting these important social developmental milestones.

In adolescence, young persons are highly focused on peers and whether they are accepted by them. Erikson (1963) describes a hyper-focus on who is "in" and who is "out" through the formation of cliques. One need only walk in the halls of a high school to see this play out. Clearly, adolescents who have SOC are at greater risk of being left out socially due to their anxiety in approaching and interacting with their peers. In young adults, a key social milestone involves forming intimate relationships or becoming isolated. One can see how social anxiety may prevent emerging adults from being in social situations where they are likely to meet potential partners and from participating in social activities like dating and coupling. School psychologists should consider the social developmental milestones that children and adolescents are expected to master when designing interventions and supports to help and support students they work with who have social anxiety, whether or not they meet the formal *DSM-5* diagnosis for it.

Functioning at Home

Children and adolescents who are diagnosed with SOC may be impacted in the home when being prompted or encouraged to interact with peers. This may arise when they are prompted to attend school and avoidant behaviors, like crying and having tantrums may be seen (APA, 2013). As an example, these students may avoid school when there is a group project that is happening or they are being required to do a public presentation or be evaluated in front of others in some way. Further, such individuals may avoid interacting with peers in the neighborhood, and engaging in routine activities like going to the grocery store or being out in public, as there is exposure to a public environment. Families will need support in helping their children cope with the anxiety associated with social situations broadly. Cognitive behavioral therapy (CBT) interventions with a parent psychoeducation component, as described in the next section (Warner et al., 2007), may be very helpful and supportive for parents as they work with their child to expose the child to fearful situations and not engage in reinforcing their anxiety. In the current context of COVID-19, parents whose children suffer from SOC will need support as transitions to face-to-face instruction occur and continual adaptations are made to classroom structure and the degree to which students are required to be in close proximity to peers changes (Loades & Reynolds, 2021).

IMPACT OF SOCIAL ANXIETY DISORDER ON LEARNING IN THE CLASSROOM

Given what has been described about the social–emotional, behavioral, and social developmental impact of SOC, school success and functioning may be impacted. The school years are marked by engaging with peers to produce and master academic tasks. Children and adolescents with SOC avoid social interactions that are the basis for learning. Even being in a classroom around other peers may be debilitating for someone with SOC. Therefore, academic performance may be harmed through the social-avoidant behaviors that are part of SOC symptoms. Attendance may also be impacted if children avoid school altogether. Therefore, monitoring of absences and academics is critical for all children, but is particularly relevant in supporting children and adolescents who have SOC.

There are many classroom situations that children and adolescents with SOC may not be adequately equipped to navigate. Some specific examples of these situations would be when children and adolescents are required to interact with peers during cooperative learning activities, engage in small-group work, and complete projects with partners and groups. Another context in which SOC symptoms may elicit social–emotional/behavioral needs would be in unstructured school activities, such as recess, lunch, coming to and from school and during crowded passing periods where peers are more likely to be present. Yet another context would be extracurricular activities, such as team sports, clubs, or community recreational activities.

In addition, it is important to note that the school shutdowns that occurred across the world in the wake of COVID-19 and the return to face-to-face instruction in many parts of the country have likely made an impact and will continue to do so in the lives of children and adolescents who suffer from SOC. As noted in two letters to the editor about school closures and the impact on children and adolescents who have social anxiety, Morrissette (2021) cautions that those with social anxiety have likely been reinforced to avoid school, which goes against effective treatments that require exposure to anxiety-producing situations. He argues that although those who have social anxiety may report feeling better, it is because they are reinforced in their avoidant behavior, and it is imperative that treatment and support continue. In their response to Morrissette, Loads and Reynolds (2021) provide multiple reasons why returning to school will be particularly challenging among those who have anxiety, including inadvertent reinforcement of anxiety described by Morrissette, triggering of already existing anxiety about danger, media messaging about COVID-19, and coping with novel COVID-19–related mitigation strategies, such as social distancing. Loads and Reynolds (2021) stress the need for school-based mental health professionals to be prepared for what is anticipated to be an increased incidence of mental health problems, which would include social anxiety. They note, "it is highly likely that school staff will observe elevated rates of distress and behavioral challenge. Schools and mental health services therefore need to be prepared for this prospect" (Loads & Reynolds, 2021, p. 7).

IMPLICATIONS FOR SCHOOL PSYCHOLOGISTS

Assessment

There are a number of tools available to school psychologists for the assessment of SOC among children and adolescents. The Anxiety Disorders Interview Schedule for *DSM-IV*: Child and Parent Versions (ADIS-IV-CP; Silverman & Albano, 1996) measures several anxiety subtypes and contains a specific subscale measuring social phobia. The ADIS-IV-CP has been described in research reviewed in this chapter. Specific to the social phobia subscale, Silverman et al. (2001) found strong reliability and also utility for use of the ADIS-IV-CP in arriving at *DSM* diagnoses using both the parent and child interview portions as well as both in combination.

Another tool that is commonly used in the assessment of all forms of anxiety, including a social anxiety subscale, is The Screen for Child Anxiety Related Emotional Disorders (SCARED; Birmaher et al., 1997). The SCARED was reduced from an 85-item parent and child rating scale to a 35-item version. Based on a meta-analysis of anxiety assessment studies conducted by Runyon et al. (2018), the social anxiety subscale has very strong psychometric properties in studies conducted in both communities and clinical settings. Runyon et al. (2018) recommend the SCARED for both diagnosing and evaluating the efficacy of interventions. Given that this is a rating scale that can be completed relatively quickly and over time, school psychologists may want to consider using the SCARED or a similar tool to evaluate how students with SOC are responding to treatment that may be occurring at school or in the community by an outside mental health clinician.

A widely used anxiety scale, which has both parent and child versions, is the Multidimensional Anxiety Scale for Children (MASC), which has a subscale that measures social anxiety. The MASC has been revised and there is a second edition available to mental health clinicians (March, 2013). The psychometric properties of the earlier version of the MASC (March et al., 1997) were evaluated by Wei et al. (2014). Their findings were positive for the use of the social anxiety subscale in that it was a strong predictor of social phobia. Social phobia (which is currently referred to as *social anxiety*) was measured by the ADIS-IV C/P (Silverman & Albano, 1996) both for whether the *DSM-IV* (APA, 1994) criterion were met and how serious the symptoms were.

There are tools that have been specifically developed to measure social anxiety. The Social Anxiety Scale for Children-Revised (SASC-R) is a rating scale consisting of 22 items that has adequate psychometrics, including internal consistency when tested in both community and clinical settings (LaGreca & Stone, 1993). In addition, a three-factor structure of the SASC-R has been derived, which includes the following: (a) a measure of fear over negative peer evaluation, (b) avoidance and distress around new social situations, and (c) general distress and avoidance of social situations (1993). Of particular importance to school psychologists is that children who had elevated levels of social anxiety reported less social acceptance, felt worse about their worth, and were less likely to be accepted by peers (1993). An adolescent version of the rating scale—Social Anxiety Scale for Adolescents—was developed, which has good psychometric properties and has the same three-factor structure as the SASC-R (Inderbitzen-Nolan & Walters, 2000).

Another tool that was developed specifically to measure social anxiety in children and adolescents is the Liebowitz Social Anxiety Scale for Children and Adolescents (LSAC-CA; Masia et al., 1999). The LSAC-CA is a 24-item tool completed by mental health clinicians, with half of the items measuring interpersonal interactions in social contexts and the other half evaluating scenarios in which performance is required. Masia-Warner et al. (2003) evaluated the psychometric properties of the LSAC-CA by administering it, along with other measures of SOC, and interviewing a sample of children and adolescents with an average age of 13.4. They found strong psychometrics when examining internal consistency and test-retest results. In addition, the LSAC-CA scores distinguished children and adolescents who had SOC from others who had other forms of anxiety or were in the control group.

There are a number of tools that are available to school psychologists to screen and evaluate children and adolescents suspected of having SOC, which include scales that measure multiple subtypes of anxiety as well as those designed exclusively for the assessment of SOC.

Consulting With Parents, Outside Agencies, and Teachers

School psychologists have a critical role consulting with parents, outside agencies, and teachers. They can consult with teachers and work in the classroom by conducting ongoing observations of social interactions with peers to determine whether interventions that are being applied are working or not, and to make ongoing adjustments as needed. Consultation with teachers could also take the form of designing and implementing behavioral and social–emotional support plans to address anxiety that children and adolescents with SOC may have in interacting with peers and engaging with others in the classroom. In addition, school psychologists can consult with teachers and other educators to create an inclusive school community but also work with students not to engage in reinforcement of avoidant behavior.

Consultation with parents and families can take the form of working with them to establish a behavior plan and implement the components of a CBT intervention that will involve strategies to support students in approaching social situations that are anxiety producing through therapeutic techniques and behavior practices rather than inadvertently reinforcing avoidance. Parents and families may also benefit from working on supportive strategies that assist their child in becoming more socially engaged in the neighborhood, community, in sporting and recreation events, as well as common childhood events like birthday parties, play dates, and so forth.

Advocacy Efforts on Behalf of the Child

School psychologists play a key role in advocating for children and adolescents who have SOC. Adults who work with individuals who have social anxiety may not have be aware of the key symptoms and how they impact social functioning and academic success. School psychologists could be integral to ensuring that children and adolescents who have SOC receive educational protections through IDEA (2004) or Section 504 (U.S. Department of Education, Office for Civil Rights, 2016). They can work with educators and discipline deans to ensure that behaviors related to social anxiety are not punished through classroom removal but met with therapeutic interventions.

EDUCATIONAL SUPPORTS

Social Skills Interventions

Children and adolescents with SOC may benefit from educational supports that could be offered along a tiered continuum aligned with MTSS, beginning with Tier 1 social–emotional learning, which has benefits for all students, including those with social anxiety, and could be offered through classroom instruction and supplements to it on a school-wide and/or classroom basis (CASEL, 2021). It is likely that children who have social anxiety, including those who may or may not meet the *DSM-5* (APA, 2013) criteria for SOC, may also require additional educational supports to address the anxiety they feel in social situations and their fear in performance-related situations, which are common in schools. One area of educational support could be social skills interventions aimed at helping children form peer relationships and gain social skills to use in all types of school situations, including unstructured play-based and social ones (i.e., lunch, recess) and during more formal group instruction. Although social skills intervention makes logical sense to implement with children and adolescents who have SOC, or the precursors to it, there is limited evidence-based research available (Olivares-Olivares et al., 2019). Olivares-Olivares et al. (2019) conducted an empirical evaluation of a group intervention with adolescents with SOC residing in Spain. They assigned participants to three conditions: (a) an intervention without social skills training that focused on CBT, such as exposure therapy to situations that produce anxiety, cognitive restructuring, challenging irrational thoughts, homework, and so forth; (b) the cognitive behavioral intervention described plus social skills training that included instruction in forming friendships, skills in having conversations, being assertive, and speaking in public; and (c) a wait-list control group. Olivares-Olivares et al. (2019) found improvement among the participants in both treatment conditions in the expression of SOC symptoms (i.e., fearfulness and avoidance of social situations), but the SOC outcomes were worse among the wait-list group. However, at a 12-month follow-up the participants who received the social skills and cognitive behaviorally based intervention had statistically better outcomes, overall, in SOC symptoms and were less likely to drop out of school. These findings are very promising for the role of social skills interventions in supporting children and adolescents who have SOC symptoms. School psychologists are well positioned to implement directly and/or support the implementation of social skills interventions and interventions to support children with SOC in gaining positive social interactions skills as well as forming friendships and social relationships with peers.

Academic Interventions

Children and adolescents with SOC may be at risk for school avoidance if their fear of social situations is so intense that they skip school or remove themselves from class and/or engage in disruptive behaviors because they are socially anxious, which may lead to classroom removal. As noted previously, children with SOC will likely avoid peer and group learning activities, which may impact their ability to complete assignments, learn important academic content, and pass their classes successfully. In the classroom, teachers can prompt students to use strategies that they may be learning as part of CBT interventions (described in more detail in the next section). For example, in the classroom, students can be taught to recognize signs of their own anxiety, and be subtly prompted to take a sensory break or use deep-breathing strategies they are practicing through outside counseling. Another strategy would be for students with anxiety to have a visual reminder under the desk (i.e., a note card) that prompts them to use coping strategies when experiencing social anxiety, such as practicing thinking of alternative healthy thoughts to replace automatic negative ones they may be having. Further, the classroom teacher can make peer group work assignments with a consideration of peers who may be optimal for students who have social anxiety to work with. School psychologists can serve as classroom consultants in designing, delivering, and evaluating the outcome of classroom supports.

In addition, school psychologists are the professionals in the building who typically have the training to engage in universal academic screening and progress monitoring aligned with combining the academic and behavioral components of MTSS, as both may be relevant for children and adolescents who have a formal diagnosis of SOC and/or the early signs of it (McIntosh & Goodman, 2016). Therefore, they can help to monitor how students who have social anxiety are doing academically, intervene early, and help to collect progress-monitoring data to determine whether academic interventions should be continued, changed, or phased out.

SCHOOL-BASED MENTAL HEALTH INTERVENTIONS AND SUPPORTS

CBT is a commonly implemented mental health intervention that has empirical support for use with children and adolescents who have a wide range of anxiety disorders, including SOC (Herbert et al., 2009; King et al., 2005). Herbert et al. (2009) conducted a randomized control trial (RCT) study comparing group CBT, individual CBT, and a third psychotherapy condition that did not incorporate CBT components. RCT methods are considered the "gold standard" of efficacy studies. The CBT components for both the individual and group condition were the same, which incorporated common components used to treat anxiety (i.e., in vivo and simulated exposure therapy to socially fearful situations, social skills training, cognitive restructuring, breathing exercise, psychoeducation). The results showed positive outcomes for all three treatment conditions that included improvement in SOC symptoms and better personal functioning. However, the CBT conditions produced better behavioral outcomes.

Despite its promise and efficacy, most children and adolescents who suffer from anxiety do not receive treatment (Chavira et al., 2004a; Warner et al., 2007). School psychologists can help to address this treatment gap by implementing CBT in schools and supporting other school-based mental health professionals in doing so. Warner et al. (2007) evaluated a school-based CBT intervention with adolescents who have an SOC diagnosis. They randomly assigned adolescents to one of two treatment conditions: (a) Skills for Social and Academic Success (SASS; Fisher et al., 2004) or (b) Attention Control: Educational Supportive Group Function (ESGF; Masia-Warner et al., 2004). The SASS condition contained specific CBT components used to treat SOC (i.e., exposure to fearful social situations, social skills intervention, psychoeducation, two sessions with parents and teachers about managing social anxiety symptoms/not reinforcing social avoidance outings with peers). The attention control condition was meant to control for therapist attention and included supportive time/relaxation training. The SASS condition was statistically better than the ESGF condition in the relief of SOC symptoms. Further, at the end of treatment, 59% of the participants in the SASS treatment no longer met criteria for SOC compared with no participants in the ESGF condition. The participants in the SASS conditions continued to do better in the outcome measures compared to the other condition at a 6-month follow-up point. These findings support the implementation of CBT in schools, which may be more efficient and possible for children and adolescents who suffer from SOC and other anxiety disorders than seeking out treatment on their own with a private provider.

CBT interventions certainly hold promise based on the research reviewed here and school psychologists have an outstanding opportunity to make these efficacious interventions possible through school-based implementation. In combination with CBT, pharmacological treatment has also been recommended for the treatment of children and adolescents who have SOC (Mohatt et al., 2014). Specifically, selective serotonin reuptake inhibitors (SSRIs) have been recommended for the treatment of anxiety (2014). The use of medication with children who have SOC is certainly a decision that must be made with sensitivity and determined by a treating physician. Families must be the critical decision makers, along with their children with careful consideration given to their developmental stage. School nurses, community health providers, pediatricians, psychiatrists, and the families themselves are critical members of a team that can support students with SOC. With respect to medication management, school psychologists could support a team by collecting school-based data about how children and adolescents with SOC are responding and providing it with proper parental consent and releases to the healthcare providers. School psychologists can be in consultation with medical providers and the family in terms of differences that are being observed at school with respect to the student's level of anxiety, behavior, and social–emotional functioning when being exposed to peers.

CBT is an efficacious treatment for children and adolescents who have SOC. Pharmacological treatments, specifically SSRIs, are sometimes used in conjunction with CBT.

Children with anxiety disorders, including SOC, do not receive the treatment they need and deserve (Chavira et al., 2004a). School psychologists are well positioned to help fill this gap by supporting children and adolescents who have SOC in social–emotional, behavioral, and academic domains. Through application of an MTSS system, school psychologists can help students with internalizing mental health issues, including persons who suffer from SOC (Doll, 2019). Evidence-supported practices, like CBT and social skills and behavioral interventions, have shown positive outcomes with those who suffer from SOC and could be embedded into MTSS practices within schools (Herbert et al., 2009; Loman et al., 2019). As many schools transition to face-to-face instruction in the midst of COVID-19, school psychologists will be needed more than ever to support students with a range of anxiety disorders, particularly those who suffer from social anxiety and may have not have received ongoing mental health treatment (Loades & Reynolds, 2021). We turn next to the case of Alexis to provide a fictional illustration of a student with SOC who is facing a transition from remote learning to face-to-face instruction.

CASE STUDY 10.1 ALEXIS: CASE OF A WHITE FEMALE WITH SOCIAL ANXIETY DISORDER

Background

Alexis is a 15-year-old female who lives with her mom, Diane. Her brother, Kevin, who is 20, attends college out of state. Alexis's parents divorced when she was 3 and her dad has not been in her life for many years. Diane works many hours as a nurse and she has been working particularly long hours due to the COVID-19 pandemic. Diane's mom, Susan, lives very close by and has always helped in caring for Alexis and Kevin, often spending weekends with them and evenings when Diane is working. Alexis is close to her mom, grandma, and Kevin. She was very sad when Kevin left for college as she felt he was the one person she could hang out with. Kevin has many friends and was active in the band, yet took time out to look out for his younger sister. Diane has had a history of depression on and off since adolescence. Recently, she has been feeling exhausted due to her work schedule and is not sure whether she is simply extremely tired or perhaps may be having a relapse of depression.

Alexis has been described as shy since she first enrolled in preschool. As a pre-K student, she would prefer to sit by herself in the corner, withdraw, and not interact with peers. She was called to the attention of a school team, who completed early-childhood screening and subsequently enrolled her in an early-childhood program. At that time, Diane attributed Alexis's withdrawal behavior as related to the divorce and her need to work many hours to support her family. However, Alexis's social withdrawal behavior continued throughout elementary and middle school. She frequently became extremely anxious when leaving for school, particularly on days when she was required to work on a group project or give a presentation in front of the class. Her anxiety would show up as crying at times to avoid social interactions and as symptoms of extreme distress, frequently manifested in physical symptoms like sweaty palms, racing heart, stomachaches, and dry mouth. She reported feeling as if other kids were always judging her. In elementary school, she missed many school days. She is a very capable student and is able to keep up with her classes for the most part, but her school attendance has been very inconsistent over the years and she has sometimes missed completing assignments. There were times in middle school when she would simply take a zero for a group project. When group projects were required, she asked to do the entire project on her own and was frequently accommodated by her teachers in middle school. She is an exceptional artist and has become close with her art teachers over the years. She has not received any formal services over the years, except for the early-childhood services. She has visited the social worker at times when it gets to be too much to be around other kids her age. She also has avoided places where her peers are by eating lunch with her art teachers or on her own in the corner of the cafeteria.

Currently, Alexis is a sophomore in high school. She has spent the vast majority of her time in remote online instruction due to the COVID-19 pandemic. She has done well academically during remote instruction and prefers this to being in school. However, she has learned that her school will be transitioning back to face-to-face instruction. She refuses to go back face-to-face and says that she would rather drop out of school. Diane and Susan are very worried about her and afraid that she will withdraw from school. Alexis doesn't have any close friends, but she does go online and plays video games with others at times. She says she simply prefers being alone or spending time with her family and doesn't feel the need to make friends. She spends a great deal of time on her own, drawing, sketching, painting, and writing. Alexis thought she might want to go to art school after high school, but she doesn't want to be around other people. She is also fearful that her art work will be judged as being bad by others and, therefore, she has put the idea of art school out of her mind. She also likes to write and keeps a journal about her experiences. She thinks she will just live with her mom indefinitely.

Discussion

Alexis shows many of the classic *DSM-5* symptoms of SOC (APA, 2013). She is fearful about entering situations where she may encounter her peers and avoids social interactions with

(continued)

CASE STUDY 10.1 ALEXIS: CASE OF A WHITE FEMALE WITH SOCIAL ANXIETY DISORDER (continued)

others besides her immediate family. She shows physical symptoms of anxiety and avoidant behavior in social scenarios. She also feels like others are negatively evaluating her. One might argue that Alexis is performing adequately in school and therefore special education or Section 504 (1973) services are not warranted. What is concerning is that Alexis has likely been inadvertently reinforced to avoid social situations in the midst of the pandemic and she is vowing not to return to school (Morrissette, 2021). She also appears to be limiting herself from pursuing postsecondary education even though she is a very gifted artist. As the school psychologist, there are several recommendations that could be made. Alexis may benefit from a behavioral support intervention that would prioritize her transitions back to face-to-face instruction. She could also benefit from a CBT intervention that is focused on supporting her with exposure therapy to social situations that involve peers. The art teacher could be consulted to be a supportive individual to her as she makes this transition. Diane and Susan would also benefit from consulting with the school psychologist about family mental health supports they could receive in the community, given the stress that they are all under due to COVID-19. Diane may want to seek out referrals for her own mental health counseling. As Alexis is supported through CBT and gains coping skills in managing her anxiety in social situations, she could be encouraged to join the art club, which could be a component of treatment once she is ready.

SUMMARY POINTS

- SOC in children and adolescents is marked by extreme fear, anxiety, and avoidance of a variety of social situations, specifically those that involve peers (APA, 2013). Persons with SOC fear being negatively evaluated by others (APA, 2013).
- *DSM-5* criteria now have a performance-only specifier when making the SOC diagnosis (APA, 2013; Center for Behavioral Health Statistics and Quality, 2016).
- Individuals with SOC may be at risk for acquiring a number of comorbid *DSM* (APA, 2013) disorders, such as depression, anxiety, personality disorders, and alcohol abuse/dependence.
- Females may have higher rates of SOC compared with males.
- School psychologists should consider the cultural norms and beliefs that a student and their family have about what is considered acceptable in social interactions and relationships.
- CBT and social skills training has strong empirical evidence to support its use in clinical and school settings in treating children and adolescents who have SOC.
- SSRIs are pharmacological interventions that are sometimes used with children and adolescents who have SOC.
- As children and adolescents with SOC and other anxiety disorders return to school following school shutdowns due to COVID-19, they will need mental health supports and should have continued access to appropriate treatment, particularly exposure therapy as part of CBT.

TEST YOUR KNOWLEDGE

1. Based on the *DSM-5* criteria, SOC has a performance-only specifier.
   a. True
   b. False

2. The following interventions have empirical evidence in treating children and adolescents who have SOC:
   a. Cognitive behavior therapy
   b. Psychodrama
   c. Humanistic therapy
   d. Psychodynamic therapy

3. Most children and adolescents who have SOC are diagnosed and treated.
   a. True
   b. False

4. Children with SOC may receive educational services through the following:
   a. IDEA—Other Health Impaired
   b. IDEA—Emotional Disturbance
   c. Section 504 of the Rehabilitation Act of 1973
   d. All of the above

5. Gender and racial/ethnic differences have been found in epidemiological studies of SOC.
   a. True
   b. False

Answers: (1) a, (2) a, (3) b, (4) d, (5) a.

DISCUSSION QUESTIONS

1. Describe the *DSM-5* (APA, 2013) criteria for SOC and how it has changed from the *DSM-IV-TR* (APA, 2000).

2. Discuss how social development could be impacted by SOC.

3. Outline a support at each tier within MTSS (Tier 1, Tier 2, and Tier 3) that could be offered for students suspected of or diagnosed with SOC.

4. Outline how school psychologists can use family collaboration skills (NASP, 2020a) in working with families who have a child or adolescent who has SOC.

5. Describe how family history may predict the onset of SOC in children and adolescents.

CHAPTER RESOURCES

American Academy of Child and Adolescent Psychiatry: www.aacap.org/aacap/Families_and_Youth/Resource_Centers/Anxiety_Disorder_Resource_Center/Home.aspx
Anxiety and Depression Association of America: https://adaa.org/understanding-anxiety/social-anxiety-disorder
Child Mind Institute *Social Anxiety Disorder Basics*: https://childmind.org/guide/social-anxiety-disorder
National Institute of Mental Health *Social Anxiety Disorder: More Than Just Shyness*: www.nimh.nih.gov/health/publications/social-anxiety-disorder-more-than-just-shyness
National Social Anxiety Center *Resources*: https://nationalsocialanxietycenter.com/resources

KEY REFERENCES

Only key references appear in the print edition. The full reference list appears in the digital product on Springer Publishing Connect: connect.springerpub.com/content/book/978-0-8261-3587-2/part/part04/chapter/ch10

Chavira, D. A., Stein, M. B., Bailey, K., & Stein, M. T. (2004b). Comorbidity of generalized social anxiety disorder and depression in a pediatric primary care sample. *Journal of Affective Disorders, 80,* 163–171. https://doi.org/10.1016/S0165-0327(03)00103-4

Collins, T. A., Dart, E. H., & Arora, P. G. (2019). Addressing the internalizing behavior of students in schools: Applications of the MTSS model. *School Mental Health, 11,* 191–193. https://doi.org/10.1007/s12310-018-09307-9

Festa, C. C., & Ginsburg, G. S. (2011). Parental and peer predictors of social anxiety in youth. *Child Psychiatry Human Development, 42*(3), 291–306. https://doi.org/10.1007/s10578-011-0215-8

Grant, B. F., Hasin, D. S., Blanco, C., Stinson, F. S., Chou, P., Goldstein, R. B., Dawson, D. A., Smith, S., Saha, T. D., & Huang, B. (2005). The epidemiology of social anxiety disorder in the United States: Results from the national epidemiologic survey on alcohol and related conditions. *Journal of Clinical Psychiatry, 66,* 1351–1361. https://doi.org/10.4088/jcp.v66n1102

Herbert, J. D., Gaudiano, B. A., Rheingold, A. A., Moitra, E., Myers, V. H., Dalrymple, K. L., & Brandsma, L. L. (2009). Cognitive behavior therapy for generalized social anxiety disorder in adolescents: A randomized controlled trial. *Journal of Anxiety Disorders, 23,* 167–177. https://doi.org/10.1016/j.janxdis.2008.06.004

Hofmann, S. G., Asnaani, A., & Hinton, D. E. (2010). Cultural aspects in social anxiety and social anxiety disorder. *Depression and Anxiety, 27,* 1117–1127. https://doi.org/10.1002/da.20759

Inderbitzen-Nolan, H., & Walters, K. S. (2000). Social Anxiety Scale for Adolescents: Normative data and further evidence of construct validity. *Journal of Clinical Child Psychology, 29*(3), 360–371, https://doi.org/10.1207/S15374424JCCP2903_7

Kerns, C. E., Comer, J. S., Pincus, D. B., & Hofmann, S. G. (2013). Evaluation of the proposed social anxiety disorder specifier change for *DSM-5* in a treatment-seeking sample of anxious youth. *Depression and Anxiety, 30,* 709–715. https://doi.org/10.1002/da.22067

LaGreca, A. M., & Stone, W. L. (1993). Social Anxiety Scale for Children-Revised: Factor structure and concurrent validity. *Journal of Clinical Child Psychology, 22*(1), 17–27. https://doi.org/10.1207/s15374424jccp2201_2

Olivares-Olivares, P. J., Ortiz-Gonzalez, P. F., & Olivares, J. (2019). Role of social skill training in adolescents with social anxiety disorder. *International Journal of Clinical and Health Psychology, 19,* 41–48. https://doi.org/10.1016/j.ijchp.2018.11.002

Runyon, K., Chestnut, S. R., & Burley, H. (2018). Screening for children anxiety: A meta-analysis of the Screen for Child Anxiety Related Emotional Disorders. *Journal of Affective Disorders, 240,* 220–229. https://doi.org/10.1016/j.jad.2018.07.049

Sulkowski, M. L., Joyce, D. K., & Storch, E. A. (2012). Treating childhood anxiety in schools: Service delivery in a response to intervention paradigm. *Journal of Child and Family Studies, 21,* 938–947. https://doi.org/10.1007/s10826-011-9553-1

CHAPTER 11

Selective Mutism

LEARNING OBJECTIVES

- Summarize the diagnostic features for the *Diagnostic and Statistical Manual of Mental Disorders* (5th ed.; *DSM-5*; American Psychiatric Association [APA], 2013) diagnosis of Selective Mutism (SM).
- Highlight the risk factors for SM in children and adolescents.
- Describe common school and home concerns for children with SM.
- Understand the classroom challenges for students with SM.
- Identify effective mental health supports for students with SM.

INTRODUCTION

Within the *Diagnostic and Statistical Manual of Mental Disorders,* Fifth Edition (*DSM-5*; American Psychiatric Association [APA], 2013), Selective Mutism (SM) is classified among the Anxiety Disorders. The disorders within this category are characterized by excessive fear and worry that goes beyond what is considered typical in most situations. Examples of other Anxiety Disorders include Separation Anxiety Disorder, Social Anxiety Disorder, and Generalized Anxiety Disorder. The Anxiety Disorders differ from one another in the focus of the fears and the thoughts related to the anxiety associated with the fear (APA, 2013).

DIAGNOSTIC ISSUES: *DSM-5* AND SCHOOL-BASED SERVICES

DSM-5 Diagnosis

Children with SM often appear shy due to their refusal to speak and because of their social anxiety. This refusal to speak tends to be especially prevalent in school settings, which negatively impacts both their academic and social functioning in that environment. Although children with SM choose to severely limit their verbal communication, they often use methods like pointing, writing, or gesturing to convey information to others (APA, 2013; Crundwell, 2006; Sharp et al., 2007). On occasion, they may even communicate with barely audible whispers (Crundwell, 2006). When in their own homes with immediate relatives, they will often communicate orally (and at typical volume) but may not do so even with nonhousehold family members or family friends (APA, 2013; Muris & Ollendick, 2021a; Viana et al., 2009). This contrast between the behavior shown at school and at home may lead some parents to believe that the issue is the result of something adverse that is happening with the child in the school setting (Mulligan et al., 2015). However, it has been noted that SM frequently emerges at times of change for the child (e.g., school entry, parental divorce, or death in the family; Podgorska-Jachnik, 2020; Standart & Le Couteur, 2003; Wong, 2010).

> The contrast between the child speaking at home but not at school may lead some parents to believe that the issue is the result of something adverse that is happening with the child in the school setting (Mulligan et al., 2015).

Recent research investigated the triggers for mute behavior in children. Schwenck et al. (2021) found that the most common situations known to elicit mutism include engaging in new activities, visiting unfamiliar settings, and interacting with people who are demanding of the child or insensitive to the child's psychological needs. It is interesting to note that these researchers indicate that it is easier for a child with SM to engage verbally with a new person who is not pressuring the child to speak than for the child to break the pattern of silence with someone with whom the child has previously been selectively mute (Schwenck et al., 2021). With adults with whom the child with SM is familiar and comfortable, the child may appear clingy to a degree that would not be considered developmentally appropriate and become distressed if that person leaves the child's presence (Crundwell, 2006).

According to the *DSM-5*, there are five criteria for the diagnosis of SM. The first criterion describes an individual's continual refusal to speak in expected circumstances although that person will communicate orally in other settings. The second criterion relates to the impairment caused by the refusal to speak. It must be demonstrated that the lack of communication is negatively affecting school, work, or social adjustment. The third criterion notes that the person must have failed to speak in a particular setting for at least 1 month, but this criterion does not apply if the refusal to speak is in the academic environment, and that month is the first month of a school year. The fourth criterion excludes diagnosis if the choice to remain silent is due to lack of knowledge or comfort with the language being used in that particular setting, and the fifth criterion indicates that the failure to speak cannot be associated with another disorder (e.g., communication disorder, autism spectrum disorder [ASD], or a psychotic disorder) in order to apply the diagnosis of SM (APA, 2013).

As noted previously, the psychiatric condition of SM is categorized with the Anxiety Disorders within the *DSM-5* (APA, 2013). However, this represents a change from the prior version, the *DSM-IV-TR* (APA, 2000), where it was clustered under the umbrella of Disorders of Childhood and Adolescence. Although the actual diagnostic criteria were not altered, Holka-Pokorska et al. (2018) contend that this change represents more than just an organizational artifact. Rather, it highlights the anxiety component of SM and opens the possibility of diagnosis in adulthood. This focus on anxiety is critically important in that the early description of disorders akin to what is now SM suggested that the refusal to speak was a manifestation of oppositional behavior or the result of excessively controlling parents as opposed to a form of anxiety (Holka-Pokorska et al., 2018; Muris & Ollendick, 2021a; Sharp et al., 2007; Viana et al., 2009). Muris and Ollendick (2021a) contend that the basis of SM as an issue of anxiety is supported by research that highlights its high co-occurrence with other anxiety disorders, research that explores the thoughts of children with SM that are focused on social anxiety themes, and research on the shy and reserved temperaments of children with SM. In fact, the role of temperament in SM is evidenced in infancy as people who exhibit SM often demonstrate extreme behavioral inhibition even at the youngest ages (Gensthaler et al., 2016). Given this collective evidence, some scholars have even suggested that SM may be a variant of social anxiety disorder as opposed to its own unique disorder (Bogels et al., 2010).

However, the focus on anxiety as the impetus for SM is not without controversy. Some researchers contend that current evidence does not support a link to social anxiety. They point to research that shows that the age of onset of SM is younger than what is evidenced in social phobia and to data that indicates lower social anxiety among children with SM than social phobia, suggesting that the link between anxiety and SM is not wholly supported by data (Holka-Pokorska et al., 2018). In fact, the *International Classification of Diseases, Eleventh Revision* (an alternative diagnostic system to the *DSM*), categorizes SM as a speech expression disorder (Podgorska-Jachnik, 2020). In addition, Muris and Ollendick (2021b) propose that SM may not be solely a disorder of anxiety but that it also features significant symptom characteristics with ASD. This is supported through research by Steffenberg et al. (2018) that found significant symptom overlap between the two disorders.

The controversy over the heterogeneity of SM has led some researchers to propose that it is indeed its own disorder, but it may have a number of subtypes. Mulligan et al. (2015) believe that their research supports the presence of five subtypes of SM. The first subtype would be the Emotional/Behavioral subtype, which has a large anxiety component. The second proposed subtype is Sensory/Pathology, which is a combination of mute behaviors combined with developmental delays and learning problems. The third subtype supported by their research is the Anxiety/Language category, which is marked by early speech and language challenges. The fourth identified subtype is the Low Functioning subtype, which is characterized by more significant academic problems, and the final subtype is the Global subtype, which encompasses children with greater self-esteem issues (Mulligan et al., 2015). Despite their findings, more research is needed to validate the possible delineation of SM subtypes. Also, regarding the heterogeneity of SM, Kearney and Rede (2021) suggest that it may be more appropriately classified as a Neurodevelopmental Disorder by the *DSM* due to its complex combination of behavioral, cognitive, emotional, and developmental symptomatology.

With regard to prevalence, SM is a relatively rare psychiatric disorder. Most estimates suggest that is occurs in 0.03% to 1% of the population (APA, 2013; Viana et al., 2009) and with greater frequency in girls as opposed to boys (Capozzi et al., 2018; Kristensen, 2001; Steffenberg et al., 2018). Despite these estimates, Viana et al. (2009) contend that the actual prevalence of SM is difficult to establish due to the lack of an agreed upon approach to etiology, assessment, and treatment of this mental health condition. In addition, research has found significantly higher prevalence when conducted with school-based samples as opposed to clinical populations (Standart & Le Couteur, 2003). The onset of SM is typically before 5 years of age, and its complications become more pronounced as the child starts school (APA, 2013; Viana et al., 2009). Research indicates a range of onset from 2.7 to 4.1 years old (Viana et al., 2009). An encouraging fact is that the prevalence of SM declines as children age; children are thought to outgrow this disorder although it is not clear why this might be the case (Starke, 2018; Wong, 2010).

> The onset of selective mutism is typically before 5 years of age, and its complications become more pronounced as the child starts school (APA, 2013; Viana et al., 2009).

In relation to comorbidity, there is an especially elevated co-occurrence of SM with other anxiety disorders, with rates of comorbidity as high as 100% in some research (Dummit et al., 1997). Social phobia and separation anxiety disorder tend to be particularly prevalent in children with SM (Arie et al., 2006; Kristensen, 2001). SM also frequently co-occurs with ASD and obsessive-compulsive disorder (Wong, 2010). Other comorbidity concerns with SM include tics, enuresis, and encopresis among a small subset of children with this psychiatric condition (Black & Uhde, 1995; Kristensen, 2001). In addition, even into adolescence, individuals with SM may display agoraphobic tendencies (Schwenck et al., 2021). Finally, children who are selectively mute express more somatic complaints than their typically developing peers (Cunningham et al., 2004).

School-Based Eligibility

Under the auspices of the Individuals with Disabilities Education Improvement Act (IDEA), federal law has established protections for students with disabilities, and children with SM may be eligible for additional supports and services in the school setting according to IDEA mandates (U.S. Department of Education, n.d.). With IDEA, schools must establish evaluation teams (which include the parents of the child under review) to determine which students meet eligibility requirements to receive special education and related services to assist them in progressing in the academic environment. IDEA outlines 13 disability categories. The evaluation team is charged with determining whether the child meets criteria under one (or more) of those categories and whether they also demonstrate a need for services. If the team determines that both of these conditions are met, then an individualized (and legally binding) plan is developed to provide the child with needed services.

It should be noted that the diagnosis of SM is neither necessary nor sufficient in determining IDEA eligibility; however, the team may seek to qualify the child under the IDEA disability category of Emotional Disturbance. The law states that "Emotional disturbance means a condition exhibiting one or more of the following characteristics over a long period of time and to a marked degree that adversely affects a child's educational performance" (U.S. Department of Education, n.d., Section 300.8 (c) (4)). Those characteristics include the following: challenges with educational attainment not due to other cognitive or medical conditions, difficulty in establishing and keeping social relationships, atypical emotional and behavioral responses under normal circumstances, frequently depressed mood, and somatic symptoms associated with individual problems. The criteria also explain that children and adolescents diagnosed with schizophrenia are eligible for certification under the category of Emotional Disturbance, but a child who demonstrates socially maladjusted behaviors is ineligible for services under the Emotional Disturbance criteria. It is possible for a student with SM to exhibit all five of the characteristics that denote Emotional Disturbance.

However, if the evaluation team does not find supporting evidence of the presence of Emotional Disturbance, they may seek to provide the child with additional supports and services under a different federal law—Section 504 of the Rehabilitation Act of 1973 (Office of Civil Rights, n.d.). This piece of civil rights legislation aims to give individuals with disabilities equal access to government services, organizations, and entities, including public schools. According to this law, a student may be found eligible under its mandates if the child has an impairment that "substantially limits one or more major life functions" (Office of Civil Rights, n.d.) such as caring for oneself, performing manual tasks, walking, hearing, seeing, speaking, breathing, learning, and working. In the case of a child with SM, it is highly probable that a team may determine that the symptomatology of the diagnosis negatively impacts their ability to both speak and learn. Therefore, the child would be eligible for academic, social, emotional, and behavioral supports necessary to maintain their progress in the school environment.

CULTURAL ISSUES RELATED TO SELECTIVE MUTISM IN YOUTH

Risk Factors for Selective Mutism

At present, a number of correlates have been associated with the development of SM in children, but no consensus has been reached regarding etiology of this psychiatric disorder (Viana et al., 2009). Both environmental and genetic risk factors have been highlighted as possibly contributing to SM in children; however, the most consistent finding is related to familial psychopathology. One such risk factor is having a first-degree relative diagnosed with an anxiety disorder. Black and Uhde (1995) found that 70% of children with SM have a close relative with social phobia, and 37% had a relative with similar SM symptomatology. Other studies have found high rates of differing forms of psychopathology in parents of children with SM. These disorders include depression, anxiety, social phobia, and personality disorders (Capozzi et al., 2018; Chevira et al., 2007; Remschmidt et al., 2001; Steinhausen et al., 2006). Finally, in a recent study of parental psychopathology and SM, Koskela and colleagues (2020) found that when both parents have any psychiatric diagnosis, it nearly triples the probability of them having a child with SM. The authors suggest that this is evidence of a shared etiology across mental health conditions. Of note, when only one parent has a psychiatric disorder, then the study found stronger effects for maternal psychopathology on SM in the child than for paternal psychopathology (Koskela et al., 2020).

Beyond parental issues with mental health, research has also pointed to a number of other factors in relation to SM. One relatively new finding relates to paternal age. Koskela et al. (2020) found that having a father over the age of 35 at the birth of the child was related to future development of SM in that child and having a father over the age of 40 represented even greater probability of SM in the child. In this same study, the researchers found that lower socioeconomic status of the family and living in a single-parent home with a mother were also related to increased odds of having a child with SM (Koskela et al., 2020). In sum, although research has identified a variety of correlates of SM, the evidence of etiology is far from definitive at this point in time.

Cultural Considerations

One particular challenge for clinicians in the diagnosis of SM relates to bilingual children and the application of the criterion related to insufficient knowledge and comfort with the language as an exclusionary issue. To be specific, it is challenging to determine at what level language acquisition is adequate for diagnosis (Toppelberg et al., 2005). Although the *DSM-5* states that prevalence of SM does not vary by race/ethnicity (APA, 2013), some researchers suggest that its occurrence in immigrant children who speak English as a second language may be as high as 3 times that of the native-speaking population (Elizur & Perednik, 2003; Toppelberg et al., 2005). However, the group of immigrant children for whom this is the case appear to have higher levels of social anxiety as well (Elizur & Perednik, 2003). In fact, a recent study found that anxiety was the greatest predictor of SM for bilingual children, although parents' level of cultural adaptation was also negatively related to their child's silence in preschool (Starke, 2018).

> Although the *DSM-5* states that prevalence of SM does not vary by race/ethnicity (APA, 2013), some researchers suggest that its occurrence in immigrant children who speak English as a second language may be as high as 3 times that of the native-speaking population (Elizur & Perednik, 2003; Toppelberg et al., 2005).

Nonetheless, researchers in this area contend that it is common for new language learners to go through a silent period, and research evidence supports its normalcy as a development stage (Le Pichon & de Jonge, 2016; Toppelberg et al., 2005). According to Toppelberg et al. (2005), "It typically starts when children realize that their home language is not understood at school and their second language skills are insufficient or absent. They then stop speaking completely in that setting" (p. 593). Empirical studies suggest that these developmental silences among English-language learners are relatively common in children ages 3 to 8 and usually persist for a duration of 1 to 6 months (Tabors, 1997). Thus, understanding and correctly applying the language exclusion criterion with immigrant and/or English-language learning children prevents overdiagnosis of SM within this population. However, scholars contend that there are certainly circumstances within which an SM diagnosis should be considered for immigrant children, such as when children fail to progress through the silent phase, when the child's discomfort with the language is disproportionate to the level of acquisition, when the child demonstrates predisposing shyness and anxiety, or when the child displays SM in both their native and newly acquired/acquiring language (Toppelberg et al., 2005).

IMPACT OF SELECTIVE MUTISM ON SOCIAL–EMOTIONAL AND BEHAVIORAL FUNCTIONING IN SCHOOL AND HOME ENVIRONMENTS

Social–Emotional and Behavioral Functioning in School

Given the significant comorbidity of SM and social anxiety and/or social phobia, it is not surprising that both parents and teachers of children with SM rate them as higher than even peers with social phobia in their levels of social distress, particularly in the school setting (Yeganeh et al., 2003). In addition, parents and teachers rate the verbal and nonverbal social skills of children with SM as deficient as compared to their typically developing peers (Cunningham et al., 2006; Klein et al., 2019). Similarly, Cunningham et al. (2004) found that children with SM are rated as less socially assertive, meaning that they are less likely to engage in behaviors like joining groups or introducing themselves to others. Their parents also note that they are shyer than peers and more likely to withdraw in social situations (Capozzi et al., 2018; Milic et al., 2020). Although both parents and teachers indicate that children with SM are withdrawn, parents rate them as significantly more so in relation to teacher ratings (Klein et al., 2019). Yet, it is interesting to note that children with SM do not view themselves as distinct from their peers in their level of social skills (Cunningham et al., 2006). Some research indicates that children with SM are of equal social status as classmates (Longobardi et al., 2019), but other studies show that children with SM struggle with forming friendships and have fewer friends than children without SM (Milic et al., 2020). When children with SM do make friends, their parents report that they are able to maintain those relationships in a manner consistent with peers (Milic et al., 2020). Empirical evidence does not support that children with SM are victimized by their peers at higher rates than typically developing children. However, as selectively mute children display more oppositional or anxious behaviors, their probability of victimization by peers increases (Cunningham et al., 2004).

Parents and teachers rate the verbal and nonverbal social skills of children with SM as deficient compared to their typically developing peers (Cunningham et al., 2006; Klein et al., 2019).

Beyond peer experiences, research has shown that the relationships between teachers and students is critically important to children's adjustment and school success in a variety of domains (Collins et al., 2017; O'Connor et al., 2012; Ruzek et al., 2016). Yet, despite their reticence to engage socially at all, children with SM are more likely to engage with peers than they are with teachers or other individuals of authority in the school setting (Schwenck et al., 2021). This may be why teachers rate their relationships with typically developing students as closer than their relationships with children with SM even though teachers endorse equivalent levels of conflict in their relationships with both sets of students (Longobardi et al., 2019). Therefore, the social and behavioral functioning of children with SM in the school setting is often marked by both challenges and inconsistencies in their adaptation.

Social–Emotional and Behavioral Functioning at Home

With regard to the home environment of children with SM, strained conditions have been reported in the literature. According to Capozzi et al. (2018), parents of children with SM report higher incidences of stressful life events relative to other families. In addition, researchers suggest that these homes are marked by higher levels of conflict than other homes. This conflict includes the marital relationship of the parents as well as the parent–child relationships (Remschmidt et al., 2001). Perhaps adding to familial discord, parents of children with SM rate them as less cooperative and compliant than children without SM (Cunningham et al., 2004). In fact, when parents and teachers are asked to rate the behaviors of children with SM, parents are often more negative regarding the children's behavioral symptoms than are teachers (Klein et al., 2019). Parents also report their belief that their children with SM are more demanding at home than they are in the school environment (Klein et al., 2019). And children with SM report feeling less warmth and acceptance from their parents compared to children who have other types of social anxieties (Yeganeh et al., 2006).

Finally, the families of children with SM may be more socially isolated than other families (Remschmidt et al., 2001). This may, in turn, lead to an underreporting of SM overall due to a lack of comparison to other children and a lack of opportunity for parents to observe their children's silence outside the home (Mulligan et al., 2015). Thus, although the children with SM may speak more inside the home environment than in other settings, the home environment may (in some circumstances) contribute to and/or exacerbate SM symptomatology.

IMPACT OF SELECTIVE MUTISM ON LEARNING IN THE CLASSROOM

One of the prevailing theories regarding the etiology of SM relates its occurrence to language deficits and auditory processing impairment in children (Arie et al., 2006; Holka-Pokorska et al. 2018). Some research suggests that up to 38% of children with SM also have forms of speech and/or language disorders, including issues with articulation and language expression (Kristensen, 2001). In addition, even when their language issues are not significant enough to warrant a diagnosis, children with SM have been found to have impaired performance on language tasks as compared to their typically developing peers and in relation to children with other forms of anxiety (Manassis et al., 2003, 2007). Also, in regard to communication, children with SM have been found to use shorter and less detailed sentences (McInnes et al., 2004) and speak less overall (Milic et al., 2020) even when they do not have a language disorder. All of the aforementioned issues have a significant probability of negatively impacting both academic and social performance in the classroom as teachers struggle to assess children's knowledge and progress despite their impaired communication and as peers have difficulty developing relationships with a student whose communication is not on par with their classmates.

> Children with SM have been found to use shorter and less detailed sentences (McInnes et al., 2004) and speak less overall (Milic et al., 2020), even when they do not have a language disorder.

Children with SM tend to avoid all classroom situations in which speech would be expected (Crundwell, 2006). Interesting research explored the fear-related thoughts of children with SM. Vogel et al. (2019) found that 59% of their sample of children with SM described social fears as a reason for their silence, whereas 28% expressed fears of making mistakes, 8% endorsed fears associated with language-related mistakes, and 5% noted voice-related fears. Beyond their issues with speaking aloud, research has also found that children with SM struggle to engage in classroom activities even when they do not involve speech such as working problems on the board (Martinez et al., 2015). All of these issues may be related to the perfectionism that is often reported for children with SM (Vogel et al., 2019).

Beyond the issues with communication, researchers have also identified other factors among children with SM that may represent challenges for the classroom. Some of those deficits relate to memory. Studies have noted that children with SM demonstrate impairments in both visual memory and nonverbal working memory (Manassis et al., 2007). In addition, although there have been few studies in this area, researchers have also found that students with SM may have a greater prevalence of fine and gross motor delays relative to their typically developing peers (Kristensen, 2002). According to Klein et al. (2019), teachers in their study indicated that children with SM are less attentive to classroom instruction than their peers, but this may be related to their hyper-focus on their fears of being asked to respond verbally during lessons. Nonetheless, teacher ratings of the academic performance of children with SM do not differ from their typically developing peers (Cunningham et al., 2004).

Finally, a small subset of children with SM have been found to exhibit oppositional behaviors that would negatively impact classroom adjustment (Black & Uhde, 1995; Kristensen, 2001; Manassis et al., 2007; Yeganeh et al., 2006). The oppositional behavior may emerge in instances when the child with SM is being pressured to communicate verbally (Crundwell, 2006). However, recent research has failed to find a relationship between SM and challenging classroom behavior in large clinical studies (Longobardi et al., 2019).

IMPLICATIONS FOR SCHOOL PSYCHOLOGISTS

Assessment Role

Clinical researchers suggest that, due to its often problematic presentation in the school setting, the initial diagnosis of SM should include comprehensive assessment of school-based behavior (Martinez et al., 2015; Muris & Ollendick, 2021a; Ponzurick, 2012; Viana et al., 2009), and the school psychologist may collaborate with the external clinician in that assessment process. In fact, given that children with SM commonly speak within the home, school entry could represent the first manifestation of the disorder (Crundwell, 2006; Kehle et al., 2018; Mulligan et al., 2015; Sharp et al., 2007). In support of this, research shows that primary care physicians frequently fail to either accurately diagnose and/or refer children with SM for assessment despite parent-expressed concerns and clear symptomatology (Schwartz et al., 2006). Thus, information regarding verbal/nonverbal behaviors across settings and individuals in the school environment could represent data critical to the assessment and treatment process that would likely be unknowable to the clinician without the input of school personnel (Martinez et al., 2015). In addition to the aforementioned shyness, anxiety, and silence displayed by children with SM, early-warning signs also include blushing, fidgeting, avoiding eye contact, withdrawal, and bodily stiffness in social situations (Crundwell, 2006). When shyness and the associated symptoms of SM last beyond the first month of school, early intervention is needed as research has demonstrated that the longer the period between symptom onset and treatment, the less amenable SM is to effective treatment for children with this mental health disorder (Capobianco & Cerniglia, 2018; Hung et al., 2012; Kehle et al., 2018; Kovac & Furr, 2019; Mulligan et al., 2015; Schwartz et al., 2006). Therefore, school psychologists may represent a critical link in the information gathering for the initial diagnosis of SM by a community-based healthcare provider.

> Research shows that primary care physicians frequently fail to either accurately diagnose and/or refer children with SM for assessment despite parent-expressed concerns and clear symptomatology (Schwartz et al., 2006).

Beyond this type of assessment, the knowledge and skills of the school psychologist are necessary in the evaluation of a student with SM for school-based eligibility under IDEA or Section 504. When an evaluation is initiated and parent permission is obtained for that evaluation, then the team is charged with assessing a student in all areas of suspected disability. For the child with SM, these are likely to include cognitive, academic, social, emotional, behavioral, speech, and language assessments. The evaluation would likely begin with the school psychologist conducting classroom observations, a file review (grades, attendance, disciplinary, and standardized tests), interviews (student, teacher, parent), and record reviews (external providers such as counselors, psychologists, and/or psychiatrists) necessary to establish the prior and current functioning of the student. The classroom observations would be the first stage of a functional behavioral assessment conducted in the context of the evaluation to provide enlightenment on the mute behavior. Those observations could be used to identify the antecedents or setting events that trigger mutism (or conversely, the antecedents or setting events that support speech), and the consequences that support/maintain the mutism (or speech). These data are critical to intervention development. Beyond these investigations, the school psychologist would begin a testing process that would likely include assessments of intellectual functioning, academic achievement, overall behavior ratings, and specific anxiety scales. Further, the speech–language pathologist would be a necessary team member in assessing language components like receptive vocabulary, expressive vocabulary, and oral expression. After collecting the necessary data, the team would collaboratively determine whether the child met criteria as a student with a disability in a manner that necessitated supports and services in order to appropriately progress in the curriculum.

Advocacy Role

Selective serotonin reuptake inhibitors (SSRIs) are commonly prescribed by healthcare providers and used in the treatment of SM (Holka-Pokorska et al., 2018; Manassis & Tannock, 2008; Muris & Ollendick, 2021a, 2021b; Ponzurick, 2012; Schwartz et al., 2006; Viana et al., 2009; Wong, 2010). Thus, school psychologists should be well versed in their application in order to provide external professionals with objective data regarding their effectiveness for the child in question. Though SSRIs have shown success in the reduction of symptoms, research has yet to support that SSRIs will eliminate the symptoms of SM for children with this diagnosis (Black & Uhde, 1994; Manassis et al., 2016; Manassis & Tannock, 2008). In addition, it may be concerning to utilize a pharmacological approach given the young age of most children who are diagnosed with SM. Thus, Muris and Ollendick (2021a, 2021b) recommend that SSRIs may be more appropriately used when psychosocial interventions have failed to show improvement or in conjunction with therapy-based treatments. Nevertheless, school psychologists can assist families in advocating with their physicians for appropriate and effective care for the child with SM. Given the likelihood of external service providers for children with SM, Crundwell (2006) stresses the importance of continuous communication between school personnel and those professionals. The school psychologist is uniquely suited as a liaison to conduct observations, collect data, and report treatment effectiveness to counselors, psychologists, psychiatrists, and/or pediatricians who are involved in the child's treatment outside of the school setting.

Consultation Role

Individual behavioral interventions that involve shaping and modeling of behavior and systematic desensitization have been found to be effective in the treatment of SM (Oerbeck et al., 2020; Ponzurick, 2012; Schwartz et al., 2006; Viana et al., 2009). In particular, graduated exposure to new settings and child-initiated communication with new people show promise as behavioral techniques used to increase the verbal communication of children with SM (Schwerck et al., 2021). These behavioral interventions are often the result of consultation and collaboration between a school psychologist and teacher, and they are designed based on information gathered through a functional assessment process from a basis of behavioral observation. With regard to behavioral observation of SM, Shriver et al. (2011) state, "For the purposes of treatment planning, behavior observation is conducted for two primary purposes; 1) to identify the settings and situations in which the child does and does not speak, and 2) within each setting and situation, to identify what the child does to communicate" (p. 392). The school psychologist may then use this information to design, implement, and evaluate the success of interventions for the child with SM in the school and/or classroom setting.

Further, Kovac and Furr (2019) specifically recommend that educators seek information and support from their building's assigned school psychologist with regard to children with SM. They suggest that teachers and administrators would benefit from the provision of in-service offerings that improve the identification, understanding, and support of children with SM. School psychologists are perfectly suited to address these training needs. With their background in both education and psychology, school psychologists can provide both knowledge and practical strategies aimed at improving the effectiveness of educators to address the needs of these students with SM within their care.

> Kovac and Furr (2019) specifically recommend that educators seek information and support from their building's assigned school psychologist with regard to children with SM.

Counseling/Therapy Role

Cognitive behavioral therapy is a primary treatment method used for children with SM (Holka-Pokorska et al., 2018; Muris & Ollendick, 2021a; Oerbeck et al., 2018; Viana et al., 2009). The use of cognitive behavioral therapy has consistently corresponded with improvements in its symptomatology for those who struggle with this mental health condition (Capobianco & Cerniglia, 2018; Cohan et al., 2006; Muris & Ollendick, 2021a), and school-based treatments have shown overall effectiveness in this regard (Oerbeck et al., 2018; Schwartz et al., 2006). School psychologists are specially trained professionals with the expertise to deliver these therapeutic interventions to children within the academic environment. Providing these services will minimize the need for additional family resources devoted to the issue in regard to financial and time commitment. However, and more powerful, the interventions can be delivered in the environment where children with SM often experience significant adjustment issues due to their symptomatology. Therefore, upon identification of a student with SM, school psychologists should seek information to determine what external supports are already in place and how these can be complemented within the school setting.

EDUCATIONAL SUPPORTS

Researchers suggest that there are conditions within the school environment that may increase the probability of vulnerable bilingual students developing SM. Those include tenuous relationships between parents and school personnel, biased views regarding the child's culture, and insufficient education support for English-language learning. Given the association between language acquisition and risk for SM (particularly in the presence of anxiety), it is important for school personnel to understand and support second-language acquisition. According to Starke (2018), simultaneous bilingual children are those who are exposed to both languages before the age of 3. Simultaneous bilingual children typically demonstrate knowledge and access to both languages in a manner similar to single-language children. In contrast, sequential bilingual children are exposed to the second language after the age of 3 when the first language is already solidly established for the child. The acquisition of the second language may then proceed more slowly and represent greater stigma for the child. If the child also evidences a shy temperament and higher levels of anxiety, then that student may be at risk for the development of SM (Starke, 2018). As such, it would behoove school personnel to provide culturally appropriate academic supports while also determining need for psychosocial interventions.

For all children with SM (regardless of mono- or multilingual status), researchers suggest that it is critical to avoid situations that increase the child's anxiety in the classroom and attempts at pressuring the child to speak as these situations often reinforce and exacerbate silence (Crundwell, 2006). Crundwell (2006) offers further recommendations for assisting children with SM in the classroom. One recommendation is to have a private conversation between the teacher and the child during which the teacher expresses understanding and empathy regarding the child's silence and anxiety in that setting. The child should be given an open invitation to speak when they are comfortable to do so. In addition, teachers can carefully observe the child in a variety of classroom situations to assess which of those appear most anxiety provoking and strive to create a safer classroom experience for the child (Crundwell, 2006; Kehle et al., 2018). However, it is essential that the classroom teacher does not remove all expectations for speech in the classroom for the child with SM. When it is too easy for the child to use alternative communication methods, it can unwittingly reinforce their lack of verbal communication, thereby reducing the probability of increased oral participation and effective treatment outcome (Kehle et al., 2018).

> Teachers can carefully observe the child in a variety of classroom situations to assess which of those appear most anxiety provoking and strive to create a safer classroom experience for the child with SM (Crundwell, 2006; Kehle et al., 2018).

Finally, Kehle et al. (2018) remind school personnel that although it is critical to engage in supportive classroom strategies for the student with SM, these supports alone are unlikely to alleviate all SM presentation and symptomatology. Nonetheless, Kehle et al. (2018) recommend a number of practical strategies to offer safety and encouragement for the child with SM. These include continuing verbal engagement with the student and offering ideas and observations without expecting a similar verbal response from the student. They suggest that it can also be helpful to increase opportunities to interact with the child in small-group settings. If the child whispers a response or answer, then it is appropriate for the teacher to offer praise for the verbalization and repeat it more loudly for the larger group (Kehle et al. 2018). Further, the teacher should avoid posing direct open-ended questions to the student but attempt to use either/or questions that prompt a simple verbal response without being overly intimidating in the manner of a question that would require a multi-word interaction. Also, if the child does not answer a direct question, wait 5 seconds before moving on with the discussion. Creating alternate ways to evaluate assignments and projects that require speaking may be appropriate for a time (Kehle et al., 2018; Kovac & Furr, 2019). These strategies and supports are child-friendly, and they are a bridge to successful initiation of speech for the student with SM.

SCHOOL-BASED MENTAL HEALTH INTERVENTIONS AND SUPPORTS

SM continues to be confusing and misunderstood even among mental health professionals. As late as 2018, Holka-Pokorska et al. wrote, "A comprehensive and uniform theory about the diagnosis and treatment of this disorder does not exist" (p. 323). Nonetheless, individual cognitive behavioral therapy and individual/group behavioral therapy have shown promise in the treatment of children with SM (Cohan et al., 2006; Stone et al., 2002).

According to Muris and Ollendick (2021a), cognitive behavioral therapy for children with SM should include the following core components: psychoeducation to improve the understanding of SM as an issue of anxiety, relaxation training to target symptoms of anxiety, modeling and exposure to increase comfort in social situations, cognitive restructuring to combat unhelpful thoughts, and parent training. Kehle et al. (2018) suggest pairing cognitive behavioral therapy with praise and reinforcement as the child moves toward more verbal means of communication. These scholars note that the clinician should monitor the child's response to praise conditions and slowly incorporate peers in also reinforcing the child for speech. According to Oerbeck et al. (2018), positive gains for their school-based cognitive behavioral treatment of SM are even shown at 5 years post-treatment with many children experiencing complete symptom remission by that time. Finally, an exposure-based therapy (with reinforcement and parent collaboration) called *Integrated Behavior Therapy for Selective Mutism* has shown initial success in increasing functional communication for children with SM with gains that were sustained for at least 3 months' time (Bergman et al., 2013). Similar results were attained by Catchpole et al. (2019) with a parent–child interaction therapy in which parents were taught effective communication strategies and utilization of exposure techniques in novel settings. This can be implemented in the school setting as long as the school psychologist has had appropriate training in this technique. As an alternative, the school psychologist may have a more collaborative role with a clinical psychologist who provides this type of therapy.

On the surface, group therapy may seem counterintuitive in the treatment of children for whom social situations create anxiety. However, recent research has supported its use with children with SM. One treatment protocol that included a group for children with SM and a separate group for their parents demonstrated effectiveness in increasing the children's speaking behaviors across settings and also in reducing parents' levels of anxiety. The children's group focused on psychoeducation regarding SM, graduated exposure to anxiety-producing stimuli, and a system of rewards. The parent group also included psychoeducation and provided practical strategies for managing their children's symptomatology (Sharkey et al., 2008). Although the Sharkey et al. (2008) therapy lasted for a number of weeks, Lorenzo et al. (2021) have developed an Intensive Group Behavioral Treatment that uses a week-long, camp-type format to deliver behavioral therapy with exposure-based strategies, parent training, and school outreach in a significantly concentrated format. The authors contend that the camp atmosphere better simulates school experiences in which students with SM often struggle and allows therapists to intervene naturally for improved outcomes (Lorenzo et al., 2021). Although implementation of the protocol developed by Lorenzo et al. (2021) may not be feasible for the school setting, school psychologists may consider a more intensive treatment schedule (as opposed to the typical one session per week) to boost opportunities for skill practice and gains in a group format for children with SM.

Due to the rarity of this disorder, research regarding effective treatment is scant and often relies on case studies or small sample sizes. Nonetheless, data are emerging regarding the effectiveness of the aforementioned treatments, many of which are applicable within the school environment for delivery by the appropriately trained school psychologist.

CASE STUDY 11.1 RYAN: A CASE OF A MALE WITH SELECTIVE MUTISM

Background

Ryan is a 5-year-old boy who lives at home with his dad, stepmom, and baby brother, who just turned 2. Ryan has not always lived with his dad. From birth until he was 4 months old, he lived with his mother. At 4 months, he went to live with his grandmother, who was also taking care of two other children belonging to his aunt (mother's sister), while his mother attended rehab. At age 2, he lived with his father for a year. His father had several women who lived with him during this time, but none who lived there for more than a few weeks. At 3, Ryan went back

(continued)

CASE STUDY 11.1 RYAN: A CASE OF A MALE WITH SELECTIVE MUTISM (continued)

to live with his mother for a few months. She returned to rehab, and he was moved to foster care until his father was located. Ryan's dad has some college education but did not complete his degree. He joined the army after college and served for 5 years and currently works as a mechanic. Ryan's stepmother considers herself the primary caregiver as she has more days off to spend with the boys. The family's daily schedule is "hectic," but the stepmom tries to keep some consistency, because Ryan struggles without it. Ryan's stepmom is a medical technician who works three 10-hour shifts a week to be able to spend more time with the boys, and Ryan's dad has a typical 9 to 5 job.

Ryan is in kindergarten. He stayed home with his stepmother and did not attend preschool. It was in kindergarten that the concerns with speaking began. When Ryan started school he blushed, avoided eye contact with the teacher, and spoke in a barely audible whisper. As school progressed, he would only communicate with gestures. It was also noted that Ryan was quite shy, struggled in transitions, and seemed to shut down during any new activities. He rarely participated in group activities that involved speaking or singing. Ryan would play in groups of children, but it was parallel in nature. He would make eye contact with peers and even smile and laugh but only gestured and did not speak. In class, he would often use methods like pointing, writing, or gesturing to convey information to others. As school went on, his academic skills have been heavily affected by his lack of willingness to speak at school. His teacher stated it was impossible to determine his academic skills due to his unwillingness to speak. The school and his parents have met several times to address his lack of verbal communication. This has also been a source of tension between the school and home.

At home, he spoke to his parents and brother but became very shy in public places and did not speak to other people. His parents struggled with the seriousness of the behaviors, because he did speak at home. His stepmother indicated that their routine needs to be discussed beforehand. She believes Ryan's reactions to change or transitions are age appropriate or typical, but they can be challenging. Besides Ryan's struggles with transitions and changes, his stepmom indicates that his demeanor is appropriate for his age. He is generally happy but gets very anxious and shy. She also noted that he seems to get frustrated quickly when he is unable to do something "perfectly."

Ryan's stepmom states that Ryan is excellent at communicating his needs at home. He will ask for things when he wants or needs them and even asks for permission to go to the bathroom, despite being able to go independently. He likes to be independent and tries to work things out without assistance but, similar to his behavior at school, can get frustrated quickly if he cannot do something. Ryan often cries when he is frustrated. Ryan's stepmother believes that he was delivered without any complications and has no history of major illness. He has no noted visual or auditory problems. The stepmom stated that Ryan reached typical milestones as expected.

Discussion

Given that children with SM commonly speak within the home, school entry could represent the first manifestation of the disorder and can be frustrating to parents and educators. Therefore, a thorough assessment should be conducted. Information regarding verbal/nonverbal behaviors across settings and individuals in the school environment could represent critical data to the assessment and treatment process. Communication disorders and ASD must be ruled out. Ryan speaks at home and communicates at school. Early on, he spoke in a whisper, but currently he only communicates with gestures and writing. He also exhibits shyness, anxiety, and the early warning signs of SM which include blushing, fidgeting, avoiding eye contact, withdrawal, and bodily stiffness in social situations. Given all this, it would seem that SM matches the symptoms more closely than communication disorders or ASD. However, a good assessment by a speech pathologist would be needed as well. In addition, his anxiety and memory should be fully explored. Memory issues and anxiety are both very common in children with SM.

His verbal and nonverbal social skills could possibly be delayed. Working on social skills could be a less threatening way to begin intervening with Ryan. This can help to bridge the

(continued)

CASE STUDY 11.1 RYAN: A CASE OF A MALE WITH SELECTIVE MUTISM (continued)

divide between school and home that the parents are experiencing. Some consultation with the parents about how to deal with his shyness and reactions to change or transitions may also help to build back the school–home relationship. It may be necessary to work as an advocate with his primary medical provider. It is common for the primary medical provider not to have a clear picture of the symptoms due to the disorder being more evident at school than at home. Once they have a clear picture of the symptoms and know whether other interventions are not as effective as expected (especially as Ryan gets older), they may choose to use SSRIs, which are commonly prescribed in the treatment of SM.

The school psychologist may want to consider individual behavioral interventions that involve shaping and modeling of behavior, and systematic desensitization. These have shown positive outcomes. Providing clear information to the educators and parents about SM also helps individuals understand the complexity of the disorder and makes the interventions more relevant. The use of cognitive behavioral therapy has consistently corresponded with improvements in symptomatology of SM. School psychologists are specially trained professionals with the expertise to deliver these therapeutic interventions to children within the academic environment. Providing these services in the school will minimize the need for additional family resources devoted to the issue in regard to financial and time commitments and continue to help rebuild the relationship between the school and family.

It is critical to engage in supportive classroom strategies for the student with SM. This assists and reinforces the ongoing interventions. These strategies include continuing verbal engagement with the student and offering ideas and observations without expecting a similar verbal response from the student. It can also be helpful to increase opportunities to interact with the child in small-group settings. The school personnel can model appropriate communication and if the child whispers a response or answer, then it is appropriate for the teacher to offer praise for the verbalization and repeat it more loudly for the larger group.

SUMMARY POINTS

- SM is often first observed when a child enters school.
- The *DSM-5* outlines five criteria for diagnosis of SM.
- A child with SM often speaks normally within the home.
- SM is thought to be associated with anxiety and/or language issues rather than oppositional behavior.
- School psychologists can engage in many roles and functions to support the needs of students with SM, including assessment, advocacy, consultation, and counseling and/or therapy.
- Behavioral and cognitive behavioral therapy may be effective in the treatment of SM although the evidence base is limited to small sample sizes and single case studies.

TEST YOUR KNOWLEDGE

1. When can SM NOT be diagnosed?
   a. During the first month of school
   b. During preschool
   c. In the teen years
   d. In adulthood

2. As a child ages, the child is more susceptible to developing SM.
   a. True
   b. False

3. It is developmentally appropriate for children who are learning a second language to go through a period of silence in some settings.
   a. True
   b. False

4. Which of the following is associated with the development of SM in children?
   a. Parental psychopathology
   b. Parental education level
   c. Sibling depression
   d. Sibling conflict

5. Bilingual children are excluded from diagnosis of SM.
   a. True
   b. False

Answers: (1) a, (2) b, (3) a, (4) a, (5) b.

DISCUSSION QUESTIONS

1. Describe the *DSM-5* diagnostic criteria for SM.
2. Explain the cultural considerations for diagnosis of a bilingual child with SM.
3. Explain why a child with SM may meet IDEA Emotional Disturbance criteria.
4. Describe the challenges for peer relationships for a child with SM.
5. Discuss the advocacy role for school psychologists for a child with SM.

CHAPTER RESOURCES

American Speech Language Hearing Association *Selective Mutism*: www.asha.org/practice-portal/clinical-topics/selective-mutism/
Cedars-Sinai *Selective Mutism*: www.cedars-sinai.org/health-library/diseases-and-conditions---pediatrics/s/selective-mutism.html
Child Mind *A Teacher's Guide to Selective Mutism*: https://childmind.org/guide/teachers-guide-to-selective-mutism/
Selective Mutism Association *Educators and School Staff*: www.selectivemutism.org/educators/
Selective Mutism *Resources: The Silence Within*: www.selective-mutism.com/sm-resources

KEY REFERENCES

Only key references appear in the print edition. The full reference list appears in the digital product on Springer Publishing Connect: connect.springerpub.com/content/book/978-0-8261-3587-2/part/part04/chapter/ch11

American Psychiatric Association. (2013). *Diagnostic and statistical manual of mental disorders* (5th ed.). https://doi.org/10.1176/appi.books.9780890425596

Holka-Pokorska, J., Pirog-Balcerzak, A., & Jarema, M. (2018). The controversy around the diagnosis of selective mutism—A critical analysis of three cases in the light of modern research and diagnostic criteria. *Psychiatria Polska, 52*(2), 323–343. https://doi.org/10.12740/PP/76088

Kovac, L. M., & Furr, J. M. (2019). What teachers should know about selective mutism in early childhood. *Early Childhood Education Journal, 47*, 107–114. https://doi.org/10.1007/s10643-018-0905-y

Lorenzo, N. E., Cornacchio, D., Chou, T., Kurtz, S. M. S., Furr, J. M., & Comer, J. S. (2021). Expanding treatment options for children with selective mutism: Rationale, principles, and procedures for an intensive group behavioral treatment. *Cognitive and Behavioral Practice, 28*(3), 379–392. https://doi.org/10.1016/j.cbpra.2020.06.002

Muris, P., & Ollendick, T. H. (2021a). Current challenges in the diagnosis and management of selective mutism in children. *Psychology Research and Behavior Management, 14*, 159–167. https://doi.org/10.2147/PRBM.S274538

Podgorska-Jachnik, D. (2020). Selective mutism and shyness. Differential diagnosis and strategies supporting child development. *Interdisciplinary Contexts of Special Pedagogy, 30*, 125–149. https://doi.org/10.14746/ikps.2020.30.07

Ponzurick, J. M. (2012). Selective mutism: A team approach to assessment and treatment in the school setting. *Journal of School Nursing, 28*(1), 31–37. https://doi.org/10.1177%2F1059840511422534

Schwenck, C., Gensthaler, A., Vogel, F., Pfeffermann, A., Laerum, S., & Stahl, J. (2021). Characteristics of person, place, and activity that trigger failure to speak in children with selective mutism. *European Child & Adolescent Psychiatry*. https://doi.org/10.1007/s00787-021-01777-8

Toppelberg, C. O., Tabors, P., Coggins, A., Lum, K., & Burger, C. (2005). Differential diagnosis of selective mutism in bilingual children. *Journal of the American Academy of Child and Adolescent Psychiatry, 44*(6), 592–595. https://doi.org/10.1097/01.chi.0000157549.87078.f8

U.S. Department of Education. (n.d.). *Individuals with Disabilities Education Improvement Act*. https://sites.ed.gov/idea

UNIT 5

MENTAL HEALTH DISORDERS IN CHILDREN AND ADOLESCENTS: MOOD DISORDERS

CHAPTER 12

Major Depressive Disorder

LEARNING OBJECTIVES

- Summarize the diagnostic features for the *Diagnostic and Statistical Manual of Mental Disorders* (5th ed.; *DSM-5*; American Psychiatric Association [APA], 2013) diagnosis of Major Depressive Disorder (MDD).
- Highlight the risk factors for MDD in children and adolescents.
- Describe common social–emotional and behavioral concerns for children with MDD.
- Understand the classroom implications for students with MDD.
- Identify effective social, emotional, and behavioral interventions for students with MDD.

INTRODUCTION

The *Diagnostic and Statistical Manual of Mental Disorders*, Fifth Edition (*DSM-5*; American Psychiatric Association [APA], 2013), classifies Major Depressive Disorder (MDD) under the category of Depressive Disorders. MDD and the other disorders in this diagnostic category feature issues related to chronic sadness, deflated mood, and/or moodiness. Although it is normal for people to experience brief or even prolonged episodes of sadness in response to challenging life circumstances, the Depressive Disorders are distinguished from these instances by their pervasiveness and intensity, which impairs the individual's ability to engage in daily activities. According to the *DSM-5*, MDD represents the most characteristic disorder among the mental health conditions clustered within this category. Some examples of other Depressive Disorders include Disruptive Mood Dysregulation Disorder and Persistent Depressive Disorder (APA, 2013).

DIAGNOSTIC ISSUES: *DSM-5* AND SCHOOL-BASED SERVICES

DSM-5 Diagnosis

The *DSM-5* defines five criteria for the diagnosis of MDD (APA, 2013). The first criterion includes a list of nine symptoms. Of those nine, the individual must have experienced a minimum of five symptoms that occur during the same 2-week period in order to warrant diagnosis. In short, the nine symptoms of the first criterion are depressed mood (or irritability in youth clients) that lasts throughout the day for most days (as noted by self or others), decreased pleasure in activities that were previously of interest, change in body weight (or failure to reach typical weight benchmarks in children), persistent difficulty in sleep patterns, alterations in movement patterns, diminished energy, self-degradation, difficulty in focus or decision-making, and perseverative thoughts of death and dying. Across the nine symptoms of criterion one, the *DSM-5* further notes that either the first (depressed mood) or second symptom (decreased pleasure) must be present within the identified five to meet that criterion. The second criterion elaborates on the first to establish that the identified symptoms of criterion one must be significant enough to negatively impact the individual's daily functioning or be dismaying to the individual. The third criterion denotes that the depressive symptoms experienced by the individual are not due to another medical condition or substance usage. The *DSM-5* explains that the first three criteria define a major depressive episode.

The fourth criterion requires other psychological conditions be ruled out, and the fifth excludes manic/hypomanic episodes (APA, 2013).

Beyond the diagnostic criteria, Rush (2007) describes four symptom-based subgroups. One such subgroup is referred to as *melancholia*. It is marked by a depressed mood that is not dependent on external circumstances and a particular struggle with feeling pleasure. A second is psychotic depression. Psychotic depression appears to occur most frequently in severely depressed individuals and is denoted by hallucinations. People with psychotic depression often have poorer overall outcomes and responsiveness to treatment. A third subgroup of MDD is described as *anxious depression* and features symptoms of anxiety. Members of this subgroup are more likely to experience suicidal ideation (Rush, 2007). Finally, atypical depression is characterized by a mood that will improve in relation to positive events, but also by weight gain, hypersomnia, and feelings of heaviness in the limbs (Thase, 2007). Neurological evidence supports the distinction among these subgroups of depression (Rush, 2007).

Research indicates that MDD among children and adolescents is frequently underdiagnosed, with as many as 50% of adolescents reaching adulthood before receiving proper identification and care (Birmaher & Brent, 2007; Zuckerbrot et al., 2018). This underdiagnosis is likely due to a differential presentation of symptoms between youths with MDD as compared to adults with MDD (Mullen, 2018). Researchers suggest that children with depression are more likely to present with irritability, behavioral issues, and somatic complaints than adolescents and adults with MDD (Clark et al., 2018; Dopeheide, 2006). In addition, Gehlawat and Gehlawat (2020) note that diagnosis of MDD in children and adolescents often takes more time than diagnosis in adults due to the challenges they have describing their moods and internal states.

> The underdiagnoses of MDD in children and adolescents is likely due to a differential presentation of symptoms between youths with MDD as compared to adults with MDD (Mullen, 2018).

One critical issue for the clinician considering a diagnosis of MDD is distinguishing the disorder and its features in the presence of grief or bereavement associated with traumatic loss (APA, 2013; Friedman, 2012; Parker et al., 2015; Wayment & Vierthaler, 2002). The *DSM-5* indicates that grief may come in waves, but it typically lessens over time. The associated feelings of grief are of "emptiness and loss," and the thoughts are centered around the source of the grief (APA, 2013, p. 161). In contrast, a major depressive episode is related to chronic and invasive sadness generally without a specific target for thoughts other than self-focused critiques and overall negativity. In regard to thoughts about death, those individuals experiencing grief will focus on being reunited with the deceased, whereas people who are struggling with a major depressive episode will demonstrate suicidal ideation (APA, 2013). On this topic, Parker et al. (2015) elaborated that (in a study of people who had experienced depressive states at one time) grief was described as more natural, externally focused, and expected than major depressive episodes. They also found that those who suffered through major depressive episodes were more likely to report physical symptoms, greater symptom severity, and lesser control over symptoms than was experienced with bereavement. The authors suggest that these features should be used in disentangling the impacts of grief from a major depressive episode (Parker et al., 2015). Although most of the empirical work in this area is based on adults, Dillen et al. (2009) report evidence confirming the distinction between grief and depression in their sample of 14- to 18-year-old adolescents in Belgium. Despite the distinguishing features, under some circumstances, the *DSM-5* notes that grief associated with bereavement may represent a major depressive episode if the other conditions of the disorder are met based on the clinical judgment of the examiner using the context of the individual's cultural expression of grief and their prior history (APA, 2013).

Lee et al. (2016) refer to MDD as the most prevalent mental health disorder in the world and a significant public health concern. The World Health Organization (WHO) reports that over 264 million people worldwide experience depression (WHO, n.d.), and based on the National Survey of Children's Health (NSCH), the Centers for Disease Control and Prevention (CDC) notes that approximately 1.9 million children and adolescents between the ages of 3 and 17 in the United States have depression (CDC, n.d.). This represents 3.2% of the youth in America (CDC, n.d.; Ghandour et al., 2019). Of those children and adolescents with current depression, their parents rate 9.7% as being severely impaired by this mental health condition, and another 45% were noted as struggling with moderate impairment from depression. Some preliminary data also suggests that MDD may be increasing in frequency across the globe, although further exploration is needed to confirm the validity of this finding (Ferrari et al., 2013). This is in contrast to the CDC data, which demonstrate that rates of depression among children and adolescents in the United States has remained relatively constant since 2007 (CDC, n.d.).

According to the *DSM-5*, the overall 1-year prevalence of MDD across the population in the United States is about 7%. *Twelve-month prevalence* refers to the percentage of people who report experiencing MDD in the prior year. Brody et al. (2018) report that from 2013 to 2016, 8.1% of Americans over the age of 20 had experienced depression. The prevalence of MDD varies around the world, with the lowest reported rates in East/Southeast Asia (point prevalence 4.0) and the highest rates in Africa/Middle East (point prevalence 6.6), and South Asia (point prevalence 8.6). The authors indicate that the higher rates among Middle Eastern countries may be due to the significant conflicts experienced in that region over the past few decades (Ferrari et al., 2013).

The *DSM-5* and a number of researchers report higher prevalence of MDD among females than males (APA, 2013; Bennett et al., 2005; Brody et al., 2018; Eaton et al., 2008; Ferrari et al., 2013; Lee et al., 2016). According to a global study by Ferrari et al. (2013), the 12-month prevalence for females is 7.2%, whereas for males it is 3.9%. In the United States from 2013 to 2016, the prevalence of MDD in women was reported at 10.4%, and was noted for men at 5.5% (Brody et al., 2018). Among children and adolescents with MDD, some gender differences are also reported in symptom expression (Bennett et al., 2005). Relative to boys with MDD, girls with the diagnosis are significantly more likely to indicate feelings of excessive guilt and self-blame. Girls also note that they feel unattractive, unable to work, and experience greater sleep problems than their male counterparts. Boys with MDD are more likely to indicate difficulty with morning fatigue and an inability to experience pleasure (Bennett et al., 2005). Finally, with respect to gender differences in MDD, females demonstrate a longer duration of depressive episodes than males (Eaton et al., 2008).

According to data from the NSCH, during the ages of 3 to 17, depression is most commonly present from 12 to 17 years of age (Ghandour et al., 2019). Likewise, the *DSM-5* explains that although MDD may arise in any developmental period, the probability of emergence increases markedly during puberty (APA, 2013; Kessler et al., 2003). Despite its significant prevalence in puberty, depression is present in younger children as well. CDC data note an incidence of 0.5% in children ages 3 to 5 and 2% in the period from 6 to 11 years of age (Perou et al., 2013). With regard to the course of depression and age, in their meta-analysis, Twenge and Nolen-Hoeksema (2002) found that depression did not correlate with age for boys outside of a brief increase in symptoms at age 12. However, from childhood into adolescence, girls demonstrate significant increases in their depressive symptoms. Similar to boys, girls also show a significant increase in symptoms at age 12, but their level of symptoms is even higher at ages 14 to 16 (Twenge & Nolen-Hoeksema, 2002).

Earlier ages of onset of MDD are correlated with far more negative life outcomes than later ages of onset (Fergusson & Woodward, 2002; Kovacs et al., 2015; Zisook et al., 2007). Based on research by Zisook et al. (2007), individuals with a younger age of onset have a greater probability of future social struggle, employment instability, poorer quality of life, more medical/psychiatric comorbidities, negative self-perception, suicidality/suicide attempts, and depressive episodes. In addition, people with earlier onset are less likely to marry in adulthood (Zisook et al., 2007). These findings are supported by other researchers as well (Hammen et al., 2008; Rohde et al., 2013). Despite the apparent differences in outcome for individuals with early onset, Zisook et al. (2007) fortunately did not find that this severity was related to lessened treatment response. Finally, Eaton et al. (2008) found that as age of onset for individuals with MDD increases, the risk of recurrence of depressive episodes decreases. However, Wilson et al. (2015) argue that it is not simply the early age of onset that is predictive of poorer psychosocial outcomes but rather the recurrence of MDD that yields these negative future life circumstances. Their data and that of others (Hammen et al. 2008) support that the deleterious outcomes are equivalent with adolescent and adult onset when depressive episodes are recurrent in the life span.

> Based on research by Zisook et al. (2007), individuals with a younger age of onset have a greater probability of future social struggle, employment instability, poorer quality of life, more medical/psychiatric comorbidities, negative self-perception, suicidality/suicide attempts, and depressive episodes.

Recurrence of depressive episodes is common for individuals with MDD, and some individuals experience persistent symptoms over the course of their lifetimes. The *DSM-5* notes that people with chronic depressive symptomatology are more likely to have the negative life-functioning issues noted previously (APA, 2013). Although some individuals with MDD struggle with this type of ongoing symptom expression, others may go months or even years between depressive episodes. As the length of time between episodes increases, the probability of recurrence of a depressive episode decreases (APA, 2013). As compared to adult-onset MDD, children and adolescents with MDD are more likely to experience recurrence of symptoms and progress into bipolar disorder in adulthood (Birmaher & Brent, 2007).

With regard to comorbidity, the *DSM-5* lists the following diagnoses as frequently co-occurring with MDD: substance-related disorders, panic disorder, obsessive-compulsive disorder, anorexia nervosa, bulimia nervosa, and borderline personality disorder (APA, 2013). However, some variation exists in the most common comorbid conditions for children and adolescents. According to Kovacs et al. (1989), those are attention deficit hyperactivity disorder, anxiety disorders, disruptive disorders, substance abuse issues (alcohol and nicotine), enuresis/encopresis, and separation anxiety. Among children and adolescents, the CDC indicates that 73.8% of youths with depression also have issues with anxiety, and over 47% have co-occurring behavioral issues (CDC, n.d.; Ghandour et al., 2019). When depression and anxiety are comorbid in youth, data from Avenevoli et al. (2001) suggest a temporal sequence with anxiety disorders preceding the development of depression symptoms in children and adolescents. Kessler et al. (2003) also found anxiety to precede MDD in adult populations as well. Other research from adult populations notes that when MDD is comorbid with generalized anxiety disorder, there is a significant negative impact on physical and psychological quality of life (Zhou et al., 2017). There is also significant comorbidity between MDD and posttraumatic stress disorder (PTSD) with poor psychosocial outcomes and high treatment attrition. However, some scholars suggest that this may actually represent a trauma-induced subtype of PTSD rather than comorbid disorders (Flory & Yahuda, 2015). Finally, MDD is associated with increased risk of a number of physical health conditions, including heart attacks, strokes, diabetes (Rush, 2007), and obesity (Anderson et al., 2007).

Perhaps the most dire concern related to MDD is the considerable risk for suicidal ideation and death by suicide (Mullen, 2018). Suicide is the second leading cause of death for adolescents between the ages of 12 and 17, and approximately 8% of adolescents diagnosed with MDD die by suicide (O'Connor et al., 2016). MDD is also the most common mental health condition in suicidal adolescents (Wilkinson et al., 2011). For these reasons, Gehlawat and Gehlawat (2020) recommend that any assessment of depression in children and adolescents should be accompanied by an additional evaluation of suicide risk.

School-Based Eligibility

The Individuals with Disabilities Education Improvement Act (IDEA) is federal legislation that provides support for school-age children and adolescents with disabilities (U.S. Department of Education, n.d.). Under the tenets of this law, over 7.5 million students in the United States are assured a free and appropriate public education in the least restrictive environment. The *least restrictive environment* requirement mandates that youth with disabilities are educated to the maximum extent possible in settings with their typically developing peers. The law defines criteria for 13 categories of disability under which children and adolescents may qualify for special education and related services as needed to allow them to progress in the school environment despite their disabilities. Qualification for these supports is based on a two-pronged eligibility decision made by school personnel and the student's parent(s). After a thorough evaluation, this team of individuals determines whether the child meets criteria under one of the disability criteria and whether the student demonstrates a need for services in order to properly advance in their education. If the team decides that both prongs can be answered affirmatively, then the student will be provided with an Individual Education Program (IEP; U.S. Department of Education, n.d.).

With regard to the evaluation process, the first step is the referral. Either the school personnel or the parent may initiate the referral for an IDEA evaluation, and the parent must provide written consent for the process to begin. Upon receipt of parent permission, the school personnel have 60 school days to complete the process and initiate the provision of services (if the child or adolescent is found eligible). IDEA mandates that the student must be assessed in every area of suspected disability.

In the case of a child or adolescent with MDD, the most probable category for eligibility will be that of Emotional Disturbance. IDEA defines this category as follows: "Emotional disturbance means a condition exhibiting one or more of the following characteristics over a long period of time and to a marked degree that adversely affects a child's educational performance" (U.S. Department of Education, n.d., Section 300.8 (c) (4)). The five characteristics under consideration are challenges with educational attainment not due to other cognitive or medical conditions, difficulty in establishing and keeping social relationships, atypical emotional and behavioral responses under normal circumstances, frequently depressed mood, and somatic symptoms associated with individual problems. The criteria also denote that children and adolescents diagnosed with schizophrenia are eligible for certification under the category of Emotional Disturbance, but a child who demonstrates only socially maladjusted behaviors is ineligible for services under the criteria for Emotional Disturbance. Regarding these characteristics and their overlap with the symptomatology for MDD, there is likelihood that a student may experience all of the aforementioned issues. However, the second prong of eligibility requires that these concerns have a direct impact on classroom performance. In circumstances where that is the case, the eligibility team makes a determination that the student may receive services under IDEA. These services would include special education support and could include services such as counseling with the school psychologist or school counselor, and school nurse involvement with medication management.

If the student's education is not impacted adversely by their symptoms of MDD, then school personnel have the option of pursuing services (other than special education) in an alternate manner. Section 504 of the Rehabilitation Act of 1973 is a federal law that protects the rights of individuals with disabilities. It mandates that a person may not be discriminated against on the basis of their disability, and the law applies to any entity or organization that is the recipient of any form of federal funding. Thus, schools are required to apply its tenets in the educational environment for students who have or are suspected of having a disability. The evaluation for Section 504 eligibility is similar to that of IDEA, and students may receive services and educational modifications and accommodations if a school-based evaluation demonstrates that the child has an impairment that "substantially limits one or more major life functions" (Office of Civil Rights, n.d., Section 104.3 (2) (iv)). Although the legislation notes that the list is not exhaustive, the major life functions specified in the law include caring for oneself, performing manual tasks, walking, hearing, seeing, speaking, breathing, learning, and working (Office of Civil Rights, n.d.). Thus, children and adolescents with MDD could obtain beneficial academic, social, emotional, and/or behavioral assistance in the school setting that allows for more successful adjustment within that environment.

CULTURAL ISSUES RELATED TO MAJOR DEPRESSIVE DISORDER IN YOUTH

Risk Factors for Major Depressive Disorder

In the research literature, a consistent relationship is found between poverty and depression (Kessler et al., 2003; Rice et al., 2017). Based on data from the NSCH, depression is significantly higher among children and adolescents living below the poverty line as opposed to those from higher income households. Rice et al. (2017) also found a direct relationship between MDD in adolescents and socioeconomic disadvantage. Brody et al. (2018) had similar findings among adults studied in the United States. At the poverty level, rates of depression rise to nearly 16% of the adult population but steadily decrease as income rises. In addition, a large-scale Taiwanese study found the highest incidence of MDD among low- income individuals under the age of 65 (Lee et al., 2016). In their study, Riolo et al. (2005) noted the incidence of MDD to be 1.5 times higher among participants living in poverty, but indicated that this finding only applied to their White participants and did not hold for individuals of other races. In contrast, Twenge and Nolen-Hoeksema (2002) noted no relationship between socioeconomic status and ratings of depression symptoms among children and adolescents on a measure of childhood depression. However, their investigation was limited to a single measure of depressive symptomatology.

> Rice et al. (2017) found a direct relationship between MDD in adolescents and socioeconomic disadvantage.

Beyond demographic variables, research also supports that childhood anxiety is a risk factor for the development of depression in children and adolescents (Axelson & Birmaher, 2001; Ghandour et al., 2019; Rice et al., 2017). Axelson and Birmaher (2001) explain that the evidence from twin studies indicates a common genetic etiology for both anxiety and depression, and that shared biological components may explain the negative affect common with those two mental health conditions. Perhaps due to the genetic issues, NSCH data support that among youth who are rated as having fair or poor physical health, the incidence of depression is 18%, and 13% of children and youth who live with a primary caregiver in fair/poor health show symptoms of depression (Ghandour et al., 2019). Similarly, in their study of children of depressed parents, Rice et al. (2017) found that symptoms of irritability and anxiety in the children often preceded the development of the first depressive episode of their own MDD.

Aside from the previously noted comorbid disorders, researchers have also found a high cooccurrence of MDD and PTSD within individuals with a history of trauma (Afzali et al., 2017; Vallati et al., 2020). Studies have also shown a relationship between sexual abuse and MDD in adolescents (Fergusson & Woodward, 2002; Vallati et al., 2020). Widom et al. (2007) did not find sexual abuse to be related to MDD, but their data did support that children who were physically abused or suffered multiple forms of abuse were at increased likelihood of lifetime MDD. Children who were neglected had an elevated probability of current MDD. In addition, both abused and neglected children had an early age of onset of MDD and greater comorbidity with other mental health conditions as compared to children who were not abused or neglected. Finally, abused and neglected children with MDD experience increased risk of substance abuse issues in adulthood (Widom et al., 2007). Similarly, Chorot et al. (2017) found a relationship between neglectful parenting and childhood depression. Recent research by Vallati et al. (2020) noted that greater MDD severity was noted in adolescence and adulthood among those who suffered from emotional maltreatment in childhood. This was particularly true when the perpetrator of the emotional abuse was the child's mother. When the perpetrator of emotional abuse was the child's father, then that individual was more likely to experience PTSD as an adolescent or adult. Emotional abuse was measured as hostility, criticism, and rejection. Other findings from Vallati et al. (2020) support that victims of emotional or nonrelative sexual maltreatment in youth have a greater probability of MDD diagnosis and more incidents of depressive episodes in later life than victims of physical abuse. Aside from the trauma of abuse and neglect, the loss of a parent or loved one has also been associated with the development of MDD in children and adolescents (Gehlawat & Gehlawat, 2020).

Cultural Considerations

Although earlier research found higher incidence of MDD in Hispanic children in this country (Twenge & Nolen-Hoeksema, 2002), more recent data among children and adolescents within the United States are indicative of lower incidence of MDD among African American and Hispanic youth as compared to their White counterparts, based on the NSCH. However, researchers are unclear regarding the nature of this difference in prevalence. Ghandour et al. (2019) note that this may be due to lack of access to healthcare providers for diagnosis or bias in diagnosis in which providers are more likely to diagnose racial minority individuals with conduct disorders. This theory may be supported by research from Wang et al. (2013), Williams et al. (2007), and Riolo et al. (2005), and sadly, data indicate that when African Americans and Caribbean Black individuals do have MDD, they are more likely to rate their symptoms as severe and disabling relative to White people (Williams et al., 2007). Yet, the authors also posit a competing (and more encouraging) hypothesis for the lower prevalence of depressive symptoms among African American and Hispanic children and adolescents in the United States. Ghandour et al. (2019) explain that research by O'Donnell et al. (2004) may indicate that it is greater resiliency among African American and Hispanic families that offers protection for their youth with regard to some internalizing disorders.

IMPACT OF MAJOR DEPRESSIVE DISORDER ON SOCIAL–EMOTIONAL AND BEHAVIORAL FUNCTIONING IN SCHOOL AND HOME ENVIRONMENTS

Social–Emotional and Behavioral Functioning in School

In general, school appears to be a significant stressor for children with depression. In their study, Garaigordobal et al. (2017) found that (in comparison to typically developing peers), children aged 7 to 10 who report depressive symptoms also indicate that they have issues with negative attitudes toward school and teachers, low academic performance, problem behaviors, high emotional reactivity, and high stress. Further, they report that their stress is related to teachers, peers, and academic performance.

Peer relationships are a critical factor for social–emotional and behavioral functioning for children and adolescents in the school environment, and Garaigordobal et al. (2017) found that children with depression also struggle with poor social skills and high social stress. In that regard, Herman et al. (2019) investigated the relationship between students' likability, academic competence, and depressive symptoms. They found that likability is a mediating variable. Thus, a developmental pathway was revealed whereby low academic skills in first grade and higher depressive symptoms in third grade were explained by lower likability ratings in second grade. Other empirical work has also found relationships between social incompetence and depression as well (Cole et al., 2001). In addition, childhood loneliness (from poor peer relationships) predicts adolescent social impairment and adult depression (Katz et al., 2011). The social relationship issues noted in children and adolescents with MDD may be related to concerns with self-esteem. Research consistently demonstrates lower self-esteem among children and adolescents with depressive symptoms than their typically developing peers (Bos et al., 2010). Conversely, Jaureguizar et al. (2018) report that in their sample of children ages 7 to 10, self-concept, social skills, and resiliency moderated the relationship between school stress and depression, thus, providing evidence of their role as possible protective factors for childhood depression.

> Childhood loneliness (from poor peer relationships) predicts adolescent social impairment and adult depression (Katz et al., 2011).

These relationship issues combined with academic concerns (discussed in the section titled "Impact of Major Depressive Disorder on Learning in the Classroom") may lead to adolescents dropping out of school. However, the research in this area is somewhat conflicting. Some studies have found that there is no relationship between depression and withdrawing from school (Briere et al., 2017; Melkevik et al., 2016). Yet, Dupere et al. (2018) produced research to support that internalizing issues are linked to the risk of not graduating from high school and that conflicting research is due to underreporting during retrospective studies. Their findings indicate that dropping out of high school is a concern during episodes of depression. In fact, the risk of school withdrawal was approximately doubled among adolescents with recent depressive symptoms as compared to their typically developing peers. It is plausible that the increased likelihood of dropping out of school in close proximity to depressive episodes is a result of the impulsive tendencies seen among individuals with MDD as found by Dekker and Johnson (2018).

Social–Emotional and Behavioral Functioning at Home

According to Rice et al. (2017), the most common risk factor for the development of MDD in a child or adolescent is having a parent who is diagnosed with MDD, and statistics in the United States note that approximately 15 million children in this country live with a depressed parent (National

Research Council, 2009). Some research even suggests that adolescent depression may be reinforced through greater attention in homes where a parent also struggles with depressive episodes (Davis et al., 2000). Beyond that, Bresland et al. (2016) and Hammen et al. (2004) found that the impact of parental depression on their offspring's development of depression is exacerbated when there is also conflict between parents. And research on adult relationships demonstrates that individuals with MDD have significantly fewer positive interactions with their significant others than people without mental health diagnoses (Zlotnick et al., 2000).

These issues and the children's and adolescent's mental health condition often combine to strain family functioning. According to Garaigordobal et al. (2017), children with depression report significantly higher concerns in the following areas as compared to control participants: lack of parental affection, feelings of loneliness in the home, sibling disputes, and parental demandingness. These perceptions by children with depressive symptomatology equate to high familial stress (Garaigordobal et al., 2017). These findings are consistent with other research in this area. Parenting practices influence children's and adolescents' social–emotional and behavioral functioning at home. Chorot et al. (2017) found significant relationships between childrearing styles and the development of depression in youth. To be specific, parental aversiveness and neglectfulness toward their offspring and low levels of communication and warmth are related to increased levels of depressive symptomatology in children.

> According to Garaigordobal et al. (2017), children with depression report significantly higher concerns in the following areas as compared to control participants: lack of parental affection, feelings of loneliness in the home, sibling disputes, and parental demandingness.

IMPACT OF MAJOR DEPRESSIVE DISORDER ON LEARNING IN THE CLASSROOM

Research by Fergusson and Woodward (2002) indicates that adolescents with depression show a significantly elevated risk of school failure and a reduced probability of pursuing education beyond their high school experience. Riglin et al. (2014) and Jaureguizar et al. (2017) similarly report data from their research indicative of lower grades among adolescents with depression. Poirier et al. (2019) also found low academic skills to be correlated with depressive symptoms, but the authors suggest that gender may play a role in the association since this finding related to girls but not to boys in their study. However, longitudinal research by Hishinuma et al. (2012) and McArdle et al. (2014) is indicative of a causal relationship between depressive symptoms and decreased academic achievement. In their study of Hawaiian high schools, they noted that the depressive symptoms impaired academic achievement but lowered academic achievement did not lead to depressive symptoms. Further, they note the importance of monitoring students' grade point averages (GPAs) for declines that may be an early indicator of the development of depression. They explain, "At the very least, decreases in GPA, especially dramatic ones, should be potential markers to educators, school counselors, and parents that youths experiencing such GPA declines may already be experiencing affective difficulties, including depressive symptoms and disorders" (McArdle et al., 2014, p. 1338). Garaigordobal et al. (2017) found low interest in schoolwork (among other variables) to be a predictor of depression in children. Similarly, Herman et al. (2019) suggest that low academic competence be considered a flag for screening for internalizing concerns.

With regard to cognitive abilities, in relation to typically developing peers, children and adolescents with MDD have been found to have decreased cognitive processing speed based on paper/pencil measures (Favre et al., 2008). Due to other assessments within their research, the authors did not believe that the impaired processing speed performance was related to diminished attention and concentration but rather slowed physical movements that are associated with MDD (Favre et al., 2008). Nonetheless, the research offers important findings for the classroom. Given that as children age, more academic tasks require writing, it is probable that students with MDD may demonstrate slower assignment completion and note-taking in their classrooms. In turn, this slower performance may compound over time to create academic gaps and performance concerns as the child or adolescent struggles to keep up with the pace of instruction and expectations to produce work.

Further complicating the classroom environment for students with MDD, research indicates that active MDD is associated with concerns in memory (Owens et al., 2012; Vance & Winther; 2020), attention, and executive functioning as well (Allott et al., 2016; Morey-Nase et al., 2019; Wagner et al., 2015). Deficits have been noted in verbal and visual memory among adolescents with MDD (Goodall et al., 2018). In addition, Vance and Winther's (2020) research found a correlation between MDD and deficits in spatial working memory (a component of executive functioning). Other studies have also supported a link between spatial working memory and inattention (Barnett et al., 2001). Likewise, the data from Owens et al. (2012) demonstrated that higher negative affect impairs working-memory performance. Perhaps associated with the working-memory issues, Stack and Dever (2020) noted a relationship between depression symptoms and math achievement. In their study of low-income elementary students and elementary students from primarily Latin heritage, self-reported subclinical levels of depression predicted underachievement in math. However, Romano et al. (2010) discovered that depressive symptoms in kindergarten were predictive of increased math achievement at third grade. The differing results between Stack and Dever (2020) and Romano et al. (2010) may be due to age of participants, measurement issues, and/or cultural distinctions. Regardless, the preponderance of evidence suggests that the relationship between academic functioning and depression bears monitoring by personnel in the school environment.

IMPLICATIONS FOR SCHOOL PSYCHOLOGISTS

Assessment Role

One role for school psychologists with regard to the identification of emotional concerns like depression in the school system relates to universal screening. Medical practitioners recommend the annual screening of adolescents ages 12 and up for signs of depression (U.S. Department of Health and Human Services, 2010; U.S. Preventive Services Task Force [USPSTF], 2009; Weare & Nind, 2011; Zuckerbrot et al., 2018), and these efforts could easily be incorporated into a school's Multi-Tiered Systems of Support (MTSS; Weist et al., 2018). School psychologists should play integral roles in school-based mental health screenings for the improved academic, social, emotional, and behavioral adjustment for all students within their learning environments.

Beyond their role in MTSS, school psychologists are also critical to school-based evaluations for special services for children and adolescents with MDD. As previously noted, students with MDD could be eligible for such supports under two different forms of federal legislation—IDEA and Section 504 of the Rehabilitation Act of 1973. The training and experiences of the school psychologist offer the greatest competence among school personnel for the administration of assessments related to the child's or adolescent's cognitive, academic, and psychological functioning. The school psychologist could also conduct the observations, file reviews, interviews, and record reviews necessary to establish the prior and current functioning of the student. The multidisciplinary team would utilize the collected data to make any determination of IDEA or Section 504 eligibility and make appropriate data-based decisions for the child or adolescent with MDD to be able to function most effectively in the academic curriculum and school environment.

Advocacy Role

The CDC reports an encouraging statistic: Nearly 80% of children and adolescents aged 3 to 17 in the United States receive treatment when diagnosed with depression (CDC, n.d.; O'Connor et al., 2016). However, children and adolescents living in poverty or near poverty are less likely to receive treatments for their symptoms than children and adolescents in higher income households (Ghandour et al., 2019). Untreated depression in youth is related to the risk of substance abuse, poor employment outcomes, and suicidal tendencies in adulthood (Mullen, 2018). According to Mullen (2018) and the USPSTF (2009), treatment options for mild to moderate depression include psychoeducation and psychotherapy. However, the most effective treatment combination for children and adolescents with more severe forms of MDD is cognitive behavioral therapy and the prescription drug fluoxetine (Cipriani et al., 2016; Mullen, 2018). Fluoxetine is in the class of drugs referred to as selective serotonin reuptake inhibitors (SSRIs). Mullen (2018) contends that antidepressant drug therapy alone should not be used in the treatment of childhood depression, but Gehlawat and Gehlawat (2020) recommend that medication be used as a frontline treatment when symptoms are so severe that they would prohibit effective psychotherapy. Mullen (2018) further recommends that when symptoms have abated, treatment should be tapered for 6 months to 1 year. Although drug treatment alone is not a recommended strategy for the treatment of MDD, a large study of adolescents with depression indicates that older adolescents were 4 times more likely to receive antidepressants as their only treatment (O'Connor et al, 2016). It is also critical to note the increased probability for suicidal ideation at the outset of pharmacological treatment (Birmaher & Brent, 2007; Clark et al., 2018; USPSTF, 2009). Nonetheless, school psychologists should assist families in accessing community-based services for depression assessment and medication provision when necessary.

> Untreated depression in youth is related to the risk of substance abuse, poor employment outcomes, and suicidal tendencies in adulthood (Mullen, 2018).

Consultation Role

In a consultation role, school psychologists may be called upon to work with the parents of children and adolescents with MDD, and, due to the increased risk of suicide with MDD, assisting parents in safety planning for their children is a critical role. When parents or professionals suspect the child or adolescent may be suicidal (even without confirmation of such thoughts), it behooves those involved to take steps to ensure their safety. First, school psychologists should advise parents to remove any lethal weapons or means from the child's or adolescent's environment. Second, the family should be instructed in other factors (beyond depression) related to suicidality, including sexual orientation, other clinical diagnoses, and medical concerns. Third, the family should be encouraged to pursue or continue engaging in treatment for the child or adolescent. Fourth, the child or adolescent should be provided with contact information for emergency use, and finally, a plan for continuous monitoring and follow-up should be established (Zuckerbrot et al., 2018). For many years, the use of suicide prevention contracts was a standard of practice with children, adolescents, and adults experiencing suicidal ideation, but these have become controversial due to the lack of evidence supporting their effectiveness and warnings regarding the legal ramifications of their use (Garvey et al., 2009; Zuckerbrot et al., 2018). However, it is important to note that there is little evidence to indicate that the use of a suicide contract causes harm for an individual who is struggling with suicidal thoughts when used in conjunction with other suicide assessment and therapeutic interventions (Garvey et al., 2009).

Aside from the safety issues, researchers suggest that psychoeducation with families should be utilized to help them comprehend the significance of depression (Morey-Nase et al., 2019), and school psychologists are positioned through their training and experience to offer this component. According to Morey-Nase et al. (2019), psychoeducation has the probability of promoting empathy toward the child or adolescent struggling with MDD and reinforcing the need for seeking and maintaining a course of treatment.

Counseling/Therapy Role

According to Cheung et al. (2013), Clark et al. (2018), and Hopkins et al. (2015), both cognitive behavioral therapy and interpersonal therapy have shown equivalent effectiveness in the treatment of MDD in children and adolescents, although it appears that cognitive behavioral therapy has become more common and may be more amenable to the school setting. Social skills training and play therapy have also produced positive results in youths with MDD (Gehlawat & Gehlawat, 2020). Regardless of the type of intervention, research has shown that increasing school-based mental health services is associated with reductions in adolescent depressive episodes and suicide risk (Paschall & Bersamin, 2018). Overall, evidence suggests that school-based services have the greatest likelihood of reaching the children and adolescents with the most need for those interventions (Kern et al. 2017). The training of school psychologists as mental health professionals gives them the competence and credibility to implement a broad base of supports for students who are struggling with social, emotional, and behavioral needs. Therefore, school psychologists should lead the efforts in the development of mental health programs within schools and also in the provision of counseling and therapy interventions for children and adolescents with MDD. Finally, research by Atkins et al. (2006) found that therapy attendance for children and adolescents is significantly higher when the intervention is delivered within the school setting than when services are provided at a separate community-based facility (Atkins et al., 2006).

> Regardless of the type of intervention, research has shown that increasing school-based mental health services is associated with reductions in adolescent depressive episodes and suicide risk (Paschall & Bersamin, 2018).

EDUCATIONAL SUPPORTS

Poirier et al. (2019) indicate that academic competency may be a protective factor against both depressive symptoms and conduct problems. They suggest that academic intervention may be beneficial in mediating depressive symptoms in children and adolescents, and this is supported by a growing body of literature (Herman et al., 2019; Kellam et al., 1994). Thus, engaging students with MDD with fundamental academic supports and/or intervention may reap benefits beyond the resulting educational gains.

As previously noted, the research supports a correlation between depression in children and adolescents and executive functioning deficits. In practical application, Vance and Winther (2020) theorize that intervening to build working memory skills may lead to associated improvements in depressive symptoms. Thus, advancing students' executive functions in the classroom could show benefits for children and adolescents with MDD. Fortunately, a recent meta-analysis of 90 research studies demonstrates that it is possible to train executive functions in children and adolescents. The meta-analysis found significant improvements in functioning through the use of explicit training with working-memory programs, physical activity, mindfulness practices, and self-regulation strategies (Takacs & Kassai, 2019). Olive et al. (2019) also found that physical activity produced short-term improvements for students with depression, including a decrease in depressive symptoms and ratings of body dissatisfaction. The use of physical activity, mindfulness practices, and self-regulation strategies are easily incorporated as classroom strategies, can be delivered efficiently as a group intervention, are inexpensive, and have the probability of improving functioning in children throughout the learning environment.

> Olive et al. (2019) also found that physical activity produced short-term improvements for students with depression, including a decrease in depressive symptoms and ratings of body dissatisfaction.

Based on the scholarly literature and empirical studies, Hart et al. (2018) offer a number of practical strategies to help students with depression improve their adjustment and functioning in the classroom setting. The strategies include creating a classroom that feels safe for all students and normalizing adjustment and mental health issues through group and individual discussions. It is further suggested that school personnel should get to know students on an individual level and also seek connections to their lives beyond the classroom. Building relationships and making connections between students and adult school personnel can help to ensure that every child and adolescent feels included within the educational environment. In addition, classroom journaling activities and collaborative exercises can be used with both academic and social–emotional content to make connections and foster relationships with teachers and peers for students with depression (Hart et al., 2018).

SCHOOL-BASED MENTAL HEALTH INTERVENTIONS AND SUPPORTS

The importance of intervening on depression in children and adolescents to promote their individual and school-based adjustment was highlighted by Hishinuma et al. (2012). They state,

"Emphasis must also be made on screening, identification, and treatment of depressive symptoms and disorders, not only to ameliorate the ill effects of depressive symptoms but also to potentially prevent lower GPAs" (p. 1337). MTSS offer the opportunity to address these issues through increasing levels of intensity as student need dictates. According to Weist et al. (2018), the most effective system will likely be an interconnected systems framework (ISF) that combines positive behavioral interventions and supports with school mental health initiatives. In short, "The ISF implementation follows an evidenced-based protocol including school-wide social-emotional-behavioral skills training at Tier 1 and interventions at Tiers 2 and 3, with ongoing fidelity monitoring and correction throughout implementation" (Weist et al., 2018, p. 175). School and community stakeholders in this system collaborate to identify or create evidenced-based interventions that are delivered and monitored for effectiveness. At Tier 1, behavioral expectations and the evidenced-based practices are intentionally interconnected and often applied through manualized interventions. At Tier 2, students who are identified as at risk for concerns like depression participate in interventions that build on skills taught at Tier 1 and offer additional opportunities for instruction, coaching, practice, and reinforcement. For Tier 3, the students represented are already experiencing significant impairment in functioning due to their internalizing issues. A functional analysis of the issue is undertaken to select interventions for the development of new skills (Weist et al., 2018). The ISF design offers promise for students with MDD to receive necessary intervention in the school setting.

> MTSS offer the opportunity to address issues of depression among students through increasing levels of intensity as student need dictates.

Research in this area notes the need and effectiveness of both universal and targeted prevention efforts in the schools for childhood and adolescent depression (Dupere et al., 2018; Herman et al. 2019; Lee et al., 2017; Merry et al., 2012; Weare & Nind et al., 2011). Herman et al. (2019) recommend the use of universal supports, such as socialemotional learning programs, to address internalizing symptoms like depression in children and adolescents within the school environment. These efforts could identify at-risk students for prevention efforts or currently struggling students for more intensive intervention. With regard to prevention, empirical evidence from adult studies indicates that prevention efforts may reduce the subsequent development of MDD by as much as 21% (Cuijpers et al., 2008; van Zoonen et al., 2014). Also, Merry et al. (2012) conducted a large-scale meta-analysis with studies of prevention of depression among children and adolescents. They report that universal prevention programs and programs targeted to at-risk students show significant benefit in the reduction of depression across participants. The positive outcomes were even evident 12 months after delivery of the programs (Merry et al., 2012). Although Werner-Seidler et al. (2017) found universal and targeted prevention programs to be effective, the targeted programs were slightly more effective. Regardless, Weare and Nind (2011) point out that compulsory schooling represents the last point at which to offer prevention and intervention to a nearly complete population of adolescents, and Dupere et al. (2018) note that school-based screening, prevention, and treatment of depression have the potential to prevent students with depressive symptomatology from dropping out of school. Further support for universal prevention programs for depression in the schools comes from Lee et al. (2017), who found these programs to be cost-effective when delivered in either face-to-face or online formats.

Research by Tang et al. (2018) provides a neural basis for the effectiveness of cognitive behavioral therapy with adolescents due to abnormalities in the cognitive control network in the amygdala. The amygdala is important to memory, the processing of emotions, and the fight-or-flight response. Peters et al. (2017) also found evidence of impairment of cognitive control in students with MDD. Within that cognitive behavioral framework, the school psychologist can implement the intervention strategies recommended by Garaigordobal et al. (2017) based on their predictive model of depression in children. They suggest the use of relaxation and cognitive training to reduce overall stress and confront negative thoughts along with social skills training to enhance peer and adult relationships. In order to build overall coping skills, they further promote the use of therapeutic techniques to enhance self-esteem, reinforce the use of an internal locus of control, and develop resiliency. According to Garaigordobal et al. (2017), addressing the affiliated anxiety is critical in therapeutic intervention with children and adolescents with depression. And, given the association between early irritability and anxiety symptoms and the later development of MDD, Rice et al. (2017) recommend that the treatment of anxiety in children and adolescents be used as a prevention effort for MDD as well.

School psychologists have an array of supports at their disposal to intervene on behalf of children and adolescents with MDD. These school-based mental health initiatives may be offered as prevention or intervention efforts and can be delivered in large-group, small-group, or individual formats based on the intensiveness of the need. Given the prevalence of MDD and the significant lifetime impacts of depressive symptomatology, it is imperative that this mental health condition be addressed on multiple levels with comprehensive evidenced-based protocols.

CASE STUDY 12.1 JEREMY: A CASE OF MAJOR DEPRESSIVE DISORDER

Background

Jeremy is a 16-year-old male who lives with his mother. According to Jeremy, his father lives in another state, and he has no contact with him. His mother has a vocational diploma from a technical college. Jeremy's mother works 3 days a week as a certified nursing assistant. She typically works three 12-hour overnight shifts during the week. Due to his mother's work schedule, Jeremy is often alone at home.

His mother describes him as sad. She goes on to say he is almost always irritable and moody. Jeremy reports that he has lost weight and sleeps more than he used to sleep. Jeremy states that he is not suicidal but has had some dark thoughts about his mother being better off without him. He is not very interested in being around people much. He would prefer to stay in his room. His mother believes that if he wasn't so negative, he would get along better with others and get better grades. He has recently become more withdrawn and stays in his room, frequently listening to music. He used to play online video games with his friends, but his mother states he is not really interested in that anymore. She also notes that he used to enjoy school but now gets very agitated when she brings it up.

According to Jeremy and his mother, he has adapted to high school well but struggles in English Language Arts (ELA). This is evident in report cards and progress reports from ninth through 11th grade. Currently, he is passing all of his classes; however, he is on the verge of failing ELA. Jeremy's mother stated that he becomes irritated and angry when asked about ELA. Jeremy describes biology as his favorite subject and ELA as his least favorite subject. He stated that if not for ELA, he would be on the honor roll.

Jeremy does not always ask for guidance when something seems too difficult to navigate on his own. For example, if he needs assistance academically, he does not communicate that to his teachers. When his mother confronted him about his ELA homework, he stated that he did not understand the assignments but did not want to ask for help during class and did not have the time to stay after school. When asked how he deals with frustration and failure, Jeremy stated that does not like to fail, because he wants to be successful and make his mother proud. He stated that when he is frustrated or fails at homework and exams, he just shuts down and wants to hide.

Discussion

Jeremy has a depressed mood and is irritable. This lasts throughout the day for most days. He has decreased pleasure in activities that were previously of interest, such as school and video gaming. He notes that he has lost weight and sleeps more often than he used to. He is showing diminished energy, self-degradation, and some difficulty in focus or decision-making. His friendships and school work are suffering due to his MDD.

The multidisciplinary team should develop a clear battery of assessments to explore the elements of his depression and how this is affecting his academic life to include social issues. Emphasis should be placed on his emotions and memory. Visual and verbal memory can be an issue with depression. Social skills should also be examined. Interventions should be designed around Jeremy's specific needs.

(continued)

CASE STUDY 12.1 JEREMY: A CASE OF MAJOR DEPRESSIVE DISORDER (continued)

The school psychologist could work with Jeremy in many capacities. In an advocacy role, the school psychologist could help connect the family to programs that deal with households in or near poverty, risk of substance abuse, and suicidal tendencies. As a consultant, the school psychologist may work with the school and/or family to develop safety plans and protective watch ideas to keep Jeremy safe. The school psychologist may also provide some direct service in the form of therapy.

Academically, school personnel should get to know students on an individual level and also seek connections to their lives beyond the classroom. Building relationships and making connections between students and adult school personnel can help to ensure that every child and adolescent feels included within the educational environment. Classroom journaling activities and collaborative exercises may also be helpful.

SUMMARY POINTS

- In order to apply a *DSM-5* diagnosis of MDD, an individual must exhibit either depressed mood or inhibition of pleasure along with other symptom criteria.
- With regard to risk factors, the school psychologist should remember that both poverty and trauma are associated with the development of MDD in children and adolescents.
- There is a high co-occurrence of childhood depression in homes in which a parent also struggles with depression.
- Improving academic functioning may contribute to a decrease in depressive symptomatology in children and adolescents.
- School psychologists can engage in many roles and functions to support the needs of students with MDD, including assessment, advocacy, consultation, and counseling and/or therapy.
- Cognitive behavioral and interpersonal therapy have demonstrated effectiveness in the treatment of children and adolescents with MDD.

TEST YOUR KNOWLEDGE

1. A student with MDD may qualify for special education services under which IDEA category?
   a. Anxiety Disorders
   b. Emotional Disturbance
   c. Specific Learning Disability
   d. Intellectual Disability

2. Childhood abuse has not been shown to have a relationship to adult depression.
   a. True
   b. False

3. There is a high comorbidity between anxiety and depression in children and adolescents.
   a. True
   b. False

4. Which of the following is NOT associated with the development of MDD in children and adolescents?
   a. Poverty
   b. Trauma
   c. Parental depression
   d. Sibling conflict

5. Cognitive behavioral therapy and SSRIs are more effective together than cognitive behavioral therapy alone in the treatment of children and adolescents with MDD.
   a. True
   b. False

Answers: (1) b, (2) b, (3) a, (4) d, (5) a.

DISCUSSION QUESTIONS

1. Describe the *DSM-5* diagnostic criteria for MDD.
2. Highlight the IDEA criteria for eligibility under the category of Emotional Disturbance.
3. Explain the relationship between trauma and the development of MDD.
4. Describe the relationship between academic functioning and MDD.
5. List some evidenced-based social–emotional interventions for students with MDD.

CHAPTER RESOURCES

American Academy of Child and Adolescent Psychiatry *Depression in Children and Teens*: www.aacap.org/AACAP/Families_and_Youth/Facts_for_Families/FFF-Guide/The-Depressed-Child-004.aspx

American Academy of Child and Adolescent Psychiatry *Depression Resource Center*: www.aacap.org/aacap/Families_and_Youth/Resource_Centers/Depression_Resource_Center/Depression_Resource_Center.aspx

American Psychiatric Association *What Is Depression?*: www.psychiatry.org/patients-families/depression/what-is-depression

American Psychological Association *Resources for Clinicians for the Treatment of Depression in Children and Adolescents*: www.apa.org/depression-guideline/resources/children-adolescents

Anxiety and Depression Association of America *Clinical Practice Review for Major Depressive Disorder*: https://adaa.org/resources-professionals/practice-guidelines-mdd

Anxiety and Depression Association of America *Depression*: https://adaa.org/understanding-anxiety/depression

Merck Manual *Depressive Disorders in Children and Adolescents*: www.merckmanuals.com/professional/pediatrics/mental-disorders-in-children-and-adolescents/depressive-disorders-in-children-and-adolescents

National Alliance on Mental Illness *5 Things You Can Do to Help Your Child with Depression*: www.nami.org/Blogs/NAMI-Blog/December-2018/5-Things-You-Can-Do-to-Help-Your-Child-with-Depression

National Association of School Psychologists *Depression: Supporting Students at School*: www.nasponline.org/Documents/Resources%20and%20Publications/Handouts/Families%20and%20Educators/Depression_Supporting_Students_at_School.pdf

National Institute of Mental Health *Depression*: www.nimh.nih.gov/health/topics/depression/

Stanford Children's Health *Major Depression in Children*: www.stanfordchildrens.org/en/topic/default?id=major-depression-in-children-90-P02569

Stanford Children's Health *Major Depression in Teens*: www.stanfordchildrens.org/en/topic/default?id=major-depression-in-adolescents-90-P01614

KEY REFERENCES

Only key references appear in the print edition. The full reference list appears in the digital product on Springer Publishing Connect: connect.springerpub.com/content/book/978-0-8261-3587-2/part/part05/chapter/ch12

American Psychiatric Association. (2013). *Diagnostic and statistical manual of mental disorders* (5th ed.). https://doi.org/10.1176/appi.books.9780890425596

Birmaher, B., & Brent, D. (2007). Practice parameter for the assessment and treatment of children and adolescents with depressive disorders. *Journal of the American Academy of Child and Adolescent Psychiatry*, 46(11), 1503–1526. https://doi.org/10.1097/chi.0b013e318145ae1c

Brody, D. J., Pratt, L. A., & Hughes, J. (2018). Prevalence of depression among adults aged 20 and over: United States, 2013–2016. In *NCHS Data Brief, no 303*. National Center for Health Statistics.

Kessler, R. C., Berglund, P., Demler, O., Jin, R., Koretz, D., Merikangas, K. R., Rush, A. J., Walters, E. E., & Wang, P. S. (2003). The epidemiology of major depressive disorder: Results from the National Comorbidity Survey Replication (NCSR). *Journal of the American Medical Association*, 289(23), 3095–3105. https://doi.org/10.1001/jama.289.23.3095

Lee, C., Chiang, Y., Huang, J., Tantoh, D., Nfor, O. N., Lee, J., Chang, C., & Liaw, Y. (2016). Incidence of major depressive disorder: Variation by age and sex in low income individuals: A population based 10-year follow-up study. *Medicine*, 95(15), e3110. https://doi.org/10.1097/MD.0000000000003110

Parker, G., McCraw, S., & Paterson, A. (2015). Clinical features distinguishing grief from depressive episodes: A qualitative analysis. *Journal of Affective Disorders*, 176(1), 43–47. https://doi.org/10.1016/j.jad.2015.01.063

Rice, F., Sellers, R., Hammerton, G., Eyre, O., Bevan-Jones, R., Thapar, A. K., Collishaw, S., Harold, G. T., & Thapar, A. (2017). Antecedents of new-onset major depressive disorder in children and adolescents at high familial risk. *Journal of the American Medical Association Psychiatry*, 74(2), 153–160. https://doi.org/10.1001/jamapsychiatry.2016.3140

Riolo, S. A., Nguyen, T. A., Greden, J. F. & King, C. A. (2005). Prevalence of depression by race/ethnicity: Findings from the National Health and Nutrition Examination Survey III. *American Journal of Public Health*, 95(6), 998–1000. https://doi.org/10.2105/AJPH.2004.047225

Zisook, S., Lesser, I., Stewart, J. W., Wisniewski, S. R., Balasubramani, G. K., Fava, M., Gilmer, W. S., Dresselhaus, T. R., Thase, M. E., Nierenberg, A. A., Trivedi, M. H., & Rush, A. J. (2007). Effect of age of onset on the course of major depressive disorder. *American Journal of Psychiatry*, 164, 1539–1547. https://doi.org/10.1176/appi.ajp.2007.06101757

Zuckerbrot, R. A., Cheung, A., Jensen, P. S., Stein, R. E. K., & Laraque, D. (2018). Guidelines for adolescent depression in primary care (GLAD-PC): Part I. Practice preparation, identification, assessment, and initial management. *Pediatrics*, 141(3), e20174081. https://doi.org/10.1542/peds.2017-4081

CHAPTER 13

Disruptive Mood Dysregulation Disorder

LEARNING OBJECTIVES

- Summarize the diagnostic features for the *Diagnostic and Statistical Manual of Mental Disorders* (5th ed.; *DSM-5*; American Psychiatric Association [APA], 2013) diagnosis of Disruptive Mood Dysregulation Disorder (DMDD).
- Highlight the risk factors for DMDD in children and adolescents.
- Describe common school and home concerns for children with DMDD.
- Understand the classroom challenges for students with DMDD.
- Identify effective mental health supports for students with DMDD.

INTRODUCTION

Within the *Diagnostic and Statistical Manual of Mental Disorders*, Fifth Edition (*DSM-5*; American Psychiatric Association [APA], 2013), Disruptive Mood Dysregulation Disorder (DMDD) is categorized as one of the Depressive Disorders. The commonality that binds these disorders under this umbrella relates to feelings of sadness, emptiness, or, in the case of DMDD, pervasive irritability. The intensity, duration, and functional impairment of these feelings in the context of the Depressive Disorders is what distinguishes them from short-term mood problems experienced by all people. Other Depressive Disorders include Major Depressive Disorder and Persistent Depressive Disorder (APA, 2013).

DIAGNOSTIC ISSUES: *DSM-5* AND SCHOOL-BASED SERVICES

DSM-5 Diagnosis

Within the *DSM-5*, there are 11 diagnostic criteria associated with DMDD. The first criterion relates to the rageful behaviors seen among children with this disorder. It denotes the presence of excessive verbal or physical outbursts inconsistent with any perceived provocation. The second criterion states that those behaviors would not be consistent with expectations for the child's age, and the third criterion quantifies their occurrence at an average of a minimum of three times per week. The fourth criterion describes the behavior between the rageful episodes as irritated or mad on a nearly constant basis. According to the fifth criterion, all of the aforementioned symptoms must have persisted for at least 1 year, with no more than 3 consecutive symptom-free months. Criterion six relates to the settings in which the outbursts of temper and irritable moods occur. It says that they must occur in a minimum of two of the following three settings: home, school, and social situations. Further, the demonstration of the symptoms must be considered severe in one of those three settings. The seventh criterion specifies that initial diagnosis must occur between the ages of 6 and 18, and criterion eight further expounds that the presence of the symptoms must have been noted prior to 10 years of age. Criterion nine through criterion eleven serve to rule out other situations or conditions. The ninth criterion excludes the presence of mania. If an individual's behavior could meet criteria for mania or hypomania for a period of time that is longer than one day, then the DMDD diagnosis cannot be applied. The tenth criterion precludes application of the diagnosis if the symptoms occur solely during a major depressive episode or are consistent with another psychiatric condition. And the eleventh criterion explains that the diagnosis may not be applied if the characteristics of the disorder are actually the result of substance abuse or a medical issue.

According to the *DSM-5*, DMDD was created as a response to researchers and practitioners who feared that bipolar disorder was being diagnosed too frequently among children. This represented a legitimate concern as bipolar diagnoses in youths skyrocketed by approximately 40 times their previous diagnostic rate in just under a decade, from 1994 to 2003 in the United States (Moreno et al., 2007). Although Moreno et al. (2007) noted a need for further research to determine whether this exponential increase in diagnoses was related to prior underdiagnosis or current overdiagnosis of bipolar disorder, Lochman et al. (2015) surmised that it was likely the latter. They explained that the risk factors for bipolar disorder had not changed nor had the rest of the world seen a similarly rapid increases in the diagnosis. Thus, they attributed the diagnostic increases to changes in clinical practice that likely reflected overdiagnosis due to a lack of comprehension of the true markers of bipolar disorder in children or the presence of more significant symptoms of emotional dysregulation (Lochman et al., 2015). Rao (2014) argued that there simply was not a place for children with this type of chronic irritability (as characterized by the current diagnosis of DMDD) prior to the *DSM-5*. In addition, Roy et al. (2014) note that misdiagnosing a disorder of chronic irritability as bipolar disorder was particularly problematic at the treatment phase as many youths were being prescribed medications for bipolar disorder that were likely ineffective for their non-episodic condition. Finally, in support of the addition of DMDD to the *DSM-5*, Chen et al. (2016) suggest that early data (since its inception) is indicative of a reduction in bipolar diagnoses with the introduction of DMDD.

> According to the *DSM-5*, DMDD was created as a response to researchers and practitioners who feared that bipolar disorder was being diagnosed too frequently among children.

Through the creation of DMDD, the *DSM-5* was attempting to address a serious concern in practice and treatment, but the solution was not without controversy as researchers and scholars in this area argued that there was insufficient scientific evidence to support the new disorder and that it might lead to greater instances of pathologizing typical behavior for children and adolescents (Lochman et al., 2015; Rao, 2014). In fact, Axelson (2013) explained that at the time of the publication of the *DSM-5*, there had been no empirical work that used the diagnostic criteria as written. In addition, *DSM-5* field trials related to DMDD proved to have limited test–retest reliability (Regier et al., 2013). Due to these challenges to its legitimacy, another classification system, the *International Statistical Classification of Diseases and Related Health Problems, 11th Revision*, chose not to include DMDD as a diagnosis but rather included a chronic irritability specifier under the diagnosis of oppositional defiant disorder (ODD; Srinath et al., 2018). In fact, in support of this approach, research by Mayes, Mathiowetz, et al. (2015); Mayes, Waxmansky, et al. (2015); and Mayes et al. (2019) indicates that the diagnoses of DMDD and ODD may not be meaningfully different. In contrast, and in support of the legitimacy of DMDD as a separate mental health condition, Coccaro's (2018) data supports that though there are similarities between DMDD and the similar outbursts associated with intermittent explosive disorder, the two diagnoses are distinct based on the irritability that persists between rageful episodes for children and adolescents with DMDD. Additional concerns have been raised about the differentiation of DMDD from bipolar disorder (Noller, 2016). Nonetheless, although care must be taken to distinguish the two diagnoses (DMDD and bipolar disorder), the *DSM-5* describes DMDD as significant and persistent (non-episodic) irritability versus bipolar disorder in which symptom presentation is episodic in nature (APA, 2013). Further, its distinction from bipolar disorder is supported by the fact that the conversion from DMDD in youth to adult bipolar disorder has been demonstrated to be low (Agarwal & Tiwari, 2013), and research by Wiggins et al. (2016) has supported a distinction between youth with DMDD and youth with bipolar disorder in the neural mechanisms of their symptoms of irritability.

Beyond the criticisms related to the development of this new mental health condition for the *DSM-5*, other concerns have been raised about the criteria themselves. One such issue is highlighted regarding the age criterion. As previously noted, a child or adolescent must be between the ages of 6 and 18 to have the diagnosis applied, thereby excluding children under the age of 6. Unlike most disorders of childhood, its prevalence (based on criteria, not diagnosis) appears to be the highest during the preschool years where issues related to outbursts of temper are more common (Copeland et al., 2013; Mayes et al., 2017, 2019). In fact, prevalence of symptomatology in preschool has been noted as 2 to 3 times that of rates in older children despite the fact that the diagnosis is not allowed (per criteria) for this age group. Scholars in this area note that adequate justification is not given by the *DSM-5* for excluding this developmental period from DMDD diagnosis. They suggest that empirical data support that DMDD can be reliably diagnosed for children under 6 years of age and that comorbidity data indicate similarity between younger and older youths with DMDD (Copeland et al., 2013). Wiggins et al. (2021) express dismay that age-based limiting of the diagnosis in this manner may prevent the most effective early intervention. They contend that at even very young ages, normal irritability can be distinguished from abnormal or excessive irritability in children. Beyond their concerns about excluding preschoolers from DMDD diagnosis, Wiggins et al. (2021) further note that the quantitative criteria associated with the frequency of outbursts was not empirically derived. Based on their research, they recommend that early childhood criteria for DMDD be developed and centered around the following bases: irritable mood with rapid onset that is challenging to de-escalate over two assessment periods, dysregulated tantrum behavior in situations that would not be considered typical for such outbursts, and low frustration tolerance. In sum, the problems of DMDD led Mahli and Bell (2019) to state "DMDD has added to existing diagnostic confusion and likely distracted researchers and clinicians from more meaningful exploration of the mechanisms underlying irritability in children and adolescents" (p. 706).

In an effort to understand the symptomatology of DMDD, Meyers et al. (2017) offer a conceptualization based on their analysis and synthesis of research across a number of domains. They believe that children with DMDD experience higher levels of physiological arousal (as measured by heart rate) in response to frustration, which, in turn, leads to outbursts of temper. In addition, they posit that youth with DMDD may struggle to adapt to changing environmental conditions, which exacerbates frustration and increases the probability of an explosive tantrum. Further, an increased amygdala activation with frustration lends itself to chronic irritability, and children with DMDD exhibit reduced emotional regulation capacity. This impairment in emotion regulation is related to their inability to control their irritability and rageful episodes (Meyers et al., 2017), and research by Vidal-Ribas et al. (2018) supports the association between emotional regulation deficits and irritability. The difficulty in emotion regulation could be related to cognitive issues with attention shifting (or an inability to do so) and/or language development concerns that inhibit the ability of the individual to use self-regulation strategies. Although Meyers et al. (2017) offer this explanation, they strongly note that more research is needed in all of the aforementioned areas in order to truly conceptualize the symptoms and characteristics associated with DMDD in children and adolescents.

Fortunately, the prevalence of DMDD is considered to be quite low (Copeland et al., 2013; Grau et al., 2017; Lin et al., 2021; Munhoz et al., 2017). According to Copeland et al. (2013), the overall prevalence of DMDD by age 16 is approximately 1% when applying all DMDD criteria. This is consistent with retrospective data by Grau et al. (2017) that notes prevalence at 0.79% in a population-based study. In contrast, the *DSM-5* reports the 12-month prevalence of DMDD to be from 2% to 5% (APA, 2013). Data regarding the prevalence also indicate that the expression of DMDD appears to lessen with age (Bruno et al., 2019; Copeland et al., 2013) and that its occurrence is relatively infrequent past the early childhood years (Copeland et al., 2013). Finally, with respect to gender, higher prevalence is noted among males (APA, 2013; Benarous, Renaud, et al., 2020; Copeland et al., 2013; Lin et al., 2021; Mayes et al., 2019) with at least one study noting the ratio of diagnosis to be as high as 3:1 male to female. Despite the consistency of these gender findings, one study with a juvenile justice population found a higher prevalence among females, but the authors related this difference to the distinctive population under study rather than a finding as related to DMDD in general (Mroczkowski et al., 2018).

Regarding comorbidity, children and adolescents with DMDD are at risk of co-occurrence of a number of concerns across the life span (Bruno et al., 2019; Grau et al., 2017; Lin et al., 2021). According to Bruno et al. (2019), the majority of children and adolescents with DMDD are diagnosed with at least one other psychiatric condition. The significantly elevated comorbidity of DMDD with other mental health diagnoses has caused some researchers to question whether it is in fact a separate condition or perhaps its primary symptoms should be considered specifiers for other psychiatric disorders (Grau et al., 2017). The most common diagnoses to co-occur with DMDD are those with central facets related to externalizing behaviors, including ODD, attention deficit hyperactivity disorder (ADHD), and conduct disorder. Mulraney et al. (2016) also found that of children who have both ADHD and DMDD diagnoses, 89.7% could also meet criteria for ODD (though that is not permitted per the *DSM-5*), and 41% meet criteria for anxiety. In addition, youth with DMDD are at significantly higher risk for experiencing both anxiety and depression in adulthood (Copeland et al., 2014; Grau et al., 2017). They also have a greater likelihood of participating in high-risk and/or illegal activities, including smoking, unprotected sexual encounters, sexual contacts with strangers, physical altercations, and breaking and entering (Bruno et al., 2019; Copeland et al., 2014). Although parents of DMDD children also report that they experience sleep disturbances (Waxmonsky et al., 2017) and sleep studies have shown significantly fragmented sleep (Delaplace et al., 2018), research has found that this is probably due to other behavioral issues (such as hyperactivity or impulsivity) rather than the DMDD itself (Waxmonsky et al., 2017). Children and adolescents with DMDD are also more likely to engage in self-injurious behaviors and experience suicidal ideation even in relation to peers who have psychiatric diagnoses other than DMDD (Althoff et al., 2016; Bruno et al., 2019). Suicide attempts among DMDD children and adolescents are frequently unplanned and impulsive (Benarous, Renaud, et al., 2020). Finally, according to the National Institute of Mental Health (NIMH, n.d.), youth with DMDD have higher overall rates of hospitalizations as compared to typically developing children and adolescents.

According to Bruno et al. (2019), the majority of children and adolescents with DMDD are diagnosed with at least one other psychiatric condition.

With regard to adulthood, Copeland et al. (2014) found that psychosocial outcomes include a greater likelihood of serious health problems, emotional distress, financial concerns, and social isolation. Similarly, adults who report experiencing DMDD symptoms in childhood are more likely to be childless and unemployed in comparison to individuals who have never struggled with DMDD symptomatology (Grau et al., 2017). Specifically, this research is indicative of life-long and persistent negative impacts of DMDD on the daily functioning of individuals (Grau et al., 2017), and Copeland et al. (2014) surmise that dire outcomes in adulthood for youths with DMDD may be more significant than other psychiatric diagnoses.

School-Based Eligibility

In light of the nature of this psychiatric condition, it is highly probable (and noted by research) that children and adolescents with DMDD will experience adjustment issues in the school setting. As such, federal law provides a pathway for specialized support when students meet criteria as having a disability that impairs their ability to function and/or progress adequately through the curriculum due to academic or emotional needs. The Individuals with Disabilities Education Improvement Act (IDEA) outlines 13 disability categories within its confines (U.S. Department of Education, n.d.). Of those 13, the two most likely to apply for a student with DMDD would be Emotional Disturbance or Other Health Impairment. These categories have specific criteria for eligibility. When a disability such as these is suspected within the school environment, then a multidisciplinary team is charged with determining whether the child or adolescent does qualify as a student with a disability. The eligibility evaluation is designed to answer two questions: (a) Does the student meet criteria under one of the 13 categories? and (b) Does the student demonstrate a need for special education services in order to fully participate in the curriculum (U.S. Department of Education, n.d.)?

With regard to the Emotional Disturbance category, the criteria under consideration are difficulty with educational progress not due to other cognitive or medical conditions; challenges in making and keeping friendships; atypical emotional and behavioral responses under normal circumstances; depressed mood; and physical symptoms associated with individual problems. The criteria also indicate that a child or adolescent diagnosed with schizophrenia is eligible for certification under the category of Emotional Disturbance, but a child who demonstrates behaviors that could be characterized as primarily socially maladjusted are excluded from services under the Emotional Disturbance criteria. It is required that the student demonstrate one or more of the aforementioned characteristics for an extended period of time and in a manner that precludes educational progress (U.S. Department of Education, n.d.).

In the case of DMDD and in consideration of its symptomatology, it is probable that the student may struggle with social relationships, atypical emotions and behaviors under normal circumstances, and perhaps even depressed mood at times. Thus, a team could likely answer in the affirmative to question 1 for a child or adolescent with DMDD. The more complex question under consideration would be question 2. The team would need to collect sufficient data to determine whether the symptoms of DMDD for the child are preventing the student from progressing in the curriculum in a manner that demonstrates a need for special education supports.

The second category that could be considered for special education eligibility under IDEA is that of Other Health Impairment. According to IDEA, Other Health Impairment refers to "having limited strength, vitality, or alertness, including a heightened alertness to environmental stimuli" that negatively impacts the educational performance of the child or adolescent (U.S. Department of Education, n.d., Section 300.8 (c) (9)). IDEA further specifies a number of health conditions that should be considered here. Those include the following: asthma, diabetes, epilepsy, a heart condition, hemophilia, lead poisoning, leukemia, nephritis, rheumatic fever, sickle cell anemia, and Tourette syndrome. Although DMDD is not one of the listed health concerns, the law also states that other diagnoses should be considered if the criteria are otherwise met (U.S. Department of Education, n.d.). Regarding DMDD, one could certainly conceptualize it as a heightened alertness to environmental stimuli, but, again, the team would need to determine whether adverse educational impacts exist that are due directly to the DMDD symptomatology.

Beyond IDEA regulations, there exists another potential pathway for providing some specialized services and supports for students with DMDD within the school setting. That federal legislation is referred to as *Section 504 of the Rehabilitation Act of 1973*. This law was passed in order to provide equal access to any services for individuals with disabilities into any services organizations that receive federal funding. Public schools are just one of the many government entities that are subject to the mandates of Section 504. Section 504 indicates that a student who has (or is suspected of having a disability may receive special supports if their disability "substantially limits one or more major life functions" (Office of Civil Rights, n.d., Section 104.3 (2) (iv)). Among the major life functions are caring for oneself, performing manual tasks, walking, hearing, seeing, speaking, breathing, learning, and working. In the case of DMDD, if the student's symptomatology is shown (through appropriate evaluation) to limit the ability to learn, then the child or adolescent with DMDD may receive services within the school setting according to their need.

CULTURAL ISSUES RELATED TO DISRUPTIVE MOOD DYSREGULATION DISORDER IN YOUTH

Risk Factors for Disruptive Mood Dysregulation Disorder

As with most psychiatric conditions, the risk for development of DMDD is likely a combination of both genetic and environmental conditions (Bruno et al., 2019; Moore et al., 2019). However, Roberson-Nay et al. (2015) found genetic factors to outweigh environmental risk factors in the development of irritability (a primary symptom of DMDD) in their analysis. Among the biological factors, people with DMDD show abnormal amygdala activation (consistent with irritability) in response to images of facial expressions depicting a range of emotions (Wiggins et al., 2016). In addition, parental depression and other forms of psychopathology in parents have been indicated as a risk factor for the development of DMDD in children and adolescents (Bruno et al., 2019; Matijasevich et al., 2015; Propper et al., 2017; Tufan et al., 2016). Specifically, Munhoz et al. (2017) found that mood symptoms among mothers during pregnancy and maternal depressive symptoms during early childhood are particularly related to the development of DMDD in their children and the severity of irritability in those offspring. However, Perich et al. (2017) and Propper et al. (2017) did not find evidence of DMDD in the offspring of parents with bipolar disorder as had been suspected in other research (Sparks et al., 2014). Paternal substance abuse has been found to be related to DMDD diagnosis in offspring (Bruno et al., 2019; Dougherty et al., 2014).

> As with most psychiatric conditions, the risk for development of DMDD is likely a combination of both genetic and environmental conditions (Bruno et al., 2019; Moore et al., 2019).

With regard to environmental conditions, a higher prevalence for DMDD has been noted among children who come from both low-income and single-parent households (Bruno et al., 2019; Copeland et al., 2013; Mayes et al., 2019) as well as homes in which the mother has a low level of education (Lin et al., 2021; Munhoz et al., 2017). Finally, the experience of trauma has been noted as significantly higher among youth with DMDD as compared to children and adolescents with no psychiatric disorders (Benarous, Renaud, et al., 2020). Overall, research by Moore et al. (2019) indicates that it is environmental conditions that are especially salient in the development of irritability, which is central to the diagnosis of DMDD.

Cultural Considerations

Given the newness of the diagnosis, little is currently known regarding influences of race, ethnicity, or cultural issues with respect to DMDD. In one large study of Medicaid recipients in one state, the authors found that children who were given the DMDD diagnosis were more likely to be older, Black, male, and from rural homes. However, these researchers explain that children in their dataset who offered no racial information were excluded from their analysis. They indicate that this may have skewed their findings related to race (Le et al., 2020). In contrast to the findings by Le et al. (2020), other researchers have surmised that race has not been found to be related to DMDD symptoms (Dougherty et al., 2014, 2017; Mayes et al., 2019). Certainly, more research is warranted to elucidate whether there are cultural issues related to the DMDD diagnosis. In the meantime, it behooves clinicians always to strive for cultural competence in their assessment, conceptualization, and treatment of all children and adolescents with DMDD.

IMPACT OF DISRUPTIVE MOOD DYSREGULATION DISORDER ON SOCIAL–EMOTIONAL AND BEHAVIORAL FUNCTIONING IN SCHOOL AND HOME ENVIRONMENTS

Social–Emotional and Behavioral Functioning in School

Children with DMDD experience significant issues of concern within the school setting (Benarous, Renaud, et al., 2020; Dougherty et al., 2017; Lin et al., 2021; NIMH, n.d.). These include frequent suspensions due to behavioral infractions (Bruno et al., 2019; Copeland et al., 2013; Dougherty et al., 2017) and difficulty with peer relationships (Benarous, Renaud, et al., 2020; Lin et al., 2021). In fact, youths with DMDD are 3 to 4 times more likely to display physical and verbal aggression toward peers even in comparison to children and adolescents with other psychiatric disorders and are also more likely to engage in relational aggression than typically developing peers (Dougherty et al., 2017). These children also have a greater likelihood of being victims of aggressive behaviors by peers (Benarous, Renaud, et al., 2020) and being socially excluded (Dougherty et al., 2017). In addition, children with DMDD may sometimes present as withdrawn in social situations, thereby increasing their probability of social rejection. Researchers suggest that this may be due to children with DMDD being particularly sensitive to their social challenges (Cimino et al., 2020). Finally, these issues with peer relationships may be related to the challenges that children with DMDD face in recognizing emotion. Although they tend to improve in these skills with age, research has found that children and adolescents diagnosed with DMDD often misinterpret happy faces as fearful (Vidal-Ribas et al., 2018).

> Youths with DMDD are 3 to 4 times more likely to display physical and verbal aggression toward peers even in comparison to children and adolescents with other psychiatric disorders (Dougherty et al., 2017).

Social–Emotional and Behavioral Functioning at Home

Within the home, children and adolescents with DMDD symptomatology have been found to have strained relationships, frequent conflict with both parents and siblings, and a greater number of behavioral issues as compared to youth without DMDD (Bruno et al., 2019; Cimino et al.,

2020; Dougherty et al., 2017; Lin et al., 2021; NIMH, n.d.; Uran & Kilic, 2020). In fact, parents of children with DMDD rate them as having higher levels of oppositional behavior, hyperactive behavior, socially challenging behavior, impulsive behavior, and emotionally erratic behavior even in comparison to ratings by parents of children with other psychiatric disorders (Uran & Kilic, 2020). Some research suggests that mothers find the irritability of DMDD to be more challenging to deal with than even the explosive outbursts (Mayes et al., 2017). Families with a child with DMDD are also marked by poorer overall functioning and higher rates of divorce than families with a child who has another mental health condition. Research by Cimino et al. (2020) further suggests that children with DMDD struggle with insecure forms of attachment with their parents, and the children rate their parents as being low in sensitivity and responsiveness.

Ramires et al. (2017) suggest that the relationship issues in the home often stem from the belief of the child or adolescent with DMDD that they do not have a problem. These scholars note that the youth with DMDD feels frequently misunderstood and that conflict in the home is related to others' misguided expectations of them. In response to this belief, the child becomes demanding and oppositional. Adults in the home respond with disapproval, and the child subsequently reacts to the disapproval with defiance of even greater intensity (Ramires et al., 2017). Perhaps intensifying this cycle, and given the relationship between DMDD diagnosis and lower parental education, Lin et al. (2021) make the following statement, "Parents with lower educational levels, relative to those with higher educational levels, may be more inconsistent in parenting and have more difficulties managing their anger and their children's emotional problems effectively due to a lack of skills or time, thereby exacerbating the children's irritability" (p. 490). Thus, parenting skills intervention is often necessitated for youth with DMDD.

IMPACT OF DISRUPTIVE MOOD DYSREGULATION DISORDER ON LEARNING IN THE CLASSROOM

Executive functioning deficits and learning challenges have been noted in children and adolescents with DMDD (Althoff et al., 2016; Benarous, Iancu, et al., 2020; Benarous, Renaud, et al., 2020; Bruno et al., 2019; Dougherty et al., 2017). In addition, Benerous, Bury, et al. (2020); Benarous, Iancu, et al. (2020); and Benarous, Renaud, et al. (2020) noted a significantly higher prevalence of written language disorders and sensory processing difficulties among children and adolescents with DMDD, which would have significant impacts on classroom performance. Sensory processing issues are challenges with organizing and comprehending information derived through the senses. In general, Sahu et al. (2020) indicate a pattern of academic decline over time for students with DMDD. As such, a diagnosis of DMDD is also associated with a greater probability of grade retention (Benarous, Renaus, et al., 2020) and qualification for special education services (Dougherty et al., 2017) among children and adolescents with this disorder in comparison to typically developing peers. Despite these findings, the understanding of DMDD in the classroom is in its infancy. It is critical to note that the relative newness of the diagnosis itself means that few studies have explored its dimensions fully and that those research findings that have been noted are often based on one (or very few) studies. Minimal large-scale work has been done in this area, and the current studies are insufficient in number for meta-analysis. Thus, even the work cited here should be interpreted with caution until researchers have had the opportunity to establish an evidence base of much greater depth and breadth.

> It is critical to note that the relative newness of the diagnosis itself means that few studies have explored its dimensions fully and that those research findings that have been noted are often based on one (or very few) studies.

IMPLICATIONS FOR SCHOOL PSYCHOLOGISTS

Assessment Role

Whether evaluating for IDEA or Section 504, school psychologists often play critical roles in the assessment processes for students with additional needs, including those who may be diagnosed with DMDD. When determining eligibility for services, the school personnel have 60 school days to complete any evaluation and implement qualifying supports. Although the school psychologist is not required (by name) in federal law as a mandated member of the multidisciplinary team, the psychologist often fills the role of the person designated to and capable of interpreting assessment results. The other members of the team include the child's parent(s), a general education teacher, a special education teacher, and an administrative representative. Also, because the law requires that the student be evaluated in every area of suspected disability, other school personnel with specific skill sets may be included in the process as well.

The evaluation itself is multifaceted in nature, and the school psychologist is central in collecting much of the data used in the eligibility determination. A likely starting point for the evaluation is the collection and review of existing data. This includes a review of school-based records for things like attendance, discipline, grades, and prior standardized test scores. If the school implements Multi-Tiered Systems of Support (MTSS), then this record review may also include a collection and analysis of all previously implemented interventions for the child. Records that exist beyond the school system would be gathered and evaluated as well. With regard to a student with DMDD, it is highly likely that external service providers would have already been involved with the child's care. These may include pediatricians, psychologists, psychiatrists, and/or counselors. The school team would seek written permission from the parents to access these records to assist in the eligibility process. It is common for the school psychologist to take the lead on collecting the internal and external records, but certainly other team members may be a part of this as well.

Aside from the collection of existing data and information, the team will also seek new information to aid in their decision-making process. One source of newly gathered assessment data is interviews. A member of the team (frequently the school psychologist) will interview the parent(s), teacher, and student about all domains of the child's functioning that is relevant to the evaluation process. At this point, new testing is usually done, and the school psychologist is often the most highly qualified and competent team member to do this type of assessment. With a student with DMDD, it is going to be essential to fully explore the child's home and school behavior in a number of ways. The school psychologist will direct both the teacher and parent to complete general and specific rating scales of the behavior and psychological functioning. The team will also need a functional behavioral assessment for the purpose of eligibility determination. The functional behavioral assessment consists of multiple, systematic observations of a target behavior. Trained professionals (like school psychologists) can then use these observations to determine what is triggering a particular behavior in a setting and what is causing it to continue. This process gives insight into the behavior itself but also lays the groundwork for future intervention. Finally, cognitive and academic components are assessed through the use of individually administered tools designed for this purpose. Upon collection of all the aforementioned data, the team is poised to determine eligibility for special services for the child or adolescent with DMDD.

Advocacy Role

Within the confines of their roles, school psychologists may be called on to collaborate with medical providers (external to the school system) to support overall functioning for children and adolescents with DMDD. This collaboration may include providing information (with appropriate parental permission) about school-based behavior at the diagnosis or treatment phase. The school psychologist can be an objective source of data about behavioral needs, symptomatology, and/or medication progress monitoring as students with DMDD are often prescribed psychotropic drugs.

Thus, school psychologists should be aware of the commonly used medications for DMDD. Although there are no U.S Food and Drug Administration (FDA)-approved treatments for DMDD, Tourian et al. (2015) note that pharmacological intervention for the irritability associated with DMDD is primarily treated with either selective serotonin reuptake inhibitors (SSRIs) or serotonin-noradrenaline reuptake inhibitors (SNRIs). The NIMH also reports that stimulant medications may be used to address irritability in youths with DMDD as well in that it has been shown to be effective in decreasing and/or alleviating irritability in children and adolescents with ADHD. Finally, antipsychotic medications have been successfully used in the treatment of children with DMDD (Averna et al., 2016).

Although there are no FDA-approved treatments for DMDD, Tourian et al. (2015) note that pharmacological intervention for the irritability associated with DMDD is primarily treated with either SSRIs or SNRIs.

Consultation Role

As previously noted, school psychologists may serve a crucial role in the development of a functional behavioral assessment for a student with DMDD. Although this functional behavioral assessment may take place in the context of an evaluation for special services, it may also be initiated at any time that a behavioral need is identified. When it comes to intervention design, school psychologists often work with teachers to use the knowledge from the functional behavioral assessment to select and implement an evidence-based intervention to replace aberrant behaviors with more adaptive classroom behaviors and functioning. This consultation process is dynamic and ongoing as the school psychologist provides indirect service to the student by applying their psychological expertise to the child's functioning within the classroom setting.

Counseling/Therapy Role

Given their training and experiences, school psychologists are uniquely suited to provide counseling and therapy services to children and adolescents with DMDD within the school setting. Though much is still to be learned about the most effective approaches and services for students with DMDD, therapeutic interventions that have been documented as successful with other disorders of similar behavioral manifestation should be considered. Specifically, school psychologists would be well served to focus intervention efforts on parent training, cognitive behavioral therapy (in particular, dialectical behavior therapy), and other programs that target aggressive outbursts and irritability. Providing these types of psychosocial intervention within the school environment may improve access and adherence for children with DMDD and their families as has been demonstrated with students with other psychiatric diagnoses (Atkins et al., 2006).

EDUCATIONAL SUPPORTS

Although researchers continue to explore the potential academic needs of children and adolescents with DMDD, until such time as a strong evidence base has been developed, it is likely that these students would benefit from classroom supports to develop executive functioning skills in the same manner as children and adolescents with similar externalizing behavioral issues (like ODD). Executive functioning deficits impair skills like attention, direction following, impulse control, and problem-solving and create challenges for both academic and behavioral functioning in the learning environment (Schaeffer et al., 2003). As such, school psychologists should assist teachers in developing a repertoire of classroom strategies to promote positive change in this area.

According to Dawson (2014), students who struggle with executive functioning can benefit from a number of simple modifications and accommodations within the classroom. Utilizing structured (as opposed to abstract or open-ended) assignments, shortening the length of classroom tasks, giving directions in multiple formats, and using direct questions can help maintain focus on the academic expectations and away from other disruptive thoughts. In addition, teachers and other school personnel can model and reinforce the use of organizational strategies and classroom engagement practices to support the development of executive functioning skills in children and adolescents (Dawson, 2014).

In addition, teachers (and their classrooms) may benefit from techniques used to prevent and respond to behavioral outbursts that feature heavily for students with DMDD. With regard to prevention, McGoey et al. (2018) recommend that classroom expectations (and consequences for not adhering to the rules) should be clear. Within that context, teachers should form directives to the child as statements rather than questions, and develop ways to offer choices when it is necessary to say no. Transition times should be carefully planned to avoid being abrupt or surprising students, and classroom tasks should be designed to be engaging and motivating. Finally, they suggest that social–emotional skills should be instructed, practiced, and reinforced within the learning environment (McGoey et al., 2018). Even when the aforementioned strategies are being utilized consistently, there is still a likelihood of behavioral outbursts with a child with DMDD in the classroom. As such, these authors also offer suggestions for effective response. They note that teachers and classroom personnel should avoid giving attention during the episode to the extent that is possible and safe, and they should also ensure that they are not reinforcing the outburst by giving the child what they desire in that moment. It is critically important for the teacher to remain calm, empathic, and assist the child in communicating their feelings when it is appropriate (McGoey et al., 2018). Beyond these general suggestions, collaboration with the school psychologist to design a behavioral intervention specific to the child or adolescent's need is also warranted to promote longer term success and build new and generalizable skills for functioning.

SCHOOL-BASED MENTAL HEALTH INTERVENTIONS AND SUPPORTS

In 2014, Roy and colleagues wrote that, "Since DMDD is a new diagnosis, there are no informative clinical trials from which to establish judicious practice" (p. 922). Although advances have been made in the interim, science can move quite slowly in this regard. Nonetheless, the authors recommended the use of evidence-based practices that have shown support with children who exhibit behavioral challenges (NIMH, n.d.; Roy et al., 2014), and since that time, research has begun to show some therapeutic interventions as effective with children and adolescents with DMDD. With regard to treatment, Rao (2014) recommended that clinicians must search for the source of the irritability in youths (e.g., family, social, or school) to appropriately tailor treatment to their needs. However, Rao warns that many children and adolescents with DMDD have behavioral outbursts that are so out of proportion in relation to their precipitants that multiple forms of treatment may be necessary to effect positive change. Thus, Bruno et al. (2019) emphasize the critical importance of both behavioral types of therapy and parent training in the treatment of children and adolescents with DMDD. Finally, the NIMH (n.d.) notes that treatment may need to change over time as anger outbursts lessen and symptoms of anxiety and depression increase.

Parent training for children and adolescents with DMDD has been shown as effective in improving symptomatology (Byrne & Connon, 2021; Noller, 2016), and Baweja et al. (2016) note that parent training should be incorporated for children with DMDD due to the similarity between DMDD and ODD and the effectiveness that has been demonstrated with the reduction of oppositional symptoms through the use of parent training. A pilot study with a DMDD population demonstrated that parents perceived improvement among their children in prosocial behaviors, aggression, and behavioral concerns, but they did not report a decrease in irritability through the use of this intervention. Nonetheless, parent training shows promise in efficacy although more research is needed to establish an evidence base with this unique psychiatric population. Through the parent training, parents are taught to recognize and circumvent triggers for extreme behaviors. They also gain skills in providing a structured environment with predictable schedules and consistent enforcement of expectations.

Parent training for children and adolescents with DMDD has been shown as effective in improving symptomatology (Byrne & Connon, 2021; Noller, 2016).

Experts in this area suggest that children with irritability (such as that seen in DMDD) are often receptive to cognitive behavioral therapy (Linke et al., 2020; Mikita and Stringaris, 2013; NIMH, n.d.; Noller, 2016). Coping skills and anger management should be essential components of this therapy for children and adolescents with DMDD. In addition, Moore et al. (2019) recommend that exposure therapy be included within the therapeutic plan to target the symptom of irritability. With exposure therapy, the child would be exposed to increasingly frustrating situations to practice coping skills and improve their frustration tolerance. Case study research has supported improvement in the symptoms of anger, aggression, and irritability through the use of cognitive behavioral therapy with children with DMDD. School psychologists could also employ strategies in schools that include psychoeducation, relaxation training, identifying anger triggers, social problem-solving, reframing intentions, social skills, conflict resolution, and parent training (Tudor et al., 2016).

It is important to note that when school psychologists engage in therapeutic interventions, research indicates rapid progress in the reduction of DMDD symptoms with children with the application of dialectical behavior therapy (Gholipour et al., 2015; Perepletchikova et al., 2017; NIMH, n.d.), which is a specific type of cognitive behavioral therapy. Dialectical behavior therapy uses a balance of acceptance of the client along with change strategies. This therapy is focused on helping children and early adolescents build a repertoire of skills to regulate their emotions and moods. It utilizes traditional strategies of cognitive behavioral therapy while incorporating aspects of mindfulness practice. There is emphasis on analyzing maladaptive behaviors for the promotion of positive change (Dimeff & Linehan, 2001).

Beyond individual mental health supports, schools may offer some group interventions through their MTSS for students who demonstrate at-risk behaviors like those associated with DMDD. According to Boxmeyer et al. (2018), three such interventions that have shown promise for students with anger and aggression issues are the Fast Track program (Bierman & Greenberg, 1996), the Anger Coping Program (Lochman et al., 2008), and the Coping Power Program (Lochman & Wells, 2003). The Fast Track program targets overall social skills training through sessions within the school environment and components that are external to the school, like home visits and parenting training. Anger Coping and Coping Power are designed to build problem-solving and anger management skills through structured group lessons within the school. The Coping Power Program also incorporates parent groups in its process. Beyond these interventions, schools are also well served to offer comprehensive social–emotional learning programs to explicitly teach and reinforce those skills for students for whom direct instruction is necessary.

Although the evidence base specific to DMDD may be sparse at this point in time, it is clear that intervention is needed to support positive progress for these children and adolescents to prevent the dire outcomes often seen within this population. Schools and school psychologists are well served to utilize the mental health supports demonstrated as effective with children who have similar diagnoses to address the challenging symptomatology and build more adaptive skills for children and adolescents with DMDD within the learning environment.

CASE STUDY 13.1 LUKE: CASE OF A WHITE MALE WITH DISRUPTIVE MOOD DYSREGULATION DISORDER

Background

Luke is an 8-year-old boy who lives with his parents. His parents state they no longer know how to deal with Luke's "explosive and destructive" behavior. They go on to say that he exhibits outbursts of temper several times a day that last approximately 10 minutes, and more intense 30-minute outbursts occur multiple times a week, during which he becomes physically aggressive. Luke's room has several holes in the drywall from him kicking it, punching it, and throwing furniture into it. The hallway has also become a broken mess. When Luke is having a "fit," his mother and father will attempt to calm him and keep him from hurting himself or the home. In this process, they frequently end up with bruises on their arms and legs from Luke. His mother reports that the family no longer attends church due to his outbursts and cursing. His mother said being in public with Luke is humiliating.

Luke's parents state that Luke had always been a difficult child. He was colicky and rarely slept through the night. They go on to say he is ill-tempered and grouchy for the better part of the day on most days. When grouchy, Luke appears agitated and does not want to be around others. His parents state that he really does not have any friends. They have tried a few play dates, but after a few outbursts, they do not think it is worth it. When playing with others, Luke has become hostile. He states that he believes that others do not like him. Once in a game of kickball, he told his parents that they were "out to get him," and everyone wanted to get him out during the game. Luke has expressed the negative thoughts that no one likes him and that his parents do not love him. When his parents try to cheer him up by suggesting a fun activity, he snaps, demanding to be left alone. Luke's outbursts and noncompliance at home increased once he entered school, as homework became a constant fight between him and his parents.

(continued)

CASE STUDY 13.1 LUKE: CASE OF A WHITE MALE WITH DISRUPTIVE MOOD DYSREGULATION DISORDER (*continued*)

In school, Luke continued to be disruptive and to have difficulty focusing, following instructions, and completing classwork. He states that he gets bored easily. His teachers state he frequently refuses to do any work and causes disruptions in class. Luke is in the second grade. He has been classified under IDEA as emotionally disturbed. The school has assigned a paraprofessional to work with Luke at all times. He has a behavior plan that they apply throughout the day. In the past year, he has been sent home several times and has been suspended four times due to destruction of school materials and violence against others, including students and school personnel. The school recognizes that his behavior is due to his condition but removes him for safety reasons. He has thrown desks, chairs, and books. On one occasion, he kicked the principal's shins multiple times while she was attempting to restrain him. His teachers describe him as smart, if you can get beyond the moodiness and aggregation. Luke struggles academically due to missing lessons frequently as school personnel deal with his behavior. Over time, Luke's academic progress has declined. His teachers noted that even on the best days, Luke often appeared to be in an irritable, agitated mood and that he rarely smiled or appeared happy. Over time, his teachers have placed fewer academic demands on him to avoid outbursts.

Discussion

Luke's temper outbursts are frequent (at least three per week), severe, and explosive, causing impairment at home and in school. Between the explosive episodes, Luke's mood is chronically irritable and grumpy. These symptoms have been present for several years without periods of amelioration. Luke fits the criteria for DMDD. He is already being served in special education under the category of Emotional Disturbance. The multidisciplinary team may want to make sure that all needs are being addressed and interventions are being applied with fidelity. Services should focus on attendance, discipline, grades, classroom management, social engagements, work completion, and any other area for which there is need. Even with the controversial diagnosis, most agree that a referral for a psychiatric evaluation would be appropriate. If services are provided, the school psychologist may work with the provider in an advocacy role. The school psychologist may collaborate with medical providers (external to the school system) to support overall functioning for children and adolescents with DMDD. There may be a place for a consultation role with the development of a functional behavioral assessment for a student with DMDD. Luke has a behavior plan, but this plan should be reassessed to ensure it is addressing the needs properly. Luke must be rewarded for specific positive behaviors in the classroom to shape his behavior. Luke's outbursts at home and in school have become a means of avoiding demands. Management training and modeling may help the teachers and parents gain specific strategies that enhance effective communication and discipline. A focus on building academic successes will help to keep him motivated to engage in schoolwork.

Given their training and experiences, school psychologists are uniquely suited to provide counseling and therapy services to children and adolescents with DMDD within the school setting. A strong cognitive behavioral or reality-based treatment has been shown to be effective with aggressive outbursts and irritability. Luke may learn how to better regulate his mood and improve his frustration tolerance. He could be taught coping skills to regulate his anger and to identify and relabel distortions that contributed to his hostile reactions.

Luke's behaviors are extremely challenging to deal with. Aggression and hostility do not typically generate a sympathetic caring response. The parents and those who work with Luke may benefit from an informative support group. This can give them a chance to vent some of their frustration and get skills and support that is needed. Clear and honest communication between the family and school will be critical throughout the treatment.

SUMMARY POINTS

- DMDD is a new disorder for the *DSM-5*.
- DMDD's most prevalent symptoms are significant behavioral outbursts with persistent irritability between the episodes of rage.
- The development of DMDD is associated with both genetic and environmental risk factors.
- Though the research is not yet clearly established, children and adolescents with DMDD may struggle with executive functioning deficits.
- School psychologists can engage in many roles and functions to support the needs of students with DMDD, including assessment, advocacy, consultation, and counseling and/or therapy.
- Parent training and forms of cognitive behavioral therapy may be effective in the treatment of DMDD, although the evidence base is sparse at this time.

TEST YOUR KNOWLEDGE

1. What is the age range for DMDD diagnosis?
   a. 3–12
   b. 6–12
   c. 6–18
   d. 12–18

2. Irritability is episodic in DMDD.
   a. True
   b. False

3. DMDD and ODD may be diagnosed together.
   a. True
   b. False

4. Which of the following is NOT associated with the development of DMDD in children and adolescents?
   a. Poverty
   b. Trauma
   c. Parental depression
   d. Sibling conflict

5. Dialectical behavioral therapy combines cognitive behavioral strategies with mindfulness practice.
   a. True
   b. False

Answers: (1) c, (2) b, (3) b, (4) d, (5) a.

DISCUSSION QUESTIONS

1. Describe the *DSM-5* diagnostic criteria for DMDD.
2. Explain why the diagnosis of DMDD was developed for the *DSM-5*.
3. Highlight the IDEA criteria for eligibility under the category of Other Health Impairment.
4. Describe the challenges of peer relationships for a child or adolescent with DMDD.
5. Discuss why parent training may be an appropriate intervention for children and adolescents with DMDD.

CHAPTER RESOURCES

American Academy of Child & Adolescent Psychiatry *Disruptive Mood Dysregulation Disorder*: www.aacap.org/AACAP/Families_and_Youth/Facts_for_Families/FFF-Guide/Disruptive-Mood-Dysregulation-Disorder-_DMDD_-110.aspx

Disruptive Mood Dysregulation Disorder *Tips for Educators*: https://disruptivemooddysregulation.weebly.com/tips-for-educators.html

Merck Manual *Depression and Mood Dysregulation Disorder in Children and Adolescents*: www.merckmanuals.com/home/children-s-health-issues/mental-health-disorders-in-children-and-adolescents/depression-and-mood-dysregulation-disorder-in-children-and-adolescents

National Alliance on Mental Illness *Beyond Growing Pains: Children and Mood Disorders*: www.nami.org/Blogs/NAMI-Blog/June-2018/Beyond-Growing-Pains-Children-and-Mood-Disorders

National Institute of Mental Health *Disruptive Mood Dysregulation Disorder*: www.nimh.nih.gov/health/topics/disruptive-mood-dysregulation-disorder-dmdd/disruptive-mood-dysregulation-disorder

National Institute of Mental Health *Disruptive Mood Dysregulation Disorder: The Basics*: www.nimh.nih.gov/sites/default/files/documents/health/publications/disruptive-mood-dysregulation-disorder/20-mh-8119-dmdd.pdf

Stanford Children's Health *Mood Disorders in Teens*: www.stanfordchildrens.org/en/topic/default?id=overview-of-mood-disorders-in-children-and-adolescents-90-P01634

KEY REFERENCES

Only key references appear in the print edition. The full reference list appears in the digital product on Springer Publishing Connect: connect.springerpub.com/content/book/978-0-8261-3587-2/part/part05/chapter/ch13

American Psychiatric Association. (2013). *Diagnostic and statistical manual of mental disorders* (5th ed.). https://doi.org/10.1176/appi.books.9780890425596

Benarous, X., Renaud, J., Breton, J. J., Cohen, D., Labelle, R., & Guile, J. (2020). Are youths with disruptive mood dysregulation disorder different from youths with major depressive disorder or persistent depressive disorder? *Journal of Affective Disorders, 265*, 207–215. https://doi.org/10.1016/j.jad.2020.01.020

Bruno, A., Celebre, L., Torre, G., Pandolfo, G., Mento, C., Cedro, C., Zoccali, R. A., & Muscatello, M. R. A. (2019). Focus on disruptive mood dysregulation disorder: A review of the literature. *Psychiatry Research, 279*, 323–330. https://doi.org/10.1016/j.psychres.2019.05.043

Copeland, W. E., Angold, A., Costello, J. E., & Egger, H. (2013). Prevalence, comorbidity, and correlates of DSM-5 proposed disruptive mood dysregulation disorder. *American Journal of Psychiatry, 170*(2), 173–179. https://doi.org/10.1176/appi.ajp.2012.12010132

Dougherty, L. R., Smith, V. C., Bufferd, S. J., Carlson, G. A., Stringaris, A., Leibenluft, E., & Klein, D. N. (2014). DSM-5 disruptive mood dysregulation disorder: Correlates and predictors in young children. *Psychological Medicine, 44*(11), 2339–2350. https://doi.org/10.1017%2FS0033291713003115

Grau, K., Plener, P. L., Hohmann, S., Fegert, J. M., Brahler, E., & Straub, J. (2017). Prevalence rate and course of symptoms of disruptive mood dysregulation disorder (DMDD). *Kinder-und Jugenpsychiatric und Psychotherapie, 46*(1), 29–38. https://doi.org/10.1024/1422-4917/a000552

McGoey, K. E., Dreste, T., & Quinn, C. (018). Temper tantrums: Helping handout for school and home. In G. G. Bear & K. M. Minke (Eds.), *Helping handouts: Supporting students at school and home*. National Association of School Psychologists.

Meyers, E., DeSerisy, M., & Roy, A. K. (2017). Disruptive mood dysregulation disorder (DMDD): An RDoC perspective. *Journal of Affective Disorders, 216*, 117–122. http://doi.org/10.1016/j.jad.2016.08.007

Moore, A. A., Lapato, D. M., Brotman, M. A., Leibenluft, E., Aggen, S. H., Hettema, J. M., York, T. P., Silberg, J. L., & Roberson-Nay, R. (2019). Heritability, stability, and prevalence of tonic and phasic irritability as indicators of disruptive mood dysregulation disorder. *Journal of Child Psychology and Psychiatry, 60*(9), 1032–1041. https://doi.org/10.1111/jcpp.13062

U.S. Department of Education. (n.d.). *Individuals with Disabilities Education Improvement Act*. https://sites.ed.gov/idea

CHAPTER 14

Persistent Depressive Disorder

LEARNING OBJECTIVES

- Summarize the diagnostic features for the *Diagnostic and Statistical Manual of Mental Disorders* (5th ed.; *DSM-5*; American Psychiatric Association [APA], 2013) diagnosis of Persistent Depressive Disorder (PDD).
- Highlight the risk factors for PDD in children and adolescents.
- Describe common school and home concerns for children with PDD.
- Understand the classroom challenges for students with PDD.
- Identify effective mental health supports for students with PDD.

INTRODUCTION

Persistent Depressive Disorder (PDD) is classified as one of the Depressive Disorders within the *Diagnostic and Statistical Manual of Mental Disorders*, Fifth Edition (*DSM-5*; American Psychiatric Association [APA], 2013). Other disorders in this category include Major Depressive Disorder (MDD) and Disruptive Mood Dysregulation Disorder (DMDD). The Depressive Disorders are characterized by chronic sadness and/or irritability that have additional negative impacts on a person's physical health and thought processes. Although it is normal for people to feel sad or irritable in relation to certain life circumstances, individuals with Depressive Disorders experience these feelings for an extended duration and beyond typical adjustment issues (APA, 2013). The debilitating impacts of the Depressive Disorders cannot be understated; as Bernaras et al. (2019) noted, "Depression is the principal cause of illness and disability in the world" (p. 2).

DIAGNOSTIC ISSUES: *DSM-5* AND SCHOOL-BASED SERVICES

DSM-5 Diagnosis

According to the *DSM-5*, the determination of PDD is based on eight diagnostic criteria. The first criterion describes the presentation of the individual under assessment as being depressed throughout the day most of the time. The *DSM-5* specifies that this pervasive appearance of depression should have been present for a minimum of 2 years in an adult, but a duration of 1 year is sufficient for diagnosis in children. The second criterion expands on the first by noting that two additional symptoms (among a list of six) must also be apparent. Those six symptoms include changes in appetite, disrupted sleep patterns, decreased energy, impaired self-esteem, challenges in focus or decision-making, and expressions of a lack of hope for the future. The third criterion states that during the period of depression, the individual has not been symptom free for a period longer than 2 months. The fourth criterion states that MDD may be apparent for the duration of the period, and the diagnosis of PDD be given. The fifth criterion indicates that the depression is unipolar in nature. The sixth and seventh criteria exclude diagnosis in the presence of schizophrenia (or other psychotic disorders), physical health concerns, and substance abuse as precipitating the symptoms. And the final criterion denotes that the symptoms of the depression must cause serious impact to the individual's ability to function in order to apply the diagnosis (APA, 2013).

Beyond the diagnostic criteria, the *DSM-5* outlines five different specifiers that may be applied with the diagnosis of PDD. The first specifier indicates additional features that may be present with the PDD. Some examples of those features include anxiety, melancholy, and psychosis. A second specifier may be added if the individual is in full or partial remission during the assessment period. A third specifier describes age of onset as either early (before 21 years of age) or late (after 21 years of age). The fourth specifier provides a descriptor of the depressive episodes themselves (i.e., pure dysthymic syndrome, persistent major depressive episode, intermittent major depressive episodes with current episode, and intermittent major depressive episodes without current episode), and the final specifier is indicative of the severity of the PDD. Through this specifier, the symptomatology may be described as either mild, moderate, or severe (APA, 2013).

PDD is a new disorder for the *DSM-5*. It is considered a combination of two other disorders in prior versions of the *DSM*. Those disorders were dysthymic disorder and chronic major depressive episode (APA, 2013). In fact, some literature and practitioners continue to refer to PDD as *dysthymia* (Melrose, 2017). According to Rodriguez-Testal et al. (2014), the inclusion of PDD in the current version of the *DSM* is a signal to users that significance is placed on the course of symptomatology in that chronic depression has become PDD as opposed to MDD. In essence, they argue that the development of PDD as a new diagnosis renders MDD as a provisional or transitional diagnosis dependent on its duration (Rodriguez-Testal et al., 2014). In addition, even by 2017, Vandeleur et al. (2017) noted that no empirical studies had explored the new diagnosis of PDD using the full *DSM-5* criteria. When they did begin these studies, they found large disparities in the presentation and severity across PDD with the various depressive episode specifiers, which caused them to further question the validity of the diagnosis given the heterogeneity of symptoms across individuals who meet the diagnostic criteria for PDD (Vandeleur et al., 2017). Finally, Kriston et al. (2014) referred to the inclusion of PDD in the *DSM-5* as premature due to conflicts about its validity in the literature.

Despite the controversy over its inclusion in the *DSM-5*, the manual reports its 12-month prevalence as approximately 0.5% in the United States (APA, 2013). With regard to lifetime prevalence, Vandeleur et al. (2017) found rates of 15.2% for PDD with major depressive episode, 3.3% for PDD with pure dysthymic syndrome, and 0.4% for PDD with intermittent major depressive episode. However, these researchers note that their prevalence estimates for PDD with major depressive episode may be inflated due to the difficulty of differentiating that form of PDD from chronic MDD. Polanczyk et al. (2015) reports the incidence of depression symptoms among school children worldwide at 3%. Prior to adulthood, higher incidence of depressive symptoms is also noted among females as opposed to males (Breslau et al., 2017; Kwong et al., 2019; Lewis et al., 2020; Tharpar et al., 2012; Vibhakar et al., 2019), with approximately 3 times as many girls as boys experiencing adolescent depression than boys (Breslau et al., 2017). These differences in prevalence between males and females may be accounted for by different developmental trajectories for boys and girls that have found support in the literature (Lewis et al., 2020). Empirical work also suggests an upward trend in the incidence of depression among adolescents (especially girls) in the United States, which may be due to economic stressors in the country and/or increases in cyberbullying (Mojtabai et al., 2016). Beyond prevalence, age of onset is a significant issue with PDD, with research suggesting that early onset (defined by the *DSM-5* as prior to the age of 21) is associated with more serious symptomatology, greater comorbidity, and more negative outcomes (APA, 2013; Wilkowska-Chmielewska et al., 2013). However, more specific research on age of onset for depression has shown greater intensity when the onset is during adolescence versus childhood (Copeland et al., 2021).

> Prior to adulthood, higher incidence of depressive symptoms is noted among females as opposed to males (Breslau et al., 2017; Kwong et al., 2019; Lewis et al., 2020; Tharpar et al., 2012; Vibhakar et al., 2019), with approximately 3 times as many girls experiencing adolescent depression than boys (Breslau et al., 2017).

Much has been written about the trajectory of depressive symptoms. Recently, Lewis et al. (2020) identified four trajectories for depression across childhood and adolescence (ages 4–14) in their large dataset. According to their research, a low and stable pattern of symptomatology was indicative of the vast majority (nearly 75%) of young people, and it was the most stable trajectory over time. This developmental pattern was followed by a decreasing trajectory (10.67%), an increasing trajectory (8.6%), and a high and rising trajectory (5.57%; Lewis et al., 2020). From late adolescence to early adulthood (ages 15–25), Schubert et al. (2017) found that 60% to 80% of people in that age range across a number of studies maintain low-level symptomatology. Protective factors for a low-level trajectory include healthy parental support, two-parent homes, greater coping skills, and higher socioeconomic status. In addition, they found that 1% to 5% have either an increasing or decreasing trajectory of symptoms, and 5% to 12% experience consistently high symptoms across the span of their lives (Schubert et al., 2017). In their research, Ames and Leadbeater (2018) identified health risks for adolescents associated with depressive symptom trajectories. They found that in comparison to youth with a low symptom trajectory, those with a high trajectory are at greater risk for sleep problems, smoking, risky sexual behavior, lowered physical self-esteem, and lessened physical activity (Ames & Leadbeater, 2018).

In relation to comorbidity, Vandeleur et al. (2017) and Copeland et al. (2021) found significant relationships between PDD and anxiety disorders, posttraumatic stress disorder, and substance abuse in adult samples. These authors also found the greatest levels of depressive symptomatology and highest comorbidities among people with PDD with major depressive episodes. Another study indicated that anxiety disorders are more frequent among children and adolescents with PDD even in comparison to youth with other depressive disorders (Benarous et al., 2020). In addition, in young adults, Wilkowska-Chmielewska et al. (2013) have noted co-occurrence between depression and irritability, suicidal ideation, and suicide attempts. According to Benarous et al. (2020) suicidal ideation is higher among youths with PDD, and suicide attempts are significantly higher among females with persistent depressive symptoms as compared to individuals with other depressive symptomatology (Breslau et al., 2017). A study of youth suicides found that depressed mood was reported prior to death in over 37% of suicides across 17 states (Schlagbaum et al., 2020). Further, Copeland et al. (2021) document comorbidity between PDD and criminal behavior in adulthood. Finally, in relation to outcomes associated with PDD, research by Alaie et al. (2021) and Philipson et al. (2020) indicates that adolescents with PDD have greater likelihood in adulthood of struggling with unemployment, lower pay in jobs, reliance on government financial assistance, and work disability in relation to typically developing peers and in comparison to adolescents with other forms of depression. The outcome-related concerns with persistent issues of depression (versus more episodic depression) have been noted in other research as well (Colman et al., 2007).

A study of youth suicides found that depressed mood was reported prior to death in over 37% of suicides across 17 states (Schlagbaum et al., 2020).

School-Based Eligibility

Although a *DSM-5* diagnosis assists individuals in accessing services outside of the school system, federal legislation dictates a separate process be used to determine eligibility for specialized supports within the public school arena. This legislation, the Individuals with Disabilities Education Improvement Act (IDEA), designates 13 disability categories for which students are eligible to receive intensive modifications and accommodations to their educational curriculum as befitting their needs (U.S. Department of Education, n.d.).

In relation to a student with PDD, the most likely category for qualification would be that of Emotional Disturbance. Emotional Disturbance is defined within IDEA according to the following criteria: difficulty with educational progress not due to other cognitive or medical conditions, challenges in making and keeping friendships, atypical emotional and behavioral responses under normal circumstances, depressed mood, and physical symptoms associated with individual problems. The criteria further state that children and adolescents diagnosed with schizophrenia are eligible for certification under the category of Emotional Disturbance, but youths who demonstrate behaviors that could be characterized as primarily socially maladjusted are excluded from services under the criteria. The aforementioned criteria must be present for an extended period of time for the child or adolescent to be considered emotionally disturbed (U.S. Department of Education, n.d.).

When a school-based eligibility team is considering a student for qualification for special services under any IDEA disability category, then two questions must be answered in the affirmative. The first question addresses whether the child does indeed meet the criteria for the disability under consideration. The second question asks whether the student also demonstrates a need for the specialized services. If the data under review support that the answer to both questions is yes, then the child is considered a student with a disability and is eligible for the supports designed to allow them to progress adequately in the least restrictive environment possible for them to attain prescribed yearly goals (U.S. Department of Education, n.d.).

If a child is found to be ineligible under IDEA, then there is also another path for the provision of supports within the school system. Section 504 of the Rehabilitation Act of 1973 is civil rights legislation designed to ensure equal access for people with disabilities to any organization or entity that receives federal funding. This includes public schools. Section 504 indicates that a student who has (or is suspected of having a disability may receive special supports if their disability "substantially limits one or more major life functions" (Office of Civil Rights, n.d.). The prescribed list of major life functions are as follows: caring for oneself, performing manual tasks, walking, hearing, seeing, speaking, breathing, learning, and working. In the case of PDD, the school-based eligibility team would collect assessment data to determine whether the depressive symptomatology does, in fact, impair the individual's ability to learn in the classroom in a manner that allows for sufficient academic progress (Office of Civil Rights, n.d.).

CULTURAL ISSUES RELATED TO PERSISTENT DEPRESSIVE DISORDER IN YOUTH

Risk Factors for Persistent Depressive Disorder

As with most forms of psychopathology, both genetic predisposition and environmental conditions play a role in the development of depression in childhood and adolescence (Bernaras et al., 2019; Kwong et al., 2019; Schubert et al., 2017). Schubert et al. (2017) explain it this way: "When individuals with genetically determined vulnerability are exposed to certain internal or external environmental risks factors, their odds of experiencing chronically elevated levels of depressive affect are further enhanced" (p. 495). Kwong et al. (2019) concur that a complex interplay of genetic and environmental variables likely contributes to the development of depression in children and adolescents.

> As with most forms of psychopathology, both genetic predisposition and environmental conditions play a role in the development of depression in childhood and adolescence (Bernaras et al., 2019; Kwong et al., 2019; Schubert et al., 2017).

A number of genetic variables have been identified as being associated with the onset of depression in children and adolescents. One such variable relates to the amygdala. The amygdala is the part of the brain that is believed to control responses to fear or threat to the individual. In relation to depression, some theorists suggest that people with depression have developed an excessive amygdala response, which causes depressive symptoms (Bernaras et al., 2019). Other researchers point to genetic anomalies in children with depression (2019) and reduced white matter in the brain as impacting the expression of depression (Vilgis et al., 2017).

One of the strongest risk factors for the development of depression in children and adolescents is a family history of depression (Tharpar et al., 2012). In particular, maternal depression is often predictive of childhood depression in both boys and girls (Chen et al., 2020; Kwong et al., 2019; Lewis et al., 2020; Rohrer et al., 2011) but appears to have a more serious impact on the development of symptomatology in their female offspring (Lewis et al., 2020). This may be particularly prevalent in the presence of a particular type of temperament. A reactive child temperament is noted as a risk factor in the development of depression. A reactive temperament is marked by emotional volatility and intensity of reactions (Lewis et al., 2020).

Finally, both trauma and adverse life experiences during childhood have been linked to the development of depression (Elmore et al., 2020; Vibhakar et al., 2019), and an increased number of adverse childhood events also increases the likelihood of the development of depression (Elmore & Crouch, 2020; Elmore et al., 2020). Adverse life experiences can range from unexpected death in the family and parental divorce (Elmore et al., 2020) to even peer bullying (Kwong et al., 2019). In fact, Sokratous et al. (2013) suggest that precipitating events may be relatively minor but still trigger depression as an adverse life event. Vibhakar et al. (2019) report that a child is 2.6 times more likely to develop depression when they have been exposed to trauma, and the prevalence rate of depression among a trauma-exposed sample of children was over 24%. Fortunately, research also demonstrates that positive parental engagement can serve as a buffer for the development of depression even in the presence of multiple adverse life experiences (Elmore et al., 2020).

> Both trauma and adverse life experiences during childhood have been linked to the development of depression (Elmore et al., 2020; Vibhakar et al., 2019).

Beyond the risk factors for the initial development of depression, risk factors have also been noted for an increasing trajectory of symptoms after initial diagnosis. According to Schubert et al. (2017), those risk factors include: being female, hailing from a low socioeconomic status home in childhood, having low self-esteem, experiencing chronic health problems, identifying with a sexual minority orientation, displaying impulsivity in adolescence, and facing psychosocial adversity (Schubert et al., 2017). Similarly, Marshal et al. (2013) also found that identifying as a sexual minority youth is associated with the development of depression.

IMPACT OF PERSISTENT DEPRESSIVE DISORDER ON SOCIAL–EMOTIONAL AND BEHAVIORAL FUNCTIONING IN SCHOOL AND HOME ENVIRONMENTS

Social–Emotional and Behavioral Functioning in School

Social issues can have significant impact in the school setting, where children and adolescents spend the majority of their waking hours during the school year. Although research is scant specific to the social functioning of children and adolescents with PDD, evidence from adults with PDD and general depression studies allow insight into some of the struggles in this area. One such study explored loneliness among adults with PDD (Nenov-Matt et al., 2020). This study found that individuals with PDD have significantly smaller social networks and significantly higher ratings of loneliness in comparison to their peers. In this study, the pattern appeared linear as well, in that greater self-reported PDD symptom severity was correlated with a higher report of loneliness among the participants. It is interesting to note that the perceived loneliness was related to a history of child maltreatment (emotional abuse and neglect) and also to rejection sensitivity. *Rejection sensitivity* is a preconceived expectation of being rejected in social situations and an overreaction when perceived rejection occurs (Nenov-Matt et al., 2020). According to Nenov-Matt et al. (2020), rejection sensitivity is one type of cognitive-affective bias. These biases often prolong feelings, such as loneliness, as they prompt the person to seek self-preservation in social situations. They also alter attention, interpretation, and memory in social situations. Further, cognitive-affective biases often negatively fulfill their own expectations in that the person anticipates being rejected in social situations and subsequently behaves in ways that lead to social rejection. The researchers note that people with PDD tend to wall themselves off in social situations. This attempt at protection from rejection then creates greater loneliness (Nenov-Matt et al., 2020).

> Rejection sensitivity is a preconceived expectation of being rejected in social situations and an overreaction when perceived rejection occurs (Nenov-Matt et al., 2020).

Theorists in this area attempt to explain the social cognition deficits for people with PDD as stemming from their adaptation of a hostile yet submissive interactional style with others. This interactional style may be the result of their early exposure to an abusive or neglectful upbringing and yields continually unsatisfactory interpersonal connections that reinforce depressive symptomatology (Negt et al., 2016). In support of this (and similar to Nenov-Matt et al., 2020), research by Struck et al. (2020) also found that social cognition challenges for individuals with PDD may be connected to earlier experiences of maltreatment in childhood. Their research further suggests that people with PDD struggle to handle tense social situations and experience emotional distress when others are feeling or expressing negative emotions. These situations become overwhelming for them and reinforce an even more avoidant interactional style (Struck et al., 2020).

Social–Emotional and Behavioral Functioning at Home

Interesting research investigated the emotion regulation of youths with depression in the context of their interactions with parents. Depression has been theorized as a disorder of emotion regulation whereby its sufferers display elevated negative affect and reduced positive affect. The ability to appropriately regulate emotions is critical to coping in stressful situations (Melero et al. 2020). Fussner et al. (2015) found that during a reward condition, adolescents with depression were less able to maintain a positive affect (even after a positive experience) than youth without depressive symptoms. They also experienced greater difficulty in avoiding negative affect when switching from a rewarding task to a nonrewarding task. The authors suggest that these findings support a context-dependent nature of emotion regulation in adolescents with depression (Fussner et al., 2015). Similarly, Melero et al. (2020) found that higher scores on depressive symptoms is predictive of the use of maladaptive strategies in regulating emotions in youth. The maladaptive strategies often adopted by children with depression in stressful situations include blaming themselves for the situation, blaming others for the situation, and catastrophizing (Melero et al., 2020).

> The maladaptive strategies often adopted by children with depression in stressful situations include blaming themselves for the situation, blaming others for the situation, and catastrophizing (Melero et al., 2020).

In addition, with regard to stressful situations, other research has indicated that children's depression introduces strain into the family relationship, and greater depressive symptomatology introduces higher levels of strain (Chan et al., 2014). Thus, the youth's disorder has a negative impact on the entire family functioning. Chan et al. (2014) wrote, "Suboptimal family functioning may limit the family's ability to promote positive coping with other stressors" (p. 39). And indeed, they further found that child chronic strain (as noted by issues such as school performance or social issues) was a predictor of persisting childhood depression at a later time. The authors suggest that this chronic strain decreases the probability of strong social support in the home (Chan et al., 2014).

Other authors have proposed that parental depression (which is linked with depression in offspring) has an indirect effect on their children being victimized at school (Chen et al., 2020). In fact, Chen et al. (2020) found support for their theory. Through their research, they learned that children of depressed parents have a greater likelihood of being depressed themselves. When those symptoms begin to manifest, the youth become more avoidant in interactions and socially isolated. In turn, this avoidance and isolation make them targets for victimization by both peers and teachers in the learning environment. However, it should be noted that greater variance was explained in the victimization by peers than by teachers (Chen et al., 2020).

IMPACT OF PERSISTENT DEPRESSIVE DISORDER ON LEARNING IN THE CLASSROOM

In relation to classroom functioning and adjustment, research suggests that both conduct problems and academic performance issues are more prevalent in adolescents with persistent depression than in comparison to their typically developing peers (Breslau et al., 2017; Cash et al., 2017). Studies demonstrate that youth with symptoms of depression often have lower classroom grades as compared to students who do not struggle with these issues (Sharar et al., 2006). Some initial research has noted a link between PDD and lower IQ (Khandaker et al., 2018) and spatial working-memory deficits (Vilgis et al., 2014) in children, although more empirical work is needed to elucidate these findings. A number of issues may manifest themselves in the classroom. As Huberty (2010) explained, children with depression often experience classroom issues, such as difficulty with focus, participation, and work completion. In addition, they struggle with academic competence and accurate perceptions of their schoolwork.

Recent research also demonstrates a concerning relationship between depression and school absences. Finning et al. (2019) found that students with depression have higher rates of overall absences, unexcused absences/truancy, medical absences, and absences due to school refusal. Further, the authors noted that their meta-analysis determined that (when it could be evaluated), the symptoms of depression preceded the higher rates of absenteeism among students. Even when absences were excused, the researchers propose that these could be related to the common somatic symptoms associated with depression like headaches, stomachaches, and excessive fatigue (Finning et al., 2019).

> Finning et al. (2019) found that students with depression have higher rates of overall absences, unexcused absences/truancy, medical absences, and absences due to school refusal.

In addition, the risk of dropping out of school is markedly higher for adolescents who have experienced psychiatric issues (Breslau et al., 2011), particularly depression (Quiroga et al., 2013). According to research by Quiroga et al. (2013), self-reported depressive symptoms in the seventh grade are related to dropping out of school in future academic years. Students who report depressive symptoms are 23% more likely to withdraw from school than peers without depression, but the relationship between the depressive symptoms and dropping out is mediated by the student's perceptions of their own academic competence (Quiroga et al., 2013). Thus, it is critically important to provide appropriate academic supports in the classroom in order to boost the perceived competence of children and adolescents who are experiencing symptoms of depression.

IMPLICATIONS FOR SCHOOL PSYCHOLOGISTS

Assessment Role

Within the school setting, school psychologists are integral to the eligibility processes (noted earlier) that are associated with qualification for students with disabilities under both IDEA and Section 504 of the Rehabilitation Act of 1973. When multidisciplinary teams are seeking to determine whether a student with PDD is, in fact, eligible for special services per these pieces of federal legislation, then the school psychologist features prominently in the data collection, data interpretation, and decision-making processes. The school psychologist administers assessments of the child's or adolescent's cognitive, academic, and psychological functioning to determine present levels of performance in each of the areas and any impacts of the depression on the child's school performance. The psychological assessment would likely include general behavior rating scales as well as measures specific to depression. The school psychologist also conducts the classroom observations, file reviews (attendance, grades, discipline, and prior standardized test results), interviews (teacher, parent, and student), and record reviews (external service providers like counselors, psychologists, psychiatrists, and/or pediatricians) necessary to establish the prior and current functioning of the student. The collected data is interpreted and analyzed in accordance with eligibility criteria. If the child or adolescent is found to be eligible for special services, then the team determines what supports are necessary to provide the student with an appropriate educational experience in the context of their disability. These services might include special education, counseling or therapy with the school psychologist, and/or medication management with the school nurse.

Aside from their role in the eligibility determinations for individual students, school psychologists might also provide vital assessment at the larger school level as well. Many schools use Multi-Tiered

Systems of Support (MTSS) for the screening, identification, and intervention of students at risk for mental health conditions like PDD. As a part of these processes, school psychologists may assist in the design or application of screening tools to select students who may benefit from programs used to prevent or remediate symptoms associated with depression.

Advocacy Role

For children and adolescents with PDD, pharmacological treatment is often used. School psychologists can be powerful allies for students and their families in offering advocacy in seeking treatment for the symptoms associated with PDD and in monitoring any impacts (positive or negative) of the drug treatment as observed in the school setting. As such, school psychologists may offer objective data regarding any apparent side effects or progress monitoring of symptom reduction.

Antidepressants are commonly used for the purpose of symptom suppression or alleviation, but their use is not without controversy (Bernaras et al., 2019). One critical concern with the use of antidepressants in children and adolescents has been the documented risk of suicide reported with their use (Cipriani et al., 2016). Fluoxetine is the only selective serotonin reuptake inhibitor (SSRI antidepressant) with Food and Drug Administration approval for the treatment of depression in youths in the United States. Due to the risks involved, Bernaras et al. (2019) recommends that they only be prescribed for children and adolescents with moderate or severe cases of depression, and they should be used in combination with other therapeutic interventions. Cash et al. (2017) further note that this combination of therapies should be used particularly when the child's or adolescent's depression is considered to be moderate to severe. Given these potential critical impacts, school psychologists may assist families in advocating for the best care scenario for the child or adolescent with depression in conjunction with their external care providers.

> One critical concern with the use of antidepressants in children and adolescents has been the documented risk of suicide reported with their use (Cipriani et al., 2016).

Consultation Role

With their knowledge and expertise in both realms of education and psychology, school psychologists are often called upon to offer consultative support to teachers regarding issues occurring within the classroom. In the case of students with PDD, the depressive symptomatology may produce a number of classroom impacts, including issues related to attention, assignment completion, and social connection. School psychologists can offer strategies to build rapport and relationships between the student and teacher to help them be more successful in the classroom. In addition, school psychologists can help teachers understand the difference between a chronic mental health condition (and its affiliated symptomatology) like PDD and the occasional sadness or moodiness associated with typically developing children and adolescents.

Counseling/Therapy Role

The need to address depression with interventions within the school setting may be dire in that research demonstrates that fewer than 20% of children and adolescents with depression in the United States receive any form of treatment (Merikangas et al., 2010); however, the provision of school-based mental health services has been shown to reduce depressive episodes and suicidal ideation in adolescents (Paschall & Bersamin, 2018). In addition, therapy attendance for children and adolescents is significantly higher when the intervention is delivered within the school setting than when services are provided at a separate community-based facility (Atkins et al., 2006). Thus, given their training and experience, school psychologists are uniquely positioned to offer effective intervention for a particularly vulnerable population in a manner that is resource- and cost-efficient. School psychologists should seek opportunities to incorporate counseling and therapy services into their practices with depressed children and adolescents within their charge for their potential emotional, social, and academic benefits to students.

EDUCATIONAL SUPPORTS

Children and adolescents with PDD can benefit from a number of simple educational supports. Huberty (2010) suggests that one of the first things that a teacher can do to support youths with depression in their classroom is to establish a caring relationship. This should be marked by encouragement and positivity rather than any form of sarcasm or belittling of them or their situation. Teachers should feel comfortable in talking with students with depression about their thoughts and feelings in a manner that conveys empathy. It is especially beneficial to provide opportunities for success in the classroom and/or make modifications and accommodations that support their growth. These may include offering additional academic support, shortening assignments, assisting them with organizational strategies, or implementing a peer mentoring program (Huberty, 2010).

Beyond the recommendations by Huberty (2010), Hart et al. (2018) offer additional strategies for supporting children and adolescents with depression within the classroom setting. They note that educational personnel should strive to design the classroom in a manner that feels safe for all students by normalizing adjustment and mental health issues through group and individual discussions. Teachers should get to know students on an individual level and seek to form meaningful connections to their lives both within and outside the walls of the classroom. By establishing these supportive relationships, teachers can help to ensure that every child and adolescent feels included within the educational environment. One simple way to do this is to use classroom journaling activities and collaborative exercises that foster relationships with teachers and peers for students with depression (Hart et al., 2018). Educational personnel should be mindful that even academic content can be melded into relationship building social and emotional learning for the classroom environment for the benefit of all students.

SCHOOL-BASED MENTAL HEALTH INTERVENTIONS AND SUPPORTS

Many scholars in this area strongly recommend the use of prevention programs to combat early manifestations of depressive symptoms before the development of PDD, and both universal programs for a widespread school audience and targeted programs for those children and adolescents at risk for the development of depression may show benefits when the programs are delivered with fidelity. The majority of these evidence-based programs are cognitive behavioral in orientation (Bernaras et al., 2019; Bodicherla et al., 2021). The universal programs that have shown promise include the Penn Resiliency Program (Gilham et al., 1990), the Aussie Optimism Program (Rooney et al., 2000), the Resourceful Adolescent Program (Shochet et al., 2001), FRIENDS (F = Feelings, R = Remember to Relax, I = I can try my best, E = Explore coping step plans and strategies for finding helpful solutions, N = Now reward yourself for trying your best, D = Don't forget to practice, S = Stay calm; Barrett & Turner, 2001), Problem Solving for Life (Spence et al., 2003), and Fortius (Mendez et al., 2013). The targeted programs that demonstrate effectiveness include Coping with Course (Clarke et al., 1995), Interpersonal Psychotherapy-Adolescent Skills (Young et al., 2010), and Adolescents Coping with Emotions (Sheffield et al., 2006). For a brief overview of each of these prevention programs, see the review by Bernaras et al. (2019). Of note, a recent review and meta-analysis by Feiss et al. (2019) found that targeted prevention programs were more effective in reducing depressive symptomatology than universal prevention programs.

Aside from these programs, research also suggests the value and efficacy of social and emotional learning programs in the prevention of adolescent depression (Reicher & Matischek-Jauk, 2017), but Baughman et al. (2020) note that it would be especially advantageous to begin prevention efforts at preschool to head off the long-term consequences of depression in children and adolescents. In that vein, they offered a comprehensive review of effective social and emotional learning programs for the prevention of depression that are developmentally appropriate in early childhood. As such, programs with demonstrated efficacy include the Preschool PATHS Program (Domitrovich et al., 2007), Fun FRIENDS (Barrett, 2007), and Play Skills for Shy Children (Coplan et al., 2010). For a more thorough review of these programs, see Baughman et al. (2020). With regard to all types of prevention programs for depression, Bodicherla et al. (2021) and Feiss et al. (2019) urge that schools invest in a long-term approach as their results indicate that the effects of said programs are often lost over time. These prevention programs may be implemented as a part of a school's MTSS program.

> With regard to all types of prevention programs for depression, Bodicherla et al. (2021) and Feiss et al. (2019) urge that schools invest in a long-term approach as their results indicate that the effects of said programs are often lost over time.

Beyond the aforementioned prevention programs, one of the most commonly used and heavily researched psychosocial treatments for depression in children and adolescents is cognitive behavioral therapy (Cash et al., 2017; Das et al., 2016). In their meta-analysis of cognitive behavioral therapy (CBT) in the treatment of depression, Crowe and McKay (2017) found that programs that incorporate psychoeducation, emotional awareness, coping skills, and reinforcement techniques show benefit for children and adolescents with depression. In a systematic review and meta-regression analysis by Oud et al. (2019), it was demonstrated that CBT is not only effective in the treatment of depression, but it is particularly so when components include behavioral activation, challenging thoughts, and incorporation of the child's or adolescent's primary caregiver. Research also suggests the effectiveness of technologically delivered CBT when a traditional format is not feasible (Bodicherla et al., 2021; Das et al., 2016; Grist et al., 2019).

Finally, the risk of suicide with chronically depressed children and adolescents cannot be ignored, and school personnel must be appropriately attuned to these risks for students. Aside from the provision of group and individual support services, schools must have crisis plans in place in the event that a child or adolescent is suspected of or expresses suicidal ideation. School psychologists are trained and experienced in the identification of at-risk students, the assessment of suicide risk, and the application of safe and effective crisis protocols. As such, school systems should lean in to school psychologists' expertise for the benefit of all students who may be contemplating the most dire of responses in reaction to their depressive symptomatology.

CASE STUDY 14.1 CASE OF EMMA: AN ADOLESCENT FEMALE WITH PERSISTENT DEPRESSIVE DISORDER

Background

Emma is a 14-year-old girl who is in the ninth grade. She appears sad, making poor eye contact and demonstrating poor social skills. Her affect is flat and apathetic. Emma lives in a household with her mother, younger sister, and grandmother. Her mother is divorced and is the primary caregiver for the children. Her mother is a victim of domestic violence, and her mother stated that the father is an alcoholic and in treatment. He has no parental rights and no contact with the children. Emma's younger sister is currently in elementary school, and her grandmother is unemployed. Her grandmother recently moved in with them, and Emma reported that, due to this, her depression had worsened in the past 2 weeks. She states her sister is the favorite child and is very aggressive toward her. In one instance, her sister choked her for using her phone. Emma believes her grandmother does not punish her sister appropriately, and her mother is too busy at work to notice.

Emma reports that she does not sleep much. She typically sleeps 2 to 3 hours a night. She has thoughts that are racing in her head, and she just cannot relax. She states that it has always been that way for her, and it is no big deal. Emma is significantly overweight and self-conscious about it. Her sister is not overweight and makes frequent comments about Emma's weight. Three years ago, Emma took dance, but she felt the other girls judged her, and she quit. At dinner, she attempts to eat but struggles. She then sneaks food later and throughout the night.

Emma's mother states that as a child Emma was cheerful and smiling. However, at some point in elementary school, she became a different person. She rarely smiles and is very agitated. This has been going on for years. Emma reports that she doesn't like herself and feels worthless. She has felt this way throughout elementary school. She goes on to say she worries frequently but cannot really say what she worries about. She states that she is not suicidal but has wondered what the world would be like without her. She doesn't think about this often and has not entertained a plan ever. She said that her aunt is in an institution, and her cousin has tried to commit suicide, and she doesn't want to be like that.

Emma's mother noted that there is not usually a set routine on weekends in their household, but on weekdays, the family has a routine schedule. Emma gets up for school at 5 a.m., gets dressed and has breakfast, and then leaves her home to catch the school bus. However, Emma states that she doesn't sleep well and listens to music and looks at social

(continued)

> **CASE STUDY 14.1 CASE OF EMMA: AN ADOLESCENT FEMALE WITH PERSISTENT DEPRESSIVE DISORDER (*continued*)**

media frequently throughout the night. Emma rides the bus home and usually arrives home at 3:30. Frequently, Emma goes to her room to rest and do homework until dinner. Her mother states they all do their own thing in the evening, and the kids go to bed around 11 p.m.

Emma notes that she has a small circle of friends. She mostly connects with them digitally. She states that relationships are not really worth it. People just use other people to get what they want and then discard them. She goes on to say it can be lonely, but it is better than rejection.

Discussion

Emma is depressed and has lost interest in daily activities. She feels sadness, emptiness, and hopelessness; has low self-esteem; is self-critical; and has difficulty sleeping, decreased energy, irritable mood, and poor appetite. She also reported significant feelings of worthlessness and helplessness. Emma seems to remember things differently than do others in social situations, blaming others for the situation and catastrophizing. She then has a tendency to wall herself off from others. This has been going on for well over 2 years.

The assessment should focus on her depressive symptoms, their frequency, and, specifically, their duration. Because her attention and thought process may be affected, a complete cognitive assessment should be conducted. A good assessment of social skills would be helpful as well. For children and adolescents with PDD, pharmacological treatment is often used. School psychologists can be powerful allies for students and their families in offering advocacy in seeking treatment for the symptoms associated with PDD and in monitoring any impacts. The depressive symptomatology may produce a number of classroom impacts, including issues related to attention, assignment completion, and social connection. With their knowledge and expertise in both realms of education and psychology, school psychologists are often called upon to offer consultative support to teachers regarding these issues within the classroom. Addressing depressive symptoms with therapeutic interventions is critical and therapy attendance for children and adolescents is significantly higher when the intervention is delivered within the school setting. Thus, given their training and experience, school psychologists are uniquely positioned to offer effective therapeutic intervention. CBT has been demonstrated to be effective in alleviating symptoms.

Children and adolescents with PDD can benefit from a number of simple educational supports. One of the first things that a teacher can do to support youth with depression in their classroom is to establish a caring relationship. This should be marked by encouragement and positivity rather than any form of sarcasm or belittling of them or their situation. Emma is particularly sensitive to situations. She has a tendency to blame others for the situation and then has a tendency to wall herself off. Creating a positive atmosphere in which everyone is comfortable talking about their thoughts and feelings in a manner that conveys empathy is helpful to all students. By establishing these supportive relationships, teachers can help to ensure that every child and adolescent feels included within the educational environment.

SUMMARY POINTS

- PDD is chronic in nature and must be evident for a period of at least 1 year for diagnosis in children or adolescents.
- PDD is a new (but somewhat controversial) diagnosis in the *DSM-5*.
- Both genetic and environmental factors are associated with the development of PDD in children and adolescents.
- School psychologists can engage in many roles and functions to support the needs of students with PDD, including assessment, advocacy, consultation, and counseling and/or therapy.
- Universal and targeted prevention programs in schools show promise for preventing depression in children and adolescents, but schools should take a long-term approach in order to maintain any gains associated with these programs.

TEST YOUR KNOWLEDGE

1. Which IDEA eligibility category is most probable for a child with PDD?
   a. Emotional Disturbance
   b. Specific Learning Dsability
   c. Traumatic Brain Injury
   d. Section 504

2. PDD may not be diagnosed when an adolescent displays symptoms of MDD.
   a. True
   b. False

3. Parental depression is associated with the development of depression in offspring.
   a. True
   b. False

4. Adolescents with depression often show which social cognition deficit?
   a. Attribution bias
   b. Pathological avoidance
   c. Cyberbullying
   d. Rejection sensitivity

5. Universal and targeted prevention programs have shown promise for combatting the development of depression in youth.
   a. True
   b. False

Answers: (1) a, (2) b, (3) a, (4) d, (5) a.

DISCUSSION QUESTIONS

1. Describe the *DSM-5* diagnostic criteria for PDD.
2. Explain the environmental risk factors associated with PDD.
3. Explain why a child with PDD may meet IDEA criteria for Emotional Disturbance.
4. Describe how rejection sensitivity impacts peer relationships for a child with PDD.
5. Discuss the consultation role of school psychologists for a child with PDD.

CHAPTER RESOURCES

Harvard Health *Persistent Depressive Disorder (Dysthymia)*: www.health.harvard.edu/a_to_z/dysthymia-a-to-z
Johns Hopkins Medicine *Dysthymia*: www.hopkinsmedicine.org/health/conditions-and-diseases/dysthymia
Mayo Clinic *Persistent Depressive Disorder (Dysthymia)*: www.mayoclinic.org/diseases-conditions/persistent-depressive-disorder/symptoms-causes/syc-20350929
Merck Manual *Depressive Disorders in Children and Adolescents*: www.merckmanuals.com/professional/pediatrics/mental-disorders-in-children-and-adolescents/depressive-disorders-in-children-and-adolescents
National Alliance on Mental Health *Understanding Dysthymia*: www.nami.org/Blogs/NAMI-Blog/January-2018/Understanding-Dysthymia
National Institute of Mental Health *Persistent Depressive Disorder (Dysthymic Disorder)*: www.nimh.nih.gov/health/statistics/persistent-depressive-disorder-dysthymic-disorder
Stanford Children's Health *Persistent Depressive Disorder in Children*: www.stanfordchildrens.org/en/topic/default?id=persistent-depressive-disorder-in-children-90-P01600

KEY REFERENCES

Only key references appear in the print edition. The full reference list appears in the digital product on Springer Publishing Connect: connect.springerpub.com/content/book/978-0-8261-3587-2/part/part05/chapter/ch14

American Psychiatric Association. (2013). *Diagnostic and statistical manual of mental disorders* (5th ed.). https://doi.org/10.1176/appi.books.9780890425596

Baughman, N., Prescott, S. L., & Rooney, R. (2020). The prevention of anxiety and depression in early childhood. *Frontiers in Psychiatry, 11*, 517896. https://doi.org/10.3389/fpsyg.2020.517896

Bernaras, E., Jaureguizar, J., & Garaigordobil, M. (2019). Child and adolescent depression: A review of theories, evaluation instruments, prevention programs, and treatments. *Frontiers in Psychology, 10*, 543. https://doi.org/10.3389/fpsyg.2019.00543

Hart, S. R., Varahamurti, N., & Huang, L. V. (2018). Depression: Helping handout for school. In K. M. Minke & G. G. Bear (Eds.), *Helping handouts: Supporting students at school and home*. National Association of School Psychologists.

Kwong, A. S. F., Lopez-Lopez, J. A., Hammerton, G., Manley, D., Timpson, N. J., Leckie, G., & Pearson, R. (2019). Genetic and environmental risk factors associated with trajectories of depression symptoms from adolescence to young adulthood. *JAMA Network Open, 2*(6), e196587. https://doi.org/10.1001/jamanetworkopen.2019.6587

Lewis, A. J., Sae-Koew, J. H., Toumbourou, J. W., & Rowland, B. (2020). Gender differences in trajectories of depressive symptoms across childhood and adolescence: A multi-group growth mixture model. *Journal of Affective Disorders, 260*, 463–472. https://doi.org/10.1016/j.jad.2019.09.027

Nenov-Matt, T., Barton, B. B., Dewald-Kaufmann, J., Goerigk, S., Rek, S., Zentz, K., Musil, R., Jobst, A., Padberg, F., & Reinhard, M. A. (2020). Loneliness, social isolation and their difference: A cross-diagnostic study in persistent depressive disorder and borderline personality disorder. *Frontiers in Psychiatry, 11*, 608476. https://doi.org/10.3389/fpsyt.2020.608476

Tharpar, A., Collishaw, S., Pine, D. S., & Tharpar, A. K. (2012). Depression in adolescence. *Lancet, 379*, 1056–1067. https://doi.org/10.1016/S0140-6736(11)60871-4

U.S. Department of Education. (n.d.). *Individuals with Disabilities Education Improvement Act*. https://sites.ed.gov/idea

Vibhakar, V., Allen, L. R., Gee, B., & Meiser-Stedman, R. (2019). A systematic review and meta-analysis on the prevalence of depression in children and adolescents after exposure to trauma. *Journal of Affective Disorders, 255*, 77–89. https://doi.org/10.1016/j.jad.2019.05.005

UNIT 6

MENTAL HEALTH DISORDERS IN CHILDREN AND ADOLESCENTS: OBSESSIVE-COMPULSIVE DISORDERS

CHAPTER 15

Obsessive-Compulsive Disorder

LEARNING OBJECTIVES

- Summarize the *Diagnostic and Statistical Manual of Mental Disorders* (5th ed.; *DSM-5*; American Psychiatric Association [APA], 2013) diagnostic features of Obsessive-Compulsive Disorder (OCD).
- Identify common obsessions and compulsions across ethnic groups.
- Describe how OCD can impact a child's social–emotional and behavioral functioning.
- Understand how OCD can influence a child's classroom performance.
- Describe ways in which school psychologists can help provide educational and psychological support for students who experience symptoms of OCD.
- Gain knowledge of school-based mental health interventions designed for children with OCD.

INTRODUCTION

Obsessive-compulsive disorder (OCD) is a neurobiological disorder that can have a significant impact on a child's social–emotional functioning, behavior, and classroom performance. It can also have an adverse influence on the functioning of the child's family. This disorder is characterized by unwanted, persistent obsessive thoughts and/or compulsive behaviors. The obsessive thoughts are intrusive and can lead to much anxiety and distress for the child. As a means of alleviating the distress, the child may engage in compulsive behaviors or rituals (Adams, 2011; Beauchaine & Hinshaw, 2017; Pontillo et al., 2020). Stressful situations, such as the COVID-19 pandemic, can worsen the severity of OCD symptoms (Davide et al., 2020). Although the impact of this disorder can be debilitating for many children and adolescents, it has been reported that as many as 90% of youths experiencing symptoms do not receive treatment (Geller & Marsh, 2012).

Although OCD was once thought not to occur frequently in youth because symptoms were often hidden, it is now considered to be a common mental health disorder in children and adolescents (Adams, 2011; American Academy of Child & Adolescent Psychiatry [AACAP], 2018; Walitza et al., 2011). In the literature, it has been estimated that OCD impacts 1% to 4% of children and adolescents in the United States (Helbing & Ficca, 2009; Leininger et al., 2010), whereas others report that the disorder occurs in approximately one in 200 youth (AACAP, 2018; Beauchaine & Hinshaw, 2017; Kraynak & Hart, 2017). Although the reported age of onset varies among sources, OCD has been found to begin typically during puberty or adolescence and has even been reported to begin as young as 6 or 7 years of age by some sources (AACAP, 2018; Barton & Heyman, 2016; Beauchaine & Hinshaw, 2017; Kraynak & Hart, 2017). Research studies have indicated that approximately 30% to 50% of adults diagnosed with OCD experienced an onset of symptoms in childhood (Pauls et al., 2014). Stewart (2008) reports that a first peak generally occurs between the ages of 10 and 12, and a second peak occurs during early adulthood. It is interesting to note that both of the time periods for these peaks of OCD seem to coincide with developmental and/or stress-related transitions. For example, the first peak occurs around the onset of puberty-related neurobiological changes in the brain and more academic-related stress, whereas the second peak that occurs in early adulthood may be associated with stress related to transitioning into an emerging adult (Adams, 2011).

With regard to gender and age of onset, most studies tend to indicate that early onset of OCD in childhood typically occurs more in boys, whereas onset in late adolescence and early adulthood tends to occur more frequently in females (Adams, 2011; American Psychiatric Association [APA], 2013; International OCD Foundation [IOCDF], n.d.-a, n.d.-b; Walitza et al., 2011). During the rest of the life span, the prevalence of OCD is about the same between genders (Walitza et al., 2011).

DIAGNOSTIC ISSUES RELATED TO OBSESSIVE-COMPULSIVE DISORDER

When working with children who are exhibiting obsessions and compulsions, it is important to keep in mind that typically developing children may exhibit obsessive thinking and/or compulsive behaviors such as following bedtime rituals. It is common for young children to have a bedtime routine such as having a particular story read to them each night or making sure they have a favorite stuffed animal with them before falling asleep. As Adams (2011) notes, such rituals may be soothing to young children and provide a sense of consistency in the environment in which they live. These early rituals eventually cease as the child matures and may be replaced with different interests such as collecting certain items like toy dinosaurs or learning as much as they can about a particular topic of interest. Typical development also includes children and adolescents experiencing fears—such as the fear of strangers, which usually occurs around 9 months of age, as well as fear of the dark and of monsters during early childhood.

> It is common for young children to engage in developmentally appropriate rituals such as having a story before bedtime and/or having fears such as fear of the dark.

Adams (2011) has identified several characteristics that differentiate typical rituals and fears seen in childhood from those observed in children with OCD. One distinguishing factor is whether the content of the rituals or fears is one that typically occurs in childhood. For example, a child's wanting to sleep with a favorite stuffed animal every night is developmentally appropriate and very different from a child who insists that the stuffed animals be placed in a specific order each night and who then becomes emotionally distressed if the stuffed animals are not placed in that particular order. A second factor is whether the ritual or fear is age appropriate. For example, a young child asking a parent to check under the bed for monsters before going to sleep would be viewed as age appropriate, whereas an adolescent in high school who will not go to bed unless their parent checks their room five times to make sure it is safe would seem unusual. Another distinguishing factor between typical rituals and fears of childhood and those associated with OCD is that typical childhood rituals and fears often provide a sense of comfort for the child, whereas children with OCD are often distressed emotionally and experience much anxiety if they are not able to engage in the ritual because they fear something dreadful will happen if the ritual is not carried out (Adams, 2011). In addition, unlike rituals and fears related to OCD, typical childhood rituals do not consume a lot of time, nor do they negatively impact a child's daily functioning. Children and adolescents with obsessions and compulsions associated with OCD can spend hours engaged in a repeating cycle of obsessive thoughts that trigger anxiety, which results in their performing compulsions to relieve the anxiety, but the relief is only temporary and reinforces the compulsion, which maintains the obsessive thought (Adams, 2011; Kyrios et al., 2014; Pauls et al., 2014). Perpetuation of the cycle can lead to more time spent on the obsession and compulsion, which can adversely impact the child's social–emotional, behavioral, and academic functioning. The final factor noted by Adams (2011) is that children with typical childhood rituals and fears will respond to reason and stop the rituals, whereas children with OCD believe that they must engage in the compulsion after experiencing the obsessive thought.

Understanding the distinction between obsessive thinking and compulsive behaviors observed in typical development and those exhibited by children with OCD is imperative for professionals working with children and adolescents. For school psychologists working with students who may be experiencing obsessions and compulsions, it is also important to understand factors related to the etiology of OCD and classification issues based on the medical model using the *Diagnostic and Statistical Manual of Mental Disorders*, Fifth Edition (*DSM-5*; APA, 2013), and the educational model using the Individuals with Disabilities Education Improvement Act (IDEA; 2004) disability categories that some students with OCD might be served under in their schools. Knowledge of factors contributing to the onset of OCD and its symptoms can lead to early recognition of the disorder, which is important since some youths may attempt to hide their symptoms because of embarrassment, poor insight about how the symptoms are impacting their functioning, and/or lack of awareness that there is treatment for the disorder (Barton & Heyman, 2016).

Etiological Considerations

Within the OCD literature, no conclusive evidence of a specific cause of OCD has been identified. However, it is generally accepted that the etiology of OCD is multifactorial. Research studies indicate that OCD most likely results from neurobiological, genetic, cognitive, behavioral, and environment factors that initiate the onset of symptoms (Adams, 2011; Pauls et al., 2014; Wilmshurst, 2014). Neurobiological factors linked to OCD include neurotransmitters, which are chemicals in the brain that relay messages from neurons to specific target cells. It is thought that OCD symptoms are related to an abnormal metabolism of three neurotransmitters: serotonin, dopamine, and glutamine (Adams, 2011; Johnco, 2017; Pauls et al., 2014; Wilmshurst, 2014). Serotonin helps to modulate mood, anxiety, behavior, cognition, and other brain functions and has been found to be associated with OCD and other mental health disorders (Sinopoli et al., 2017). Dopamine has also been found to be linked to OCD, and it has been found to be involved in adaptation of behavior, motor control, motivation, learning, working memory, long-term memory, and cognitive flexibility (Bhandari, 2019; Pauls et al., 2014). The third neurotransmitter thought to be involved with OCD, glutamine, is involved with cognition, memory, and learning (Karthik et al., 2020). Research studies on neuroimaging of individuals with OCD have revealed evidence of abnormal activity in the cortico–striatal–thalamic–cortical circuits (Pauls et al., 2014; Salles Andrade et al., 2019). This neural circuit is involved in executive functioning and regulation of behavior (Salles Andrade et al., 2019).

> The etiology of OCD includes neurobiological, genetic, cognitive, behavioral, and environmental factors.

Genetics is another factor linked to OCD, and research evidence of its involvement in the etiology of this disorder has been established from twin and family studies (Grados & Wilcox, 2007; Pauls, 2008; Pauls et al., 2014; van Grootheest et al., 2005). In comparison to fraternal twins, an increased likelihood of OCD has been found among identical twins (Grados & Wilcox, 2007). Family studies indicate that OCD occurs more frequently in relatives among youths with OCD in comparison to control groups (Grados & Wilcox, 2007; Pauls et al., 2014). First-degree relatives are 3 to 12 times more likely to have the disorder when compared to the general population (Walitza et al., 2011). In addition, an increased risk for OCD is associated with a family history of tics (Adams, 2011).

Cognitive models of OCD address factors such as dysfunctional beliefs and misinterpretations of those beliefs (Adams, 2011; Taylor, 2002). Although many individuals experience intrusive thoughts or "pop-up" thoughts and do not develop OCD, misinterpretation of the importance or significance of these thoughts can result in obsessive thinking (Adams, 2011; Frost et al., 1997; Taylor et al., 2012). Dysfunctional thoughts associated with OCD have been identified (Obsessive Compulsive Cognitions Working Group, 1997) and discussed in the literature by OCD professionals (Adams, 2011; Frost et al., 1997; Taylor et al., 2012). These beliefs include the following:

1. *Excessive responsibility*—The belief that one is responsible for causing and/or preventing unfavorable outcomes.
2. *Overimportance of thoughts*—The belief that the presence of the thought itself makes the thought important.
3. *Extreme concern regarding control of thoughts*—The belief that it is critical and possible to have complete control over one's thoughts.
4. *Overestimation of threat*—The belief that negative events are likely to occur and will be dreadful.
5. *Perfectionism*—The belief that mistakes and imperfections are unacceptable.
6. *Intolerance for the uncertainty*—The belief that it is imperative and possible to be absolutely sure that adverse events will not occur.

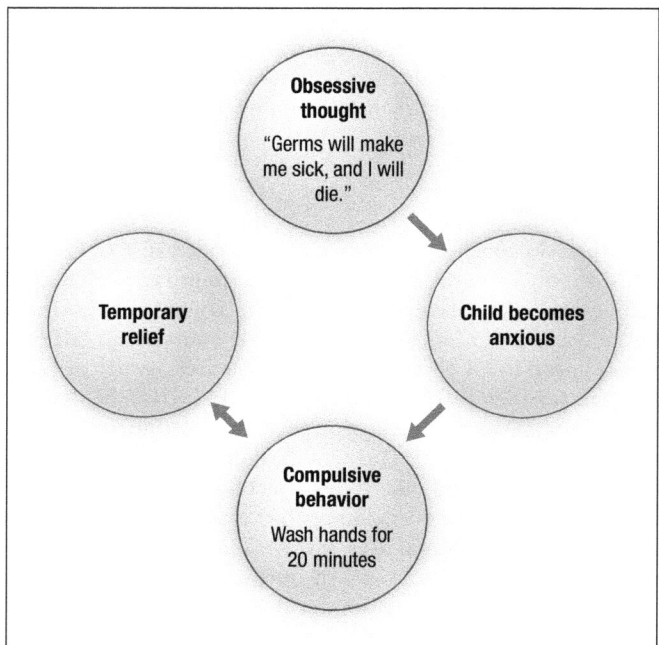

FIGURE 15.1 Cycle of obsessive thoughts and compulsive behaviors.

As noted by Walitza et al. (2011), the result of dysfunctional beliefs and misinterpretation of intrusive thoughts can lead to a sense of danger and subjective urgency to cease the thoughts by avoiding them or engaging in some other type of aversive action. Through these actions, the child gets temporary relief of the distress caused by the intrusive thoughts and learns to engage in compulsive behaviors in an effort to get relief. This pattern results in behavioral conditioning in that it leads to a preoccupation of the intrusive thought, which increases its subjective importance and, thus, reinforces the compulsive behavior (Adams, 2011; Pauls et al., 2014; Walitza et al., 2011). This results in a cycle of obsessive thoughts and compulsions as illustrated in Figure 15.1.

In addition to the factors just described, research has demonstrated several environmental factors that have been linked to the onset and continued expression of OCD symptoms. For example, negative life events, such as divorce, changing schools, and other events that are traumatic or stressful, may render a child or adolescent at risk for OCD (Adams, 2011; Gothelf et al., 2004; Grisham et al., 2008; Lochner et al., 2002). A study conducted by Gothelf et al. (2004) indicated that children diagnosed with OCD reported significantly more adverse life events in the year prior to the onset of symptoms when compared to a control group. Other research studies have found a link between OCD and a history of abuse and neglect (Lochner et al., 2002) and significantly greater severity of symptoms among individuals having a diagnosis of OCD who have experienced one or more traumatic events (Cromer et al., 2007). Moreover, a history of psychological trauma may be overrepresented in children and adolescents with OCD as suggested in a study by Lafleur et al. (2011), which indicated a higher rate of posttraumatic stress disorder (PTSD) among children diagnosed with OCD compared to a matched control group having no OCD symptoms. The study also revealed that children diagnosed with PTSD and OCD experienced more intrusive thoughts and emotional distress as well as less control over their rituals when compared to a control group of children diagnosed with OCD alone (Lafleur et al., 2011). Other negative life events, such as injuries and infections among individuals with OCD, have been reported in the literature. One study found that 30% of youths with a history of a traumatic brain injury (TBI) exhibited OCD symptoms within a year of the injury, and girls having TBI within the sampled group experienced symptoms more frequently than boys (Grados et al., 2008).

Over the past 2 decades, attention in the literature has been given to a possible connection between OCD and streptococcal infection (Adams, 2011; Grisham et al., 2008). Some professionals have proposed that exposure to streptococcal infection can lead to a sudden onset of OCD symptoms in some children (Swedo, 2002). This condition is known as *Pediatric Autoimmune Neuropsychiatric Disorders Associated with* Streptococcus *(PANDAS)*. However, there is much controversy about the link between early-onset OCD and PANDAS among OCD researchers, with some professionals contending that there is enough evidence to support the connection, and other professionals who believe that more research is needed on PANDAS before a clear, definitive link between the two can be made (Adams, 2011; Grisham et al., 2008).

DSM-5 Diagnostic Criteria

Although OCD was classified as an Anxiety Disorder in the *DSM-IV* (APA, 1994), it was placed in a new category of disorders, Obsessive-Compulsive and Related Disorders, newly added to the *DSM-5* (APA, 2013). This category includes OCD, Hoarding Disorder, Body Dysmorphic Disorder, Trichotillomania (hair pulling), and Excoriation (skin-picking). Common features among all of the disorders in this category are repetitive thoughts, compulsive behaviors, anxiety, and distressing emotions (APA, 2013). *DSM-5* diagnostic criteria and related issues specifically for OCD will be the focus of this section.

For both children and adults, the primary diagnostic features of OCD include obsessive thoughts, compulsive behaviors, or both. Based on *DSM-5* (APA, 2013) diagnostic criteria for this disorder, obsessions include unwanted, intrusive, and persistent thoughts, urges, images, or ideations that can trigger anxiety and fear in a child or adolescent. In an effort to alleviate the anxiety and fear, an individual may attempt to ignore the thoughts, neutralize them with another thought, or engage in a behavior such as a compulsion. It is important to note that obsessions are defined in the *DSM-5* (APA, 2013) as the presence of both intrusive thoughts and efforts to neutralize the intrusive thoughts. Examples of obsessive thoughts in youths include obsessions about getting germs and becoming sick if they touch certain items, such as a TV remote controller or a cell phone, which they may perceive as dirty.

As noted before, compulsions are repetitive and persistent behaviors, rituals, or mental acts that are intended to alleviate emotional distress or anxiety or prevent an adverse event even though the behaviors or mental acts may not realistically be linked to what they are intended to neutralize (APA, 2013). Individuals with OCD may experience excessive repetitive compulsive behaviors that are triggered by an obsessive thought or engage in behaviors conducted in a ritualistic manner that serve as a means to lower anxiety or prevent a dreaded event (Beauchaine & Hinshaw, 2017). According to the diagnostic criteria of *DSM-5* (APA, 2013), an individual must exhibit repetitive behaviors or mental acts and engage in these acts to alleviate anxiety or prevent a fearful event. Examples of repetitive observable compulsive behaviors in which children or adolescents might engage include repeatedly washing one's hands for a specified amount of time if they think their hands are contaminated after touching an object that they consider to have germs or avoid touching objects that they consider to be dirty. An example of a mental act might include counting or saying a prayer repeatedly. It is important to note that, although the aim of compulsions is to alleviate anxiety associated with the obsessive thought, young children may not be able to explain why they are engaging in compulsive behaviors. Although most children and adults experience both obsessions and compulsions (Beauchaine & Hinshaw, 2017; Adams, 2011), some children with early age of onset who also have a tic disorder tend to exhibit compulsions only (Beauchaine & Hinshaw, 2017).

> Obsessions are unwanted, intrusive thoughts, urges, or images that can trigger distress or anxiety, whereas compulsions are repetitive and persistent behaviors or mental acts that are intended to alleviate distress or anxiety.

Based on diagnostic criteria, the child's obsessive thoughts or compulsive behaviors must occur for more than 1 hour daily or cause significant distress or impairment in the child's functioning (APA, 2013). The child or adolescent may experience excessive, time-consuming obsessions and/or compulsions that can impact their quality of life. Studies have found that the overall quality of life for children with OCD was significantly reduced in comparison to children who did not have OCD based on self-reports and parent reports (Weidle et al., 2014). In particular, social competence and school functioning were significantly lower in youths with OCD (2014). Other diagnostic criteria include ruling out effects from substance use or a medical condition and determining whether the symptoms exhibited by the child are not better explained by another mental health disorder (APA, 2013).

SYMPTOM DIMENSIONS

Within the OCD literature, there are generally four obsessive-compulsive symptom dimensions that are typically reported. These include the following obsessive thought/compulsion symptoms: (a) symmetry obsessive thoughts and ordering, repeating, and counting compulsions; (b) sexual, aggressive, religious (scrupulosity), and somatic obsessive thoughts and checking compulsions; (c) contamination obsessive thoughts and cleaning compulsions; and (d) hoarding obsessive thoughts and hoarding obsessions (Adams, 2011; Alvarenga et al., 2015; Bloch et al., 2008; Mataix-Cols et al., 2005; Pauls et al., 2014). Obsessive thoughts involving symmetry may be related to an urge to have things in a certain order to avoid an adverse event from occurring. Sexual obsessions might include intrusive thoughts of being involved in sexual acts, whereas religious obsessions might include thoughts such as not praying enough or committing sins. Contamination obsessions may be related to a fear of germs and becoming sick. Adams (2011) notes that the subtype symmetry/ordering, repeating, counting occurs more frequently in males, whereas the contamination/cleaning, washing subtype occurs more frequently in females. In addition, sexual obsessions have been more frequently reported by boys (Mataix-Cols et al., 2005). In comparison to the other subtypes, hoarding has been more frequently associated with poor insight (Adams, 2011). Children and adolescents with OCD who also exhibit hoarding tend to have an earlier age of onset, more severe lifetime symptoms, and experience more difficulty making decisions when compared to those with OCD only (Samuels et al., 2014). It is important to note that hoarding is now a distinct disorder in the *DSM-5*, and there are differences between OCD hoarding and non-OCD hoarding. According to Adams (2011), OCD hoarding is characterized by obsessions, such as fear of contamination if certain items are touched or a fear that something bad will happen if particular objects are thrown out, whereas non-OCD hoarding is not driven by obsessions. OCD hoarding can be distressing, whereas non-OCD hoarding does not generally cause distress (Adams, 2011).

LEVEL OF INSIGHT

Diagnostically, it is important to assess the individual's level of insight in understanding that their obsessive thoughts are irrational and compulsive behaviors are excessive, because it can influence an individual's response to treatment. Although the *DSM-IV* (APA, 1994) included a criterion that individuals must recognize that their obsessive thoughts and compulsive behaviors were excessive or irrational and only had one insight level (poor) as a specifier, this is not the case with the *DSM-5*. The criterion requiring recognition of the excessive nature of obsessions and compulsions was removed in the *DSM-5*, and three levels of insight specifiers were added: (a) "good or fair insight," (b) "poor insight," and (c) "absent insight/delusional beliefs" (APA, 2013, p. 237; Kraynak & Hart, 2017, p. 25). *Good or fair insight* indicates that the individual realizes that the obsessive thoughts most likely are not true, whereas the specifier *poor insight* indicates that the individual thinks that the obsessive thoughts are probably true. The specifier *absent insight/delusional beliefs* indicates that the individual believes fully that the obsessive thoughts are true. Individuals with absent insight/delusional beliefs typically tend to have a worse outcome (APA, 2013). Although adolescents may recognize that their obsessions and compulsions are irrational and/or excessive, younger children may not have much insight in understanding the irrationality and excessiveness of their obsessive thoughts and compulsions (APA, 2013; Beauchaine & Hinshaw, 2017). Research studies have examined levels of insight and other characteristics among children and adolescents diagnosed with OCD (Lewin et al., 2010; Storch et al., 2008). For example, Lewin et al. (2010) found that, in a sample of treatment-seeking youths who had a diagnosis of OCD and were between the ages of 8 and 17 years old, participants with low insight tended to be younger, had lower intellectual functioning, and reported reduced perception of control over their environment. Youths with low insight also reported more depressive symptoms and lower levels of adaptive functioning (Lewin et al., 2010). In addition, an earlier study conducted by Storch et al. (2008) found that, in comparison to youths with good insight, those with poor insight had significantly more severe OCD symptoms, higher levels of internalizing behaviors, and more impairment related to school, family, and social contexts. The authors concluded that children and adolescents with OCD who have little insight may experience more difficulty resisting OCD symptoms, which could potentially impact cognitive behavior therapy (CBT) treatment (Storch et al., 2008).

Comorbidity

In addition to experiencing OCD-related symptoms, children and adolescents with OCD may also experience other mental health disorders. Research studies have indicated comorbidity in 70% to 75% of children diagnosed with OCD (Coluccia et al., 2017; Walitza et al., 2011). Coexisting disorders can impact the severity of OCD symptoms as well as the course of the disorder, which is chronic in approximately 40% to 75% of youths who have OCD (Weidle et al., 2015). Studies have found that, the more severe the OCD symptoms are in a child, the more likely the child may experience one or more other mental health disorders (Walitza et al., 2011). Some of the disorders that been found to coexist with OCD are anxiety disorders, including social phobia, separation anxiety, and specific phobia; depressive disorders; attention deficit hyperactivity disorder (ADHD); disruptive behavior disorders such as oppositional defiant disorder and conduct disorder; eating disorders; autism spectrum disorder, and tic disorder/Tourette syndrome (Adams, 2011; APA, 2013; Beauchaine & Hinshaw, 2017; Nazeer et al., 2020; Walitza et al., 2011; Weidle et al., 2015). It should be noted that treatment for children and adolescents with OCD can also be influenced by the presence of coexisting disorders (Adams, 2011).

> Research studies have shown that the more severe the OCD symptoms are in a child, the more likely the child will have one or more other psychiatric disorders (Walitza et al., 2011).

School-Based Eligibility

Research studies have found that children diagnosed with OCD often have difficulties in their academic, behavioral, and social functioning (Adams et al., 2007; Paige, 2007; Piacentini et al., 2003). Although some children with OCD may have their educational needs met with school-based accommodations through Section 504 of the Rehabilitation Act of 1973, others may need special education services under the IDEA of 2004, depending on the outcome of a psychoeducation evaluation and other data reviewed (Adams, 2011). As noted by Adams et al. (2007), disability categories that might be considered by school psychologists and their school-based teams include Emotional Disturbance (ED) or Emotional Behavioral Disorder (EBD; depending on the state) or Other Health Impairment (OHI). Much concern has been expressed by professionals, such as Adams et al. (2007), about using the classification *ED* or *EBD* for students diagnosed with OCD because of the stigma associated with the term *emotional disturbance,* which is sometimes used to refer to individuals with aggressive backgrounds. Another concern identified is the fact that OCD is a neurobiological disorder rather than an emotionally based disorder (Adams et al., 2007), and, hence, OHI should be considered over ED or EBD. As Adams notes (2011), other disorders having a neurobiological basis, such as ADHD and Tourette syndrome, are now included in the list of health impairments considered for OHI as a result of advocacy efforts by professional organizations supporting these disorders.

CULTURAL ISSUES RELATED TO OBSESSIVE-COMPULSIVE DISORDER IN YOUTH

Although OCD symptoms have been described in the literature for a number of decades, cultural differences in the presentation of OCD symptoms have received little attention in the literature, particularly in regard to OCD in children and adolescents. One explanation for this is that few participants from diverse cultural backgrounds are included in research studies (Williams & Jahn, 2017; Williams, Sawyer, et al., 2017). A recent study by Hunt (2020) reviewed 51 studies with child and adult samples to examine the demographic differences in the frequencies of OCD presentations from the Yale-Brown Obsessive-Compulsive Scale Symptom Checklist (Y-BOCS) across cultural regions that included the United States and Europe, South America, South Africa, Asia, and the Middle East. The study found that, although the frequencies of the presentation of symptoms varied across cultures, no significant differences in the frequencies of the symmetry obsession and ordering compulsion were found across cultures. Findings also revealed that the OCD content varied across cultures, but the differences were modest. Hunt (2020) concluded that, overall, the findings indicated that OCD subtypes are fairly universal.

Given that cultural factors may influence the presentation of OCD symptoms, cross-cultural manifestation of OCD at an international level has been examined by researchers (de Bilbao & Giannakopoulos, 2005; Hunt, 2020; Sharma et al., 2021; Williams, Chapman, et al., 2017). Within the Jewish culture, individuals with OCD may experience scrupulous (religious) obsessions. These obsessions are often accompanied by compulsive behaviors that include excessive handwashing, praying, and consulting with religious leaders about their religious concerns (Williams, Chapman, et al., 2017). Similarly, religious content related to prayers, faith, purity, contamination, washing, and ordering has been reported in OCD symptomatology in Islamic Middle Eastern cultures, which emphasize religion, purity, and cleanliness (Hunt, 2020; Williams, Chapman, et al., 2017). Other studies have noted that clinical samples from Muslim and Jewish Middle Eastern countries in which religion is a primary focus of the culture report more OCD symptoms related to religion in comparison to clinical samples from Western countries (de Bilbao & Giannakopoulos, 2005). Among Eastern Asian countries of Japan, Taiwan, and China, OCD symptomatology related to contamination, symmetry, doubts, and aggression were the most frequently reported obsessions, whereas compulsions of washing, checking, repeating rituals, and orderliness were the most frequently reported (Williams, Chapman, et al., 2017). Studies examining OCD symptoms in India revealed common obsessions of contamination, religious concerns, symmetry, aggression, sexual thoughts, and pathological doubt (Williams, Chapman, et al., 2017). Among a sample of children and adolescents having a primary diagnosis of OCD seeking treatment at various centers in India, symptom presentation included the following five obsessions/compulsions factors: (a) religious obsessions/checking, counting, and repeating compulsions; (b) magical thing-superstitious obsessions/superstitious games and arranging compulsions; (c) hoarding and saving obsessions and compulsions; (d) contamination obsessions/washing compulsions and somatic obsessions; and (e) aggression and sexual obsessions/harm prevention compulsions (Sharma et al., 2021). Finally, in Hispanic and South American cultures, contamination and aggression were the most commonly reported obsessions (Williams, Chapman, et al., 2017).

Within the United States, little is known about OCD prevalence and symptom presentation in African Americans. The importance of researching OCD symptom presentation in African Americans has been emphasized by Williams, Proetto, et al. (2012) for several years. As Williams, Proetto, et al. (2012) point out, it is essential that information about cross-cultural differences be obtained because individuals who do not exhibit common OCD symptoms may not be identified, and African Americans with severe OCD and less common symptoms may be misdiagnosed. Most of what is known about OCD and African Americans comes from epidemiological studies, which have indicated that OCD in African Americans occurs at rates equal to the general population (Williams, Proetto, et al., 2012). Himle et al. (2008) examined data from the National Survey of American Life that focused on three groups: African Americans, Blacks of Caribbean descent, and non-Hispanic Whites. Himle and colleagues (2008) found that approximately 1.6% of African American and Caribbean Blacks met diagnostic criteria for OCD and experienced high rates for at least one other mental health disorder. They also found that, among African Americans and Caribbean Blacks, OCD is persistent, coexists with other mental health disorders, and is associated with high severity and functional impairment. These factors, along with limited access to treatment and reduced response to treatments that have not been tested with African Americans, help to maintain the high persistence of OCD in African Americans.

In response to a critical need for more clinical research on OCD in African Americans and to better understand the phenomenology of OCD among this group, Williams, Domanico, et al. (2012) conducted a study in which the Y-BOCS was given to a sample of African American adults who were experiencing OCD symptoms or who had experienced symptoms in the past. The authors compared the data from a sample of African Americans with OCD symptoms who were recruited at a university to a sample of African Americans and Caribbean Blacks who participated in the National Survey of American Life. The findings from the university sample indicated six separate symptom dimensions, which included: (a) contamination/washing, (b) hoarding, (c) sexual thoughts/reassurance, (d) aggression/mental compulsions, (e) symmetry/perfectionism, and (f) doubt/checking. The results from both samples also indicated that African American participants reported more symptoms related to contamination than their White counterparts and were twice as likely to report concerns related to animals (Williams, Domanico, et al., 2012). As indicated by the authors, cultural relevance of increased contamination concerns among African Americans may be linked to individuals with low incomes who may be concerned about contamination exposure or to historical practices of segregation in which African Americans were forced to use separate water fountains and restaurants out of White Americans' fear of contamination through close interactions or exchanges. The authors also noted that increased concerns about animals may be linked to a fear of animals or historical use of dogs to track slaves (Williams, Domanico, et al., 2012).

Research studies have found that African Americans with OCD are more likely to report contamination symptoms than their White counterparts and twice as likely to report animal concerns.

Efforts to better understand OCD in African American youth are needed given that African American youth, like their adult counterparts, are underrepresented in research studies and treatment centers (Williams et al., 2016). In an effort to gather more information about OCD among African American youth, Williams and Jahn (2017) reviewed potential sociocultural protective factors that may contribute to resilience in some African American children and risk factors that may be barriers to treatment. Potential protective factors identified by Williams and Jahn (2017) included the following: (a) a positive ethnic identity and racial socialization, which help to promote a sense of belonging and is associated with well-being and resiliency during adverse situations; (b) authoritarian parenting typically present in African American families that may avert family accommodation of OCD behaviors; (c) social support from family members and peer support, which can sometimes be challenged in youth having OCD; (d) African Americans' tendency to focus on the present rather than the future (which is sometimes the focus of some obsessions); and (e) the reliance of religious coping and faith during adverse times if it does not become a religious obsession. Potential risk factors include the following factors: (a) possible variation in OCD symptom presentation or unusual symptoms that could potentially lead to misdiagnosis; (b) low income and lack of insurance that are financial barriers to seeking treatment; (c) limited access to treatment influenced by a lack of therapists being proficient in treatment of OCD among African Americans and limited knowledge of where to seek treatments among some African Americans; (d) lack of trust of the medical profession due to past racist and discriminatory practices in clinical research and current racism in our society; (e) the stigma of mental health and negative view of needing help for mental health problems; and (f) negative family communication style that could potentially increase the risk of OCD in children and adolescents.

IMPACT OF OBSESSIVE-COMPULSIVE DISORDER ON SOCIAL–EMOTIONAL AND BEHAVIORAL FUNCTIONING IN SCHOOL AND HOME ENVIRONMENTS

Impact on Social–Emotional Functioning

Managing anxiety associated with OCD can render a child emotionally and socially vulnerable, which can impact their social–emotional functioning. The emotional toll of seeking relief from anxiety related to obsessions and performing compulsions can be debilitating in youths with OCD, who may have difficulty regulating their emotions, which subsequently leads to other emotional difficulties. In addition to experiencing OCD symptoms, many youth experience feelings of shame (Tangney & Dearing,

2002; Veale & Roberts, 2014; Weingarden and Renshaw, 2015), depression (Peris et al., 2010; Storch, Jones, et al., 2012; Storch, Lewin, et al., 2012), anxiety (Langley et al., 2010), loneliness (Storch et al., 2006), low self-esteem and self-doubt (Canavera et al., 2010), emotional dysregulation (Jacob et al., 2012), and increased risk of suicide (Goodwin et al., 2002). This section focuses on the emotional distress and social functioning impairments experienced by many children and adolescents with OCD.

Emotional Distress

The emotional toll of OCD on children and youth can be significant. Some youth with OCD may be embarrassed that they have the disorder, because they fear that their obsessions and compulsions might be noticed by others and/or fear that their OCD symptoms indicate that they are "crazy" (AACAP, 2018). The concern that they may be "crazy" may also stem from some children with OCD reporting that they experience hearing an inner voice that tells them to perform compulsions such as rituals (Vera & Vera, 2010). A sense of shame and viewing themselves negatively may be experienced, which may lead to efforts to hide their compulsions from others (Barton & Heyman, 2016; Helbing & Ficca, 2009; Leininger et al., 2010). This shame and tendency to hide symptoms can result in a delay in disclosing symptoms to parents, leading to a delay in seeking treatment (Veale & Roberts, 2014). In addition, fear that others will notice their compulsions can contribute to secondary, school-related anxiety and school avoidance in an effort to prevent others from discovering their compulsions (Fischer-Terworth, 2013).

> A sense of shame and negative self-view may lead youths with OCD to not disclose their symptoms and attempt to hide them, which can delay treatment.

In general, shame can be a painful emotion that is often associated with different mental health disorders and can negatively impact interpersonal relationships, serving as a motivating factor in social isolation (Tangney & Dearing, 2002). Therefore, it is important to examine the role of shame in children and adolescents with OCD. In a conceptual review of shame in obsessive-compulsive related disorders, Weingarden and Renshaw (2015) found different types of shame. Although not just limited to OCD, shame related to having a mental illness was reported in several OCD studies reviewed by Weingarden and Renshaw (2015). This type of shame was associated with being viewed as "abnormal" by others when compulsions were displayed in public. Symptom-based shame among individuals with OCD was also identified in the review, indicating that the content of obsessions related to sexual and/or aggressive thoughts or images was shame inducing. As noted by Veale and Roberts (2014), shame associated with such obsessions can prevent disclosure in individuals with OCD, because they fear that others will misunderstand them and view them negatively. This type of shame was conceptualized as a treatment barrier in that avoidance of disclosing obsessions and compulsions can prevent one from seeking treatment for their OCD (Weingarden & Renshaw, 2015).

Emotional regulation, the ability to manage one's emotional experiences, can positively influence psychological well-being and adapting to emotional situations. When children and adolescents have difficulty regulating their emotions, they may experience psychological maladjustment. McGuire and colleagues (2013) found that youths with OCD who had emotional dysregulation experienced more symptom severity than youths with OCD who were able to regulate their emotions. Likewise, youths with anxiety disorders have been found to have difficulty regulating their emotions (Suveg & Zeman, 2004). To compare emotional regulation among youths with OCD and youths with other anxiety disorders, Jacob and colleagues (2012) conducted a study that examined emotional regulation among youths with OCD and youths with anxiety disorders that frequently coexist with OCD, namely, generalized anxiety disorder, social phobia, and separation disorder. Their findings indicated that those with OCD experienced more difficulty in regulating their emotions in comparison to the those diagnosed with other anxiety disorders. As noted by the authors (Jacob et al., 2012), intrusive thoughts and obsessions may render youths with OCD less able to tolerate emotional experiences, which may lead to ineffective coping when they experience negative emotions. Emotional dysregulation may be manifested in severe anxiety, depressed mood, or fluctuating mood changes (McGuire et al., 2013).

Children and adolescents with OCD may experience feelings of depression and non-OCD anxiety. As noted earlier, OCD often coexists with depressive disorders. Peris et al. (2010) examined clinical and cognitive correlates of depression in youths having a primary diagnosis of OCD. The results of their study indicated that greater levels of depressive symptoms were linked with greater levels of cognitive distortions, older age, and more severe symptoms of OCD. In addition, depressive symptoms were linked to low perceived control and self-competence as well as high OCD severity (Peris et al., 2010). Based on their findings, Peris et al. (2010) noted that, over time, OCD may have an emotional toll on youths, which can place them at risk of developing depression, and that youths who are ineffective in controlling their symptoms or whose symptoms persist despite their efforts to control them may view themselves as incompetent, which can increase the risk of depression. Other studies have found similar results and indicated that girls with OCD are more likely to have a depressive disorder than boys (Storch, Jones, et al., 2012; Storch, Lewin, et al., 2012). Coexistence of OCD and depression can render children and adolescents vulnerable to self-doubt and low self-esteem, which can impact peer relations and possibly lead to social isolation (Canavera et al., 2010). Similarly, youths with OCD may experience non-OCD anxiety, which can impact symptom severity and functioning. Langley et al. (2010) found that those with OCD and a coexisting anxiety disorder experienced more OCD symptom severity than youths with OCD and those who had OCD and a coexisting externalizing behavior.

Other types of distress experienced by youths with OCD include distress from the tendency to be a perfectionist. Many individuals with OCD strive to be perfectionists (Ye et al., 2008). In a clinical sample of youths with OCD, Ye and colleagues (2008) found that perfectionism was associated with more severity of OCD symptoms, contributed to depressed mood, and negatively impacted interpersonal relationships. As Ye et al. noted, those with OCD often have an overinflated sense of responsibility (as demonstrated from prior research) and believe that flawlessness is a way to prevent adverse events. This unrealistic goal of being "perfect" further intensifies their stress and worries (Ye et al., 2008). The findings of their study also indicated that sensitivity to mistakes was a maladaptive domain of perfectionism, whereas self-esteem was found to be an adaptive domain. Self-criticism associated with a sensitivity to mistakes and low self-esteem were associated with the severity of psychological distress (2008) and negatively impacted interpersonal relationships.

Social Functioning Impairment

The importance of peer relationships on children's well-being and social development is well documented in the literature (Asher & Weeks, 2018; Glick & Rose, 2011; Rose & Asher, 2000). Social functioning and peer relationships can be negatively impacted among children and adolescents with OCD as evidenced by difficulties engaging in social interactions and establishing friendships (Leininger et al., 2010). Borda and colleagues (2013) found that, in comparison to a nonpsychiatric control group, preadolescent children diagnosed with OCD reported significantly more difficulties in social functioning, more fearfulness of negative evaluations, and more peer victimization. Preadolescents with OCD also reported less bullying behaviors (bullying others) and prosocial behaviors compared to the control group. Their findings also revealed that preadolescents with OCD were significantly more likely to experience difficulties in their relationships with peers such as having fewer friends compared to their peers, difficulty making friends, and wanting more friends. Borda et al. (2013) concluded that parents and teachers may need to help encourage positive social interactions with peers and mental health providers working with children diagnosed with OCD may need to be attentive to their clients' difficulties with peer relationships.

> Research studies have found that preadolescents with OCD report more difficulties in social functioning, fearfulness of negative evaluations, and peer victimization when compared to a control group.

Although preadolescents with OCD have reported significantly less bullying and prosocial behaviors in comparison to peers with no psychiatric history (Borda et al., 2013), many children and adolescents with OCD experience peer victimization. Storch et al. (2006) examined peer victimization among youth with OCD and found that approximately 25% of participants in the study had experienced victimization by their peers, which occurred in the form of being ridiculed and teased, socially excluded, and physically mistreated. Peer victimization was positively associated with feelings of loneliness, depression, and internalizing as well as externalizing behaviors (Storch et al., 2006). Moreover, the severity of symptoms was positively associated with peer victimization, indicating that the more severe the symptoms the more those with OCD were victimized, which increased feelings of loneliness and depression (2006).

Difficulties in social functioning have also been reported at an international level. A study among Turkish adolescents with OCD found lower social comparison scale scores and higher shyness scores compared to a control group (Sen & Memik, 2020). Parents of adolescents with OCD reported that their children had more difficulty in making friends and were more likely to be excluded by their peers. The parents also indicated that their children had fewer friends and reported higher levels of shyness, but this was not a significant difference when compared to the control group (Sen & Memik, 2020). The authors concluded that the higher levels of shyness may be related to the tendency of adolescents with OCD to avoid social interactions in an effort to hide their symptoms, whereas lower social comparison scale scores may reflect their tendency to be perfectionists and perceiving themselves as not being good enough (Sen & Memik, 2020). Another study examined functional impairments in a clinical sample of Norwegian and Swedish youth diagnosed with OCD and found that the majority of those in the clinical sample exhibited impairments in psychosocial development (Valderhaug & Ivarsson, 2005).

Behavioral Functioning

As noted earlier, disruptive behaviors can coexist with OCD. Externalizing behaviors in youths with OCD have been reported in the literature. Jacob et al. (2012) contend that children and adolescents with OCD may be prone to externalizing behaviors given that they often attempt to control family members so that their compulsive behaviors can be maintained. In their study, Jacob and colleagues (2012) examined externalizing behaviors between a group of preadolescent youth (ages 7–12) who had a diagnosed anxiety disorder and a group of youths whose primary diagnosis was OCD. The results of their study indicated that youths with OCD exhibited more parent-reported oppositional behavior than those diagnosed with an anxiety disorder. The authors pointed out that this finding may be related to the child's attempt to involve the family in their compulsions. Alternatively, it may reflect the parents' frustration at the rigidity associated with maintaining compulsive behaviors when they attempt to intervene, thus increasing the child's anxiety associated with their obsessions and compulsions, which may lead to oppositional behaviors (Jacob et al., 2012). Other studies have examined coercive–disruptive behaviors in youths with OCD. In a study by Lebowitz et al. (2015), *coercive–disruptive behaviors*, defined as "forceful attempts to impose symptom accommodation on family members" (p. 2589) were common among a group of youths with a primary diagnosis of OCD based on reports by the mothers. Clinically, coercive–disruptive behaviors were found to be associated with the severity of OCD symptoms and linked to anxiety, hyperactivity, and oppositional behavior based on mothers' reports. With regard to the family, coercive–disruptive behavior was associated with family accommodation of the child's OCD symptoms and parental distress (Lebowitz et al., 2015).

> Coercive–disruptive behaviors may be related to the child's or adolescent's attempts to have family members accommodate their OCD symptoms.

Rage has also been reported in children and adolescents with OCD. Storch, Jones, et al. (2012) and Storch, Lewin, et al. (2012) examined rage attacks among youths with a primary diagnosis of OCD. The results of their study indicated that rage was relatively common within the sample of participants and associated with the severity of OCD symptomatology. Rage attacks were often linked with a disruption of compulsive behaviors but were not found to be triggered by an obsession. Storck and colleagues noted that children reported feeling calm after a rage attack and that the rage might be negatively reinforced by serving as an escape from the OCD-related stimuli or decreased internal distress. The findings also indicated that the rage attacks occurred in the home with family members and may be triggered by a situation such as the parents' setting limits with the child or the child's attempt to avoid a stimulus that causes the child to become anxious (Storch, Jones, et al., 2012; Storch, Lewin, et al., 2012). Another explanation for why the rage attacks occur at home rather than school may be due to disciplinary actions that are implemented by the school or fear of exhibiting such behavior in the presence of their peers (Storch, Jones, et al., 2012; Storch, Lewin, et al., 2012).

Finally, greater functional impairment has been found in children and adolescents who have a diagnosis of OCD and an externalizing behavior disorder. Langley et al. (2010) found that, in comparison to youths with OCD and youths who have OCD and anxiety disorder, youths with OCD and an externalizing disorder exhibit more OCD-specific functional impairment at home, school, and other familiar settings. Langley and colleagues (2010) also found that those with OCD and an externalizing behavior disorder experienced more attentional difficulties, delinquent behaviors, and aggression compared to the other two groups. In addition, greater family impairment was reported in youths with OCD and an externalizing behavior disorder (Langley et al., 2010).

Family Functioning at Home

As shown in the previous section, externalizing behaviors in children and adolescents with OCD can influence family involvement in maintaining OCD symptoms (Storch, Jones, et al., 2012; Storch, Lewin, et al., 2012) and family conflict (Langley et al., 2010). As a means of attempting to reduce the child's OCD-related distress, family members may accommodate the child's OCD by engaging in the child's compulsions. For example, parents may provide gloves for their child or open doors for their child, because the child fears that such objects have germs. Similarly, a parent, in an effort to reduce their child's distress, may provide reassurance to a child who continuously seeks reassurance. Parents and other family members engage in such accommodations as a way to protect their child from anxiety-inducing situations that might result in emotional distress for the child or to prevent the child from becoming disruptive at home or in public situations in which the child's anxiety might be triggered (Kagan et al., 2017).

Research studies have been conducted to examine the frequency with which family accommodations occur, the types of accommodations used by families, and whether the accommodations are associated with greater symptom severity. A study conducted by Wu et al. (2019) examined family accommodations within a clinical sample of youths with OCD and their caregivers, which revealed that almost all of the parents (99.3%) reported that family accommodation had occurred in the past week and almost 83% reported that it had occurred on a daily basis and/or in an "extreme" manner. Another finding of their study indicated that verbal reassurance and refraining from participating in certain behaviors were the most commonly reported types of family accommodation. In a similar study, Pontillo et al. (2020) reported 100% of the parents in their study reported family accommodation and indicated that reassurance and avoidance were the most frequently used types of accommodations. Family accommodation has also been found to be associated with higher severity of symptoms and functional impairment (Pontillo et al., 2020; Wu et al., 2019).

Family accommodation has been recognized as a factor in sustaining OCD compulsions (Kagan et al., 2017; Pontillo et al., 2020; Wu et al., 2019). By accommodating the child's compulsions through reassurance or allowing them to escape or avoid anxiety-inducing situations, family members inadvertently reinforce the importance of the obsessive thought that triggered the compulsion, which, in turn, strengthens the child's belief that one should respond to that obsession (Pontillo et al., 2020). Hence, the family inadvertently negatively reinforces the child's anxiety, which maintains the OCD symptoms (Kagan et al., 2017).

Accommodating the child's compulsions can also be negatively reinforcing for the parent in that the accommodation can relieve the parent's distress related to managing the child's anxiety (Kagan et al., 2017). However, the relief, as noted, is only temporary for the child and for the parent as well (2017). Family members who provide accommodation may experience emotional distress, and there may be decreased overall family functioning (Pontillo et al., 2020). Moreover, research studies indicate that high levels of family accommodation were associated with more depressive symptoms among family members of youths with OCD and have an adverse impact on the quality of life among family members (Pontillo et al., 2020; Wu et al., 2018).

Family members who accommodate the child's OCD symptoms may experience emotional distress.

Given the fact that family accommodation has been found to be a factor in maintaining OCD symptoms and can have an adverse impact on the emotional well-being of family members and family functioning, it is important that the family understands how to manage their child's OCD symptoms and to recognize the role that family accommodation can have on the child and individual family members (Barton & Heyman, 2016). Barton and Heyman (2016) contend that one way in which families can help manage the child's OCD symptoms is to externalize the problem by naming the OCD. This enables the family to understand that the OCD compels the child to engage in the obsessions and compulsions, which can help to avoid placing blame on the child (Barton & Heyman, 2016). It is imperative that treatment for OCD in children and adolescents also involves working with the family to address family accommodation.

IMPACT OF OBSESSIVE-COMPULSIVE DISORDER ON LEARNING IN THE CLASSROOM

Although youths with OCD may attempt to hide their OCD symptoms from their peers and others, the influence of their symptoms may extend into the classroom. School-related stress, such as academic pressures or changing schools, can trigger the onset of OCD symptoms or exacerbate existing symptoms (Fischer-Terworth, 2013). OCD's influence on a child's school functioning can be significant. Students with OCD often perform well below their potential on academic work (Leininger et al., 2010). Academic difficulties may stem from concentration difficulties and reduced productivity as well missed instruction due to school refusal and school avoidance (Fischer-Terworth, 2013).

Difficulties Related to Obsessive-Compulsive Disorder Symptoms

In a study that examined the impact of OCD on social, family, and school functioning, Piacentini and colleagues (2003) found that the most common problems reported by participants were difficulty concentrating on school assignments and completing homework. OCD may initially appear to be inattentiveness when, in fact, a child with OCD may be focused on an obsessive thought or mental ritual, such as counting to a certain number, before they start a task (Adams, 2011). Obsessive thoughts or mental rituals may interfere with concentration and completion of homework (Anxiety and Depression Association of America [ADAA], n.d.; Beauchaine and Hinshaw, 2017; Leininger et al., 2010; Piacentini et al., 2003). In addition, compulsions in the classroom can involve rereading text passages, rewriting words, and rechecking math calculations, which can result in loss of time to complete schoolwork (Fischer-Terworth, 2013). Efforts to manage OCD symptoms in the classroom so that others do not detect the compulsive behaviors can utilize much mental energy within the child, which may leave the child mentally and emotionally depleted and, subsequently, interfere with the child's ability to focus and complete classwork (Adams & Burke, 1999).

Chronic tardiness and school avoidance can also have a negative impact on the academic performance of youths with OCD (Adams, 2011). As noted earlier, compulsions and rituals can be time-consuming, which can interfere with getting enough sleep, because they have bedtime rituals that they engage in prior to going to sleep. This may result in their waking up late, which can lead to a delayed start in the morning and being tardy to school. Not getting enough sleep could also leave the child feeling tired during the day at school, which may make it difficult to concentrate. Compulsions that occur in the morning can interfere with getting to school on time, resulting in chronic tardiness. For example, a child who insists on washing their hands for a set number of times or checking every door in their house prior to leaving home to go to school may arrive late at school and miss classroom instruction and activities. Some children who have contamination obsessions and fear touching objects at schools that have been touched by their peers may attempt to avoid going to school, which results in missed instruction (Leininger et al., 2010). School avoidance may also occur if the child fears being teased about their compulsions by their peers (Adams, 2011). Hence, chronic tardiness and school avoidance can result in missed instructional time, which can have an adverse impact on academic performance.

Executive Functioning and Neuropsychological Impairments

Difficulties in executive functioning may also impact the academic performance of a child with OCD. As discussed earlier in the chapter, neuroimaging studies of individuals with OCD have indicated that the neural cortico-striatalthalamic-cortical circuit is involved in OCD. Hyperactivity of the neural circuits in these areas of the brain could potentially contribute to neuropsychological impairments such as executive functioning difficulties (Pauls et al., 2014). Executive functioning skills are involved in goal-directed and problem-solving behaviors that are essential to academic success. Executive functioning encompasses skills in planning, organizing information and materials, setting goals, self-monitoring, transitioning from one task to another, and regulating emotions (National Center for Learning Disabilities, 2005). Although research in adults has demonstrated difficulties in executive functioning, there have been, overall, fewer studies on neuropsychological impairments in children and adolescents with OCD. Of the studies that have been conducted, concerns have been expressed about inconsistent findings and methodological issues such as small sample sizes, which make it difficult to draw meaningful conclusions (Lewin et al., 2014; Zandt et al., 2009). Another concern noted in the literature is that executive functioning difficulties in children with OCD may not occur as often as in adults, because the structure of the brain that is associated with executive functioning (prefrontal cortex) is not fully developed in children (Adams, 2011; Savage & Rauch, 2000). Hence, deficits may become more apparent as the prefrontal cortex matures.

Some researchers attempted to address these concerns so that more conclusive findings about executive functioning in youths with OCD could be drawn. Lewin et al. (2014) examined neuropsychological functioning in a sample of 96 children and adolescents between the ages of 7 and 17. The findings of this study indicated deficits in executive functioning, particularly in set shifting, and visuospatial memory. The authors suggested that although it may be possible that organizational strategies may be involved with visuospatial memory, it is probably more likely that orbito-frontal cortex abnormalities contribute to the visuospatial memory encoding deficits observed in OCD. The results also revealed that the deficits were not associated with the severity of OCD symptoms (Lewin et al., 2014).

To compare neurocognitive performance in children and adolescents with anxiety disorders, Kim et al. (2019) conducted a study with a total sample size of 127 participants whose ages ranged from 7 to 17 years. The study investigated neuropsychological impairment in youths with OCD, youths with generalized anxiety disorder (GAD) but not OCD, and a typically developing control group. Working memory, visuospatial memory, planning ability/efficiency, and cognitive flexibility were assessed. Results indicated that, relative to typically developing peers, those with OCD and those with GAD had deficits in planning ability/efficiency, visual processing, and cognitive flexibility. Specifically, the findings revealed that youths with OCD had significant impairment in planning ability compared to the other two groups, whereas those with GAD demonstrated delayed visual processing and more cognitive inflexibility compared to youths with OCD and typically developing youths. The authors indicated that these findings could potentially indicate that the planning ability for children and adolescents with OCD may become more strained as problems become more complex (Kim et al., 2019). This finding may have diagnostic and treatment implications in that it could differentiate youths with OCD from other clinical diagnoses and that those with OCD may benefit from training in structured problem-solving when distressed, which could potentially reduce their engagement in compulsive behaviors to manage the anxiety related to OCD. The authors indicate that further research studies with larger sample sizes are needed (Kim et al., 2019).

Cognitive sequelae and neuropsychological impairment across symptom dimensions have been examined by McGuire et al. (2014) in a sample of 93 treatment-seeking children and adolescents between the ages of 7 and 17 years who had a primary diagnosis of OCD. Neuropsychological areas assessed included nonverbal memory and fluency, verbal memory, verbal fluency, verbal learning, processing speed, and inhibition/switching. The findings of the study revealed that youths with hoarding symptoms and symmetry/ordering symptoms had more occurrence of cognitive sequelae compared to other dimensions of OCD. Compared to hoarding symptoms, symmetry/ordering symptoms were reported more frequently among youths in the sample. In addition, youth exhibiting symmetry/ordering symptoms also had a larger magnitude of neuropsychological impairment, specifically in the areas of nonverbal fluency, processing speed, and inhibition and switching. The authors conclusions regarding the findings included the following: (a) the discrepancies of neuropsychological impairments among research studies may be related to the type of symptoms experienced, (b) the findings support the neural-structuring studies that certain symptom dimensions may be related to distinctive changes in brain functioning, and (c) those with hoarding or symmetry/ordering symptoms may benefit from neuropsychological testing to identify strategies to address academic needs.

A recent study by Negreiros and colleagues (2020) examined neurocognitive markers in children and adolescents with OCD. The sample was composed of 233 children and adolescents between the ages of 6 and 18 years and consisted of three groups: (a) youths with OCD, (b) non-OCD siblings of youths with OCD, and (c) healthy youths. Areas of neuropsychological functioning that were assessed include cognitive flexibility, decision-making, planning, response inhibition, spatial working memory, attention, recognition nonverbal memory, and cognitive functioning. Findings indicated that youths with OCD and their non-OCD siblings demonstrated significantly lower scores on planning in comparison to the healthy control group. No other significant group differences were found, leading the authors to conclude that planning is a pre-existing trait marker for pediatric OCD (Negreiros et al., 2020).

Overall, research findings related to executive functioning and neuropsychological impairments in youths with OCD appear to be inconclusive, and more research is needed in the future. It is, however, important for school psychologists to be aware that children and adolescents with OCD may have difficulties in some areas related to executive and neuropsychological functioning. Consideration for neuropsychological testing may be warranted.

Noncompliant Behavior

A child or adolescent with OCD who struggles to manage the anxiety related to their OCD symptoms may seem to appear inattentive in the classroom, and the teacher may think that the child is not listening or following instructions (Adams, 2011). For the child, the intrusive thoughts and associated anxiety (along with the urge to engage in compulsive behaviors) can totally encompass them in such a way that they cannot focus on what is going on in the classroom. To the teacher and others, it may appear that the child is being noncompliant and/or unmotivated when, in fact, they are just trying to manage the symptoms related to the OCD. The child's not following through on instructions could influence the teacher's view of the child, which could impact their relationship. Therefore, it is important that teachers are aware of how OCD can impact the child or adolescent in the classroom and that what may appear as noncompliance is actually the child's efforts to manage their OCD symptoms, which could deplete the child's mental energy, making it difficult to focus in the classroom (Adams, 2011).

IMPLICATIONS FOR SCHOOL PSYCHOLOGISTS

Given that OCD behaviors may be misunderstood and early recognition of symptoms can lead to providing interventions and supports in the school as well as possible clinical treatment outside of the school setting (Leininger et al., 2010), school psychologists can be instrumental in addressing the needs of children with OCD by (a) promoting awareness and knowledge of childhood OCD among parents and educators; (b) engaging in consultation with school personnel, parents, and any outside professionals involved in providing services to the child; and (c) assessing OCD behaviors and coexisting symptoms. School psychologists' delivery of services targeted to children with OCD falls within the National Association of School Psychologists (NASP) 2020 Professional Standards domain of Mental and Behavioral Health Services and Interventions (National Association of School Psychologists, 2020), which encompasses school psychologists' addressing emotional and behavioral impacts on learning and implementing evidence-based strategies that support social–emotional well-being.

Promoting Awareness and Knowledge of Obsessive-Compulsive Disorder Symptoms

Feeling misunderstood by others and even perhaps ashamed of their symptoms, children and adolescents with OCD may experience disappointment with themselves and frustration that they cannot better manage their symptoms. It is imperative that parents and educators have an awareness of OCD and gain knowledge of the symptoms of OCD and how this disorder can impact a child's functioning at home and in the classroom. Given their training in education and mental health, school psychologists are in a unique position to promote awareness and knowledge of OCD among parents and educators. This section of the chapter focuses on ways in which school psychologists can be a resource for parents and teachers in better understanding the impact of OCD on youth.

Parent Awareness and Knowledge of Obsessive-Compulsive Disorder Symptoms

School psychologists can be a valuable resource for parents to help them better understand OCD symptoms and the impact of OCD on their child's academic performance, social interactions with peers, emotional well-being, and their behavior at home and school. Developing a brochure or information packet is one way in which school psychologists can provide parents with information about OCD. Information about possible causes of OCD; how symptoms may present in the home; and how OCD impacts the child academically, emotionally, socially, and behaviorally could be included in the brochure or information packet. It would also be important for parents to have information about the impact of OCD on the family and the stress association with family members attempting to accommodate the child or adolescent's obsessions and compulsions.

Possible resources from which to gather information include the NASP resource, *Obsessive-Compulsive Disorder: Information for Parents and Educators* (Paige, 2004), which provides some basic information about OCD, such as prevalence, symptoms, and possible treatments. This handout also addresses how the family and school can provide support to the child. Another helpful NASP resource is the handout *Obsessive-Compulsive Behavior: Helping Handout for School and Home* (Malone, 2018), which provides an overview of OCD symptoms, available treatments, and recommendations for the home, such as helping parents understand the importance of not enabling OCD behaviors in the home. These NASP resources are available free on the NASP website to its members. In addition, school psychologists may find handouts from the International OCD Foundation (IOCDF) helpful in preparing information packets for parents. For example, the handout *What Is OCD?* (IOCDF, n.d.-a, n.d.-b) provides a brief overview of OCD, whereas the handout *OCD in Children and Teenagers* (Wagner, 2009) includes a description of OCD symptoms and how OCD impacts the child and family, as well as treatment options. Another IOCDF resource for parents is *Living With Someone Who Has OCD: Guidelines for Families* (van Noppen & Pato, n.d.), which addresses how to recognize the signs of OCD, modify expectations, make private time for oneself to avoid getting overly stressed, and create a supportive environment for the child within the home. In addition, the Obsessive-Compulsive Foundation of Metropolitan Chicago's guide *How to Help Your Child: A Parents' Guide to OCD* (2006) provides basic information about OCD and how it impacts the child at school, the impact of the family, treatment and medication considerations, and the importance of seeking support. Please note that these online resources and their URL links along with other resources for parents are provided at the end of this chapter.

Videos and webinars on OCD are also available online that parents could view to learn more about OCD. The video series *OCD Kids Speak Out* is available on YouTube and features children and adolescents with OCD who share their experiences and the challenges presented by OCD. From viewing some of the episodes of this series, parents can see the impact of OCD on children struggling with the disorder and learn about ways in which these youths manage their symptoms. Parents may also want to consider sharing this series with their own child so that their child sees that there are others like them challenged by OCD. There are also videos by Dr. Aureen Wagner, an OCD expert, which address issues about OCD such as what OCD is and how to recognize it as well as a video on how to talk to children about OCD. These videos, *Advice for Parents* and *Explaining OCD*, are available on YouTube. For parents who want to gain more in-depth information about OCD, the webinar developed by ADAA provides coverage on diagnostic elements, symptoms, age-appropriate interventions, and treatment options that parents may want to consider. The webinar can be viewed on the ADAA website. The links for these video resources are provided in the Chapter Resources section at the end of this chapter.

Educator Awareness and Knowledge of Obsessive-Compulsive Disorder

Throughout the literature on OCD, professionals have noted the importance of teachers and school personnel having knowledge of specific information related to OCD and how it may present in the classroom (Adams, 2004, 2011; Adams & Burke, 1999; Chaturvedi et al., 2014; Fischer-Terworth, 2013; Leininger et al., 2010). Given that students with OCD spend most of their day at school and many of them attempt to hide their symptoms while at school, teachers can have a role in recognizing OCD-related behaviors and inform school psychologists and parents about their observations of the child in the classroom, which can lead to early identification. Early identification can lead to the implementation of educational supports and school-based interventions as well as the attainment of clinical treatment for the child. By understanding how OCD impacts a child academically, emotionally, and socially, the teacher is better able to create a learning environment that is supportive for the child and one in which the child feels safe. Moreover, being knowledgeable about OCD and recognizing whether OCD symptoms are interfering with the child's performance in the classroom enables the teacher to know when to seek help from the school psychologist.

One way in which school psychologists can promote awareness and knowledge about OCD among teachers and other school personnel is by providing an in-service training opportunity or developing an OCD information packet. School psychologists are encouraged to provide the following content for teachers:

- General overview of OCD that includes how OCD is defined; an explanation of obsessions and compulsions, symptoms, and how severity of symptoms can vary; views on possible causes; and brief information about prevalence; and
- Specific information that addresses the difference between rituals that occur in typically developing children and debilitating rituals that occur in youth with OCD that cause much emotional distress; how OCD impacts the child's academic, social–emotional, and behavioral functioning; how OCD can impact the family; and possible educational supports and interventions that could be provided in the classroom.

There are several resources that school psychologists may find helpful in preparing an in-service training or OCD information packet. NASP has available resources that are designed for educators, such as *Obsessive-Compulsive Behavior: Helping Handout for School and Home* (Malone, 2018), and *Obsessive-Compulsive Disorder: Information for Parents and Educators* (Paige, 2004), that have useful information about OCD in youth. In addition, the book *Students With OCD: A Handbook for School Personnel* by Gail Adams (2011) has thorough coverage of OCD as it relates to schools and would be a helpful resource for school psychologists who are preparing an in-service training or preparing a brochure to be included in an informational packet for teachers and other school personnel. School psychologists may also want to consider the resource *Teachers' Guide to OCD*, by the Child Mind Institute (https://childmind.org/guide/a-teachers-guide-to-ocd-in-the-classroom), which provides OCD information targeted specifically to educators. A list of common OCD symptoms that may be exhibited in school settings can be obtained from the ADAA webpage *OCD at School* (ADAA, n.d.) at the link https://adaa.org/understanding-anxiety/obsessive-compulsive-disorder/ocd-at-school. In addition, an article titled *What Does OCD Look Like in the Classroom?* (Burbrick, n.d.) can be found at the Child Mind Institute website (https://childmind.org/article/what-does-ocd-look-like-in-the-classroom). These lists provide examples of how OCD symptoms may be manifested in the classroom, which could help teachers learn to recognize signs of OCD-related compulsions.

Other resources that school psychologists may want to consider when preparing professional training materials for educators include brief video clips that could provide a picture for the teacher of the challenges experienced by children with OCD. One video developed by ADAA, *OCD Facts*, provides a brief overview of OCD that provides basic information about symptoms, causes, common obsessions and compulsions, and types of treatment. There is another brief video by ADAA, *OCD in Children*, which describes how OCD may present in children and challenges experienced by those with OCD (ADAA, 2009). Both of these videos are brief and easily accessible for viewing. These online resources are listed with their associated URL links at the end of this chapter.

Consultation on Obsessive-Compulsive Disorder–Related Issues

Beyond promoting an awareness of OCD among parents and teachers, school psychologists can have a consultative role in helping youth with OCD better function at home and school. School personnel, such as teachers, can be a valuable resource in identifying OCD symptoms in children and adolescents because they spend a great deal of time with their students each day. Consultative efforts with a teacher who has expressed concerns about a student's behavior could include gathering information about the teacher's concerns and whether the behaviors impact the child's performance in the classroom. If the behaviors appear to be related to OCD, the school psychologist could share information about how OCD behaviors may be manifested in the classroom and how it may impact the child's academic, social–emotional, and behavioral functioning. Consultation may address difficulties in the classroom such as difficulty paying attention and completing classwork, appearing distressed and anxious at times, and troubling interactions with peers such as other students bullying the child with OCD. It is imperative that the teacher understands that often children with OCD have low self-esteem (Leininger et al., 2010) and struggle with managing their OCD anxiety but may be working hard to attempt to complete assigned tasks (Adams, 2011). Efforts should be made to create a classroom environment in which the child with OCD feels safe and supported (Chaturvedi et al., 2014). In addition, the school psychologist may want to consult with both the teacher and school nurse if there is any concern about side effects of OCD medications that the child might be taking (Leininger et al., 2010).

Consultation with parents also would be important to gather information about their concerns regarding their child's functioning at school, consultation with parents is also important. Parents may want to share information about the child's functioning at home and how the child attempts to manage their symptoms. If the child has been exhibiting OCD-related behaviors at home but has not yet received a diagnosis, the parents may seek guidance as to where to find a clinical psychologist or psychiatrist so that the child can be evaluated for OCD. They may also seek advice from the school psychologist regarding what to expect in such an evaluation and what types of questions to ask during the interview with the clinician. It would be important for the school psychologist to share information about OCD in children and adolescents and the importance of obtaining appropriate treatment, cognitive behavioral therapy with exposure and response prevention, for the child if a diagnosis of OCD is confirmed. This type of treatment involves exposure to the obsessive thought and the child selecting not to engage in the compulsive behavior. The school psychologist could work with the parent and the teacher to monitor the child's functioning at home and school so that any concerning behaviors could be addressed.

If an outside mental health professional is providing services to the child, it is important for the school psychologist to communicate with the professional as long as the parents give consent. Information about the child's behavior at school and how OCD may be impacting the child's functioning at school could be shared with the outside professional. A plan for how to help the child manage symptoms and possible interventions that could be provided at school might be considered. Clear communication among all parties involved with the child is essential.

Assessment of Children and Adolescents With Obsessive-Compulsive Disorder

Although a formal diagnosis of OCD may be made by a clinical child psychologist or psychiatrist, school psychologists can have an instrumental role in gathering information about the functioning of the child or adolescent in the school setting to share with the parents and professionals working with the child. Several assessment methods and specific assessment instruments can be used to gain an understanding of how OCD may be impacting the child's functioning at school.

Behavioral Observations

Observations of the child's behavior can be a useful tool in determining whether possible OCD-related behaviors are impacting the child's functioning in the classroom. School psychologists may be asked to conduct a behavioral observation if the teacher notices a concerning behavior or an outside clinical professional seeks information about the child's functioning at school. It is important to find out what concerns the teacher or outside professional may have about the child's behavior.

The teacher may notice that the child tends to avoid touching objects in the classroom or the outside professional may wonder whether any OCD-related behaviors or signs of anxiety may be exhibited in the classroom. Specific examples of concerning behaviors should be included in a written report. It would be helpful to include details such as any antecedents that may have triggered a possible OCD-related behavior and what happened after that behavior. As Adams (2011) notes, collecting this type of information is useful in determining whether a pattern of behavior becomes evident such as the child's frequently using hand sanitizer in the room after touching objects in the room or becoming distressed if the child asks to go wash their hands but is not allowed to leave the room to do so. If concerning behaviors are observed, it would be important to determine whether the behavior has an adverse impact on the child's functioning and to possibly conduct additional observations to determine whether the severity of the behavior worsens.

ASSESSMENT OF EXECUTIVE FUNCTIONING SKILLS

Given that some research studies have reported poor executive functioning in individuals with OCD and that self-regulation may be difficult in youth with OCD, consideration may be given to assessment of executive functioning skills. The Behavior Rating Inventory of Executive Function—Second Edition (BRIEF-2; Gioia et al., 2015) measures executive function in children and adolescents between the ages of 5 and 18 years. Three primary areas of regulation are assessed and include behavioral regulation, emotional regulation, and cognitive regulation. Executive functioning skills assessed include working memory, planning, inhibition, organization, self-monitoring, task-monitoring, shifting, emotional control, and initiation. Parent, teacher, and self-report versions of the BRIEF-2 are available.

ASSESSMENT OF SOCIAL–EMOTIONAL AND BEHAVIORAL FUNCTIONING

As noted earlier, OCD can have an adverse impact on a child's social–emotional and behavioral functioning and the child may have coexisting disorders. If a child with OCD is exhibiting possible signs of anxiety or depression as well as other signs of emotional distress, school psychologists may want to consider using parent and teacher rating scales. The Behavior Assessment System for Children—Third Edition (BASC-3; Reynolds & Kamphaus, 2015) consists of parent, teacher, and self-report versions that assess a variety of behavioral and emotional problems. The BASC-3 also includes a means of conducting a systematic observation and developmental history. Another instrument to consider is the Child Behavior Checklist for Ages 6 to 18 (Achenbach Empirically-Based Assessment, 2001), which assesses externalizing and internalizing behaviors. It also has parent, teacher, and self-report versions.

There may be times a specific measure of anxiety and/or depression is needed. The Multidimensional Anxiety Scale for Children—Second Edition (MASC-2; March, 2012) is a multi-rater instrument that measures various types of anxiety such as obsessive-compulsive behaviors, social anxiety, separation anxiety/phobias, harm avoidance, and somatic symptoms of anxiety in children between the ages of 8 and 19 years. If a measure of depression is needed, the Children's Depression Inventory—Second Edition (CDI-2, Kovacs, 2010) could be considered. This multi-rater screening instrument measures emotional and functional problems associated with depression in youth.

ASSESSMENT OF OBSESSIVE-COMPULSIVE BEHAVIORS

The Children's Yale–Brown Obsessive-Compulsive Scale (CY-BOCS; Goodman et al., 2011) was developed for those between the ages of 6 and 17 years. It was designed to be administered in a semi-structured interview by a mental health professional or trained individual. The instrument focuses on OCD-related behaviors that have occurred over the past week. Another instrument, the Child Obsessive-Compulsive Impact Scale (Piacentini et al., 2007), can be utilized to assess the presence and severity of OCD symptoms in youths. It has both a parent and child version and assesses functional impairment related to OCD.

EDUCATIONAL AND SOCIAL–EMOTIONAL SUPPORTS

Given that OCD-related behaviors can interfere with the child's ability to focus and complete work in the classroom, school psychologists can serve as an advocate for students with OCD to ensure that they get the educational and social–emotional support needed to function efficiently in the classroom.

Adams (2011) has identified factors that can be taken into consideration when determining supports and accommodations for children and adolescents with OCD. First, it is important for supports and accommodations to be as discrete as possible so that the child with OCD is not singled out. This might be done by selecting a support that could involve the whole class so it is not obvious to others that the support is for the child with OCD. Also, consideration needs to be given to supports and accommodations that can be provided consistently over a period of time. Another factor identified by Adams (2011) is involving the child directly in selecting supports or accommodations, because they learn to advocate for themselves and are more likely to use the supports or accommodations if they are involved in selecting them. Involving the child in this process also enables them to see how they may benefit from the accommodation. After determining specific supports, it is suggested that they are used on a trial basis to see whether the child is benefitting from the accommodation. Therefore, it is important to collect data to determine whether the accommodation is effective. Keep in mind that supports and accommodations may need to be adjusted. Finally, if the child with OCD has an IDEA (2004) disability and is receiving special education services, the accommodations should be included in the child's Individual Education Program (IEP). Likewise, children receiving a Section 504 plan should have accommodations documented on the 504 plan.

Educational Supports

As noted previously, youths with OCD may struggle academically in the classroom as a consequence of their OCD symptoms interfering with concentration and completion of school work. Leininger et al. (2010) suggest several types of support that might help students with OCD to be successful in the classroom. One strategy is helping the child transition from one task to another as they often get stuck and want their work to be perfect. One way of doing this may be having them complete the work within a certain amount of time before transitioning to another task or assigning tasks that are not too time-consuming. Another classroom support is to help the child set short-term goals that can be completed successfully and to acknowledge the child's success in reaching the goal. It may be helpful to provide simple directions and to break down tasks so that the child is more likely to be successful at completing the tasks. In addition, the child may need more time to complete tasks since they may have stayed up late performing rituals before bedtime and may have difficulty concentrating in the classroom because of intrusive thoughts (Leininger et al., 2010).

In her book *Students With OCD: A Handbook for School Personnel*, Adams (2011) provides an extensive list of supports and accommodations to support children with OCD. Examples of some of the educational supports recommended by Adams are provided here. For a more thorough discussion of educational supports, see Adams's book.

- *Concentration*: To address difficulties in concentrating, the teacher could frequently check the child's work and provide feedback to help the child get their work completed. It might be helpful to have the child work with a partner as a means of preventing the child from engaging in OCD symptoms. It is helpful to use materials that require a lot of engagement from the child.
- *Class participation*: Since the child with OCD often becomes anxious about making a mistake or saying something wrong, it would be helpful for the teacher to ask the child's opinion about a subject during class discussions rather than a question that requires a specific answer. It might also be helpful to avoid asking open-ended questions and, instead, ask the child close-ended questions. Work with the child to develop a signal to indicate that they want to be called on and a different signal when they do not want to be called on.

- *Reading*: Given that some children with OCD are compelled to re-read words and sentences if they make a mistake, it might be helpful to provide the child with a photocopy of a reading assignment and have them mark the words as they read them to prevent them from reading the words again. Also, shorter reading assignments might help the child complete the assigned reading. If certain words cause the child anxiety, the child could place a small notecard over any words that might trigger anxiety.
- *Writing*: For some children with OCD, writing can be challenging because they feel compelled to erase or rewrite words if they make a mistake. The use of a computer for written assignments or an audio recorder to record the teacher's lecture might be helpful so that the child is not compelled to rewrite their work.
- *Taking tests*: Allow extra time for students with OCD to take tests and perhaps offer a break during the test. It might be helpful to provide oral tests rather than written tests if the child tends to get stuck while writing. Consideration might be given to assess the child's knowledge of a topic through an alternative means rather than a test.

Social–Emotional and Behavioral Supports

Social–emotional and behavioral support may need to be provided in the classroom. Adams (2004, 2011) has recommended several types of support to promote social–emotional and behavioral functioning in the classroom. Examples of supports recommended by Adams (2004, 2011) are listed here. For a more thorough discussion of social–emotional and behavioral supports and accommodations, it is recommended that the reader refer to Adams's book *Students With OCD: A Handbook for School Personnel* (2011).

- Children and adolescents with OCD often are tardy to school, because they feel compelled to engage in rituals before they leave their homes. Teachers should not hold the child accountable for being late since the compulsion is out of the child's control and penalizing them would only create more anxiety for the child.
- It is important to focus on the child's strengths as a way to help the child gain more self-confidence and build up their self-esteem.
- Promote opportunities in the classroom in which the child can interact positively with other students in the classroom. This might include incorporating cooperative learning opportunities and refraining from having a group leader select who will be in the group.
- Develop a sign or signal through which the child can let the teacher know that they are feeling overwhelmed by their OCD obsessions so that they can go to someone in the school with whom they feel safe. The designated person should be agreeable to having the child visit them when they are feeling overwhelmed by the anxiety related to their OCD.
- Teach social skills if the child needs help in establishing friendships and interacting with peers and provide strategies for how to respond to others in negative situations.
- Be supportive of the child's parents and communicate frequently with them to keep them informed about the child's functioning in the classroom.
- Monitor any changes in the child's behavior that could possibly be related to a worsening of OCD symptoms or possible side effects of medication.

Leininger and colleagues (2010) also offer various supports to promote social–emotional and behavioral functioning in the classroom. These are highlighted here.

- Techniques to alleviate anxiety might include teaching learning strategies in which the child is likely to succeed rather than fail, demonstrating how to accept mistakes, and identifying a person to whom the child can go when they experience intense anxiety.
- Avoid providing reassurance. Oftentimes, youths with OCD will seek reassurance from others, which is a compulsion that should not be reinforced. Instead of accommodating the child's reassurance seeking, the teacher can provide praise for staying on tasks and completing schoolwork.

SCHOOL-BASED MENTAL HEALTH INTERVENTIONS FOR OBSESSIVE-COMPULSIVE DISORDER

As noted by Gallant and colleagues (2007), there are advantages to providing mental health interventions for students with OCD in the schools. School personnel have daily contact with students with OCD and can closely monitor OCD-related behaviors and social–emotional status. Given that school psychologists are mental health providers, they are in a unique position to help youth with OCD by providing mental health interventions in the school and working collaboratively with outside mental health professionals who may be providing treatment for the child's OCD. This section focuses on the use of the Response to Intervention (RtI) model, CBT for children with OCD, and anxiety-management techniques.

Response to Intervention

Adams et al. (2007) proposed a three-tier RtI model for schools to consider when working with students who have OCD. The first tier includes universal screening for social–emotional and behavioral problems that might interfere with learning in the classroom. An instrument that school psychologists may want to consider as a Tier 1 screening tool is the Behavioral and Emotional Screening System (BESS; Kamphaus & Reynolds, 2007), which could help to identify any students struggling with social–emotional difficulties. Interventions designed to address social–emotional and behavioral difficulties that youths with OCD often experience could be implemented at this tier level. Tier 1 interventions might include teaching all students in the classroom ways to manage anxiety and stress, such as mindfulness exercises that include breathing techniques and guided imagery to help create a sense of calmness and reduce stress. In addition, it is important that the teacher creates a calm, positive classroom so that the child with OCD feels safe and supported. At Tier 2, the school psychologist could become involved to address the educational, social–emotional, and behavioral needs of any children who are exhibiting OCD-related behaviors. The school psychologist might consider additional assessment that addresses social–emotional or behavioral difficulties. As Adams and colleagues (2007) note, the school psychologist could work collaboratively with parents and any clinicians outside the school who may be providing services to the child regarding evidence-based interventions that could be implemented in the school. These interventions might include anxiety-management techniques or CBT techniques. At this level, the school psychologists could also monitor any effects of treatments that the child may be receiving from professionals outside the school (CBT with exposure and response prevention or medication for OCD). If more intensive interventions or services are needed in the school, the child may move up to Tier 3 to receive more individualized interventions. It is possible that an evaluation for special education services might be considered at Tier 3 (Adams et al., 2007).

Cognitive Behavioral Therapy

CBT is an evidence-based therapy that has been found to be an effective form of treatment for youths with OCD (Geller & March, 2012; Sloman et al., 2007). It consists of three components: (a) exposure, which involves directly exposing the individual to a feared object or situation that elicits anxiety and an urge to engage in a compulsion; (b) response prevention, in which the person avoids or refrains from engaging in the compulsive behavior; and (c) cognitive therapy, which involves becoming aware of distorted thoughts and changing them (Sloman et al., 2007). This therapeutic approach typically begins with educating the child and parent about OCD and encouraging them to view the OCD as an external entity (2007). Children are often encouraged to talk to the OCD and have statements prepared to say to the OCD when an obsessive thought urges them to engage in a ritual, such as "Get out of my head, OCD." Sometimes, the child is encouraged to name their OCD so that when they "talk back to the OCD" they refer to it by name (e.g. "I'm not going to listen to you, [OCD's name], so just get out of my head!"; Sloman et al., 2007).

A rank-ordered list or hierarchy of fears or situations that are likely to trigger the child's OCD symptoms is developed with the child (Adams, 2011; Sloman et al., 2007). The child is gradually exposed to each item on the hierarchy, starting with situations that cause the least amount of distress and working up the hierarchy to situations that cause the most distress for the child. After the child is exposed to the fear object or situation, they are encouraged to resist engaging in the ritual or other compulsive behavior for a certain amount of time so that their anxiety begins to decrease. Over time, the child learns that their anxiety will decrease on its own without engaging in compulsive behavior such that they become habituated to the situation that had previously caused them anxiety. In addition, the child is taught cognitive restructuring, which involves challenging irrational beliefs. For example, a child who fears that touching the sink faucet will cause them to get sick may change the irrational thought from "I will get sick and have to go to the hospital if I touch the faucet" to "My family touches the faucet and they don't get sick afterward so I won't get sick if I touch the faucet." As Sloman et al. (2007) note, the child's participating in the exposure and response prevention therapy could be reinforced by setting up a reward system in which the child receives a point for each exposure and, after a set number of exposures, the child gets to play video games or some other desired activity for a set amount of time.

Family involvement is critical in the therapeutic process for the child in order for the treatment to be successful (Adams, 2011; Sloman et al., 2007). Family members need to be encouraged not to accommodate the child's OCD symptoms by enabling them to participate in rituals. The family also needs to assist the child in the exposure session and have a supportive role when the child becomes distressed during exposure to anxiety-inducing situations (Adams, 2011; Sloman et al., 2007).

Understanding this treatment approach and what it entails enables school psychologists to work collaboratively with the outside therapist and to have a role in supporting the child's treatment. As Adams (2011) notes, school professionals may provide CBT interventions in collaboration with the outside therapist. It would be important to develop a plan that is agreed upon by the child, parents, school professional, and the outside therapist. Wagner (2002) has identified specific issues that need to be addressed before beginning any interventions in the school. These issues include identifying who will implement and monitor the intervention, setting up specific parameters for the interventions, deciding what role each person involved in the plan will have and what resources might be needed, determining whether the school psychologist or other school professional need training, preparing the child for the interventions, determining where and when the interventions will occur, identifying what will happen once the intervention is done, deciding on how the child's response will be recorded, and determining whether modifications will be needed and how changes will be made.

Anxiety-Management Techniques

If an outside therapist is not involved, school-based interventions that may be helpful to a child with OCD include anxiety management, which could be provided by the school psychologist. One technique includes deep-breathing exercises that involve diaphragmatic breathing in which the child takes a deep breath through the nose, holding it until the count of three, and exhales slowly. Relaxation techniques used for anxiety management involve muscle relaxation. This technique uses deep breathing as a first step, which is followed by tensing muscles while counting to five and then relaxing the muscles. Typically, the child would begin by tensing their shoulders, which would be followed by their arms, abdomen, legs, and feet. Another technique used to reduce anxiety is visualization and guided imagery, which involves having the child picture a place in their mind where they feel peaceful. Through guided imagery, the child visualizes sounds associated with the peaceful place or other details of the place. This technique can be used following the deep-muscle relaxation exercises so that the child is fully relaxed. Each of these techniques has been found to be effective in reducing anxiety in children (Adams, 2011).

As noted earlier in this chapter, individuals with OCD have distorted thoughts that maintain their OCD. Adams (2011) notes that children who are willing to talk about their OCD symptoms may benefit from the implementation of cognitive strategies involving constructive self-talk, cognitive restructuring, and cultivating detachment. Youths with OCD are often critical of themselves and may engage in negative self-talk, such as "I must be going crazy. I have to wash my hands over and over. I can't stop washing them." The school psychologist can work with the child to identify any negative self-talk and teach the child to replace it with positive, realistic statements, such as "I'm not going crazy. It's OCD, not me." Another cognitive strategy includes cognitive restructuring, which can be used to restructure the child thinking about dreaded events. For example, thoughts that the house will burn down if the child forgets to check the stove before leaving the house, such as "Oh, no! This is terrible. The house is probably going to burn down!" could be restructured to "I forgot to check the stove. But it is okay. That is just OCD talking. The house will be okay." A third cognitive strategy is cultivating detachment, which involves having the child view the OCD as external to the self (Adams, 2011). As mentioned, sometimes youths with OCD are encouraged to name the OCD so that they recognize their symptoms as OCD and do not view the symptoms as part of themselves.

Concluding Remarks

As is evident in this chapter, OCD is a debilitating disorder that challenges many aspects of a child's functioning and quality of life. Many children and adolescents try to hide their symptoms out of shame and embarrassment and therefore, may suffer in silence. Without mental health treatment, the OCD cycle of obsessions and compulsions continues and consumes the child's life. In order to stop this cyclic pattern of intrusive thoughts and compulsive behaviors, it is imperative that parents and school personnel recognize patterns of behavior that may be related to OCD so that this disorder can be recognized early and interventions can be provided. School psychologists can play an instrumental role in working with the child, parents, and school personnel to ensure that appropriate support and interventions are provided so that the quality of life improves for the child.

CASE STUDY 15.1 BOBBY: CASE OF OBSESSIVE-COMPULSIVE DISORDER IN A MIDDLE-SCHOOL PRETEEN

Background

Bobby is a 12-year-old boy who performed well academically in elementary school. He excelled in his academic work and was well liked by his teachers. Although Bobby was quiet, he had friends at school and participated in some extracurricular activities. About 4 or 5 months after starting middle school, Bobby's mother noticed that he started using disinfecting cloths to wipe his lunchbox and backpack when he came home from school. She also noticed that he did not seem as enthusiastic about school as he had during elementary school. When his mother asked him about school, Bobby just shrugged his shoulders. As a little more time went by, Bobby began to exhibit other behaviors related to cleanliness. He began to wash his hands excessively, sometimes washing them for 20-minute periods multiple times a day when he was at home. His washing would extend up to his forearms. His hands often appeared red and dry from the excessive washing. He also refused to sit on furniture in the house when he came home from school, preferring to sit on the floor instead. In addition, Bobby avoided touching doorknobs, light fixtures, and sink faucets. He used a tissue to open doorknobs and would use his elbows to turn on the light switch and the sink faucet. When asked by his mother about these behaviors, Bobby indicated that he thought the school was dirty and that, if he brought germs home from school, everyone in the family would get sick because of him and have to go to the hospital. He also indicated that he thought doorknobs, light switches, and sink faucets were all contaminated with germs. Bobby also became more distressed about attending school, sometimes not wanting to get out of bed to go to school. He also would become tearful, telling his mother that he did not want to go to school. One day upon getting in the car when his mother picked him up after school, Bobby burst into tears and exclaimed, "Please don't make me go back to that school!" Although he had excelled academically in elementary school, his grades began to decline. When discussing his grades with his mother, Bobby acknowledged that he had difficulty concentrating and relaxing in the classroom because he was constantly worrying about getting germs and becoming sick. He also acknowledged that he did not have friends at school. Concerned

(continued)

CASE STUDY 15.1 BOBBY: CASE OF OBSESSIVE-COMPULSIVE DISORDER IN A MIDDLE-SCHOOL PRETEEN (continued)

about her son, Bobby's mother contacted a clinical psychologist to schedule an appointment for an evaluation. The evaluation revealed that Bobby met diagnostic criteria for OCD, and a treatment plan was developed.

Discussion

Bobby exhibits clear signs of OCD symptoms. His fear of germs triggers much anxiety, and he attempts to reduce the anxiety by engaging in washing his hands excessively, wiping objects with disinfecting wipes, and avoiding touching objects that he thinks are contaminated with germs. His anxiety about germs has negatively impacted social interactions as evidenced by his stating that he does not have friends at the new school and has resulted in much emotional distress. It is important that the mother is seeking help from a mental health professional so that he can receive treatment to alleviate his anxiety. CBT with exposure and response therapy would be an appropriate treatment for Bobby. By learning about the connection between his thoughts and his behaviors, Bobby and his therapist can begin to set up a hierarchy of situations or objects that trigger anxiety for him. Exposure sessions could begin with the situation that elicits the least anxiety and then proceed forward with increasing anxiety-eliciting situations. In responding to these situations, Bobby will have to resist the urge to wash his hand after the exposure. With time, his anxiety will decrease during the exposure such that he will be able to tolerate touching objects that he believes are dirty. His family can have a supportive role in helping him during the exposure sessions. The family will also need to ensure that they do not accommodate his OCD by enabling him to maintain the washing compulsion.

In collaboration with his outside therapist, the school psychologist could provide support for Bobby at school if the parents give permission. A plan could be developed that addresses what type of supports and interventions might be implemented in the school. For example, it may be helpful to assess and monitor Bobby's symptoms at school. His teacher could keep the outside therapist, school psychologist, and parents informed about any OCD-related behaviors observed in the classroom. The teacher could also monitor his interactions with peers to make sure that he is not teased if his compulsions begin to be exhibited at school. In addition, the school psychologist could monitor Bobby's social–emotional functioning and perhaps work directly with Bobby to help him manage his anxiety. The school psychologist could also teach him deep-breathing and relaxation techniques that Bobby could use if a situation triggers anxiety. It might also be helpful to have a designated safe spot in the classroom or elsewhere in the school where Bobby can go if he becomes overwhelmed by his anxiety. Communication among all professionals and parents regarding his progress is needed to ensure that his compulsions are not maintained so that he can function effectively in the home and at school.

SUMMARY POINTS

- OCD is a neurobiological disorder that occurs more often than initially thought and can be debilitating without treatment. It involves obsessions and/or compulsions that consume more than 1 hour per day.
- Academic, social–emotional, and behavioral functioning can be negatively impacted by OCD so it is important that support is provided in the school to promote the child's functioning in these areas.
- School psychologists can have an instrumental role in helping a child with OCD through consultation with school personnel, parents, and clinical providers outside the school and with assessment of social–emotional and behavioral functioning as well as OCD behaviors.
- Mental health interventions can be provided in the school using an RtI model. Other interventions include CBT with exposure and response prevention, which may be provided by a clinician outside the school with some collaborative efforts among the clinician, parents, and school psychologists. Anxiety-management strategies could be utilized in the school to reduce stress and help the child manage anxiety.

TEST YOUR KNOWLEDGE

1. Which of the following therapies has been found to be an effective treatment of OCD?
   a. Psychoanalytic therapy
   b. Interpersonal therapy
   c. Cognitive behavioral therapy with exposure and response prevention
   d. Brief-solution therapy

2. Two of the most common types of problems reported by family members of youths with OCD are difficulty concentrating and completion of homework.
   a. True
   b. False

3. Based on the cognitive model of OCD, which of the following are dysfunctional beliefs associated with OCD?
   a. Excessive responsibility and overimportance of thought
   b. Extreme concern regarding control of thoughts and overestimation of threat
   c. Perfectionism and intolerance for uncertainty
   d. All of the above

4. It is estimated that OCD impacts ____% of children and adolescents in the United States.
   a. 1–4
   b. 5–10
   c. 11–15
   d. 16–20

5. A sense of shame and negative self-view may lead children and adolescents with OCD to not disclose their symptoms and attempt to hide them, which can delay treatment.
   a. True
   b. False

Answers: (1) c, (2) a, (3) d, (4) a, (5) a.

DISCUSSION QUESTIONS

1. Describe the *DSM-5* diagnostic features of OCD.
2. Describe the cycle of obsessions and compulsions associated with OCD and address the difference between an obsession and a compulsion as well as the role of anxiety in the continuation of the cycle.
3. Discuss the three components associated with CBT with exposure and response prevention.
4. Identify and discuss common obsessions/compulsions that occur across two different ethnic groups.
5. Discuss ways in which school psychologists may be involved in providing therapeutic services for students with OCD in the school.

CHAPTER RESOURCES

Books and Guides

FOR CHILDREN AND ADOLESCENTS

- *What to Do When Your Brain Gets Stuck: A Kid's Guide to Overcoming OCD* by Dawn Huebner (2007)
- *Up and Down the Worry Hill: A Children's Book About Obsessive-Compulsive Disorder and Its Treatment* by Aureen Pinto Wagner, PhD (2004)
- *A Thought Is Just A Thought: A Story of Living With OCD* by Leslie Talley (2004)
- *Mr. Worry: A Story About OCD* by Holly L. Niner and Greg Swearingen (2003)
- *Blink, Blink, Clop, Clop: An OCD Storybook* by E. Katia Moritz, PhD (2011)

- *Take Control of OCD: The Ultimate Guide for Kids With OCD* by Bonnie Zucker (2010)
- *Talking Back to OCD: The Program That Helps Kids and Teens Say "No Way"—and Parents Say "Way to Go* by John S. March, MD; and Christine Benton (2006)
- *Touch and Go Joe: An Adolescent's Experience of OCD* by Joe Wells (2021)
- *Being Me With OCD: How I Learned to Obsess Less and Live My Life* by Alison Dotson (2014)

For Parents
- *What to Do When Your Child Has Obsessive-Compulsive Disorder: Strategies and Solutions* by Aureen Pinto Wagner, PhD (2002)
- *Freeing Your Child From Obsessive-Compulsive Disorder: A Powerful, Practical Program for Parents of Children and Adolescents* by Tamar E. Chansky (2001)
- *When a Family Member Has OCD: Mindfulness and Cognitive Behavioral Skills to Help Families Affected by Obsessive-Compulsive Disorder* by Jon Hershfield, MFT; and Jeff Bell (2015)
- *Loving Someone With OCD: Help for You and Your Family* by Karen J. Landsman, PhD; Kathleen M. Rupertus, MA; and Cherry Pedrick, RN (2005)
- *Understanding OCD: A Guide for Parents and Professionals* by A. B. Lewin and E. A. Storch (2017)
- *How to Help Your Child: A Parents' Guide to OCD* by the Obsessive Compulsive Foundation of Metropolitan Chicago (2006): https://beyondocd.org/uploads/pdf/parents-guide.pdf
- *Parents' Guide to OCD* by the Child Mind Institute: https://childmind.org/guide/parents-guide-to-ocd/

For Educators
- *Students With OCD: A Handbook for School Personnel* by Gail B. Adams (2011)
- *Teaching the Tiger: A Handbook for Individuals Involved in the Education of Students With Attention-Deficit Disorders, Tourette Syndrome or Obsessive-Compulsive Disorder* by Marilyn P. Dornbush, PhD; and Sheryl K. Pruitt, MEd (1995)
- *Teaching Kids With Mental Health and Learning Disorders in the Regular Classroom: How to Recognize Understand and Help Challenged (And Challenging) Students Succeed* by Myles L. Cooley, PhD (2007)
- *Teachers' Guide to OCD* by the Child Mind Institute: https://childmind.org/guide/a-teachers-guide-to-ocd-in-the-classroom/

For School Psychologists
- *OCD in Children and Adolescents: A Cognitive-Behavioral Treatment Manual* by John S. March, MD; and Karen Mulle Friesen (1998)
- *Cognitive-Behavioral Treatment of Childhood OCD: It's Only a False Alarm Therapist Guide (Treatments That Work)* by John Piacentini, Audra Langley, and Tami Roblek (2007)
- *Handbook of Child and Adolescent Obsessive-Compulsive Disorder* edited by Eric A. Storch, PhD; Gary R. Geffken, PhD; and Tanya K. Murphy, MD (2007)
- *Treatment of OCD in Children and Adolescents: A Cognitive-Behavioral Therapy Manual* by Aureen Pinto Wagner, PhD (2003)
- *Students With OCD: A Handbook for School Personnel* by Gail Adams (2011)
- *OCD Is Not the Boss of Me Manual* by K. McKenney, A. Simpson, and S. E. Stewart (2020)
- Leininger, M., Dyches, T. T., Prater, M. A., Heath, M. A., & Bascom, S. (2010). Books portraying characters with obsessive-compulsive disorder: Top 10 list for children and young adults. *Teaching Exceptional Children, 42*(4), 22–28. https://doi.org/10.1177/004005991004200403

Fact Sheets/Handouts
- National Association of School Psychologists (NASP) Handouts: The following articles are available on the NASP website: www.nasponline.org
  - *Obsessive-Compulsive Disorder: Information for Parent and Educators* by Leslie Z. Paige (2004)
  - *Obsessive-Compulsive Disorder* by Leslie Z. Paige (2007)
  - *OCD: Helping Handout for School and Home* by Celeste M. Malone (2018)
- The American Academy of Child and Adolescent Psychiatry *OCD Fact Sheet*: www.aacap.org/AACAP/Families_and_Youth/Facts_for_Families/FFF-Guide/Obsessive-Compulsive-Disorder-In-Children-And-Adolescents-060.aspx

- The Child Mind Institute *Quick Facts on Obsessive-Compulsive Disorder*: https://childmind.org/article/quick-facts-on-obsessive-compulsive-disorder-ocd
- The International OCD Foundation
  - *OCD Myths Versus Facts Handout*: https://anxietyintheclassroom.org/wp-content/uploads/2018/09/OCDMyth-Handout-092313.pdf
  - *OCD in Children and Teenagers* (Wagner, 2009): https://iocdf.org/wp-content/uploads/2014/09/OCD-in-Kids-and-Teens.pdf
  - *What Is OCD?*: https://iocdf.org/wp-content/uploads/2021/01/What-Is-OCD-Brochure.pdf
  - *What You Need to Know About OCD*: https://iocdf.org/wp-content/uploads/2014/10/What-You-Need-To-Know-About-OCD.pdf

Tips for Working With OCD in Diverse Populations by the International OCD Foundation

- *Tips for Clinicians Working With African Americans With OCD*: https://iocdf.org/wp-content/uploads/2017/08/Tips-for-Clinicians-when-working-with-African-Americans-with-OCD-1.pdf
- *Tips for Clinicians Working With Asian Americans and Indian Americans With OCD*: https://iocdf.org/wp-content/uploads/2020/05/Tips-For-Clinicians-When-Working-with-Asian-and-Indian-Americans-with-OCD.pdf
- *Tips for Clinicians Working With Hispanic and Latinx Americans With OCD*: https://iocdf.org/wp-content/uploads/2013/12/Tips-for-clinicians-when-working-with-Hispanic_Latinx-Americans.pdf
- *Tips for Clinicians Working With the Transgender OCD Community*: https://iocdf.org/wp-content/uploads/2013/12/Tips-for-Clinicians-Working-with-the-Transgender-OCD-Community.pdf

Online Support

- Parents of Children With OCD (Facebook): www.facebook.com/groups/60524071859/
- International OCD Foundation Support Groups: https://iocdf.org/ocd-finding-help/supportgroups/
- Peace of Mind Foundation Support Groups: https://peaceofmind.com/resources/support-groups/

Videos

- *Unstuck: An OCD Kids Movie*: www.ocdkidsmovie.com/familypurchase
- *The Touching Tree*: www.youtube.com/watch?v=mv9-r2quPos
- *OCD Kids Speak Out*: www.youtube.com/playlist?list=PLed8YlFAGOUhT6T6ocP8QvgbMXFabN4_e
- American Academy of Child and Adolescent Psychiatry *OCD Resource Center*: www.aacap.org/aacap/families_and_youth/resource_centers/Obsessive_Compulsive_Disorder_Resource_Center/Home.aspx#video
- Anxiety and Depression Association of America (ADAA): https://adaa.org/resources-news/from-adaa-experts/videos

Webinars

- Anxiety and Depression Association of America *Helping Kids and Teens Who Have OCD*: https://adaa.org/webinar/consumer/helping-kids-and-teens-who-have-ocd
- International OCD Foundation *What You Need to Know*: https://kids.iocdf.org/for-parents

Websites

- Child Mind Institute: https://childmind.org
- International OCD Foundation: https://iocdf.org
- OCD in Kids website by the International OCD Foundation: https://kids.iocdf.org/
- Peace of Mind Foundation: https://peaceofmind.com/

KEY REFERENCES

Only key references appear in the print edition. The full reference list appears in the digital product on Springer Publishing Connect: connect.springerpub.com/content/book/978-0-8261-3587-2/part/part06/chapter/ch15

Adams, G. B. (2011). *Students with OCD: A handbook for school personnel*. Pherson Creek Press.
Adams, G. B., Smith, T. J., Bolt, S. E., & Nolten, P. (2007). Current educational practices in classifying and serving students with obsessive-compulsive disorder. *California School Psychologist, 12*(1), 93–105. https://doi.org/10.1007/BF03340934
American Academy of Child & Adolescent Psychiatry. (2018). *Obsessive-compulsive disorder in children and adolescents*. https://www.aacap.org/AACAP/Families_and_Youth/Facts_for_Families/FFF-Guide/Obsessive-Compulsive-Disorder-In-Children-And-Adolescents-060.aspx
American Psychiatric Association. (2013). *Diagnostic and statistical manual of mental disorders* (5th ed.). https://doi.org/10.1176/appi.books.9780890425596
Barton, R., & Heyman, I. (2016). Obsessive-compulsive disorder in children and adolescents. *Paediatrics & Child Health, 26*(12), 527–533. https://doi.org/10.1016/j.paed.2016.08.011
Geller, D. A., & March, J. (2012). Practice parameter for the assessment and treatment of children and adolescents with obsessive-compulsive disorder. *Journal of the American Academy of Child & Adolescent Psychiatry, 51*(1), 98–113. https://doi.org/10.1016/j.jaac.2011.09.019
Jacob, M. L., Morelen, D., Suveg, C., Brown Jacobsen, A. M., & Whiteside, S. P. (2012). Emotional, behavioral, and cognitive factors that differentiate obsessive-compulsive disorder and other anxiety disorders in youth. *Anxiety, Stress & Coping, 25*(2), 229–237. https://doi.org/10.1080/10615806.2011.571255
Kagan, E. R., Frank, H. E., & Kendall, P. C. (2017). Accommodation in youth with OCD and anxiety. *Clinical Psychology: Science and Practice, 24*(1), 78–98. https://doi.org/10.1111/cpsp.12186
Kraynak, A., & Hart, S. (2017). DSM-5 and school psychology: Obsessive-compulsive related disorders. *Communiqué, 45*(8). https://www.nasponline.org/publications/periodicals/communique/issues/volume-45-issue-8/obsessive%E2%80%93compulsive-and-related-disorders
Malone, C. M. (2018). Obsessive-compulsive disorder: Helping handout for school and home. In G. G. Bear & K. M. Minke (Eds.), *Helping handouts: Supporting students at school and home*. National Association of School Psychologists.
Paige, L. Z. (2004). Obsessive-compulsive disorder: Information for parents and educators. In G. G. Bear and K. M. Minke (Eds.), *Helping children at home and school II: Handouts for families and educators*. National Association of School Psychologists.
Piacentini, J., Bergman, R. L., Keller, M., & McCracken, J. (2003). Functional impairment in children and adolescents with obsessive-compulsive disorder. *Journal of Child and Adolescent Psychopharmacology, 13*(2, Suppl. 1), S61–S69. https://doi.org/10.1089/104454603322126359
Wagner, A. P. (2009). *OCD in children and teenagers*. https://iocdf.org/wp-content/uploads/2014/09/OCD-in-Kids-and-Teens.pdf
Williams, M. T., & Jahn, M. E. (2017). Obsessive–compulsive disorder in African American children and adolescents: Risks, resiliency, and barriers to treatment. *American Journal of Orthopsychiatry, 87*(3), 291–303. https://doi.org/10.1037/ort0000188

CHAPTER 16

Hoarding Disorder

LEARNING OBJECTIVES

- Summarize the diagnostic features for the *Diagnostic and Statistical Manual of Mental Disorders* (5th ed.; *DSM-5*; American Psychiatric Association [APA], 2013) diagnosis of Hoarding Disorder.
- Highlight the risk factors for children and youth with hoarding disorder.
- Describe common social–emotional and behavioral concerns for children who hoard.
- Understand the classroom implications for students with hoarding disorder.
- Identify effective social, emotional, and behavioral interventions for students who hoard.

INTRODUCTION

Clutter and mountains of stuff. This stuff encumbers your work/study space and living area. You cannot even imagine parting with these things. When you think about it, your anxiety gets the best of you. These items give you comfort to possess and you fear losing them for no apparent reason. Their actual value is questionable. This perceived need to have and not remove these items affects your education, friends, and family. This is hoarding.

The *Diagnostic and Statistical Manual of Mental Disorders*, Fifth Edition (*DSM-5*; American Psychiatric Association [APA], 2013), classifies Hoarding Disorder under the category of Obsessive-Compulsive and Related Disorders. Hoarding Disorder and the other disorders in this diagnostic category feature issues related to intensive focus on intrusive thoughts and repetitive behaviors. Hoarding Disorder and the other disorders in this category frequently overlap with one another in presentation despite having distinct features. Therefore, it is recommended in the *DSM-5* that a clinician who suspects the presence of one of these disorders should consider and assess the presence of all of the disorders within this category. Some examples of other Obsessive-Compulsive and Related Disorders include Obsessive-Compulsive Disorder (OCD; discussed in Chapter 15), Body Dysmorphic Disorder, and Trichotillomania (APA, 2013).

In the *DSM-5* diagnosis of any of the Obsessive-Compulsive and Related Disorders, it is critical for the clinician to consider both developmental appropriateness and severity to determine whether the individual meets criteria for the diagnoses. Many individuals engage in behaviors that may seem focused, sequential, or ritualistic, but individuals should only receive a diagnosis in this category if those behaviors are causing related emotional issues for the person and also impede the person's ability to complete tasks of daily living. Hoarding Disorder should be easily differentiated from the hobby of collecting items, which often results in an accumulation of possessions, but is orderly in both the act of accumulating and the organization of the items (APA, 2013).

Prior to the *DSM-5*, the act of hoarding was included as a one of the diagnostic criteria for Obsessive-Compulsive Personality Disorder and as a symptom of OCD as defined in the *DSM-IV-TR* (APA, 2000). However, experts in mental health concluded that the practice of hoarding and newer research on its individual features warranted the creation of a new diagnosis (Mataix-Cols et al., 2010). That research suggested that hoarding was in fact unique within the presentation of OCD (Bloch et al., 2008), in which only about 5% to 30% of individuals diagnosed with OCD exhibit characteristics of hoarding (Foa et al., 1995; Samuels et al., 2014). The argument for hoarding as its own disorder rests on a few principles from the research, including the fact that the act of hoarding is not distressing to the hoarder but is so for individuals with OCD (Frank et al., 2014). A related fact: The thoughts associated with hoarding are not distressing to the individual either but considered typical for the individual. In contrast to this element of hoarding, the accumulation of items is often a source of stress, and the act of decluttering or getting rid of possessions can be extremely distressing to the hoarder. Also, unlike similar disorders, individuals with Hoarding Disorder rarely experience repetitive types of behaviors like those associated with OCD (Frank et al., 2014; Mataix-Cols et al., 2010), their symptomatology tends to get progressively worse over time, and they often find joy and purpose in their hoarding (Mataix-Cols et al., 2010). Finally, in support of Hoarding Disorder as its own distinct diagnosis, researchers have found that even among those individuals who are diagnosed with OCD and engage in hoarding, the symptoms of the two disorders are often unrelated (Pertusa et al., 2008). The term *Hoarding Disorder* was suggested by Mataix-Cols et al. (2010), and, in light of these empirical findings, Hoarding Disorder was established as a new diagnostic category for the first time in the *DSM-5* (APA, 2013).

DIAGNOSTIC ISSUES: *DSM-5* AND SCHOOL-BASED SERVICES

DSM-5 Diagnosis

The *DSM-5* requires six criteria to be met in order for a person to be diagnosed with Hoarding Disorder. The first criterion describes an individual who experiences difficulty throwing away or giving away items that belong to them even when those items may be of little or no worth. The individual often describes emotional attachment to the items, fears losing items that they believe are important, or describes beliefs that the items will be needed or used at a later time. In children, this criterion must be carefully considered as parents may occasionally report developmentally appropriate collecting as hoarding behavior (Samuels et al., 2014). The second criterion, associated with the first, requires that the individual experiences a desire to save possessions and feels emotional strain when throwing away or giving away their items. The third criterion indicates that the individual's inability to part with possessions results in an excessive collection of items that often fills living spaces throughout the home and limits the ability of the individual to even access or use the items collected. The collection of items may be so extensive that utilitarian objects like beds, other furniture, or even appliances can no longer be accessed or used for their intended purposes due to the accumulation of items in, around, or placed upon them. The *DSM-5* offers a caveat that if communal living spaces are not excessively cluttered by the accumulation of items, then this may be due to the efforts of another family member to limit the encroachment of the items into their living spaces. In some cases, people with Hoarding Disorder may even store items outside their own homes or within the homes and spaces of family and friends (APA, 2013). However, researchers note that particular attention should be given to this criterion with children. Given that the living environments of children and adolescents are often controlled by their parents, guardians, or other caregivers, it may not be as easy to identify the impact of their hoarding symptoms on shared living spaces (APA, 2013; Morris et al., 2016). For children, personal storage areas, such as desks, bookshelves, backpacks, and closets, should be considered. The fourth criterion is that the accumulation of the possessions leads to distress for the individual or impairs the person's ability to function. This may become particularly evident if someone else attempts to clear clutter or discard items for the individual with Hoarding Disorder. The fifth criterion excludes other medical diagnoses that could contribute to hoarding (APA, 2013). One such medical condition is Prader-Willi syndrome. Prader-Willi syndrome is a genetic disorder that results in excessive appetite and massive obesity. Its sufferers also often experience compulsive behaviors like hoarding (Dykens et al., 1996). The sixth and final criterion for a *DSM-5* diagnosis of Hoarding Disorder simply indicates that the symptomatology cannot be better attributed to another mental disorder (APA, 2013). These criteria were derived from the work of Frost and Hartl (1996), whose original descriptors of hoarding were used in years of research prior to the publication of the *DSM-5* and its expanded criteria for Hoarding Disorder.

When diagnosing an individual with hoarding disorder, the clinician may also make use of two specifiers related to the person's condition. One specifier is known as hoarding disorder "with excessive acquisition." The *DSM-5* indicates that approximately 80% to 90% of people who experience hoarding symptoms to a degree consistent with a Hoarding Disorder diagnosis have also accumulated excessive possessions either through buying them or receiving them for free. In rarer cases, the individual may resort to stealing items in order to have them in their possession. The second specifier relates to the individual's insight into their problem behavior. The clinician may deem that the person has good/fair insight into the problems associated with their hoarding, that the person has poor insight, or that the person has either no insight into the problems associated with their behavior or has delusional thoughts regarding the hoarding (APA, 2013).

Approximately 80% to 90% of people with hoarding disorder have accumulated excessive possessions by either buying them or receiving them for free (APA, 2013).

For individuals who suffer with hoarding disorder, the initial symptoms tend to appear in childhood or adolescence. The average age of onset of symptoms is reported to be from 11 to 15 years of age (APA, 2013; Ayers et al., 2009; Fontenelle, 2004; Grisham et al., 2006; Tolin & Villavicencio, 2011). However, earlier onset of symptoms has been reported in children who have both hoarding disorder and OCD. Among their participants, Samuels et al. (2014) report an average age of onset as 7.7 years old with a range of 5 to 16 years of age. Some research has found an earlier average age of onset among females as compared to males who exhibit hoarding symptoms (Winsberg et al., 1999), but the sample sizes in that research were small and likely need further replication. Due to the significant progression of the symptoms over time, evidence suggests that functional impairment related to the hoarding typically begins in a person's 20s and is fully manifested as a clinical presentation by their 30s (APA, 2013; Mataix-Cols et al., 2010; Tolin et al., 2010).

With regard to prevalence, the *DSM-5* reports that 2% to 6% of the overall population has clinical levels of hoarding behavior (APA, 2013). In samples of children with hoarding behaviors, studies have reported prevalence rates ranging from 2% to 3% (Ivanov et al., 2013) up to 10% (Alvarenga et al., 2015); however, the higher range is unlikely due to parental overreport of typical collecting behaviors as symptomatic of hoarding (Morris et al., 2016). Gender differences in prevalence among children and adolescents with hoarding disorder are unclear in the literature. Although some research reports significantly higher prevalence among girls than boys (Ivanov et al., 2013), other researchers found a higher incidence of hoarding disorder among boys (within a sample who also had OCD; Masi et al., 2010). Still other findings suggest no gender differences in hoarding disorder prevalence among children (Hacker et al., 2016; Storch, Murdoff, et al., 2011; Testa et al., 2011).

School-Based Eligibility

Although no current literature addresses hoarding disorder in the context of special education eligibility, delving into the Individuals with Disabilities Education Improvement Act (IDEA) offers insight into possibilities for school-based support under this federal law. IDEA mandates that students may receive special education and related services if they are demonstrated to meet criteria as a student with a disability (under one of the 13 designated categories) and if they also exhibit a need for services based on the impact of that disability (U.S. Department of Education, n.d.). Two such categories in which children and adolescents with hoarding disorder could be found to meet criteria are Other Health Impairment and Emotional Disturbance.

According to this federal legislation, which applies to all public schools, *Other Health Impairment* refers to an individual "having limited strength, vitality, or alertness, including a heightened alertness to environmental stimuli" in relation to their surroundings that is due to a health-related concern and negatively impacts the student's educational performance (U.S. Department of Education, n.d., Section 300.8 (c) (9)). IDEA outlines a number of medical conditions that apply here. Although hoarding disorder is not specifically identified within the law, the legislation is explicit in its declaration that the list of conditions is in no way exhaustive and that individuals with other medical concerns who otherwise meet the criteria should also be included under its tenets (U.S. Department of Education, n.d.).

The other IDEA category of interest in relation to hoarding disorder is Emotional Disturbance. According to IDEA, a child can be considered as having a disability under this category if the child meets one or more criteria over an extended period of time and if it represents a significant detriment to the child's academic performance. The criteria are the following: difficulty in learning that cannot be attributed to intellectual, sensory, or other health concerns; challenges in establishing and continuing appropriate social relationships; atypical reactions or emotions in typical circumstances; chronic depressed mood; and/or somatic symptoms associated with school or personal challenges. The law specifically includes children and adolescents with schizophrenia, but directly excludes children who are considered to be socially maladjusted based on their behaviors.

Therefore, Other Health Impairment and Emotional Disturbance include directives related to the child's or adolescent's academic functioning. Both state that in order for a child to meet the criteria, the child's school performance must be negatively impacted. The spirit of the law seems to suggest that this negative impact should be a direct function of the disability. Although children and adolescents with hoarding disorder often have deficits in executive functioning that likely impact educational attainment, it would be challenging for a clinician to draw a direct connection between a student's hoarding disorder (particularly since it is most likely manifested in the home) and an adverse educational outcome.

Thus, another consideration for providing school-based services may be to consider eligibility under Section 504 of the Rehabilitation Act of 1973. This federal legislation applies to all entities (including public schools) that receive any form of federal funding. As with IDEA, Section 504 is a piece of civil rights legislation that requires public schools to provide a free and appropriate public education with any necessary related services and supports to students who have (or are suspected to have) a disability. Children and adolescents may receive services if a school-based evaluation demonstrates that the child has an impairment that "substantially limits one or more major life functions" (Office of Civil Rights, n.d., Section 104.3 (2) (iv)), such as caring for oneself, performing manual tasks, walking, hearing, seeing, speaking, breathing, learning, and working. However, the Section 504 explains that the list of major life functions is not considered exhaustive and other applicable life functions may apply here (Office of Civil Rights, n.d.).

Although under IDEA Other Health Impairment lists a number of specific medical conditions that may be considered for eligibility, Section 504 places emphasis on the type impairment rather than the diagnosis itself. These functional impairments include, "physiological disease or condition, cosmetic disfigurement, or anatomical loss affecting one or more of the following body systems: neurological; musculoskeletal, special sense organs, respiratory including speech organs; cardiovascular; reproductive; digestive; genito-urinary; hemic and lymphatic; skin; and endocrine; or any mental or psychological disorder, such as mental retardation, organic brain syndrome, emotional or mental illness, and specific learning disabilities" (Office of Civil Rights, n.d., Section 104.3 (2) (i)).

Given its status within the *DSM-5*, Hoarding Disorder certainly qualifies as a psychological disorder (per the impairment guidelines); however, as with IDEA, the diagnosis alone is not sufficient for eligibility for services under Section 504. The law mandates that a school-based eligibility team determine qualification for services through a comprehensive evaluation that explores whether the symptoms of that student's disability does, in fact, inhibit them in a major life function (Office of Civil Rights, n.d.). Since the requirements for eligibility for services under Section 504 do not specify that the disorder must negatively impact educational performance, it is more likely that a student with hoarding disorder would be found eligible here than under IDEA. When a student does qualify for a school-based 504 plan, then the multidisciplinary team (which includes the parent along with school personnel) can detail the necessary supports and services needed to ensure the child or adolescent's ability to fully participate in the curriculum and environment while accommodating the needs of the child's disability (Office of Civil Rights, n.d.). In the case of hoarding disorder, some probable services may include access to the school psychologist, school counselor, school social worker, and/or school nurse. The school psychologist or school counselor may be included to provide counseling or therapy services related to the hoarding disorder. The school social worker might serve as a liaison between the family and community-based services because the complications of the hoarding are likely most prevalent in the home. Finally, the school nurse could be involved with medication management if the child or adolescent with hoarding disorder is taking prescription medications for symptoms associated with the hoarding disorder.

CULTURAL ISSUES RELATED TO HOARDING IN YOUTH

Risk Factors for Hoarding

As recently as 2019, scholars who study hoarding disorder continue to contend that we do not fully understand the etiology of hoarding disorder (Hombali et al., 2019). However, Hombali et al. (2019) engaged in a thorough review of the literature to determine the current understanding as it relates to the development of hoarding disorder, and they found three probable risk factors for the development of hoarding disorder. The first risk factor relates to genetics. Several studies have found that individuals with hoarding disorder have close relatives who also exhibit hoarding behaviors (Ivanov et al., 2013; Matsunaga et al., 2010; Samuels et al., 2007; Winsberg et al., 1999). Genome studies have indicated a relationship between particular chromosomes and the development of hoarding disorder (Samuels et al., 2007), and evidence from twin studies is also indicative of the role of genetics in this mental health condition (Ivanov et al., 2013). A second risk factor highlighted by the research of Hombali et al. (2019) relates to abnormal neural activity within specific brain regions for people with hoarding disorder. This abnormal activity is also related to difficulty with decision-making and sustained attention, as is often evidenced in people with hoarding disorder. The third risk factor for hoarding disorder from this research is that of traumatic life experiences. It is theorized that people who hoard derive a sense of security from their accumulated items and that protecting their possessions is a form of protecting themselves (Frost et al., 1995; Hartl et al., 2005).

> It is theorized that people who hoard derive a sense of security from their accumulated items and that protecting their possessions is a form of protecting themselves (Frost et al., 1995; Hartl et al., 2005).

A condition of neglect appears to be a traumatic life event that represents a risk factor for the development of a specific type of hoarding behavior, and that is hoarding food (Morris et al., 2016; Tolin, Brady, et al., 2008). When a child or adolescent has suffered from neglectful conditions or early attachment issues with caregivers and subsequently fears being without a stable source of food, then the child may engage in food hoarding. Unfortunately, scant research has addressed these situations, and little empirical evidence is available. Nonetheless, as with hoarding symptoms within OCD, this hoarding behavior may be a distinct condition.

Although the child or adolescent who hoards food could meet some criteria for hoarding disorder, there are features of this act that do not fit with the theoretical construct of hoarding disorder. Although children with hoarding disorder often derive pleasure from their accumulation of the food, the impetus for the child who hoards food is fear. The child must have food on hand to ward off the fear associated with being without it. In fact, Winsberg et al. (1999) found that adults who hoard food report a fear of a food shortage, which may be related to the intolerance of uncertainty noted by Mathes et al. (2017) in people who hoard. In addition, the criteria for hoarding disorder specify that the behavior cannot be more accurately ascribed to another condition. Because food hoarding frequently results from earlier emotional or environmental conditions, this behavior may be associated with other clinical diagnoses such as reactive attachment disorder or posttraumatic stress disorder. Thus, the diagnosis of hoarding disorder would not be applied. It remains to be seen how the food shortage issues that occurred during the COVID-19 pandemic will impact food hoarding behaviors.

In addition to these risk factors, a number of other functional correlates have been associated with individuals with hoarding disorder. Many people with hoarding disorder struggle with decision-making skills, organizational abilities, and issues with working memory (Frost & Hartl, 1996). There is also high comorbidity between hoarding disorder and a number of other psychiatric conditions, including major depressive disorder, social anxiety disorder, generalized anxiety disorder, and ADHD (APA, 2013; Hacker et al., 2016; Testa et al., 2011; Tolin & Villavicencio, 2011). However, the most commonly and closely associated disorder is OCD; the *DSM-5* reports that up to 20% of people with Hoarding Disorder could also meet criteria for a diagnosis of OCD (APA, 2013).

Cultural Considerations

Many demographic dimensions have been investigated in relationship to hoarding disorder, including race and ethnicity. Most studies have found that hoarding disorder exists across cultures, and there appear to be few (if any) links to race, ethnicity, or culture beyond the aforementioned genetic factors. The presentation of hoarding disorder appears consistent within nearly all cultural contexts (APA, 2013). Research has been conducted across North American, European, Asian, and South American cultures and has found vast similarities across the populace in hoarding disorder (Hombali et al., 2019; Mataix-Cols et al., 2010; Matsunaga et al., 2010; Nordsletten et al., 2018; Timpano et al., 2013, 2015). Within the North American population, studies of African Americans with hoarding symptoms associated with their diagnoses of OCD have been conducted (Williams et al., 2012, 2017). The researchers found that 56% of African Americans with OCD exhibit hoarding, but no research has addressed the correlates of hoarding disorder with solely African American or Hispanic American samples.

IMPACT OF HOARDING ON SOCIAL–EMOTIONAL AND BEHAVIORAL FUNCTIONING IN SCHOOL AND HOME ENVIRONMENTS

Social–Emotional and Behavioral Functioning in School

Although some children and adolescents with hoarding disorder may collect an excessive number of possessions within their lockers, desks, or backpacks, the limitations of space allotted to the student will naturally inhibit the student's ability to hoard within the school setting. However, that does not mean that the school environment will be free from associated features for students with hoarding disorder. Research evidence supports that children and adolescents with hoarding disorder often experience a host of other symptoms as well. In comparison to children who do not hoard, children who do hoard are rated significantly higher (by their parents and mental health workers) on issues of anxiety and depression. They exhibit higher rates of attention, social, and thought problems, and research has also found that people with hoarding disorder have a greater intolerance for uncertainty than other individuals (Mathes et al., 2017). Finally, adults in their lives also suggest that children and adolescents with hoarding disorder engage in greater levels of rule breaking and aggression than their non-hoarding peers (Hamblin et al., 2015). The research to date has not found any pattern to the rule breaking and aggression or that the rule breaking and aggression were directly due to the hoarding behaviors. Therefore, future study is needed.

> Teachers and parents report that children and adolescents with hoarding disorder engage in greater levels of rule breaking and aggression than their non-hoarding peers (Hamblin et al., 2015).

Though their symptoms may not rise to the level needed for diagnosis of hoarding disorder, hoarding symptoms have been found among children and adolescents with learning disabilities (Testa et al., 2011) and ADHD (Hacker et al., 2016), which are both highly prevalent within school settings. One study in Australia found that over 16% of their sample of children with learning disabilities also present with some form of hoarding behavior and that those students with both learning disabilities and hoarding behaviors performed significantly worse on verbal learning tasks than those students with learning disabilities alone. Hoarding disorder, learning disabilities, and ADHD are all associated with poor ability to sustain attention, which leads to a host of academic, social, and behavioral concerns within school settings for students who struggle with these conditions, including impulse control, anxiety-provoking thoughts, and overall externalizing behaviors (Testa et al., 2011).

Social–Emotional and Behavioral Functioning at Home

Research suggests that when families seek mental health assistance for children with hoarding symptoms, it is rare that the hoarding behavior motivates them to do so. Hoarding symptoms in children are often less of a concern than other mental health symptoms (Burton et al., 2015). In addition to comorbid psychiatric disorders (such as ADHD, OCD, anxiety, and depression), people with hoarding disorder are at greater risk for negative life circumstances and outcomes than other individuals. For example, adults with hoarding disorder are at risk for obesity, alcohol and drug use, property fires, injury due to falls, property eviction, pest infestations, and poor sanitation conditions (Grisham & Norberg, 2010; Rodriguez et al., 2012; Steketee & Frost, 2003; Storch, Rahman, et al., 2011; Tolin, Frost, Steketee, Gray, et al., 2008). Adults with hoarding disorder also report missing an average of 7.7 workdays per month due to their disorder (Tolin, Frost, Steketee, Gray, et al., 2008), and their hoarding often puts them at risk for eventual homelessness (Rodriguez et al., 2012). These risks (along with the individual's distress) add to the necessity of early treatment for children who are exhibiting symptoms of hoarding (or are diagnosed with hoarding disorder) before these potential negative outcomes become a reality for them.

> Research suggests that when families seek mental health assistance for children with hoarding symptoms, it is rarely the hoarding that motivates them to do so (Burton et al., 2015).

An additional potential strain for the home environments for children and adolescents with hoarding disorder is the heritability of their diagnosis (Ivanov et al., 2013; Matsunaga et al., 2010; Samuels et al., 2007; Winsberg et al., 1999). It is estimated that approximately 50% of people who hoard also have a family member who exhibits hoarding behaviors (APA, 2013), but the evidence of the role of genetics in hoarding is stronger with boys than with girls (Steketee et al., 2003). Within a sample of boys, genetic components accounted for about 32% of the variance in hoarding behaviors, but these factors accounted for merely 2% of the variance among girls (2003). Given the evidence suggesting that genetics plays a role in the development of hoarding disorder, there is also an increased probability of another family member within the home suffering from the symptoms of hoarding disorder (Hacker et al., 2016; Morris et al., 2016). The presence of more than one individual in the home with psychiatric symptoms is complex enough with logistical, financial, and social constraints, but when those symptoms involve hoarding, the issues of space and hygiene could become particularly challenging in daily functioning and also in the pursuit of treatment.

Research by Tolin, Frost, Steketee, and Fitch (2008) explores the familial strain associated with living with an individual with hoarding disorder. Because the act of hoarding often does not cause distress to the individual who hoards (until there is an attempt at discarding items), the emotional strain of the disorder may impact those who care for them to a greater degree than it does to the individual who is actually diagnosed with hoarding disorder. Family members commonly report feeling pressure to enable the hoarding behavior because of the pleasure/relief that it brings to the hoarder. This may be particularly the case as parents support the hoarding of children and adolescents through buying their possessions or providing them the means to do so (Peris et al., 2008; Storch et al., 2012). However, Tolin, Frost, Steketee, and Fitch (2008) found that the greater the severity of the hoarding behavior, the more negative and critical the attitudes expressed by family members toward individuals with hoarding disorder. The perceived level of insight of the individual and the extent of the clutter also relate to family members' attitudes toward the person with hoarding disorder. Thus, it is imperative that therapeutic interventions for children and adolescents with hoarding disorder include a familial component to address both enabling behaviors among the family members and the negative affect directed toward the hoarder.

IMPACT OF HOARDING ON LEARNING IN THE CLASSROOM

The hoarding disorder diagnosis is primarily associated with an individual's need to accumulate possessions. According to the *DSM-5*, the most commonly hoarded items are newspapers, magazines, clothing, bags, books, mail, and paperwork (APA, 2013). Although it may be possible for a child or adolescent to accumulate some items within the school setting that may seem relatively excessive and that child may experience distress if others attempt to discard seemingly unnecessary possessions, the space limitations and the control over those spaces by school personnel will naturally limit the ability to hoard within that setting. Thus, the most direct concern regarding hoarding is unlikely to be manifested in the classroom or on the school property. However, other factors related to children and adolescents with hoarding disorder may become apparent and offer significant challenges in the school environment with regard to learning and academic achievement.

> According to the *DSM-5*, the most commonly hoarded items are newspapers, magazines, clothing, bags, books, mail, and paperwork (APA, 2013).

Although it has not yet been studied in children, one such possible concern for the school setting relates to cognitive functioning. Neuroimaging studies of brain function in adults with hoarding disorder have found evidence of information processing and executive functioning deficits (Gledhill et al., 2021; Morein-Zamir et al., 2014; Tolin et al., 2012). These deficits are often related to challenges for the individual in working memory, attention, impulse control, problem-solving, and decision-making skills (Hacker et al., 2016; Hartl et al., 2004). Among those concerns, Gledhill et al. (2021) determined that issues with attention are most consistently associated with hoarding disorder. They also found concerns related to motor inhibition and organization to be prevalent among people diagnosed with hoarding disorder.

These affiliated executive functioning deficits have obvious potential impacts for the classroom. A child or adolescent who struggles with sustaining attention to tasks will have subsequent difficulty in following classroom instruction and garnering the necessary content. These attentional issues can be exacerbated through concerns with impulse control, whereby even when the child is attempting to maintain focus, difficulty with behavioral inhibition will lead to frequent disruptions and inconsistent and/or interrupted delivery of instruction. When instruction is delivered, a child or adolescent with working memory deficits will exhibit impaired performance in tasks that require any cognitive manipulation or multistep use of information. Finally, concerns with problem-solving and decision-making create difficulty in engaging with applied academic content and also create issues with social interactions within the classroom. Thus, executive functioning deficits (like those associated with hoarding disorder) yield problems from the initiation of learning through the organization, completion, and expected performance of academic tasks and into the behavioral regulation components of the classroom.

IMPLICATIONS FOR SCHOOL PSYCHOLOGISTS

Assessment Role

The previous discussion highlighted the potential for school-based eligibility for services under the IDEA categories of either Emotional Disturbance or Other Health Impairment. However, seeking qualification under IDEA for the child with hoarding disorder may be challenging due to IDEA's requirement that any disability must result in impaired academic performance as a result of the disability. (See the discussion under "School-Based Eligibility" in this chapter for a more thorough treatment of this topic.) Thus, it is more likely that a school-based team (in collaboration with the child's parent or guardian) will seek eligibility for services under Section 504 of the Americans with Disabilities Education Act, which does not have an educational impact requirement.

If the multidisciplinary team does seek a 504 evaluation, then the school psychologist will most likely be called upon to conduct a psychological assessment. In addition to assessing the child's cognitive and academic abilities, this would also include an assessment of emotional and behavioral functioning. Depending on the specific presenting issues of the child and the referral question from the team, the school psychologist may evaluate the overall behavior of the child (through informal and formal means) as well as individual emotional and behavioral issues such as depression and/or anxiety.

There are also a variety of tools that have been developed for the assessment of hoarding symptomatology. Although most have focused on hoarding symptoms within the context of the overall symptomatology of OCD, the Children's Saving Inventory (CSI) is a psychometrically sound, parent-report instrument designed for the assessment of the extent and severity of hoarding in children and adolescents (Frost et al., 2000; Storch, Murdoff, et al., 2011). Despite its strength as an evaluation tool, the CSI may or may not be appropriate for use depending on the scope of the overall evaluation for Section 504 eligibility. In addition, it is likely uncommon for school psychologists to be trained within their graduate programs in the specific assessment of hoarding. Thus, consistent with the *Principles for Professional Ethics* (Standard II.1.1 Practice in Area of Competence) of the National Association of School Psychologists (2020), the school psychologist needs to ensure adequate preparation and competency before the use of the CSI or any other instrument. Nonetheless, the school psychologist would offer a critical service to the evaluation of the child or adolescent with hoarding disorder within the school setting for purposes of eligibility.

The CSI is a psychometrically sound, parent-report instrument designed for the assessment of the extent and severity of hoarding in children and adolescents (Frost et al., 2000; Storch, Murdoff, et al., 2011).

Advocacy Role

As with most issues involving psychiatric concerns with children and adolescents, the family plays a critical role in issues related to functioning and treatment. The school psychologist can serve as an informational source regarding community-based treatment options and support. These resources may be medical, psychological, or social-service oriented depending on the needs of the child and the family. Also, when community-based providers are involved, the school psychologist may serve as a liaison between those professionals and the work being done on behalf of the child within the school setting. The school psychologist may consult with other professionals regarding school performance, behavioral adjustment, progress monitoring, and/or medication management issues. The school psychologist can directly observe and report to others on the child or adolescent's functioning in a setting beyond the clinic or home and regarding interpersonal relationships and social adaptability with individuals other than family members. Helping school personnel understand the complexity, challenges, and strains on the individual and the family is also critical. With understanding and knowledge about hoarding behavior and how best to support children with hoarding disorder, educators and administrators can more effectively communicate and work with the individual and family.

Consultation Role

In working with the families of children and adolescents with hoarding disorder, school psychologists may provide a crucial educational component. Scholars in this area suggest that greater understanding is needed to prompt and promote empathy among family members. Family members often direct harmful, negative attitudes toward the individual who hoards, and Tolin, Brady, et al. (2008) recommend that the family members be taught that the hoarding is a symptom of illness rather than a conscious choice the person is making. When family members recognize this distinction and increase their empathy with regard to the symptomatology, it may help with overall adjustment and treatment outcomes and reduce familial strain for the child or adolescent with hoarding disorder.

School psychologists may also consult with parents regarding behavior management strategies for use within the home. Research suggests that (although well meaning) parents may inadvertently contribute to the development and maintenance of hoarding behaviors in children and adolescents. Parents may provide the financial and logistical resources for the accumulation of possessions and may enable the child in their failure to discard unnecessary items (Ale et al., 2014; Peris et al., 2008; Storch, Rahman, et al., 2011). In addition, in some cases, these problematic behaviors may have even been modeled through a hoarding family member. School psychologists can help family members to understand the nature of the hoarding—that the child may be attempting to avoid feelings of distress and ward off fears for the future through the act of hoarding. The school psychologist can also assist family members in comprehending how their own responses may be reinforcing hoarding. For example, when attempts are made to declutter the acquired items, children will frequently become immensely upset, perhaps even physically aggressive and rageful. Each time that a parent retreats from attempts to remove the items in order to avoid or stop the child's distress, they have reinforced maintenance of the possessions. Building upon this, school psychologists should help parents accumulate a more effective repertoire of responses to the child's distress while also counteracting the hoarding behaviors.

School psychologists may consult with school personnel regarding the rule breaking and aggressive behaviors. Hamblin et al. (2015) reported that teachers and parents note that children and adolescents with hoarding disorder engage in greater levels of rule breaking and aggression than their non-hoarding peers. This consultation may take many forms. The focus could be on developing a clear behavior plan to address the individual's behavior. It may also emphasize developing a way to teach the individual a new skill or ability to recognize the progression from trigger to aggressive behavior. The emphasis would depend on the individual and the expression of this behavior. Depending on the comfort and skill level of school personnel, this consultation may be more direct, with the school psychologist working directly with the child, or indirect, with the school psychologist working through the school personnel.

Counseling and Therapy Role

Within the school setting, school psychologists may offer the direct provision of intervention for children and adolescents with hoarding disorder through counseling or therapy. Providing these services during the school day and at no cost to families may help to expand mental health service provision to children with hoarding disorder while also reducing lost academic time due to travel to appointments (Creed et al., 2013, 2015). Farmer et al. (2003) found that only a small proportion of children with mental health concerns are able to access any form of intervention, and a majority of children and adolescents access services through practitioners within the schools. Given that many individuals with hoarding disorder report immediate relatives who also struggle with hoarding symptoms, providing the services in schools may also alleviate some familial stress associated with attempting to address the needs of multiple family members through community-based services that could represent a strain on economic and logistical resources.

> Farmer et al. (2003) found that only a small proportion of children with mental health concerns are able to access any form of intervention, and a majority of those access services through practitioners within the schools.

Although more research is needed, some evidence supports the use of cognitive behavioral therapy (CBT) as effective in the treatment of hoarding behaviors (Ale et al., 2014; Hojgaard et al., 2019; Morris et al., 2016; Rozenman et al., 2019; Storch, Murdoff, et al., 2011; Testa et al., 2011; Winsberg et al., 1999). And, although the research is not specific to hoarding disorder, studies have also shown the school setting to be an appropriate environment for the delivery of CBT to children and adolescents (Chiu et al., 2013; Creed et al., 2015; Ginsberg et al., 2011; Mychailyszyn et al., 2011). CBT is likely to be especially effective with the anxiety-based thoughts that are frequently experienced by students with hoarding disorder. Creed et al. (2015) note that the barriers to delivering CBT in the school setting include a lack of engagement by students and their parents and minimal time for delivery by school-based practitioners due to their other job responsibilities. However, through advocacy, collaboration, and organization, school psychologists can overcome these barriers to deliver this needed evidenced-based treatment for children and adolescents with hoarding disorder.

EDUCATIONAL SUPPORTS

Preliminary research with adults has found that individuals with hoarding disorder have a significantly greater intolerance of uncertainty compared with others (Mathes et al., 2017). Although this work has not yet been replicated for children and adolescents with hoarding disorder, it suggests that hoarding items may be associated with fears regarding future actions or circumstances. This intolerance of uncertainty could also manifest itself in classroom situations. If a child or adolescent experiences fears associated with unknown or impending events, then this could impact classroom behavior and academic performance.

To combat this intolerance of uncertainty, simple strategies could be employed in the educational environment like the use of schedules and presignals with students across grade levels. For young children, picture schedules would allow the child to identify where they are presently in the day's plan and also have clear expectations about what activities were coming and in what sequence throughout the day. As children age and are capable of reading fluently, those schedules could become written daily schedules. Presignals could also be used with or without schedules. With presignals, the teacher notifies students well in advance of changing activities, expectations, and/or locations (Chandler & Dahlquist, 2015). The students are told when the current activity will end, what the next activity will be, and when it will begin. This often serves to alleviate anxiety associated with unknown events and facilitates transition from one activity to the next.

Another area of probable academic support for children and adolescents with hoarding disorder could relate to the affiliated deficits in executive functioning. Executive functioning deficits impact attention, concentration, working memory, and problem-solving for students. These skill deficits can significantly impact learning and academic achievement and necessitate intervention for the student to fully access and progress in the curriculum. Dawson (2014) recommends that students with executive functioning concerns should be provided with explicit modeling to promote the use of metacognitive strategies. Teachers can prompt students through the use of questions that guide them to plan their efforts, organize their work, and solve problems through potential barriers to the completion of tasks. In addition, children and adolescents with executive functioning difficulties can benefit from greater levels of external structure in the classroom. Rather than intuiting organizational skills, these children may need modeling and practice of organizational strategies geared toward compensating for their deficits. They may also benefit from techniques like providing directions in both oral and written format and rehearsing how to respond appropriately in the classroom. Finally, as with any skill-building exercise, children who struggle with executive functioning should be praised for their efforts and progress toward the development of these abilities that greatly impact their current academic standing and their future adjustment in other domains (Dawson, 2014).

Dawson (2014) recommends that students with executive functioning concerns should be provided with explicit modeling to promote the use of metacognitive strategies.

SCHOOL-BASED MENTAL HEALTH INTERVENTIONS AND SUPPORTS

Early mental health intervention for children and adolescents with hoarding disorder is critical for a host of reasons. One reason that early intervention should be sought and prioritized is that hoarding becomes progressively more debilitating across the life span. Children who exhibit symptoms of hoarding become adolescents (and later adults) whose hoarding creates increasing havoc in their functioning and relationships to others (APA, 2013; Mataix-Cols et al., 2010; Tolin et al., 2010). As previously noted, one of the only known effective treatments for children and adolescents with hoarding disorder to date is CBT. Fortunately, most recently trained school psychologists have the education, experience, and competency to deliver CBT and could incorporate this into their practice to support these students.

CBT helps children to improve their thought patterns as a means of solving problems and regulating their emotions. Common techniques include role playing, journaling, relaxation, and cognitive restructuring. Because hoarding behaviors involve fears over discarding items, the techniques of CBT related to exposure may be useful and effective. Through exposure, the therapist would expose the child or adolescent with hoarding disorder to the act of discarding items while guiding them through coping strategies in the process. The exposure would proceed slowly and in small increments as the child can tolerate the act and feels less vulnerable and fearful in the process. Case study evidence with children with hoarding disorder has established this technique as effective, generalizable, and long-lasting over the course of the time under study (Ale et al., 2014).

Preliminary research has suggested that a specific form of CBT may be more effective for individuals with hoarding disorder than traditional CBT. This form combines the techniques of CBT with visits to the home (Gibson et al., 2010). The visits to the home allow for firsthand assessment of the extent of the excessive acquisition of possessions (that may not be evident in the school setting) and allows the practitioner to model and guide organizational skills in the setting where the challenges are manifested most frequently. It also allows for exposure exercises when appropriate (2010). However, caution is advised here. Although most school psychologists are trained and competent in the delivery of these therapeutic techniques, some school districts have guidelines regarding home visits. School psychologists should adhere to those protocols when they are in place. This typically involves sending more than one school professional to the home for the visit. In addition, school psychologists should take care that the overarching goals of their intervention (even if there is a home-based component) are focused on alleviating symptoms in order to facilitate adjustment within the school setting. This focus helps to further ensure that they are offering services within the bounds of their certification as it applies to school-based practice and not merging into a private practice arrangement that would more legally, ethically, and appropriately be conducted by a community-based professional. Gibson et al. (2010) further warn that any practitioner engaging in a therapeutic practice within a client's home should be wary of boundary issues, confidentiality concerns, and the prospect of dual roles.

Beyond individually based counseling and therapy for children and adolescents with hoarding disorder, it is likely that these students will benefit from a system of positive behavioral supports at school as well. Given that they frequently struggle with issues related to impulsivity, children and adolescents with hoarding disorder are likely to engage in poor decision-making at school that leads to behavioral infractions. Positive behavior support systems offer a framework to teach students what is expected of them with regard to behavior and offer reinforcement when those behaviors are exhibited (Bradshaw et al., 2012; Sugai & Horner, 2006). It offers a proactive approach to discipline whereby common triggers for misbehavior are defined and circumvented when possible. Although the emphasis is on positive behavior support as a system for prevention, there are also clearly outlined procedures and consequences when behavioral infractions do occur (McKevitt & Fynaardt, 2014). The explicitly stated and consistently enforced behavioral guidelines associated with positive behavior support will likely be effective for students with hoarding disorder in managing challenging behavior as well as reducing the anxiety associated with unknown expectations and unforeseen circumstances.

> The explicitly stated and consistently enforced behavioral guidelines associated with positive behavior support will likely be effective for students with hoarding disorder in managing challenging behavior as well as reducing the anxiety associated with unknown expectations and unforeseen circumstances.

CASE STUDY 16.1 KATIE: CASE OF A WHITE FEMALE WITH HOARDING DISORDER

Background

Katie is a 12-year-old White female in seventh grade. She currently attends public school, but her parents are considering homeschooling due to the current anxiety and behavior issues occurring at school. Katie was initially seen because of her struggles with her anxiety, indecisiveness, impulsive behaviors, and her strong will. At school, she has had several issues about being slow to follow directions, clutter in her desk, not being able to find assignments, and not completing assignments. When her teacher attempted to address the clutter in her desk, Katie had an episode. This included falling into the fetal position and hyperventilating. Her teacher believes that she is choosing not to comply. Her parents indicate that she is frequently late, cannot find things, and her room is a "pig sty." They go on to say that they cannot motivate her to get rid of anything, and her closet and room are unmanageable. They have given up fighting her over it.

Katie is an only child living with her biological parents. The family lives in a suburb of a major city in the Northeast. Her father is an engineer, and her mother is a dental hygienist. Her parents got married in their early 30s. Given their focus on their careers, they decided to have only one child. As a young child, Katie began to collect stuffed animals. She also developed individual personalities for them. She knew they were not really alive but developed a very special bond with the stuffed animals. One incident that was fairly traumatic occurred when Katie was 8 years old when a favorite stuffed pig was lost on a family trip to Disneyland. For several weeks, Katie mourned the loss of her pig. She still worries about what happened to her. Recently on a family trip to the lake, she ran from the cabin and jumped into the lake with her clothes on to rescue a discarded stuffed animal. Her parents were upset about this incident, but she still has the stuffed animal.

Katie believes that she has over 300 stuffed animals, whom she calls her friends. She keeps them in her bedroom. They are a variety of different types of animals. Katie cannot even discuss the possibility of getting rid of any of her friends. If the discussion comes up, she gets incredibly distressed. She also keeps items that she refers to as "her memories." These items can be just about anything from old movie tickets to a used lollypop stick. These items are kept in shoe boxes and other containers she keeps to house memories. This collection of memory boxes fills her closet and spills out onto the floor of her room. Katie does not seem bothered by the clutter and limited space in her room. She and her mother will make the room more orderly when it gets challenging to walk through. Her parents allow her to keep the items as long as they don't spill out into the living spaces. The last time they tried to purge the room, Katie went through the garbage and retrieved the items. Her parents are concerned about the anxiety that Katie has been exhibiting around any possibility of removing the items and with her being unable to keep the clutter boxed up. They are also concerned with her slowness in getting ready and keeping track of items.

Her school backpack is filled with numerous items, many of which are old assignments and worksheets. Her desk is cluttered with old pencils, pens, papers, erasers, paperclips, and numerous other types of items. Her teacher, Ms. Carmichael, has tried to get Katie to clean her desk but has decided that it is not worth the fight to get her to do it. The last time she required Katie to clean the desk out, it resulted in a scene. Katie began to hyperventilate and fell to the ground. Ms. Carmichael held a parent-teacher conference to discuss this incident. Katie's mother boxed up the items from Katie's desk and took them home. The school is also concerned about her slowness to get started with assignments and in completing the assignments.

Discussion

Her numerous stuffed animals and boxes of memories demonstrate Katie's difficulty with throwing away or giving away items. She describes a strong emotional attachment to the items, calling the stuffed animals her friends and giving them distinct personalities. The connection to her stuffed animals was developmentally appropriate but has gained substantial strength. The incident of jumping into the lake shows the overwhelming connection to inanimate objects and impulsivity. She relates to the scraps of papers as actual memories of past events. The act or

(continued)

CASE STUDY 16.1 KATIE: CASE OF A WHITE FEMALE WITH HOARDING DISORDER (continued)

thought of removing the items results in a panic attack. Her bedroom and play area are massively cluttered. The floor is covered with animals and toys unless the parents help her to organize the area. The parents avoid requesting that she get rid of the items to avoid her anxiety. They help her to box the items and keep them as long as it does not affect the rest of the home. This is also an issue at school. Katie's desk is full of items that have no real use. She is slow to start and has difficulty locating things due to this clutter in her desk. She either cannot find the item to turn in or has too much anxiety about releasing the item. The school has turned to the parents to try to deal with her issues. These issues are the reasons her parents are considering homeschooling her.

There are many things to consider regarding treatment in this case. Some of these are the act of hoarding, the anxiety, following directives, and work completion. The family would benefit from family therapy to gain an understanding of the issues and develop a clear plan to address the hoarding and the anxiety. The school would benefit from a multidisciplinary team exploring all elements of Katie's difficulties. There is evidence that hoarding has been associated with information processing and executive functioning deficits. These deficits are often related to challenges for the individual in working memory, attention, impulse control, problem-solving, and decision-making skills. This could explain some of her slowness to get started with assignments, completion of assignments, and refusal/inability to follow directions. Typically, hoarding doesn't have considerable academic needs and it would make more sense to consider a 504 plan. Given that there are several academic issues as well as issues at home, the IDEA categories of either Emotional Disturbance or Other Health Impairment could be considered. Receiving services under this category may assist in the types of interventions available to the school. As the assessment is developed, the school psychologist will most likely be called upon to conduct a psychological assessment, including a cognitive/achievement assessment and an emotional/behavioral functioning assessment. It may even include the CSI if the school has access to the inventory.

After the comprehensive assessment, a complete plan to address all areas of need would be developed. This would include addressing any academic, behavioral, and social–emotional needs. In addition to these, considerable education may need to be provided to the family and the school system regarding this disorder to minimize misunderstanding. As a consultant, the school psychologist may work with the family and Katie to provide this crucial educational component or the psychologist may be a liaison between the school and the private practitioner. A clear plan must be developed to deal with the hoarding behaviors at home and school while the issues on anxiety are also addressed. Again, this may be provided by the school psychologist or they may be a liaison between the school and the private practitioner. To address Katie's complex challenges, the provider of psychological services, the school, and the family must work together to ensure all facets of her condition are addressed.

SUMMARY POINTS

- In order to receive a *DSM-5* diagnosis of Hoarding Disorder, a child or adolescent must meet one of six criteria related to their accumulation of possessions.
- With regard to etiology, the school psychologist should remember that genetic factors often play a role in the development of hoarding disorder, and children with hoarding disorder may also live in homes with other family members who engage in hoarding behaviors as well.
- Homes that include an individual with hoarding disorder are at greater risk for fires, pest infestations, and homelessness.
- Students who hoard often experience executive functioning deficits that lead to academic struggle in the classroom.
- School psychologists can engage in many roles and functions to support the needs of students who hoard, including assessment, advocacy, consultation, and counseling and/or therapy.
- School-based interventions to support students who hoard may include CBT, which has been shown to have promise in treatment of hoarding symptoms.

TEST YOUR KNOWLEDGE

1. Which of the following is a specifier for the *DSM-5* diagnosis of Hoarding Disorder?
    a. Executive functioning deficits
    b. Excessive acquisition
    c. Childhood onset
    d. All of the above

2. A student with hoarding disorder automatically meets criteria for Other Health Impairment under IDEA.
    a. True
    b. False

3. Research does not support a genetic component to hoarding disorder.
    a. True
    b. False

4. Which of these skills is frequently impacted by executive functioning deficits?
    a. Problem-solving
    b. Working memory
    c. Attention
    d. All of the above

5. Hoarding symptoms often get progressively worse as a child ages.
    a. True
    b. False

Answers: (1) b, (2) b, (3) b, (4) d, (5) a.

DISCUSSION QUESTIONS

1. Describe the *DSM-5* diagnostic criteria for Hoarding Disorder.
2. Explain why the *DSM-5* included Hoarding Disorder as a separate diagnosis from OCD.
3. Outline how executive functioning deficits may impact a child or adolescent with hoarding disorder in the classroom.
4. Highlight the school psychologist's consultation role in working with children who hoard and their families.
5. Detail one evidenced-based social–emotional intervention for students who hoard.

CHAPTER RESOURCES

American Psychological Association *Treating People With Hoarding Disorder*: www.apa.org/monitor/2020/04/ce-corner-hoarding
Anxiety and Depression Association of America *Hoarding: The Basics*: https://adaa.org/understanding-anxiety/obsessive-compulsive-disorder-ocd/hoarding-basics
Child Mind Institute *Hoarding in Children*: https://childmind.org/article/hoarding-in-children/
Mayo Clinic *Hoarding Disorder*: www.mayoclinic.org/diseases-conditions/hoarding-disorder/symptoms-causes/syc-20356056

KEY REFERENCES

Only key references appear in the print edition. The full reference list appears in the digital product on Springer Publishing Connect: connect.springerpub.com/content/book/978-0-8261-3587-2/part/part06/chapter/ch16

American Psychiatric Association. (2013). *Diagnostic and statistical manual of mental disorders* (5th ed.). https://doi.org/10.1176/appi.books.9780890425596

Hacker, L. E., Park, J. M., Timpano, K. R., Cavitt, M. A., Alvaro, J. L., Lewin, A. B., Murphy, T. K., & Storch, E. A. (2016). Hoarding in children with ADHD. *Journal of Attention Disorders, 20*(7), 617–626. https://doi.org/10.1177%2F1087054712455845

Hombali, A., Sagayadevan, V., Tan, W. M., Chong, R., Yip, H. W., Vaingankar, J., Chong, S. A., & Subramaniam, M. (2019). A narrative synthesis of possible causes and risk factors of hoarding behaviours. *Asian Journal of Psychiatry, 42,* 104–114. https://doi.org/10.1016/j.ajp.2019.004.001

Ivanov, V. Z., Mataix-Cols, D., Serlachius, E., Lichtenstein, P., Anckarsater, H., Chang, Z., Hellner Gumpart, C., Lundstrom, S., Langstron, N., & Ruck, C. (2013). Prevalence, co-morbidity and heritability of hoarding symptoms in adolescence: A population based twin study in 15 year olds. *PLoS One, 8*(7), e69140. https://doi.org/10.1371/journal.pone.0069140

Mataix-Cols, D., Frost, R. O., Pertusa, A., Clark, L. A., Saxena, S., Leckman, J. F., Stein, D. J., Matsunaga, H., & Wilhelm, S. (2010). Hoarding disorder: A new diagnosis for *DSM-5*? *Depression and Anxiety, 27,* 556–572. https://doi.org/10.1002/da.20693

Office of Civil Rights. (n.d.). *Protecting students with disabilities: Frequently asked questions about Section 504 and the education of children with disabilities.* https://www2.ed.gov/about/offices/list/ocr/504faq.html

Samuels, J., Grados, M. A., Riddle, M. A., Bienvenu, O. J., Goes, F. S., Cullen, B., Wang, Y., Greenberg, B. D., Fyer, A. J., McCracken, J. T., Geller, D., Murphy, D. L., Knowles, J. A., Rasmussen, S. A., McLaughlin, N. C., Piacentini, J., Pauls, D. L., Stewart, S. E., Shugart, Y., ... Nestadt, G. (2014). Hoarding in children and adolescents with obsessive-compulsive disorder. *Journal of Obsessive-Compulsive and Related Disorders, 3,* 325–331. https://doi.org/10.1016/j.jocrd.2014.08.001

Steketee, G., & Frost, R. O. (2003). Compulsive hoarding: Current status of the research. *Clinical Psychology Review, 23,* 905–927. https://doi.org/10.1016/j.cpr.2003.08.002

Testa, R., Pantelis, C., & Fontenelle, L. F. (2011). Hoarding behaviors in children with learning disabilities. *Journal of Child Neurology, 26*(5), 574–579. https://doi.org/10.1177/0883073810387139

U.S. Department of Education. (n.d.). *Individuals with Disabilities Education Improvement Act.* https://sites.ed.gov/idea

UNIT 7

MENTAL HEALTH DISORDERS IN CHILDREN AND ADOLESCENTS: TRAUMA- AND STRESSOR-RELATED DISORDERS

CHAPTER 17

Posttraumatic Stress Disorder

LEARNING OBJECTIVES

- Summarize the *Diagnostic and Statistical Manual of Mental Disorders* (5th ed.; *DSM-5*; American Psychiatric Association [APA], 2013) diagnostic features of Posttraumatic Stress Disorder (PTSD) in young children.
- Describe how race-related traumatic stress can be manifested among youth of color.
- Describe how trauma impacts social–emotional and behavioral functioning in children.
- Explain ways in which traumatic stress can impact a child's ability to learn.
- Discuss ways in which school psychologists can provide educational and psychological support and mental health interventions for students who have been exposed to traumatic events.

INTRODUCTION

Traumatic experiences in childhood can have a significant influence on child and adolescent development. Research has indicated that approximately two thirds of youth in the United States experience a traumatic event by their 16th birthday (National Child Traumatic Stress Network [NCTSN], 2020a). *Traumatic events* have been defined as those experiences in which a child faces a direct or perceived threat of harm that can lead to their becoming overwhelmed with fear and concern about their safety (American Psychological Association, 2008; NCTSN, 2020a; Tobin, 2016). Such events can be experienced directly or as a witness and include incidents such as child abuse and neglect, exposure to violence such as school shootings and community or domestic violence, racially related stressors, natural disasters such as tornadoes and hurricanes, and the unforeseen death of someone to whom they were close. In addition, the COVID-19 pandemic poses a unique challenge for parents and schools across the world as they struggle to address the social–emotional needs of children and adolescents who have suffered traumatic grief from the loss of loved ones and/or friends who unexpectedly contracted the virus and died, leaving many children fearful and anxious that they may also become sick with the virus. Many professionals in the field of traumatic stress contend that COVID-19 is a traumatic stressor that could materialize through PTSD symptoms among those who have lost loved ones to the virus or in other forms of suffering related to the pandemic, such as increased exposure to family violence (Griffin, 2020; Humphreys et al., 2020; Zhou, 2020).

> Research has indicated that approximately two thirds of youth in the United States experience a traumatic event by their 16th birthday (NCTSN, 2020a).

A child's reaction to a traumatic event can be influenced by protective factors, such as a supportive family, as well as risk factors such as a history of mental health problems or previously experienced trauma. The child's response to a traumatic experience may be manifested in a presentation of traumatic stress reactions, which include feelings such as anger, fearfulness, sadness, guilt, a sense of helplessness, and loss of control (National Association of School Psychologists [NASP], 2016a). Although some children may respond to a traumatic event with short-term distress, such as shock and confusion, other children may experience severe traumatic stress reactions that are more significant, long-lasting, and develop into a clinical diagnosis of PTSD (American Psychiatric

Association [APA], 2013; Gould et al., 2020; Mills et al., 2019). Children and adolescents who experience traumatic stress may exhibit social–emotional and behavioral difficulties in school that can impact their performance in the classroom and their functioning at home (Diamanduros et al., 2018a). This chapter focuses on providing useful trauma-related information for school psychologists so that they can better serve traumatized children in the schools and ensure that educational and social–emotional needs are met.

DIAGNOSTIC ISSUES: PTSD AND DEVELOPMENTAL TRAUMA DISORDER

DSM-5 Diagnostic Criteria for PTSD—Pediatric Subtype

In an effort to address the unique presentation of traumatic stress symptoms in young children, the *Diagnostic and Statistical Manual of Mental Disorders*, Fifth Edition (*DSM-5*; APA, 2013), includes revisions (from previous editions) in the diagnostic criteria for PTSD that are developmentally sensitive, more attentive to behavioral symptoms particularly important for young children who may be nonverbal or have not yet developed the language skills to describe emotions or difficulties, and lowered diagnostic thresholds. A pediatric subtype of PTSD was developed for children younger than 6 years of age who experience a traumatic event by direct exposure, witnessing the event, or learning that a close relative or other loved one had experienced a traumatic event in which the actual or threatened death of that individual was the result of an accident or violence (APA, 2013). The PTSD subtype for younger children focuses on three symptom clusters: (a) re-experiencing the trauma through intrusive thoughts, (b) avoiding trauma-related stimuli and/or experiencing negative alterations in cognition and mood, and (c) experiencing increased arousal and reactivity. At least one symptom related to re-experiencing the trauma through intrusive thoughts must be evident, which may include recurring memories of the traumatic event demonstrated through reenactment of the trauma in play, recurring and distressing dreams for the child that may or may not be related to the traumatic event, dissociative reactions in which the child feels as though the trauma is reoccurring, and intense reactions (psychological or physiological) when exposed to trauma triggers. In young children, at least one symptom indicating avoidance of trauma-related reminders or one symptom of behaviors related to negative cognition and mood changes must be present. The avoidance may appear through the child's efforts to avoid triggering memories of the traumatic event (people or places). Negative cognition and mood changes include an increase in negative emotions, reduction in positive emotions, and/or social withdrawal. In addition, two symptoms of increased arousal and reactivity must be evident and may include behaviors such as severe temper tantrums, sleep difficulties, and difficulties concentrating. These symptoms must last more than 1 month following the traumatic event and significantly impact the child's functioning. In addition, the symptoms should not be the result of any medications, substance use, or medical condition (APA, 2013).

> The *DSM-5* (APA, 2013) added a new PTSD subtype for children younger than age 6, which has three cluster symptoms: (a) re-experiencing trauma through intrusive thoughts, (b) avoiding trauma-related stimuli and/or experiencing negative alterations in cognition and mood, and (c) experiencing increased arousal and reactivity.

DSM-5 Diagnostic Criteria for PTSD—Ages 6 and Older

For children who are older than 6 years of age and for adolescents, the *DSM-5* diagnostic criteria of PTSD (APA, 2013) are similar to the preschool subtype with the only difference being that criteria must be met for four symptoms clusters: (a) intrusive symptoms, (b) avoidance of trauma-related stimuli, (c) negative alterations in cognitions and mood, and (d) alterations in arousal and reactivity. Although at least one symptom must be present within the intrusive symptom and avoidance of trauma-related stimuli clusters, two or more symptoms must be present within the negative alterations in cognitions and mood cluster as well as the alterations in arousal and reactivity cluster (APA, 2013).

In addition to a pediatric subtype, the *DSM-5* (APA, 2013) includes a dissociative subtype for both age groups in which prominent dissociative symptoms are present. This subtype has two specifiers: *depersonalization,* in which a child feels detached from their body, and *derealization,* in which the child experiences their surroundings as unreal (APA, 2013). Research studies have found that, although a dissociative subtype of PTSD can be distinguished from PTSD among adolescents, it is important to assess a broader range of dissociative symptoms to fully understand traumatic stress symptoms among adolescents (Choi et al., 2017).

Prevalence Rates

To understand the extent to which children and adolescents have been diagnosed with PTSD, it is important to consider prevalence rates. As noted by Wilmshurst (2015), obtaining consistent estimates of prevalence rates of PTSD in youths can be difficult because of factors such as the variety and number of traumatic events (single episode vs. repeated episodes) children experience and whether the population sampled comes from the community or the clinic. Inconsistency is seen in various research studies. For example, it has been reported that 3% to 15% of girls and 1% to 6% of boys who experienced a traumatic event were diagnosed with PTSD (National Center for PTSD, n.d.). A study of approximately 10,000 adolescents between 13 and 18 years of age found that 5% of adolescents in the sample met criteria for PTSD and the prevalence for girls meeting PTSD criteria was 8% compared with a prevalence of 2.3% for boys (Merikangas et al., 2010). A meta-analysis of research studies on the rates of PTSD among youths found an overall rate of approximately 16% that varied based on gender and the type of trauma (Alisic et al., 2014). The study found that girls with exposure to interpersonal trauma had a rate of 32.9% compared to boys with non-interpersonal trauma exposure, who had a rate of 8.4% (Alisic et al., 2014). A more recent study investigating PTSD among a sample of adolescents who had been exposed to a traumatic event found that the prevalence of PTSD in boys was approximately 47%, whereas a prevalence rate of approximately 54% was found in girls (Astitene et al., 2020).

Complex Trauma and Developmental Trauma Disorder

Although children and adolescents who experience a single traumatic episode can experience PTSD, those who have been exposed to multiple traumatic events may experience a more complex symptom presentation that includes comorbid mental health conditions such as anxiety, depression, and disruptive behaviors (Complex Trauma Treatment Network of NCTSN, 2016; McLaughlin et al., 2012). Complex trauma in youth is characterized by an early onset of trauma that is often of an interpersonal nature and that is chronic and involves repeated exposure to traumatic events such as abuse (Spinazzola et al., 2017; Tobin, 2016; van der Kolk, 2005). It can influence the child's formation of a sense of self and the ability to establish secure attachments, regulate emotions, and manage one's behavior (Cook et al., 2003; NCTSN, 2014; Spinazzola et al., 2018; Tobin, 2016). In addition, complex trauma can influence brain development (Tobin, 2016; van der Kolk, 2003, 2005) and impact the child's ability to learn in the classroom (Complex Trauma Treatment Network of NCTSN, 2016; Tobin, 2016).

Recognizing the complexity of trauma-related symptoms among children and adolescents, van der Kolk (2005) proposed a new diagnostic disorder, developmental trauma disorder (DTD) for children with complex trauma prior to the publication of the *DSM-5* (APA, 2013). Under this proposed disorder, complex trauma in children who have experienced chronic and multiple traumatic events is viewed from a developmental perspective focused on the effects of trauma, disturbed attachment patterns, and emotional dysregulation. Children with complex trauma often experience difficulties in self-regulation and interpersonal relatedness that can be long term, extending into adolescence and adulthood (Cook et al., 2005; Spinazzola et al., 2018). Mental health problems among children with complex trauma extend beyond symptoms related to PTSD and include disorders such as anxiety disorders, mood disorders, reactive attachment disorder, and disruptive disorders such as attention deficit hyperactivity disorder (ADHD), oppositional defiant disorder (ODD), and conduct disorder (Cook et al., 2005; van der Kolk et al., 2019). Although the proposed diagnosis of DTD was not adopted for the *DSM-5*, it highlights the complexity of the influence of chronic trauma that is not captured by a diagnosis of PTSD and provides a framework for understanding the influence of complex trauma on a child's neurodevelopment (Denton et al., 2017; van der Kolk, 2005). Many trauma professionals contend that this model should be utilized by clinicians providing mental health services to traumatized children and adolescents (Bremness & Polzin, 2014; D'Andrea et al., 2012; Denton et al., 2017; DePierro et al., 2019; Spinazzola et al., 2018), and research is being pursued to support the use of DTD as a diagnosis (DePierro et al., 2019; Spinazzola et al., 2018). From a diagnostic perspective, an instrument to assess developmental trauma, the Developmental Trauma Disorder Semi-Structured Interview (DTD-SI)-Version 10, has been developed and found to have sound psychometric properties (Ford et al., 2018). Recent research examining comorbidities of DTD and PTSD has found that both disorders are highly comorbid, but DTD's comorbidity extends beyond that of PTSD to include panic disorder, separation anxiety disorder, and disruptive disorders (van der Kolk et al., 2019). The DTD diagnosis holds much promise as a diagnostic disorder that will help guide the use of therapeutic interventions to help children and adolescents struggling with the social–emotional and behavioral outcomes of complex trauma.

CULTURAL ISSUES RELATED TO POSTTRAUMATIC STRESS IN CHILDHOOD

The impact of traumatic exposure among youths of color has received little attention by professionals, yet exposure to traumatic events, such as community violence and historic and current racial discrimination, among these youths is high. Research has indicated that boys of color may experience five or more adverse childhood experiences prior to their 18th birthday and are exposed to traumatic events at a higher rate than other demographic groups (Graham et al., 2017). Community violence among African American youth has been positively linked to posttraumatic stress symptomatology (Deane et al., 2020; Paxton et al., 2004) and found to be a significant contributor of PTSD among African American youth living in urban communities (Hunt et al., 2011). The influence of community violence on the social–emotional well-being of children of color may be intensified by racial stress (Proctor et al., 2020; Saleem et al., 2020; Sanders-Phillips, 2009). Racial stress has been identified as a possible explanation for why children of color experience greater exposure to traumatic events than their Caucasian counterparts (Saleem et al., 2020). A recent study found that Black adolescents encounter racial discrimination experiences, on average, five times per day (English et al., 2020). Moreover, direct as well as vicarious exposure to trauma through police violence and brutality directed at people of color, particularly Black men and boys, can have a significant impact on children of color (Proctor et al., 2020). Indirect viewing of highly publicized police shootings, such as the shooting of Walter Scott or the brutal killing of George Floyd, could be traumatic triggers among people of color.

> According to Graham et al. (2017), boys of color experience traumatic events at a higher rate than other demographic groups and experience five or more adverse experiences in childhood before their 18th birthday.

As noted in research studies, racial stress can be manifested in traumatic stress symptoms (Saleem et al., 2020). Racial trauma, which is also referred to as *race-based traumatic stress*, results from experiencing stress related to exposure to racial discrimination (NCTSN, Justice Consortium, Schools Committee, and Culture Consortium, 2017; Williams et al., 2018). Symptoms of racial trauma include the child or adolescent being sensitive to situations in which there might be a possible threat, being hypervigilant, experiencing anxiety and depression, and exhibiting maladaptive responses such as aggressive behaviors (NCTSN, Justice Consortium, Schools Committee, and Culture Consortium, 2017; Sanders-Phillips et al., 2014). Some researchers contend that racial discrimination can be viewed as a form of chronic violence that can impact the social–emotional well-being of children of color (Lanier et al., 2017; Sanders-Phillips, 2009) and may lead to the development of PTSD (Sanders-Phillips et al., 2014; Tynes et al., 2019). Still, others point out that, although a racially motivated violent event may meet the criterion of the *DSM-5*'s definition of a traumatic event, the definition is subjective and restrictive such that it may not fully address some types of racial discrimination that can contribute to racial trauma such as ongoing covert racial discrimination, daily experiences of racism and chronic micro-aggressions that can have a cumulative impact over time (Holmes et al., 2016).

To better understand how racial stress is exhibited in trauma-related symptoms in youth of color, Saleem and colleagues (2020) developed the Developmental and Ecological Model of Youth Racial Trauma (EMYth-RT). The model provides a thorough conceptualization of the impact of racial stress across developmental periods of preschool- and elementary school-age children, middle school-age children, and high school-age adolescents and the manifestation of trauma-related symptoms during each developmental period. The model also takes into consideration the influence of the child's family and community on how the child interprets and manages racial stress and trauma at different ages. For a more detailed discussion of this model, see Saleem et al. (2020).

> Research has shown that Black adolescents are confronted with racial discrimination about five times per day (English et al., 2020).

Racial trauma may be overlooked by school and clinical professions as contributing sources of stress for children and adolescents. It is important that mental health professionals working with children and adolescents recognize the impact that racial trauma, racism, and racial discrimination can have on the development and school performance of children of color. Racial disparities in the schools are evident in the disproportionate number of African American boys being served in special education under the Individuals with Disabilities Education Improvement Act (IDEA) disability categories of Intellectual Disability and Emotional Disturbance/Emotional Behavioral Disorder (NASP, 2013; Sullivan et al., 2009). In fact, Sullivan and colleagues (2009) indicate that African American youth have been overrepresented in special education for over 30 years. Overrepresentation of racial minorities, particularly Black students, in subjective office discipline referrals, school suspensions, and expulsions have also been consistently documented since 1975 (Children's Defense Fund, 1975; Skiba et al., 2012). Although some have proposed that procedures for identifying underrepresented students with disabilities need to be reexamined (Donovan & Cross, 2002), consideration of such procedures needs to include an approach that allows the possibility that challenging behaviors exhibited by many youth of color may be related to chronic stress associated with racial trauma.

IMPACT OF CHILD TRAUMA ON SOCIAL–EMOTIONAL AND BEHAVIORAL FUNCTIONING IN SCHOOL AND HOME ENVIRONMENTS

Trauma can significantly influence a child's development and functioning at school and at home. This section examines protective and risk factors that play a role in the child's response to a traumatic event. Social–emotional and behavioral impairments related to trauma are also discussed.

Protective and Risk Factors

A child's response to a traumatic event depends on how the child perceives the threat posed by the situation as well as the child's level of resiliency and coping (Brock, 2004; Diamanduros et al., 2018a). Although some children may have effective coping skills and a strong support system that helps to lessen the influence of trauma on their functioning, other children's exposure to trauma may result in significant functional impairments if they perceive the distressing situation as threatening.

The perceived level of threat may be influenced by the nature of the situation, adults' reactions to the situation, the relationship to others involved in the situation, and individual protective/risk factors (NASP School Safety and Crisis Response Committee, 2015). Internal protective factors that may help a child manage their response to an adverse situation include a positive self-concept and effective problem-solving skills (Brock, 2004; NASP School Safety and Crisis Response Committee, 2015), whereas external protective factors include having a supportive family and strong social support system (Brock, 2004). In addition, the age of the child at the time of the traumatic event may be protective given that adolescents are less vulnerable to traumatic stress reactions compared to younger children (2004). Although protective factors may shield a child from experiencing severe traumatic stress reactions, risk factors can render a child vulnerable to the influence of traumatic situations. Vulnerability to a traumatic event can be influenced by factors such as whether a traumatic event involving violence was intentional or whether the traumatic event occurred unexpectedly (2004). The impact of trauma on a child's functioning is discussed in the following sections and summarized in Table 17.1.

Impact on Social–Emotional Functioning

Based on the protective and risk factors noted previously, children and adolescents may not all respond the same way to a traumatic event. Many children and adolescents become overwhelmed with the stress related to having experienced the trauma and may tend to experience emotional distress in one of two ways: hyper-responsive reactions or hypo-responsive reactions (Armsworth & Holaday, 1993; Diamanduros et al., 2018a). Hyper-responsive reactions are usually characterized by difficulty regulating emotions such as anger and anxiety, whereas hypo-responsive reactions are typically marked by emotional detachment and social withdrawal (Armsworth & Holaday, 1993).

Children who have hyper-responsive reactions are likely to experience emotional lability and may show signs of strong emotional distress, which is displayed as anger, rage, and irritability (Armsworth & Holaday, 1993; NASP, 2016a; NASP School Safety and Crisis Response Committee, 2015). For some children, the anger may serve as a defense mechanism in which the anger gives them a sense of control over the traumatic situation, which enables them to direct the anger toward the person responsible for the traumatic event (Diamanduros et al., 2018a; NASP, 2016a). In the classroom and at home, the child may become angry and/or irritable over events that occur and have difficulty controlling the anger, which may result in verbal or behavioral outbursts.

Other children may become overwhelmed with the stress associated with the traumatic event and feel intense anxiety and fearfulness about their safety (Ruiz, 2016). They may worry that they will be exposed to other situations that may put their safety in jeopardy. For example, school-aged children may be anxious about returning to school after a school shooting and attempt to avoid going to

Table 17.1 Areas of Functioning Impacted by Trauma

Social–Emotional Functioning	Behavioral Functioning	Learning and Classroom Performance
Emotional Distress	Aggressive behaviors	Cognitive Difficulties
Hyper-responses	Disruptive behaviors	*Decline in IQ*
Anger	Oppositional behaviors	*Processing difficulties*
Rage	Impulsivity	*Executive functioning problems*
Irritability	Self-destructive behaviors	Planning
Intense anxiety	Sleep disturbances	Memory
Fear related to safety	Eating disturbances	Attention
Intense sadness	Regressive behaviors	Emotional regulation
Guilt	*Clingy to parent*	Mental productivity
Hypo-responses	*Refusal to sleep alone*	Achievement
Emotional numbing	*Thumb-sucking*	*Decreased reading scores*
Dissociation	*Fearful of dark*	*Lower grades*
Other responses	Enuresis	*Grade retention*
Feelings of betrayal	Encopresis	*Special education*
Feelings of distrust	Reenactment behaviors	Other influences on learning
Feelings of shame	*Reenact trauma through play*	*Sleep difficulties*
Social Interactions	*Retell the traumatic event*	*Somatic complaints*
Social isolation	*Imitate the traumatic event*	*Concentration difficulties*
Insecure attachments		
Self-concept		
Low self-esteem		
Lack of self-confidence		

school, which may result in attendance problems. In addition, intense anxiety in school-age children may be exhibited as hypervigilance about their surroundings or triggered by a reminder about the traumatic event. Young children may experience separation anxiety and become distressed if they have to be away from their parents (Racco & Vis, 2015). Other internalized emotions, such as feelings of intense sadness and/or guilt, may also be experienced by a child who experienced the loss of a family member or friend during a traumatic event (Diamanduros et al., 2018a; NASP, 2016a).

On the other hand, some traumatized children react differently and experience hypo-responsive reactions, which are characterized by being detached from their emotions (Armsworth & Holaday, 1993). At home and school, they may appear to be emotionally numb and not display any emotions. A consequence of severe emotional numbing is dissociation, which can serve as a coping mechanism used by the child to compartmentalize the traumatic event and associated feelings as a way to avoid becoming emotionally overwhelmed when they suffer a traumatic event (Choi et al., 2017). However, continued use of dissociation by the child as a way to cope with intense feelings in nontraumatic situations can be maladaptive and result in psychopathology (Choi et al., 2017; Cook et al, 2003). For parents and teachers, it can be difficult to recognize dissociation in children and adolescents, because there are no clear physical signs of it. In some children, dissociation may present itself as daydreaming or the child's being in a daze and unaware of their surroundings.

Some traumatized children may detach from their emotions related to the traumatic event and appear to be emotionally numb. Severe emotional numbing can lead to dissociation, which, if used continually as a coping mechanism to deal with intense trauma-related emotions, may become maladaptive and lead to psychopathology (Choi et al., 2017; Cook et al., 2003).

IMPACT ON SOCIAL FUNCTIONING AND RELATIONSHIPS

Children's social functioning can be impacted by trauma and the intense emotions often associated with the trauma. Peers may be reluctant to attempt to connect with a traumatized child who is angry, irritable, and not easily engaged. Children and adolescents may begin to socially isolate themselves as a way to avoid having to talk about the traumatic experience and may believe that their fears about the traumatic event will be viewed as vulnerability by others. In addition, they feel ashamed about their traumatic experience and believe that others may judge them or not fully understand what they have gone through so they begin to isolate themselves from their families and friends (NASP School Safety and Crisis Response Committee, 2015). Children and adolescents who have been abused, particularly by someone they trusted, may experience feelings of betrayal and distrust, which can negatively impact their interpersonal relationships (Diamanduros et al., 2018a).

Chronic trauma, which is inflicted upon a child by a caregiver, can greatly impact a child's attachment to that caregiver and influence the child's relationship with others. Research has found that 80% of young children who are maltreated exhibit insecure attachment patterns (Cook et al., 2005). The most concerning insecure attachment pattern exhibited by maltreated children is disorganized attachment. Young children who have disorganized attachment may behave erratically toward the caregiver by being clingy at times and dismissive at other times and believe that they cannot rely on others, which can interfere with their ability to form healthy relationships (NASP School Safety and Crisis Response Committee, 2015; van der Kolk, 2005). Older children with disorganized attachment patterns exhibit behaviors that reflect helplessness or coercive control (Cook et al., 2005).

In addition, experiencing repeated traumatic events can also impact the development of competencies within the child, leaving them vulnerable and feeling ineffective. Their self-confidence may be compromised, which can influence their ability to establish relationships with others. Children who have experienced traumatic events, particularly those of an interpersonal nature, may feel unworthy and have low self-esteem (Cook et al., 2005; NCTSN, n.d.-e, 2013).

Impact on Behavioral Functioning

In addition to impacting social functioning, difficulty regulating intense emotions can influence a child's behavior. Some children may struggle to control strong feelings of anger, feel overwhelmed with these feelings, and react intensely to situations that typically would not trigger reactions like an outburst (American Psychological Association, 2008; NASP, 2016a; NCTSN, n.d.-a). Inability to control intense feelings may manifest in aggressive and disruptive behaviors, which can be observed at home and at school (D'Andrea et al., 2012; Diamanduros et al., 2018a). Such behaviors can interfere with learning in the classroom and, as noted earlier, impact the child's relationship with peers. Other traumatized children and adolescents may exhibit behaviors that are oppositional, impulsive, and self-destructive (D'Andrea et al., 2012; Diamanduros et al., 2018a; NCTSN, n.d.-a).

Regressive behaviors may be observed in young children who have experienced a traumatic event. Hence, children who had previously been sleeping through the night on their own may begin to refuse to sleep by themselves, want to sleep next to their parents, and/or have nightmares (American Psychological Association, 2008; Diamanduros et al., 2018a). Young children may begin to cling to their parents in anticipation of being separated from them (NASP, 2016b). Children who had previously been toilet-trained may begin to experience enuresis and/or encopresis (Diamanduros et al., 2018a; NASP, 2016b).

Other behaviors experienced by young children may include reenactment of the traumatic event in their play and retelling aspects of the traumatic experience, often without emotion (Diamanduros et al., 2018a; NASP, 2016b). Young children who may not yet be developmentally able to communicate the trauma and/or the feelings related to the traumatic event they experienced may use play to reenact the trauma or may imitate the traumatic event in their behavior as a way of working through what they experienced (NCTSN, n.d.-e).

IMPACT ON LEARNING IN THE CLASSROOM

Children who have experienced complex trauma may have difficulty learning in the classroom. Research has found that trauma can influence brain development and affect cognitive functioning, which can influence a child's ability to learn (Tobin, 2016; van der Kolk, 2003). For example, studies examining the link between brain development and maltreatment in children have found that traumatized children may exhibit cognitive difficulties that can negatively impact their classroom performance (Beers & De Bellis, 2002; Tobin, 2016; van der Kolk, 2003). To be specific, trauma can influence the development of the prefrontal cortex, which is associated with executive functioning skills such as planning, memory, attention, regulating emotions, and continued mental productivity (De Bellis, 2005; Tobin, 2016). Research studies have also indicated that IQ standard scores can be predicted to drop by approximately 7.5 points, and reading achievement standard scores can be expected to drop by 9.8 points in children who have been exposed to violence and trauma-related distress (Delaney-Black et al., 2002). In addition, studies have found that child maltreatment is associated with poor educational outcomes such as grade retention, special education, and lower grades (Romano et al., 2015). A recent meta-analysis of research studies revealed children exposed to various types of violence, including abuse and community violence, have a 13% probability of not graduating from high school, and children who have experienced violence tend to be less likely to perform well on standardized tests and to achieve high grades (Fry et al., 2018).

> Research evidence exists which indicates that IQ standard scores for children exposed to trauma can be expected to drop by about 7.5 points, whereas reading achievement scores can be expected to drop by approximately 9.8 points (Delaney-Black et al., 2002).

In the classroom, children and adolescents who have experienced a traumatic event may view school as an unsafe environment and be in a hyper-aroused state while in the classroom. They may have difficulty concentrating because they are preoccupied with worries about their safety and may experience difficulty processing information (Cole et al., 2005). In addition, a child who is overwhelmed with feelings of stress and anxiety may dissociate while in the classroom and not be attentive to classroom activities, which could impact their ability to process information. As noted previously, traumatized children may have memory difficulties, particularly sequential memory difficulties, which may impact their ability to organize information sequentially and solve problems (Cole et al., 2005).

Difficulty in regulating emotions and hypervigilance can manifest in behavioral problems in the classroom such as poor impulse control, aggressive behaviors, and other disruptive behaviors that may interfere with the child being able to focus on their schoolwork (Cole et al., 2005). Children with PTSD may also have difficulty identifying and expressing trauma-related feelings and, hence, express their emotions through their behavior, sometimes overreacting to conflicts in the classroom or on the playground. The traumatic experience may deplete internal resources, such as coping and the ability to manage emotions, which can result in maladaptive ways to deal with emotions that may be exhibited in their behavior (2005). It is important to note that these behaviors can be frustrating to teachers, who may view the disruptive behaviors as willful opposition and defiance, so it is important that educators and school administrators recognize that these disruptive behaviors may be trauma related and that the child may not possess the coping mechanisms to deal with strong emotions in an appropriate and effective way. Other traumatized children who have difficulty identifying feelings and communicating those feelings, may become disconnected and isolated from others, with some traumatized children dissociating from their current environment and focusing more on their internal state of being rather than classroom activities (Perry, 2003).

Difficulties in identifying and expressing emotions can also lead to other difficulties in the classroom. Psychosomatic symptoms, such as stomachaches, headaches, fatigue, and sleeping problems, have been reported in children with a history of trauma (Cole et al., 2005). These symptoms can influence not only behavior in the classroom, but also school attendance and missed instruction (Cole et al., 2005). It also is important to note that challenging trauma-related behaviors and difficulty functioning in the classroom may lead to increased school suspensions and drop-out rates (Cole et al., 2005; NCTSN, 2008a). A school's punitive responses to behavioral concerns through disciplinary referrals, suspension, and expulsion do not address the root cause of the problem. Therefore, it is important for school psychologists to understand the patterns of types of discipline referrals and responses in schools and to engage in consultation, support, and advocacy to address trauma triggers and reactions through mental health means rather than through exclusion and punishment.

IMPLICATIONS FOR SCHOOL PSYCHOLOGISTS

Given their training in education, psychology, and mental health, school psychologists can have a pivotal role in addressing the needs of traumatized children through their work in the schools. Such efforts would be aligned with several domains of the *NASP 2020 Practice Model* (NASP, 2020) including Domain 1: Data-Based Decision Making, Domain 2: Consultation and Collaboration, Domain 4: Mental and Behavioral Health Services, Domain 5: School-Wide Practices to Promote Learning, and Domain 6: Services to Promote Safe and Supportive Schools. There are several ways in which school psychologists can address the needs of children who have been traumatized, which have been identified by Diamanduros and colleagues (2018b). These efforts include: (a) raising awareness among educators, school administrators, and parents about the impact of trauma on a child's development and functioning; and (b) applying trauma-informed practice in assessments. This section of the chapter focuses on promoting awareness about child trauma and using trauma-informed practices in assessments by reviewing suggestions offered by Diamanduros et al. (2018b) and building on those suggestions. Other ways in which school psychologists can be involved in addressing the needs of traumatized children include advocating for the implementation of trauma-informed educational and social–emotional supports and provision of school-based mental health services, which are discussed in later sections of this chapter.

Raising Awareness About the Impact of Trauma

As noted earlier in the chapter, trauma can have a significant impact on a child's development and functioning. Without an understanding of how trauma affects a child's ability to regulate emotions, maintain relationships, manage their behavior, and learn in the classroom, educators and parents may be confused about their interactions with the traumatized child and observations of the child's behavior. In an effort to understand teachers' perception of providing support to traumatized children, Alisic (2012) interviewed teachers and found that uncertainty in how to provide optimal support to students exposed to trauma was a concern for teachers. A similar study investigated parents' perceptions of child trauma and found parental concerns focused on awareness of their child's needs and how best to meet those needs (Alisic et al., 2012). Therefore, it is important for school psychologists to promote awareness of the impact that trauma can have on children and adolescents so that educators and parents can better support traumatized children and adolescents. There are various online training resources that may be helpful for school psychologists as they prepare to work with educators, parents, and students. One such online resource is the NCTSN, which has free fact sheets for professionals and webinars on various aspects of child trauma such as *NCTSN Resources Related to Understanding Child Traumatic Stress* (NCTSN, n.d.-b); a list of printed and webinar resources is available on the NCTSN website (www.nctsn.org). Diamanduros et al. (2018b) have identified ways in which school psychologists can help educators and parents better understand how to help children and adolescents with a history of trauma. These are described in the next two sections.

Raising Awareness Among Educators and School Administrators

To promote a better understanding of traumatic stress reactions in children among educators and school administrators, Diamanduros et al. (2018b) encourage school psychologists to provide in-service workshops that focus on facts about trauma, factors that influence how a child may respond to trauma, traumatic stress reactions, and how best to help the child feel safe in the classroom so that the child can learn. Through such training, educators are able to recognize signs of trauma in children and better understand how to meet their needs. Diamanduros and colleagues (2018b) recommend several resources that may be helpful to teachers and school administrators. NASP resources on trauma include *Managing Strong Emotional Reactions to Traumatic Events: Tips for Families and Teachers* (NASP, 2016a) and *Trauma: Brief Facts and Tips for Children and Adolescents* (2016b). Both of these resources provide basic information about child trauma, which may be beneficial in helping educators recognize signs of trauma and learn how to support traumatized children in the classroom. School administrators may find the resource *The Role of Schools in Supporting Traumatized Students* (Rossen & Cowan, 2013) useful when considering school-wide approaches to helping students with a history of trauma. Another helpful resource for schools is *Trauma: Helping Handout for Schools* (Reeves & Brock, 2018). This handout provides information on trauma and recommended supports and strategies to address trauma in schools. Besides NASP-related resources, the NCTSN also provides a wealth of resources for educators and school administrators that include both printed resources, such as *Child Trauma Toolkit for Educators* (NCTSN, 2008a), and numerous webinars available on the NCTSN Learning Center (https://learn.nctsn.org/) that provide training on various aspects of child trauma. These online trainings would be beneficial for educators and school administrators to complete so that they gain an understanding of the educational and psychological needs of traumatized children. In addition, trauma videos, such as *Remembering Trauma: Connecting the Dots Between Complex Trauma and Misdiagnosis in Youth*, and *Remembering Trauma: Part 2*, as well as *A Video for Youth by Youth*, may be helpful in learning more about the impact of trauma on children and are available online at the Center for Trauma Assessment, Services, and Interventions (www.ptsd.va.gov/professional/assessment/child/index.asp).

To address race-related trauma, school psychologists may want to consider specific resources that are available at the NCTSN website. These include *Cultural Responsiveness to Racial Trauma* (St. Jean et al., 2020); *Addressing Race and Trauma in the Classroom: A Resource for Educators* (NCTSN, Justice Consortium, Schools Committee, & Culture Consortium, 2017); and *Select NCTSN Resources African-Americans and Race* (NCTSN, 2020b), which is a fact sheet that lists several resources related to race and trauma. Another resource that is recommended is a video, *Chronic Stress, Race-Related Stress, and Academic Outcomes Among Adolescents* (www.youtube.com/watch?v=X-DIOIn8Msw), sponsored by the American Psychological Association (2017), which addresses the impact of chronic stressors and race-related stress on children's brain development and school performance. In addition, there are several webinars/videos on race and trauma available on the NCTSN Learning Center website (https://learn.nctsn.org) that can serve as professional development opportunities for school psychologists and educators.

Raising Awareness Among Parents

In addition to promoting awareness among educators and school administrators, school psychologists can raise awareness of child trauma and its impact on children among parents. Parents may not understand that traumatized children function in "survival mode" and that disruptive or aggressive behaviors may be in response to a perceived threat; hence, their actions may be self-protective in an effort to stay safe. Diamanduros et al. (2018b) encourage the use of parent trauma-informational sessions that focus on providing basic facts about trauma, its impact on youth, children and adolescents' response to a traumatic event, and how to help the traumatized child feel safe. These sessions can help to provide parents with knowledge about the definition of trauma and traumatic stress reactions in children so that they learn how to provide emotional support to their child. It is important for the school psychologist to prepare a list of community resources that are available to provide additional support for families of traumatized children outside of the school setting. In addition, printed handouts, such as fact sheets that are available through NASP such as *Supporting Students Experiencing Childhood Trauma: Tips for Parents and Educators* (NASP School Safety and Crisis Response Committee, 2015) and NCTSN resources for parents, *Age-Related Reactions to a Traumatic Event* (NCTSN, n.d.-c) and *Understanding Child Traumatic Stress: A Guide for Parents* (NCTSN, 2008b), are helpful resources that provide parents information about how to support their child while helping the child feel safe. The Child Trauma Academy website also provides online trauma resources for caregivers, such as *Helping Traumatized Children: A Brief Overview for Caregivers* (Perry, 2012), which provides a guide for parents that has an overview about trauma and ways in which parents can help their child in adjusting to life after the traumatic event. Perry (2012) provides various ways to help parents talk to their child about the traumatic experience if the child wants to talk about it and how to help the child feel safe and protected.

Using Trauma-Informed School-Based Assessment Practices

As noted by Diamanduros and colleagues (2018b), identifying children who have been exposed to trauma can be challenging. A child's history of trauma may not be known to school personnel for a number of reasons (Tishelman et al., 2010). Children who have been abused may be reluctant to disclose their victimization to others for fear of being misunderstood or concern that harm might come to a parent or other family member if they reveal their abuse. Parents of a child who has been exposed to trauma may not inform the school, because they may not understand that their child's trauma may influence the child's behavior in the classroom and/or impact their ability to learn.

Disruptive behaviors exhibited by a child with a history of trauma may not be recognized by school personnel as being a reaction to the trauma and may be considered to be oppositional or defiant behavior (Tishelman et al., 2010). Similarly, a child who has difficulty completing tasks in the classroom because they are preoccupied with memories of the traumatic event or worries that the traumatic event will occur again may be viewed by the teacher as being unmotivated to do the required assignment. Challenges, such as not being able to identify traumatized students and trauma-related behaviors being misunderstood, can make it difficult to determine the educational and psychological needs of children who have been exposed to trauma. To better identify the needs of traumatized children, Diamanduros et al. (2018b) suggested two practices through which school psychologists could better meet the needs of children who have exposed to trauma: (a) trauma screening in schools using Eklund and Rossen's (2016) screening guide and (b) school-based evaluations using Tishelman et al.'s (2010) trauma-lens approach with evaluations.

Eklund and Rossen's (2016) *Guidance for Trauma Screening in Schools* is a useful tool that can be used to screen for trauma using a Multi-Tiered Systems of Support (MTSS) framework and is available on the NASP website.

School-Based Trauma Screening

In an effort to help schools determine the number of students who have been exposed to traumatic events and who are experiencing traumatic stress reactions or students who may be at risk of developing trauma-related symptoms, Eklund and Rossen (2016) created a guide for schools to follow so that they can better serve their students and ensure that students' educational and social–emotional needs can be met through various supports and interventions. The guide, *Guidance for Trauma Screening in Schools*, is available on the NASP website and serves as a useful resource for school psychologists who seek to implement trauma-informed screening practices within their schools. It provides information about universal screening through an MTSS framework and addresses related cautions about screening, parental consent procedures, trauma screening methods, trauma screening instruments, time considerations, and linking screening results to interventions. Informing parents about the screening and obtaining their consent would be a first step in the screening process and could be an opportunity to provide parents with more information about trauma. To ensure that accurate information is obtained, Elkund and Rossen recommend selecting self-report screening instruments rather than using instruments that are completed by some other informant, such as a parent or teacher. In selecting screening instruments, consideration should be given to the developmental appropriateness of the instrument, psychometric properties, and costs. In their guide, Elkund and Rossen provide a list of screening instruments that they reviewed and they include a brief description of the following instruments: Trauma Symptom Checklist for Children-PTSD Subscale (Briere, 1996), Traumatic Events Screening Inventory for Children: Brief Form (Ford et al., 2002), University of California at Los Angeles (UCLA) Posttraumatic Stress Disorder Reaction Index (Steinberg et al., 2013), and Childhood Trauma Questionnaire (Bernstein et al., 1998). Other potential resources for information about trauma screening instruments include NCTSN (www.nctsn.org/treatments-and-practices/screening-and-assessments/measure-reviews), the International Society for Traumatic Stress Studies (https://istss.org/clinical-resources/assessing-trauma), and the National Center for PTSD (www.ptsd.va.gov/professional/assessment/child/index.asp). Another useful resource is the *Review of Trauma Screening Tools for Children and Adolescents* (Wevodau, 2016).

School psychologists might also find the trauma screening process outlined on the NCTSN website useful when developing a plan for trauma screening in their schools. The NCTSN screening process (n.d.-d) focuses on evaluating potential exposure to trauma and traumatic stress reactions such as nightmares and hyperarousal symptoms. It also provides information about the types of trauma screening tools, such as self-report, parent report, and clinician report, and offers suggestions on how to engage families in the screening process. Their website also provides reviews on trauma-related assessment measures such as the Child PTSD Symptom Scale (Foa et al., 2001), Child Stress Disorder Checklist (Saxe et al., 2003), Child's Reactions to Traumatic Events Scale-Revised (Jones, 1994), and the Child Report of Post-Traumatic Symptoms (Greenwald & Rubin, 1999). The reviews address administration, psychometric information, translations, alternate forms, and pros and cons associated with the instrument. The reviews can be found at www.nctsn.org/sites/default/files/resources//complex_trauma_standardized_measures.pdf.

TRAUMA-INFORMED SCHOOL-BASED EVALUATIONS

Given the influence of traumatic experiences on children's development and functioning, school psychologists should consider implementing trauma-informed practices when conducting psychoeducational assessments (Diamanduros et al., 2018b). A trauma-informed approach for school-based evaluations proposed by Tishelman and colleagues (2010) addresses the need to formulate several hypotheses for the child's difficulties that include the possibility of trauma and the reason for the referral and to consider various domains of functioning impacted by trauma that may be contributing to difficulties that the child is experiencing, which led to the referral for an evaluation. Based on their "trauma-lens" approach to school-based evaluation, Tishelman and colleagues indicate that the purpose of the evaluation is to determine the impact of trauma on the child's functioning in the classroom with the goal of developing interventions that take into consideration trauma-related barriers to learning. There are four domains identified by Tishelman and colleagues with core issues in each domain that may contribute negatively to the child's level of functioning or be a relative strength for the child, which can be taken into consideration to build any deficits within the core areas of a domain. These domains have been identified earlier in this chapter as areas in which some traumatized children struggle in their daily lives and include: (a) self-regulation, (b) physical functioning, (c) relationships, and (d) academic functioning. A brief description of core issues within each domain is discussed. For a more thorough discussion of these domains and core issues, see Tishelman et al. (2010).

Self-regulation, the ability to regulate one's emotions, can be negatively influenced by traumatic exposure and is considered to be a source of many traumatic stress reactions exhibited in children who have a history of trauma. As noted by Tishelman and colleagues (2010), core issues within this domain that need to be considered in evaluations include identifying emotions, hypervigilance to potential threats, difficulty in regulating arousal, intense moods, and dissociation. The experience of trauma may render young children with chronic trauma unable to identify the emotions that they are experiencing and to recognize emotions in others around them. They may be hyper-alert to potential threats and react intensely to stimuli that remind them of their traumatic experience. In school, difficulties related to hypervigilance may be manifested in difficulty with transitions, interpersonal conflicts, and heightened reactivity to criticism and/or perceived threat. Difficulties in modulating arousal may be evident in the child's difficulty in sustaining attention and inconsistent performance in class. Further, behaviors of internal arousal levels could vary from the child being emotionally disconnected and appearing lazy to hyperarousal levels displayed through impulsive and disruptive behaviors. The child may utilize maladaptive coping strategies such as engaging in aggressive and self-injurious behaviors. Vulnerability to moods, such as depression and anxiety, may be shown through a lack of motivation to complete schoolwork, frustration when working on tasks, social withdrawal, and angry outbursts targeted at others. Dissociative behaviors may be reflected in inconsistent performance in the classroom and the child not understanding instructions due to what appears to be daydreaming in class, what may be mistaken as lying by denying behaviors that they had engaged in that were observed by others, and behaving differently with different people (Tishelman et al., 2010).

Self-regulation can be impacted by exposure to trauma and is viewed as a contributor to many traumatic stress reactions in youths who have been traumatized (Tishelman et al., 2010).

Physical functioning is another domain to be considered in the trauma-lens approach to evaluation proposed by Tishelman et al. (2010). As indicated earlier, traumatic stress reactions can include internal physiological reactions to trauma that can impact the child's physical functioning. Tishelman and colleagues point out that dissociative reactions may lessen awareness of bodily needs and functions, resulting in enuresis and encopresis as well as eating problems such as forgetting to eat or overeating. Another core issue within this domain includes the impact of stress on the body, which may result in somatic complaints, such as stomachaches and headaches, to which frequent school absences and trips to the school nurse may be attributed. A core issue related to physical functioning relates to rigid or inappropriate physical boundaries in which the child may avoid physical contact or seek inappropriate physical affection, particularly if they were physically violated or observed someone being physically violated. Other core issues identified include physical injuries associated with trauma, including skin injuries such as cuts and burns, as well as unexplained accidental injuries (Tishelman et al., 2010).

Another domain to consider when conducting evaluations is relationships (Tishelman et al., 2010). Trauma of an interpersonal nature, such as abuse by a caregiver, can influence a child's sense of self and impact their ability to establish a relationship with others. A disruption in a child's sense of self may be manifested in school by an inability to understand the consequences of one's own behavior and how it can impact other students' behavior in the classroom, the ability to communicate one's social and emotional needs, feeling empathy toward others, and the possession of a sense of confidence in one's abilities. Complex trauma occurring early in childhood can influence a child's attachment to people and the ability to develop trusting relationships. In the school setting, the child may have difficulty forming relationships with peers and may misinterpret cues from others as hostile, which may result in aggressive behavior toward others. The traumatized child may be vulnerable to betrayal by others and reluctant to seek out social interactions and support from others (Tishelman et al., 2010). Social competence is another core issue to consider when evaluating traumatized children who may exhibit a deficit in social skills and social problem-solving. Difficulties related to social skills and social problem-solving may be manifested in the classroom by social rejection by peers; misunderstanding social cues; hostile interactions with others; behavioral problems when interacting with a large group of peers; avoidance of school, which can result in poor attendance; socially withdrawing from peers; and interacting with younger children rather than same-age peers (Tishelman et al., 2010).

A child's academic functioning can be influenced by trauma's impact on brain development. As discussed earlier in the chapter, chronic trauma can affect neurodevelopment, which may influence information processing and executive functioning skills. Difficulties in processing information may be exhibited in the classroom as not following instructions and having poor auditory processing and reading comprehension skills (Tishelman et al., 2010). Trauma's impact on executive functioning may be manifested in poor organization and difficulties in concentrating, switching from one task to another, working independently, and initiating and completing tasks (Tishelman et al., 2010).

EDUCATIONAL AND SOCIAL–EMOTIONAL SUPPORTS

To address the educational and social–emotional needs of traumatized students, school psychologists can advocate for educational and social–emotional supports to foster learning in the classroom and to create an environment in which children exposed to trauma will feel protected and safe. Diamanduros et al. (2018b) contend that school psychologists can guide their schools in establishing trauma-informed supports that will help the traumatized child to feel safe. They suggest two resources, *Child Trauma Toolkit for Educators* (NCTSN, 2008a) and *Helping Traumatized Children Learn: Creating and Advocating for Trauma-Sensitive Schools* (Cole et al., 2005), both of which provide school-based trauma-informed practices and supports. These resources, along with trauma-informed teaching strategies recommended by Minahan (2019), could be effective tools in helping traumatized children feel safe in the classroom. One support that will assist the child in feeling safe at school is to maintain regular school routines and schedules so that the classroom environment has a sense of predictability and consistency (Minahan, 2019). If any unexpected event, such as a fire drill, is planned for a particular day, it would be important to let the child know in advance so they can expect it and will not be frightened by it. In addition, it would be helpful to inform the student of any upcoming transitions so that the child can anticipate the change and be prepared for it (Diamanduros et al., 2018b). To reduce negative thoughts and reactions when giving directions, it would be helpful for teachers to give the child a choice that enables the child to have a sense of control (Minahan, 2019). It also would be important to provide positive feedback when the child behaves positively, such as "I liked the way you raised your hand to let me know that you were done with the assignment" and phrase negative feedback in a supportive way, such as "You worked hard on this assignment. I see that a word is misspelled here. Let's look up the spelling of the word so you can correct it" (Minahan, 2019).

There may be times when the child might begin to feel overwhelmed in the classroom and may need to talk to someone with whom they feel safe. School psychologists could help teachers identify a specific school professional with whom the student feels comfortable so that, if the student becomes overwhelmed in the classroom and needs a break, that person would be available to talk to the child and provide support. It may also be helpful to have a specific quiet place in the classroom that the child can go to when a brief break from classroom activities is needed (Diamanduros et al., 2018b).

Also, school personnel need to be aware of any trauma-related cues in the environment that might trigger a reaction from the child. For example, a child whose trauma involved a shooting might become startled and frightened when a loud popping noise, such as intercom static or fireworks, occur. If this happens, the teacher could provide support to the child by speaking calmly to the child and letting them know that they are safe (Diamanduros et al., 2018b).

Another trauma-informed practice that teachers could implement is to allow the child extra time to turn in assignments because some traumatized children may be preoccupied with worries about the traumatic event and/or their safety and may struggle to get their work done on time. Providing additional time for them to complete assignments and tests would help them, not only an opportunity to complete their work, but to also have a sense of accomplishment without having additional stress about not getting their work done on time (Diamanduros et al., 2018b).

Social–emotional supports for traumatized children can be provided through an MTSS framework that school psychologists can help to develop in their schools. Rossen and Cowan (2013) contend that MTSS provides a universal and preventative approach to provide support for traumatized students. Through this framework, a continuum of services and supports at different tier levels can be utilized to help the traumatized child learn and function in the classroom. Tier 1 supports—provided to all students—can focus on integrating learning, social–emotional functioning, and mental health to create a school climate that promotes a sense of safety, which is vital for traumatized children who may struggle with feeling unsafe at school, and fosters learning in the classroom. Services at this level might include social–emotional learning programs, bullying-prevention programs, positive behavioral supports (PBS), and/or modified disciplinary practices. Students who are identified as being at risk or who do not respond to Tier 1 supports and services will move up the tiered system to Tiers 2 and 3, which provide more intensive and individualized services. Supports and services at these levels are typically provided in small groups of students who have similar needs (Tier 2) or to individual students who have specific needs (Tier3; Rossen & Cowan, 2013).

Social–emotional supports for children exposed to traumatic experiences can be provided through MTSS (Reinbergs & Fefer, 2018; Rossen & Cowan, 2013).

Others have also proposed the use of an MTSS framework to provide support to students who have been traumatized. Through a thorough review of the literature, Reinbergs and Fefer (2018) provide concrete examples of screenings, interventions, and practitioner support for each of the three tiers of an MTSS framework. Tier 1 screening, as suggested by Reinbergs and Fefer, might include the use of instruments such as the Child Trauma Screen (Lang & Connell, 2016) or the *Behavioral and Emotional Screening System* (BESS; Reynolds & Kamphaus, 2015a), whereas interventions for this tier might include social–emotional learning curriculums or school-wide positive behavioral interventions and support (PBIS) and practitioner support might include the use of the *Child Trauma Toolkit for Educators* (NCTSN, 2008a). According to Reinbergs and Fefer, students who move up to Tier 2 might be screened with the Behavioral Rating Scale for Children-3 (BASC-3; Reynolds & Kamphaus, 2015b), whereas the Bounce Back program (Langley et al., 2015; to be discussed in more detail later in this chapter), designed for young children, might be the intervention used. Tier 2 practitioner support might include professional training through NCTSN that is available for free through the NCTSN Learning Center (https://learn.nctsn.org/). Reinbergs and Fefer indicate that Tier 3 screening might include The Clinician-Administered PTSD Scale for *DSM-5*: Child and Adolescent Version (Pynoos et al., 2015), whereas the intervention might include trauma-focused cognitive behavioral therapy (CBT; Cohen et al., 2012). Practitioner support for Tier 3 might include a referral to an outside clinician. School psychologists are encouraged to advocate for a tiered framework within which to provide support for traumatized teachers, and Reinbergs and Fefer's (2018) model would serve as a useful guide. (For more examples of screening tools, interventions, and practitioner support for an MTSS framework, see Reinbergs and Fefer's [2018] publication.)

SCHOOL-BASED MENTAL HEALTH INTERVENTIONS

Given that traumatic stress reactions can have a significant impact on learning and social–emotional development that could develop into long-term psychological problems, it is imperative that traumatized children and adolescents receive mental health services. Diamanduros et al. (2018b) encourage school psychologists to advocate for the provision of mental health services in schools and to seek training, if necessary, in therapeutic services designed to be implemented in schools. They recommend considering three school-based mental health programs based on CBT that are designed to address traumatic stress symptoms and build coping skills in children and adolescents so that they can manage trauma-related emotions and behaviors. These are (a) Cognitive Behavioral Interventions for Trauma in Schools (CBITS; Nadeem et al., 2011), (b) Support for Students Exposed to Trauma (SSET; Jaycox et al., 2009), and (c) Bounce Back (Langley et al., 2015).

Cognitive Behavioral Interventions for Trauma in Schools

Designed to address the mental health needs of traumatized students in grades 5 to 12, CBITS (Nadeem et al., 2011) is an evidence-based therapeutic program that can be implemented by school-based mental health professionals such as school psychologists. The program is based on trauma-focused CBT and designed to reduce traumatic stress symptoms, cultivate coping skills, and improve overall well-being. CBITS can be provided in small-group settings and consists of 10 sessions with an additional few individual sessions as well as parent and teacher psychoeducational sessions if needed. It provides psychoeducation on trauma so that the child understands how traumatic events impact one's functioning and uses cognitive behavioral strategies such as relaxation techniques, cognitive restructuring, exposure, and social problem-solving. It can be used as a Tier 2 or Tier 3 intervention in an MTSS model (Hoover et al., 2018; Reinbergs & Fefer, 2018). Research studies have found that CBITS is effective in reducing PTSD and depressive symptoms (Kataoka et al., 2003; Stein et al., 2003) as well as improving academic performance (Kataoka et al., 2011). Moreover, it has been implemented in schools serving racially and ethnically diverse students, and results indicated a 90% completion rate, a significant reduction of PTSD symptoms, and an increase in functioning among the students receiving the interventions (Hoover et al., 2018). In a sample of Spanish-speaking, Latino youth, CBITS was found to be effective in lowering traumatic and depressive symptoms (Allison & Ferreira, 2017). Online training and free materials are available via the CBITS website (https://cbitsprogram.org). The CBITS manual, which is available in English, Spanish, and Arabic is available at the RAND website (www.rand.org/pubs/tools/TL272.html#download).

Support for Students Exposed to Trauma

Modeled after the CBITS program, SSET (Jaycox et al., 2009) is a nonclinical evidence-based program designed to address the emotional and psychological needs of students, ages 10 to 14 years old, who struggle with emotional distress such as anxiety or depressed mood related to trauma exposure. The program can be administered by a school professional who does not have clinical training. It can be administered in 10 sessions to middle school students in groups of eight to 10 during a 45-minute period. SSET focuses on training students about traumatic reactions and provides skill building in relaxation, coping with worries, dealing with difficult situations, problem-solving, and developing a trauma narrative. It can also be used as a Tier 2 intervention (Reinbergs & Fefer, 2018). Although online training for teachers and school counselors is available via the SSET website (https://ssetprogram.org/), school psychologists familiar with the program could also provide training and assistance regarding any clinical issues that may need to be addressed (Diamanduros et al., 2018b). The training manual, *SSET Group Leader Training Manual* (Jaycox et al., 2009), includes information about the program, lesson plans, homework assignments to practice techniques learned during the lessons, worksheets, and forms that can be used when implementing the program. The manual is available via RAND at www.rand.org/pubs/technical_reports/TR675.html and can be downloaded as a free ebook.

Bounce Back

Designed for elementary-school students who have been exposed to trauma, the Bounce Back program (Langley et al., 2015) is also adapted from CBITS. This evidence-based clinical program is designed to be implemented by a mental health professional in the school, such as a school psychologist, and focuses on reducing trauma-related distress in students who are between the ages of 5 and 11 years old. It can be administered in a group setting of four to seven students over 10 sessions that focus on emotions identification, problem-solving, coping skills, relaxation techniques, and social support. In comparison to SSET, the Bounce Back program also includes a few individual sessions but has more parental involvement so that parents can learn about trauma reactions and provide support in helping their child practice the techniques at home. It can be used as a Tier 2 intervention (Reinbergs & Fefer, 2018). Free resources and online training are available at the Bounce Back website (https://bouncebackprogram.org).

Three evidence-based interventions designed to address traumatic stress symptoms include (a) CBITS, (b) SSET, and (c) Bounce Back. These interventions can be implemented in schools.

CASE STUDY 17.1 TERRANCE: CASE OF A SEXUALLY ABUSED BOY EXHIBITING TRAUMATIC STRESS REACTIONS

Background

Terrance is an 11-year-old fifth grader who was placed in foster care at age 5. Prior to being in foster care, Terrance lived with his biological mother. His father had left the mother prior to his birth and has not been involved in Terrance's life. The mother was not in contact with any of her relatives. She shared an apartment with a friend who had two teenage sons. The

(continued)

CASE STUDY 17.1 TERRANCE: CASE OF A SEXUALLY ABUSED BOY EXHIBITING TRAUMATIC STRESS REACTIONS (continued)

mother and her friend began to use drugs and were frequently out of the home, leaving the two teenage boys to care for Terrance. The boys sexually abused Terrance and threatened to harm him if he told anyone. Terrance's mother was arrested for drug possession, and Terrance was placed in foster care. He was in three foster homes prior to being with the current foster parents because the previous foster parents indicated that his behavior was "out of control," and they could not manage his behavior. Terrance did not disclose the sexual abuse until he was placed with the current foster parents after living with them for 2 years. The parents shared the information with the school. At home, his behavior is described as impulsive and disruptive. The current foster parents report that he frequently seems "on edge," often gets angry, and is quick to lose his temper. In addition, the foster parents report that he has difficulty following rules at home and is argumentative. Although his behavior is challenging, the foster parents report that they want to help Terrance.

At school, Terrance exhibits aggressive behavior and initiates fights with his peers, which has resulted in him being suspended from school. His teacher reports he has poor social judgment and often becomes upset over minor things, which leads to him becoming aggressive with peers. For example, when a peer tried to get Terrance's attention by tapping him on the shoulder, Terrance jumped and was ready to hit the peer until the teacher intervened. According to his teacher, Terrance seems tense and guarded in the classroom and does not seek social interactions with his peers, tending to keep to himself in the classroom and on the playground. The teacher has noticed that he frequently looks around the room while he is seated at his desk and is easily distracted by what others are doing. When attempting to do classwork, he displays poor concentration and has difficulty starting and completing tasks. Transitioning from one activity to another is challenging for him as evidenced by his becoming distressed when required to change classrooms to go to special activities such as physical education. In addition, the teacher reports that he sometimes becomes visibly overwhelmed and emotionally distressed, but denies his feelings when she attempts to talk to him.

Discussion

Terrance's presentation of emotions and behaviors represents traumatic stress reactions that are characteristic of complex trauma. One of the main areas of difficulty seems to be in self-regulation. He is "on edge," frequently checking his environment, and jumping when his peer tapped his shoulder may represent an internal state of hyperarousal, which puts him on alert for potential or perceived threats that trigger his response to fight. Hence, his overreacting to the peer's tapping his shoulder may have triggered a memory of the sexual abuse that he had experienced in the past and, being in a hyper-aroused internal state, he felt threatened and attempted to protect himself. This hyperarousal may reflect that Terrance does not feel safe at school, and his fear of being vulnerable to more traumatic experiences; hence, he is guarded and tense in the classroom as observed by the teacher and feels the need to protect himself. His reluctance to seek social interactions may represent difficulty in trusting others. The act of one's body being sexually violated by someone with whom a relationship has been established can be experienced as an act of betrayal, resulting in difficulty trusting others. He seems to have perhaps developed some trust in his relationship with the current foster parents given that he disclosed his abuse to them after living with them for 2 years. However, trusting others most likely proves challenging for him. Finally, the impact of his traumatic experiences on his academic functioning is represented in the reported executive functioning deficits of poor concentration, difficulty transitioning from one activity to another, poor impulse control, and difficulty initiating and completing classwork. Moreover, his disruptive behaviors resulted in his being suspended and missing instruction in the classroom.

The school psychologist could be instrumental in helping the school address Terrance's social–emotional and educational needs. One of the first things to do would be to help the parents, teacher, and school administrators understand how trauma has impacted Terrance's functioning and how his difficulty in regulating emotions is linked to the disruptive behaviors observed at home and school. Collaboration with the teacher can focus on identifying ways

(continued)

> **CASE STUDY 17.1 TERRANCE: CASE OF A SEXUALLY ABUSED BOY EXHIBITING TRAUMATIC STRESS REACTIONS** (*continued*)
>
> to help him feel safe in the classroom and to help him start to build positive relationships with his peers. One possible way of helping him to feel safe in the classroom may be to identify possible triggers that lead to his becoming emotionally distressed as well as to have a safe spot to go to when he begins to feel overwhelmed. If he can establish a trusting relationship with a school staff member and begin to feel safe with that person, a plan could be developed that permits him to go to that person if he needs to talk to someone when he feels overwhelmed. Other ways to promote a sense of safety are to inform him ahead of time when there will be a transition from one activity to another and to let him know if there will be a change in his schedule or if something unexpected is planned, such as a fire drill. Transitioning to different classes, such as physical education, may trigger a sense of being vulnerable and unsafe as well as fear that he may be at risk of being victimized again while changing clothes in the locker room prior to participating in physical activities. It might be helpful to collaborate with the physical education teacher so that an adult walks along his side to class and arrangements are made so that he does not have to be in the locker area to change clothes. Having an MTSS framework of support in the schools would be a way of providing Terrance with classroom supports that could build social skills and develop social problem-solving skills. Finally, the school psychologist could implement an intervention, such as the CBITS program, so that Terrance could learn how to utilize various relaxation techniques, recognize and regulate his emotions, and restructure his thoughts so that he can begin to recognize stressful thoughts that trigger anxiety. In addition, the intervention could focus on helping him to recognize the link between his emotions and behavior so that he can monitor his emotions and behavior. Finally, the school psychologist and teacher could identify strategies to strengthen his executive functioning skills so that he can better manage his impulses and concentrate more in the classroom. Providing additional time to complete assignments might also be helpful to Terrance since he gets easily distracted in the classroom and has difficulty completing his work.

SUMMARY POINTS

- Childhood trauma is not an uncommon occurrence and can have a significant impact on a traumatized child's social–emotional and behavioral functioning as well as their ability to learn in the classroom.
- Some children with histories of trauma experience traumatic stress symptoms, which can lead to a diagnosis of PTSD. The DTD diagnosis for children with complex trauma provides a framework that focuses on the developmental effects of trauma, disturbed attachment patterns among children with complex trauma, and emotional dysregulation, which may not be addressed by a diagnosis of PTSD.
- Racial trauma, such as racism and discrimination, can significantly impact a child's development and functioning and needs to be taken into consideration when attempting to help support a child struggling with challenging behaviors and emotions that are related to chronic racial stress, which is being manifested in the child's behavior.
- School psychologists can play an instrumental role in helping traumatized children in schools by raising awareness among educators/school administrators and parents, applying trauma-informed practices in their assessments of students, and providing mental health services in the school.
- Educational and psychological supports using MTSS can help create a learning environment in which traumatized children feel safe and supported in the classroom. Such supports facilitate learning and promote positive social–emotional well-being.

TEST YOUR KNOWLEDGE

1. Which of the following are symptom clusters for the pediatric subtype of PTSD for children younger than 6 years of age?
    a. Re-experiencing the trauma through intrusive thoughts
    b. Avoiding trauma-related stimuli and/or experiencing negative alterations in cognition and mood
    c. Experiencing increased arousal and reactivity
    d. All of the above

2. Self-regulation is an area impacted by trauma and is considered to be a contributor to many symptoms exhibited in children, such as difficulty controlling emotions.
    a. True
    b. False

3. CBITS, SSET, and Bounce Back use a therapeutic approach that is based on CBT.
    a. True
    b. False

4. Working within an MTSS framework, which of the following tiers might the BESS be used to screen for children who may be dealing with traumatic stress symptoms?
    a. Tier 1
    b. Tier 2
    c. Tier 3

5. Executive functioning difficulties are not experienced by traumatized children.
    a. True
    b. False

Answers: (1) d, (2) a, (3) a, (4) a, (5) b.

DISCUSSION QUESTIONS

1. Compare the main *DSM-5* diagnostic features of PTSD for children younger than age 6 and the main diagnostic features of van der Kolk's proposed DTD diagnosis.

2. Discuss the ways in which racial trauma may impact youth of color.

3. Discuss the ways in which trauma can impact a child's social–emotional and behavioral functioning.

4. Discuss the ways in which trauma can impact a child's learning and functioning in the classroom.

5. Discuss how social–emotional support for trauma can be provided through an MTSS framework.

CHAPTER RESOURCES

For School Psychologists

EVIDENCE-BASED INTERVENTIONS

Bounce Back: https://bouncebackprogram.org
Cognitive Behavioral Interventions for Trauma in Schools (CBITS): https://cbitsprogram.org
Support for Students Exposed to Trauma (SSET): https://ssetprogram.org
Trauma-Focused Cognitive Behavioral Therapy Web: http://tfcbt.musc.edu/
Trauma-Focused Coping in Schools (TFC): www.nctsn.org/interventions/trauma-focused-coping-schools

Books

The Body Keeps the Score: Brain, Mind, and Body in the Healing of Trauma by Bessel van der Kolk, MD (2015)
Child Trauma Handbook: A Guide for Helping Trauma-Exposed Children and Adolescents by Ricky Greenwald (2005)
Children and Trauma: A Guide for Parents and Professionals by Cynthia Monahon (1993)
Clinical Work With Traumatized Young Children by Joy D. Osofsky (2013)
Cognitive-Behavioral Therapies for Trauma by V. M. Follette and J. I. Ruzek (2007)
Early Intervention for Trauma and Traumatic Loss by Brett T. Litz (2003)
Helping Children Cope With Disasters and Terrorism by Annette M. La Greca (2002)
Mass Trauma and Violence: Helping Families and Children Cope by Nancy Boyd Webb (2003)
Neurobiologically Informed Trauma Therapy With Children and Adolescents: Understanding Mechanisms of Change by Linda Chapman (2014)
Trauma Therapy in Context: The Science and Craft of Evidence-Based Practice edited by Robert A. McMackin, EdD; Elana Newman, PhD; Jason M. Fogler, PhD; and Terence M. Keane, PhD (2012)
Understanding and Assessing Trauma in Children and Adolescents: Measures, Methods, and Youth in Context by Kathleen Nader (2015)
Young Children and Trauma: Intervention and Treatment by Joy D. Osofsky (2004)

Online Resources

Child Trauma Academy: http://childtrauma.org/
Child Trauma Institute: www.childtrauma.com
Coping With Disaster: www.mhanational.org/coping-disaster
National Association of School Psychologists (NASP) *Trauma Resources*: www.nasponline.org/resources-and-publications/resources-and-podcasts/school-climate-safety-and-crisis/mental-health-resources/trauma
National Association of School Psychologists (NASP) *A National Tragedy: Helping Children Cope*: www.nasponline.org/resources/crisis_safety/terror_general.aspx
National Child Traumatic Stress Network (NCTSN): www.nctsn.org/
National Child Traumatic Stress Network (NCTSN) *Training Resources*: www.nctsn.org/resources/training
National Center for Children Exposed to Violence: www.nccev.org/
National Crime Victims Research and Treatment Center: https://medicine.musc.edu/departments/psychiatry/divisions-and-programs/divisions/ncvc
National Institute of Mental Health *Helping Children and Adolescents Cope With Violence and Disaster: What Parents Can Do*: www.nimh.nih.gov/health/publications/helping-children-and-adolescents-cope-with-violence-and-disasters-parents/index.shtml
Parenting After Traumatic Events: Ways to Support Children: https://psychcentral.com/lib/parenting-after-traumatic-events-ways-to-support-children
University of Minnesota Extension *Historical Trauma and Cultural Healing*: https://extension.umn.edu/mental-health/historical-trauma-and-cultural-healing
Zero to Three: National Center for Infants, Toddlers, and Families: www.zerotothree.org

For Parents

Books

Children Changed by Trauma: A Healing Guide by D. W. Alexander (1999)
Children and Trauma: A Guide for Parents and Professionals by Cynthia Monahon (1993)
Coping With Trauma: A Guide to Self-Understanding by J. G. Allen (1995)
The Grieving Child: A Parent's Guide by H. Fitzgerald (1992)
Integrative Parenting: Strategies for Raising Children Affected by Attachment Trauma by Debra Wesselmann, Cathy Schweitzer, and Stefanie Armstrong (2014)
It's Okay to Cry: A Parent's Guide to Helping Children Through the Losses of Life by H. Norman Wright (2004)
The Scared Child: Helping Kids Overcome Traumatic Events by Barbara Brooks and Paula M. Siegel (1996)

For Children

BOOKS

A Terrible Thing Happened: A Story for Children Who Have Witnessed Violence or Trauma by Margaret M. Holmes (2000)
Always and Forever by Alan Durant (2013)
Badger's Parting Gifts by Susan Varley (1992)
Bear's Last Journey by Udo Weigelt (2003)
The Dead Bird by Margaret Brown Wise (2016)
Everett Anderson's Goodbye by Lucille Clifton (1988)
Goodbye Mousie by Robie H. Harris (2004)
Jenny Is Scared: When Sad Things Happen in the World by Carol Shuman (2003)
The Next Place by Warren Hanson (2002)
The Purple Balloon by Chris Raschka (2007)
Remembering Crystal by Sebastian Loth (2010)

KEY REFERENCES

Only key references appear in the print edition. The full reference list appears in the digital product on Springer Publishing Connect: connect.springerpub.com/content/book/978-0-8261-3587-2/part/part07/chapter/ch17

American Psychiatric Association. (2013). *Diagnostic and statistical manual of mental disorders* (5th ed.). https://doi.org/10.1176/appi.books.9780890425596
National Association of School Psychologists. (2016a). *Managing strong emotional reactions to traumatic events: Tips for parent and educators.* https://www.nasponline.org/resources-and-publications/resources-and-podcasts/school-climate-safety-and-crisis/mental-health-resources/trauma/managing-strong-emotional-reactions-to-traumatic-events-tips-for-families-and-teachers
National Center for PTSD. (n.d.). *Understand PTSD: How common is PTSD in children and adolescents?* https://www.ptsd.va.gov/understand/common/common_children_teens.asp
National Child Traumatic Stress Network. (2008a). *Child trauma toolkit for educators.* https://www.nctsn.org/sites/default/files/resources//child_trauma_toolkit_educators.pdf
National Child Traumatic Stress Network. (2014). *Complex trauma: Facts for educators.* Author.
National Child Traumatic Stress Network. (2020a). *Understanding child trauma.* https://www.nctsn.org/sites/default/files/resources/fact-sheet/understanding_child_trauma_and_the_nctsn_0.pdf
Spinazzola, J., Habib, M., Blaustein, M., Knoverek, A., Kisiel, C., Stolbach, B., Abramovitz, R., Kagan, R., Lanktree, C., & Maze, J. (2017). *What is complex trauma? A resource guide for youth and those who care about them.* National Center for Child Traumatic Stress.
van der Kolk, B. A. (2005). Developmental trauma disorder: Toward a rational diagnosis for children with complex trauma histories. *Psychiatric Annals, 35*(5), 401–408. https://doi.org/10.3928/00485713-20050501-06

CHAPTER 18

Reactive Attachment Disorder

LEARNING OBJECTIVES

- Know the *Diagnostic and Statistical Manual of Mental Disorders* (5th ed.; *DSM-5*; American Psychiatric Association [APA], 2013) diagnostic criteria of Reactive Attachment Disorder (RAD).
- Describe the impact of RAD on a young child's social–emotional and behavioral functioning.
- Identify ways in which RAD may impact a young child's ability to learn in the classroom.
- Summarize how school psychologists can help to address the needs of children with RAD.
- Become familiar with educational supports and school-based mental health interventions to address the educational and mental health needs of children with RAD.

INTRODUCTION

Reactive attachment disorder (RAD) disorder is a rare, complex disorder that occurs in young children who have experienced severe social neglect that has contributed to the child's inability to establish an attachment to a primary caregiver (American Psychiatric Association [APA], 2013; Zeanah et al., 2016). The child may have experienced inconsistent and/or inadequate care from multiple caregivers as might occur with being placed in multiple foster homes or when being raised in overcrowded institutions, such as orphanages, in which there is a high child-to-caregiver ratio (APA, 2013). These types of early environments, which may be characterized by emotional deprivation, can contribute to the child's emotional needs not being met. As Zeanah and colleagues note (2016), the core feature of RAD is the lack of a selective attachment to a caregiver. As a result of not having established an emotional attachment with a primary caregiver, the child fails to engage with others on an emotional level and may experience social–emotional and behavioral difficulties (Cuyvers et al., 2020). For example, the child may display a lack of prosocial behaviors and appear to be withdrawn, resistant to being comforted by others, and reluctant to engage with others. Although the symptoms of RAD must be evident in early childhood for diagnostic purposes, these difficulties can extend into adolescence and adulthood and result in the individual having problems establishing close, trusting relationships with others (APA, 2013; Cuyvers et al., 2020; Humphreys et al., 2017; Nelson et al., 2018; Seim et al., 2020; Sonuga-Barke et al., 2017). However, despite a history of early emotional and social neglect, most children raised under these circumstances do not develop RAD, and the prognosis of the child's later development depends on the quality of caregiving provided after the period of extreme neglect (APA, 2013; Humphreys et al., 2017; Zeanah & Gleason, 2010).

Another disorder, disinhibited social engagement disorder (DSED), is also thought to be an outcome of serious social neglect and inadequate caregiving in early childhood. Although the primary identified risk factor for both RAD and DSED is severe social neglect, the presentation of symptoms differs substantially between the two disorders (APA, 2013; Zeanah et al., 2016). Although children with RAD may appear withdrawn and rarely seek comfort from others or respond to attempts by others to provide comfort, children with DSED are disinhibited and actively seek interactions with others, even those with whom they are unfamiliar (APA, 2013). Compared to DSED, RAD is considered to be a rarer disorder. Although the prevalence of RAD is not actually known, it is estimated that this disorder occurs in less than 10% of children exposed to severe social neglect in their early development (APA, 2013; Bruce et al., 2019). This chapter focuses on RAD and related diagnostic and cultural issues. It also examines the impact that RAD has on a young child's functioning. In addition, the chapter addresses the implications for school psychologists and offers suggestions for educational support and school-based mental health interventions.

DIAGNOSTIC ISSUES RELATED TO REACTIVE ATTACHMENT DISORDER

Etiological Considerations

In typical development, attachment is a biological process that is established between an infant and caregiver, which provides the infant with a sense of comfort and nurturing during times of distress (Bowlby, 1969). Prior to approximately 7 months of age, infants will seek interaction with others who may or may not be familiar to them. Between 7 and 9 months of age, infants selectively attach to a preferred caregiver with whom they have substantial interaction and become wary or apprehensive of individuals with whom they are unfamiliar (Zeanah et al., 2016). In anticipation of being separated from the primary caregiver, the child may protest and become distressed. At this point in development (after a developmental age of 7 to 9 months), selective attachment can be established between the infant and caregiver with whom they have spent much time (Zeanah et al., 2016). There are, however, environmental influences that can have an adverse impact on the process of selective attachment. Research studies have found that young children raised in conditions of extreme neglect and parental deprivation can have an adverse impact on the child's early development, placing the child's attachment to a primary caregiver at risk (Corval et al., 2017). Institutional care has been identified by many researchers as a risk factor for attachment disorders given the limited opportunities for establishing a preferred attachment to a primary caregiver (Corval et al., 2017; Zeanah et al., 2016).

Early research studies on the impact of adverse caregiving and living conditions focused on children with histories of living in institutions, being adopted after living in an institution, and living in foster care. In a uniquely designed study, Zeanah and colleagues (2009) conducted a randomized study that was known as the *Bucharest Early Intervention Project*. The purpose of the study was to determine whether young children between the ages of 6 and 30 months living in institutional care would exhibit less psychopathology after being placed in foster care at 54 months. The study included a sample of Romanian preschool children who lived in an institution in Bucharest, a sample of Romanian preschool children who had previously lived in institutional care prior to being placed in foster care, and a sample of Romanian preschoolers in the general population who had no history of institutional care. The findings of this research indicated that young children with a history of institutional care exhibited more mental health difficulties than children without a history of institutional care. Children with a prior history of living in an institution who are currently placed in a foster home were found to be less likely to experience internalizing behaviors than young children living in an institution. In addition, girls who were placed in foster homes were less symptomatic than boys, who demonstrated no reduction in symptom presentation after being placed in foster care (Zeanah et al., 2009).

A follow-up study of this same group of children was conducted 8 years later, as the children were approaching preadolescence (Humphreys et al., 2017). The purpose of the follow-up study was to examine whether signs of RAD were still evident in older children with histories of institutional care. The children with histories of abandonment and raised in institutional care were assessed for symptoms of RAD and DSED at age 12 and compared to children who were placed in high-quality foster care as well as children who had no histories of institutional care (2017). The findings of their study revealed that children who had been raised in institutions at an early age had more symptoms of RAD and DSED at preadolescence than the comparison group of children who had not been raised in an institution. The results of the study also revealed that children placed in high-quality foster care had significantly less symptoms of RAD and DSED than children raised in an institution. In addition, Humphreys et al. (2017) found that the number of disruptions in caregiving and the amount of time that the child had spent being raised in an institution significantly predicted symptoms of attachment disorder in preadolescence. The researchers concluded that, although children exposed to neglectful and inadequate caregiving early in development can exhibit signs of impaired attachment later on in life, they may show reduced signs of RAD and DSED after being placed in high-quality caregiving environments (Humphreys et al., 2017).

DSM-5 Diagnostic Criteria Related to Reactive Attachment Disorder

The *Diagnostic and Statistical Manual of Mental Disorders*, Third Edition (*DSM-III*; APA, 1980), included the first description of RAD as a mental health disorder (Leveille, 2014; Zeanah & Boris, 2000; Zeanah & Gleason, 2010). The central features of the disorder identified with this version of the *DSM* included a lack of social responsivity, failure to thrive as evident in weight loss and slow growth, and presence of symptoms noted prior to 8 months of age (Zeanah & Boris, 2000). As Zeanah and Boris (2000) note, these core features as outlined in the *DSM-III* were problematic, because selective attachment in infancy does not occur prior to 8 months of age. The revised version, *DSM-III-R* (APA, 1987), indicated that the focus of the disorder was abnormal social relatedness, and the age of onset had to be within the first 5 years (Zeanah & Boris, 2000). In addition, two subtypes of RAD, inhibited and disinhibited, were introduced. Characteristics of the inhibited subtype included internalizing behaviors such as emotional withdrawal, sadness, and fear, whereas characteristics of the disinhibited subtype included externalizing behaviors such as indiscriminate social interaction (Leveille, 2014; Zeanah & Gleason, 2010). It should be noted that the revisions in criteria at this point were not based on data from research studies (Humphreys et al., 2017). Although diagnostic criteria were similar for the *DSM-IV* and its revised version (*DSM-IV-TR*; APA, 1994, 2000), the two subtypes of RAD were presented as two individual disorders, RAD and DSED, with more extensive criteria listed for each under the Trauma- and Stressor-Related Disorders category in the *DSM-5* (APA, 2013).

The decision to present RAD and DSED as two separate disorders was based on validity data from many earlier studies that have examined young children currently and formerly in institutional care, children in foster care, and children in deprived groups who are at risk of inept parenting (Zeanah & Gleason, 2010). The studies have been reviewed in detail by Zeanah and Gleason (2010). Interested readers are encouraged to review Zeanah and Gleason's (2010) article, which is referenced at the end of this chapter. The *DSM-5* conceptualization of RAD and DSED as separate disorders has also been supported by more recent research. Lehmann and colleagues (2016) conducted a study using a sample of foster children with no prior history of institutionalization. The findings of this research study indicated that RAD and DSED were individual constructs that are distinct from other mental health disorders (Lehman et al., 2016).

> The *DSM-5* (APA, 2013) conceptualizes RAD and DSED as two separate disorders.

Based on the *DSM-5* (APA, 2013), diagnostic criteria of RAD in young children include a steady pattern of disturbed attachment behaviors that are developmentally inappropriate and reflect the child's difficulties in establishing meaningful relationships. Emotionally withdrawn behavior toward the child's caregivers is exhibited by the child's lack of or minimal effort to seek comfort under distressing conditions and the child's lack of or minimal response to efforts made by others to comfort the child when distraught. For example, typically developing young children seek out their primary caregivers for comfort, reassurance, and protection when they are upset and/or afraid. Infants and young children with RAD do not consistently demonstrate an effort to seek comfort, support, or protection when they are distressed. If an adult attempts to provide comfort, the infant or child exhibits little to no reaction to these attempts (APA, 2013).

The presence of a social–emotional disturbance is another criterion of RAD (APA, 2013; Zeanah et al., 2016). This must be a continual disturbance exhibited by the child and can be manifested in a few ways. One way is that the young child displays little to no social–emotional reaction when interacting with others. Also, there is little, if any, positive emotion shown by the young child. Also, some young children may appear afraid, depressed, or irritable in their interactions with caregivers even though there may be no explanation for these negative emotions. Hence, children with RAD may struggle to regulate their emotions (APA, 2013; Zeanah & Gleason, 2010). It should be noted that the *DSM-5* (APA, 2103) stipulates that at least two of the three indicators (little to no social–emotional responsiveness; minimal positive affect; and displays of fearfulness, sadness, and irritability in nonthreatening situations) of a social–emotional disturbance must be met.

Diagnostic criteria for RAD also specify that the child have a history of severe inadequate care (APA, 2013). This criterion may be met by continued social neglect in which the young child's basic emotional needs were not met by adults in the child's early life who were responsible for the child's care. Extreme inadequate care may also have resulted from having frequent changes in major caregivers during their early development that reduced the opportunities to bond with a primary caregiver. For example, young children in foster care may often be placed with several different foster families during the period of early development, which makes it difficult for the child to become attached to a consistent caregiver. A third way in which a young child might experience extreme inadequate care is growing up in an atypical setting, such as an institution in which there are many children and few caregivers and few opportunities to develop preferred attachments. At least one of these three ways in which inadequate care is provided in early childhood must have been experienced. The *DSM-5* (APA, 2013) also stipulates that the care provided in one of these three situations is responsible for the child's tendency to be inhibited and emotionally withdrawn. This stipulation is to ensure that, as Zeanah and Gleason point out (2010), a diagnosis of RAD is not made without a known history of social neglect or maltreatment that limits the child's ability to establish a selective attachment to a caregiver.

> A diagnosis of RAD cannot be made unless there is a known history of social neglect or maltreatment that impacts the child's ability to develop a preferred attachment to a caregiver.

Other criteria require that the social–emotional disturbance is present prior to age 5. To meet diagnostic criteria for RAD, the child must also have a developmental age of at least 9 months, which is around the age at which a child can selectively attach to a caregiver (APA, 2013; Zeanah & Gleason, 2010). As noted by Zeanah and Gleason (2010), children with selective attachment do not exhibit inhibited and emotionally withdrawn behaviors that are characteristic of RAD, and therefore, the core of RAD is most likely an absence of a selective attachment, which contributes to an impairment in social–emotional functioning. The authors, however, note that social–emotional functioning can improve if the child is later placed in a more supportive, nurturing environment. In addition, the *DSM-5* (APA, 2013) indicates that a diagnosis of RAD cannot be made if diagnostic criteria is met for Autism Spectrum Disorder (ASD), which also features impairment in social–emotional functioning. If the social–emotional disturbance has been present for more than 12 months, the disorder is noted to be persistent. When the young child's presenting symptoms meet all of the diagnostic criteria and each symptom occurs at a high level, a severe level of impairment can be noted (APA, 2013).

Based on the clinical presentation of children with RAD, it is clear that they may present with social–emotional and interpersonal difficulties that are associated with a disturbance in early selective attachment to a caregiver, which can be challenging for school personnel. Therefore, it is important that school psychologists be involved in helping address potential problems. School psychologists should be mindful of the importance of a developmental history and make efforts to gain information from children who have early histories of multiple foster care placements and/or international adoption. Knowledge of the diagnostic criteria associated with RAD enables school psychologists to better serve children who may be at risk for RAD.

Differential Diagnosis Related to Reactive Attachment Disorder

It is important that children with RAD be properly diagnosed and that professionals working with them, such as school psychologists, be aware of other disorders that may have clinical features similar to RAD. Within the literature, professionals conducting RAD research and working with young children who have been diagnosed with RAD have identified disorders that must be distinguished from RAD (APA, 2013; Zeanah et al., 2016). These disorders include ASD, intellectual disabilities/intellectual developmental delay, and depressive disorder.

As indicated earlier, one of the diagnostic criteria for RAD is that the diagnostic criteria for ASD have been ruled out (APA, 2013). Common features between RAD and ASD include odd social behaviors, diminished social reciprocity, social withdrawal, and reduced display of positive emotions (APA, 2013; Zeanah et al., 2016). Major distinguishing factors between the two disorders include: (a) children with RAD have a history of early social–emotional neglect and deprivation, whereas children with ASD typically have not experienced inadequate care that is characteristic of RAD; (b) children with RAD generally do not exhibit restricted interests and repetitive behaviors as seen in children with ASD; (c) both disorders can be associated with cognitive impairments but selective impairments in social communication are associated with ASD, whereas social communication in children with RAD is comparable to their overall cognitive functioning; and (d) children with ASD exhibit attachment behaviors to primary caregivers, whereas children with RAD demonstrate a lack of attachment to their caregivers (APA, 2013; Zeanah et al., 2016). It should be noted that stereotypic motor behaviors may be evident in both disorders, but impairments in symbolic representations (such as symbolic play) that are characteristic of ASD are not seenout of proportion to the level of cognitive functionin in children with RAD out of proportion to the level of cognitive functioning (Zeanah et al., 2016).

In order to make a diagnosis of RAD based on the *DSM-5*, the child cannot meet diagnostic criteria for ASD.

Intellectual disability/intellectual developmental delay also needs to be distinguished from RAD (APA, 2013; Zeanah et al., 2016). Although children with RAD may have cognitive delays, there are clear distinctions between RAD and intellectual disability/intellectual developmental delay. For example, children with an intellectual disability/intellectual developmental delay typically do not have emotional dysregulation or reduced expression of positive emotions as is seen in children with RAD (APA, 2013; Zeanah et al., 2016). In addition, children with an intellectual disability/intellectual developmental delay who have a developmental age of at least 9 months should have selected attachments no matter their chronological age (APA, 2013). In comparison, children with RAD do not demonstrate preferred attachments even if they have a developmental age of at least 9 months.

Finally, depressive disorders may also need to be considered in a differential diagnosis for RAD (APA, 2013). As with children with RAD, children with depression demonstrate diminished positive emotions and difficulty regulating emotions. However, the two disorders can be distinguished from one another given that a lack of selective attachment and response to being comforted by caregivers is characteristic of RAD but is not typically present in the history of most children with depression (APA, 2013; Zeanah et al., 2016).

Comorbidity Related to Reactive Attachment Disorder

Identifying coexisting disorders is important so that appropriate interventions can be planned for children with RAD (Seim et al., 2020). However, obtaining a clear understanding of comorbidity in RAD is challenging in that earlier studies that examined coexisting disorders in children with RAD used samples of participants whose diagnosis was based on the *DSM-IV* (APA, 1994) criteria. This can be limiting in that some studies did not separate participants by the inhibited and disinhibited subtypes of RAD. For example, Lehmann and colleagues (2013) examined mental health problems in a sample of Norwegian children placed in foster care who were between the ages of 6 and 12. Approximately, 19% of the children were diagnosed with the *DSM-IV* diagnosis of RAD and, of this group, about 59% had a coexisting disorder in the primary diagnostic groups of emotional disorders (such as anxiety and depression), ADHD, and behavioral disorders (such as oppositional defiant disorder and conduct disorder). However, there was no distinction between the subtypes and which disorders coexisted with each subtype. As noted earlier, the *DSM-5* (APA, 2013) now identifies the two subtypes as two separate disorders, RAD and DSED. Given that RAD is a rare disorder, the number of studies conducted on RAD is limited. Of the studies that have been published, some have used a combined sample of children with either RAD or DSED based on the *DSM-5* diagnostic criteria (Davidson et al., 2015). For example, Davidson and colleagues (2015) found that a combined sample of children with *DSM-5* diagnoses of RAD or DSED exhibited emotional and behavioral problems, but it is not clear whether the emotional or behavioral problems are associated more with RAD or DSED because a combined sample was used. Issues, such as the ones raised here, can make it difficult to fully understand which disorders may coexist with RAD as defined by the current *DSM-5* definition.

It should be noted that the *DSM-5* (APA, 2013) minimally addresses comorbidity with RAD, only noting that depressive disorders and some problems such as cognitive and language delays or impairments and stereotypical behaviors may be associated with RAD. Similarly, Zeanah and colleagues (2016) identified the same areas associated with RAD based on *DSM-5* diagnostic criteria of this disorder, namely, depressive symptoms, cognitive impairments, and language impairments. Zeanah et al. (2016) also noted that some children with histories of maltreatment have been found to exhibit symptoms of posttraumatic stress disorder (PTSD) and RAD, but an association between RAD and PTSD has not yet been documented. It is clear that additional studies are needed using the current *DSM-5* diagnosis for RAD to determine comorbidity in young children with RAD.

Given that little is known about comorbidity in young children diagnosed under the *DSM-5* criteria of RAD and comorbidity in young children may differ from coexisting disorders in adolescents diagnosed with RAD, Seim and colleagues (2020) conducted a study examining comorbidity in a sample of Norwegian youth who lived in residential care and were between 12 and 20 years in age. Their study revealed that a majority of adolescents diagnosed with RAD also had at least one to two co-occurring disorders. Specifically, anxiety and depressive disorders were the most common coexisting disorders in children diagnosed with RAD, whereas conduct disorder and oppositional defiant disorder were found in a minority of adolescents with RAD. As the researchers pointed out, this finding of behavioral as well as emotional disorders in youth with RAD is contradictory to previous studies (Corval et al., 2019) in preschoolers that indicated emotional problems are more associated with RAD than behavioral problems. However, Seim and colleagues contend that their findings are consistent with the results of other studies focusing on school-aged children and early adolescents (e.g. Zimmermann & Iwanski, 2018). The authors concluded that evidence of behavioral problems in school-aged children and adolescents diagnosed with RAD may reflect developmental changes that occur from early childhood to adolescence (Seim et al., 2020).

School-Based Eligibility

Although RAD is a rare disorder, a school psychologist may get a referral to conduct an assessment on a child with an early developmental history of social neglect and deprivation who appears to have a social–emotional disturbance. Concern has been voiced in the literature that children with RAD may not be identified readily in early childhood educational settings (Bosmans et al., 2020). It is important that school psychologists are familiar with possible social, emotional, and behavioral indicators of RAD so that young children can be identified and their social–emotional, behavioral, and educational needs can be addressed either through special education services or accommodations provided in the general educational setting.

To determine whether the child is eligible for special education and related services under the federal legislation, Individuals with Disabilities Education Improvement Act (IDEA) of 2004, the multidisciplinary team would need to determine whether the child has a disability and is in need of special education services (Salvia et al., 2016). The team also needs to determine whether the child's difficulties are having an adverse impact on their academic performance (IDEA, 2004).

Given that a social–emotional disturbance is a diagnostic feature of RAD, a disability category that would most likely be considered for a child who exhibits difficulties associated with RAD is Emotional Disturbance (ED) or Emotional Behavioral Disorder, depending on the term used by individual states. Under Section 300.8 (c) (4) of IDEA (2004), an ED is considered a condition that the child has experienced for a long time that has a negative impact on the child's educational performance. A medical diagnosis of RAD is not required in order to determine eligibility for an ED (Losinski et al., 2016). However, one or more of the following characteristics must be present in order to meet criteria for an ED: an inability to learn that cannot be attributed to any intellectual, sensory, or health factors; an inability to develop and keep satisfactory relationships with teachers and peers; inappropriate emotions and behaviors exhibited under typical situations; a pervasive state of being unhappy and sad; and a tendency to develop fear or physical symptoms related to school or personal difficulties (IDEA, 2004). It is important to note that under IDEA (2004), ED includes children and adolescents with schizophrenia, but does not include youths with social maladjustment unless the child also experiences an ED.

Depending on the child's needs and the assessment data, the multidisciplinary team may decide that the child does not meet eligibility requirements for special education but would benefit from accommodations to address the child's educational needs. For example, the child may exhibit some socialemotional or behavioral difficulties but they are not having an adverse impact on the child's educational performance. It may be that the child's need for additional supports or services can be met through the civil rights legislation Section 504 of the Rehabilitation Act of 1973. This legislation protects the rights of individuals with disabilities or a suspected disability and stipulates that the disability negatively impacts at least one or more major life function. Establishing a 504 plan may be an option for the multidisciplinary team to consider as a means of ensuring that the child's educational, social–emotional, or behavioral needs are met so that the child can function in the classroom.

CULTURAL ISSUES RELATED TO REACTIVE ATTACHMENT DISORDER IN YOUTH

It should be noted that the *DSM-5* cautions clinicians when making a diagnosis of RAD in a person whose culture has not been fully studied with regard to attachment. Within the developmental psychology and attachment literature, attachment patterns in North American and European countries have been well documented (Ainsworth et al., 1978; Main & Solomon, 1986). Cross-cultural patterns of attachment in non-Western cultures have also been studied (Keller, 2013; Mesman et al., 2016; Sagi, 1990; van Ijzendoorn & Sagi-Schwartz, 2008). Mesman and colleagues (2016) reviewed studies of attachment beliefs and patterns across several countries and concluded that the findings of these studies are consistent with "the bold conjectures of attachment theory about the universality of attachment, the normativity of secure attachment, the link between sensitive caregiving and attachment security, and the competent child outcomes of secure attachment" (p. 809). They also emphasized the need for more research that focuses on attachment beliefs and patterns in countries such as India and many Islamic countries as well as parts of Africa, Latin America, and Asia. Readers who are interested in learning more about attachment patterns across various cultures are encouraged to review work by Keller (2013), Mesman et al. (2016), and van Ijzendoorn & Sagi-Schwartz (2008).

> The *DSM-5* cautions clinicians when making a diagnosis in persons whose making a diagnosis of RAD in culture has not been fully studied with regard to attachment.

According to the *DSM-5* (APA, 2013), attachment behaviors similar to RAD have been noted in young children in various countries and, as seen earlier, is associated with institutional care and/or multiple placements in foster care that disrupt the child's ability to selectively attach to a primary caregiver (APA, 2013; Spangler et al., 2019; Zeanah et al., 2016). Dozier and colleagues (2012) studied institutional care for young children, noting that "Millions of infants and toddlers are in institutional care around the world, care that is poorly suited to meet young children's developmental needs" (p. 1). In fact, it is estimated that the number of children living in institutional care falls in the range of 2 to 4 million (Dozier et al., 2012). As Dozier et al. (2012) point out, most children are placed in institutional care because of parental instability and poverty. Although over the years, there has been an effort in North America and Western Europe to move away from institutional care and to utilize foster care, Dozier and colleagues point out that institutional care is still commonly used in many countries in Eastern Europe, Central and South America, Africa, Asia, and the Middle East. Institutional settings are often associated with factors that can impact a young child's psychological development such as "generally high child-to-caregiver ratios; caregivers with low wages and little education or training who work rotating shifts; regimented and non-individualized care; and a lack of psychological investment in the children" (p. 4). These factors are linked to social neglect and inadequate care, which can impact the young child's ability to selectively attach to a caregiver, which is a core feature of RAD (Dozier et al., 2012).

It is estimated that the number of children living in institutional care falls in the range of 2 to 4 million (Dozier et al., 2012).

Evidence of RAD symptoms exhibited in children living in institutional and foster care has been reported in many different countries such as the United States (Zeanah et al., 2004), United Kingdom (Bruce et al., 2019), Finland (Upadhyaya et al., 2019), Georgia and Germany (Spangler et al., 2019), Portugal (Corval et al., 2017), Romania (Guyon-Harris, Humphreys, Degnan, et al., 2019; Guyon-Harris, Humphreys, Fox, et al., 2019; Zeanah et al., 2009), Norway (Seim et al., 2020), and Korea (Hong et al., 2018). However, as noted earlier, many studies consist of samples based on the *DSM-IV* definition of RAD, whereas other studies use a combined sample of RAD and DSED based on the definition provided by *DSM-5* or *International Classification of Diseases, Tenth Revision (ICD-10), Classification of Mental and Behavioural Disorders* (World Health Organization, 1992). In addition, RAD is a rare disorder so recruiting enough participants to conduct a study can be challenging. Given these methodological issues, cross-cultural research on children diagnosed with the current *DSM-5* criteria of RAD is limited.

IMPACT OF REACTIVE ATTACHMENT DISORDER ON SOCIAL–EMOTIONAL AND BEHAVIORAL FUNCTIONING IN SCHOOL AND HOME ENVIRONMENTS

Research on social–emotional and behavioral difficulties in children with a *DSM-5* diagnosis of RAD is limited, and inconsistent findings among various studies provide challenges in understanding the impact of RAD on a child's psychosocial development. Issues related to inconsistent findings include small sample size, which set of *DSM* (*DSM-IV* versus *DSM-5*) diagnostic criteria was used, and different age levels of participants in the samples (Bruce et al., 2019). Despite these problematic issues among many of the published research studies, the findings can provide an examination into the type of social–emotional and behavioral difficulties in children exhibiting RAD behaviors. Given that an association between the parent–child relationship and psychopathology in early childhood has been demonstrated in the literature, it is likely that children with RAD will experience mental health difficulties (Bruce et al., 2019). The discussion that follows focuses on the major areas of difficulties exhibited in children with RAD in the school and home settings.

Social–Emotional and Behavioral Difficulties at School

As noted earlier, children diagnosed with RAD have a persistent social–emotional disturbance that is characterized by limited positive emotion; little social–emotional response to other people; and/or exhibiting unexplained fearfulness, unhappiness, or irritability in situations that do not warrant such negative emotions (APA, 2103). A young child with RAD may look withdrawn and unhappy, not smile in response to other people smiling at them, and/or seem uninterested in others around them. They may have difficulty interacting with others and, although they may find it hard to calm down when they become upset, they tend not to seek comfort from others (American Academy of Child and Adolescent Psychiatry [AACAP], 2014). Early social neglect and inadequate care can render a child unable to develop an attachment to a preferred caregiver (Zeanah et al., 2016), which could influence their ability to trust others and establish interpersonal relationships later on in life such as with teachers and peers at school. It is important that school psychologists understand the impact that RAD can have on a child's social, emotional, and behavioral functioning throughout their development and how it may impact their functioning in the school.

SELF-ESTEEM

Self-esteem has been studied in children with disturbed attachment behavior. Vacaru and colleagues (2018) conducted a study that examined self-esteem in children living in institutions in South Africa. The sample consisted of 33 institutionalized children between the ages of 4 and 12. The findings indicated that disturbed attachment among institutionalized children was associated with low self-esteem and that there was no difference between the children's self-reported ratings of global self-esteem and teacher ratings of global self-esteem. The only domain of self-esteem in which a difference was found was physical self-esteem, for which the children's ratings were higher than the teachers' ratings. Another study conducted by Zimmermann and Iwanski (2018) examined self-esteem among a sample of German children between the ages of 5 and 10 that was composed of a high-risk RAD group of 32 children living in some form of institutional care and a community control group, which consisted of 32 children living with at least one biological parent. The findings revealed that increased RAD symptoms were linked to lower self-esteem (Zimmermann & Iwanski, 2018).

Increased RAD symptoms are linked to lower self-esteem (Zimmermann & Iwanski, 2018).

To gain a better understanding of children with RAD and how they may differ from children with other emotional–behavioral problems, Bosmans and colleagues (2019) conducted a study that examined the interaction of children with RAD and their teachers. The basis of their study was grounded on the *DSM-5*'s diagnostic criteria of limited positive emotion expressed by children with RAD and their inhibited behavior toward caregivers under distressing conditions. The authors also contended that, given documented evidence that children with secure attachments tend to feel valued by their caregivers and have high self-esteem (Verschueren et al., 2012), it could be expected that children with RAD tend to have negative expectations of others and a negative self-view (Bosmans et al., 2019; Zimmermann & Soares, 2019). In their study, Bosmans et al. (2019) hypothesized that, in comparison to children with other emotional–behavioral problems, children with RAD would have (a) lower levels of emotional security and positive affect in "challenging and nonthreatening" situations (p. 193), (b) demonstrate less trust in their caregiver and teacher, and (c) report lower self-esteem.

To conduct their study, Bosmans and colleagues (2019) recruited children between the ages of 6 and 10 attending schools in Belgium that provide special education for children with emotional–behavioral problems. The sample included 67 students of whom 21 students exhibited RAD behaviors. The findings of the study revealed that, in comparison to children with other emotional–behavior problems, children with RAD exhibited less emotional security, positive emotion, and trust in their interactions with their teachers in challenging situations. Children with RAD also reported less trust in their teacher's ability to provide support. However, the authors' hypothesis that children with RAD would demonstrate lower global self-esteem was not supported by the findings. The comparison group consisted of school-aged children with other emotional–behavioral problems who, therefore, may also struggle with low self-esteem. As the Bosmans et al. (2019) point out, this finding contradicts research studies which have found that children with less secure attachment have lower self-esteem. However, it is important to keep in mind that children with RAD were compared to children with other emotional–behavioral problems who also may struggle with low self-esteem. Some scholars contend that low self-esteem is a risk factor for emotional–behavioral difficulties, whereas other scholars consider low self-esteem an outcome of psychopathology (Orth et al., 2012; Zeigler-Hill, 2011). It is plausible to speculate that, if a comparison group consisting of children with no prior psychiatric history had been included in the study, a difference may have perhaps been found between this comparison group and the group of children with RAD. Based on the findings of their research study, Bosmans and colleagues (2019) concluded that children with RAD may lack social resources needed to cope in challenging or distressing situations, and may be unable to depend on teachers as a "secure base for autonomous exploration at school" (p. 199). This could negatively impact learning opportunities, which, in turn, could have an adverse impact on their academic achievement (Bosmans et al., 2019).

Other studies have examined self-esteem in adolescents with RAD or DSED. Seim and colleagues (2020) investigated global and domain-specific self-esteem among adolescents between the ages of 12 to 20 who lived in a residential youth center in Norway. Youths exhibiting RAD were compared to others living in the residential center who did not exhibit RAD and youths in the general population of Norwegian adolescents. The findings of the study indicated that, in comparison to youths in the general population, those with RAD had lower scholastic self-esteem and slightly higher close friendship self-esteem. Lower scholastic self-esteem was also found in all adolescents living in the residential center compared to youths in the general population. This may suggest that the lower scholastic self-esteem may be associated with other factors common to all youths in the residential youth center. This information is important information for educators so that adequate educational support can be provided to children not only with RAD but also with histories of residential living. Regarding the slightly higher close friendship self-esteem in youths with RAD, the authors propose that this finding might represent a false high self-esteem that serves as a psychological defense utilized by those with RAD to protect a vulnerable sense of self that stems from disrupted relationships in early life (Seim et al., 2020). Hence, children with RAD may view others in the residential center as close friends no matter the quality of the relationship, because it protects them from feeling alone (Seim et al., 2020).

EMOTIONAL AND BEHAVIORAL DIFFICULTIES

As noted by Bruce et al. (2019), there are limited studies on the development of emotional and behavioral difficulties in children with RAD. Still, there is research evidence documenting the presence of emotional and behavioral difficulties that could potentially impact the child's functioning at school. It should be noted that there is some inconsistency in the results among some research studies, which may stem from some of the methodological problems described in an earlier section of this chapter.

Research studies have found an association between RAD and internalizing symptoms, which is not surprising given RAD's clinical presentation of limited expression of positive emotion and emotionally withdrawn behavior. In their review of the literature on RAD, Zeanah and Gleason (2015) report that some studies have indicated modest to moderate associations between RAD and internalizing behaviors such as depression and anxiety. In a study of Romanian children living in institutional care (part of the Bucharest Early Intervention Project described earlier in the chapter), Gleason and colleagues (2011) examined depression symptoms in children who lived in institutional care and those who initially lived in an institution but were later placed in foster care. The findings of the study indicate moderate to high associations between signs of inhibited RAD and depressive symptoms at various time points from when the children were approximately 22 to 54 months' old. However, it should be noted that some children with RAD no longer met diagnostic criteria for major depressive disorder at 54 months.

Elovainio and colleagues (2015) examined internalizing (such as anxiety and depression) and externalizing behaviors (such as aggressive behaviors and conduct problems) among international school-aged children adopted through three main adoption agencies in Finland. The findings of their study revealed that adoptees with RAD symptoms had more internalizing and externalizing behaviors than adoptees with DSED symptoms and a comparison group of children having no attachment-related symptoms. Although the authors note that these findings may suggest that children with RAD may have a worse outcome than children with DSED, this is inconsistent with those of other authors (Fox et al., 2017; Rutter et al., 2009), who contend that nurturing caregiving can lead to a more positive outcome for children with RAD. Elovainio and colleagues (2015) also found that hyperactive behaviors were associated with RAD and DSED symptoms, which, as the authors point out, is inconsistent with other studies (Gleason et al., 2011) that found hyperactive and impulsive behaviors were associated more with DSED symptoms than RAD symptoms. However, inattention was not linked to RAD or DSED symptoms (Elovainio et al., 2015).

To better understand emotional and behavioral difficulties experienced by adolescents with RAD, Seim and colleagues (2020) conducted a study that focused on adolescents. The findings of the study indicated that the prevalence of emotional and behavioral problems, such as anxiety, depression, oppositional defiant behaviors, and conduct problems, were present in adolescents diagnosed with RAD. Moreover, rates of self-harm, suicidality, and psychosocial problems—such as bullying victimization, police contact, risky sexual behavior, and alcohol or substance abuse—were found to be high. Findings from the study also revealed that the odds of anxiety and depression as well as self-harm increased as the signs of RAD increased. As the authors pointed out, it is interesting that both emotional and behavioral problems were present in adolescents with RAD, whereas other studies had found only emotional problems in preschoolers (Spangler et al., 2019).

In adolescents diagnosed with RAD, rates of self-harm, suicidality, and psychosocial problems, such as bullying victimization, police contact, risky sexual behavior, and alcohol or substance abuse, were found to be high (Seim et al., 2020).

EMOTIONAL DYSREGULATION

Diagnostic features of RAD, irritability and limited positive emotions, may reflect difficulties in emotional regulation (Rutter et al., 2009; Zeanah & Smyke, 2008). Infants who are securely attached have nurturing caregivers who help them regulate their emotions so that they can learn to manage stressful situations (Schwartz & Davis, 2006). For example, a nurturing caregiver helps to comfort them when they are distressed and crying by holding them and attempting to soothe them. Children with RAD lack this modeling of emotional regulation by a responsive caregiver. Hence, they may have difficulty managing strong emotions when they are distressed. Difficulty in regulating their emotions can be manifested in their behavior. Expectations for self-regulation in schools pose challenges for children with RAD (Floyd et al., 2008). Hence, it is important that school psychologists are aware of the difficulties in emotional regulation experienced by children with RAD so that they can guide teachers and school administrators in understanding challenges associated with RAD.

Difficulties in emotional regulation may be reflected in diagnostic features of RAD, namely, irritability and limited positive emotion.

INTERPERSONAL RELATIONSHIPS

Early bonding with a primary caregiver during infancy sets the foundation for a young child's ability to interact with and build relationships with others. The quality of the relationship with the caregiver is important and can influence the interpersonal relationships later on in the child's development (Guyon-Harris, Humphreys, Degnan, et al., 2019; Guyon-Harris, Humphreys, Fox, et al., 2019). According to the AACAP (2014), children who have a diagnosis of RAD are "less likely to interact with other people because of the negative experiences with adults in their early years" (para. 4). Children with RAD are characteristically socially withdrawn in their interactions with others (Guyon-Harris, Humphreys, Fox, et al., 2019) and do not seek comfort from their caregivers when they are upset (AACAP, 2014). RAD is associated with disturbed social–emotional functioning, which is persistent, and children with RAD do not seek to engage in a back and forth interaction with others, which is known as *social reciprocity* (Corval et al., 2017). Guyon-Harris, Humphreys, Fox, et al. (2019) contend that the social difficulties experienced by children who have a history of early institutional care or multiple foster care placements may be attributed to the disordered attachment that the children experienced early in their development.

To explore the social functioning of preteen children with a history of institutional care, Guyon-Harris, Humphreys, Fox, et al. (2019) conducted a study with a sample of 110 children who had been raised in a Romanian institution and a community comparison group of 50 participants. Participants were 12 years old. The results of the study indicated that symptoms of RAD and DSED were linked to lower general social functioning and social competence (Guyon-Harris, Humphreys, Degnan, et al., 2019; Guyon-Harris, Humphreys, Fox, et al., 2019). It is interesting to note that the manifestation of social difficulties differed between children with RAD and those with DSED. Although children with DSED were rated by their caregivers as victims and as having conflictual peer relationships, children with RAD were not reported by their caregivers to have such difficulties. Guyon-Harris, Humphreys, Degnan, et al. (2019) and Guyon-Harris, Humphreys, Fox, et al. (2019) contend that this difference may be related to the tendency of children with RAD to be inhibited and withdrawn, whereas children with DSED tend to seek out interpersonal relationships with others and can be intrusive and even socially inappropriate at times. The authors concluded that youths with RAD and DSED in early adolescence may be at risk for difficulties in social functioning.

Scholars have indicated that children with attachment disorders may use socially maladaptive and aggressive behaviors to communicate their needs (Spilt et al., 2016). According to Spilt and colleagues (2016), social–behavioral development in children with RAD can be impaired for a number of reasons. One reason is that children with RAD are thought to have a low self-concept as a result of inadequate care in early development, which may lead to feelings of unworthiness and a sense of not belonging. It can also lead to a lack of trust with caregivers, including teachers, which has been supported by research studies (Bosmans et al., 2019). Hence, they may use maladaptive behaviors, such as aggression and manipulation, when seeking social proximity as a means of self-protection against social rejection (Spilt et al., 2016). Such behaviors can influence the child's ability to establish relationships with peers and teachers upon starting school. Spilt and colleagues also contend that, as a result of unresponsive caregiving in early life, children with RAD experience difficulty in regulating their emotions, which can influence social–behavioral development. Another factor identified by Spilt and colleagues that negatively influences social–behavioral development in children with RAD is that they have (a) learned harsh, maladaptive social behaviors via modeling the behavior of their inadequate caregivers and (b) had limited opportunities to observe prosocial behaviors.

> Children with RAD may use maladaptive behaviors, such as aggression and manipulation, when seeking social proximity as a means of self-protection against social rejection (Spilt et al., 2016).

To explore whether teachers have an influence on social–behavioral development of children with RAD, Spilt et al. (2016) conducted a study in which they observed teachers' interactions with children with RAD who were placed in special education classrooms in Belgium. The researchers focused on teacher sensitivity as a protective factor that impedes maladaptive social behaviors among RAD children in special education. The results of the study indicated that teacher sensitivity was associated with heightened levels of RAD. To be specific, children with RAD exhibited less overt and relational aggression when teacher sensitivity was high and more of these behaviors when teacher sensitivity was low. The findings of the study also revealed that teacher sensitivity was not associated with prosocial behaviors. Given that the social–behavioral problems exhibited by children with RAD can be challenging and teachers may not understand the influence that their response to the child can have on the social–behavioral development of the child (Spilt et al., 2016). Spilt and colleagues recommend that support be provided to teachers of children with RAD so that they understand the connection between the child's behavior and their underlying social–emotional needs and are sensitive to the ways in which they can respond to the child (2016).

Social–Emotional and Behavioral Functioning at Home

International adoptions can pose many challenges for families that adopt a child who has lived in institutional care for the early part of their childhood. Young children who have histories of institutional care may exhibit RAD behaviors. Attempts by the adoptive parents to build a relationship with the child can trigger distressing memories for the child, and negative self-evaluations may emerge as the child questions their self-worth during the process of beginning to feel connected and safe in their new environment (Vasquez & Stensland, 2016). Therefore, it is imperative that parents are aware of the social–emotional and behavioral challenges associated with RAD and receive support as they work to establish a relationship with their newly adopted child.

Vasquez and Miller (2018) conducted a qualitative study using a small sample of five families with adopted children with RAD between the ages of 9 and 11. The study involved interviews with the individual child with RAD, the parents, and the child's siblings. The findings of the study revealed that the children with RAD experienced extreme temper tantrums that were described as rages. According to the interviews by the child and their parents, the rages seemed uncontrollable. Another finding was that parents reported that their child was inconsolable during these rage episodes, which seemed to be triggered by difficulties in adapting to their environment. The findings also revealed that the child's rages tended to be targeted at the caregiver with whom they had a close relationship. According to the authors, this seems to suggest inhibitory control even though the children reported that they did not have control over their rages. Inhibitory control of the rages would suggest that the child may be able to suppress feelings of rage when they are in school or in other situations, but release that rage later on toward the caregiver with whom they feel safest. Vasquez and Miller (2018) suggested that the rages serve as a means of emotional regulation for the adopted children. In addition to a small sample size, there are other concerning issues with the study, namely, the children had prior diagnoses of RAD based on the *DSM-IV* (APA, 1994), and there was no indication of the subtype (inhibited or disinhibited). Therefore, it is not fully clear whether the rages are unique to children having inhibited/emotionally withdrawn RAD.

Taft and colleagues (2015) conducted a qualitative study that explored experiences of parents caring for children with RAD. Through interviews with 10 families having children with RAD either through adoption or foster care, the researchers identified two main patterns of behavior that their children exhibited at home. These types of behaviors included inappropriate and unpredictable behaviors and threatening behaviors. In the interviews, parents described bizarre behaviors and "proactive planning of inappropriate behaviors to maximize response" (Taft et al., 2015, p. 241) Examples of inappropriate and unpredictable behaviors included one child's hiding bodily waste in the home, stealing, and making false accusations of abuse. Examples of threatening behavior reported by the parents included threats to harm a family member, rage-like behaviors involving physical aggression, biting a teacher at school, exhibiting more threatening behavior toward one parent, and planning to burn a building. Similar to the study conducted by Vasquez and Miller (2018), which was discussed in the previous paragraph, it is not clear whether the children with RAD had a diagnosis based on diagnostic criteria based on the *DSM-IV* or *DSM-5*. More research is needed on aggressive behaviors among children diagnosed with RAD based on *DSM-5* diagnostic criteria.

IMPACT OF REACTIVE ATTACHMENT DISORDER ON LEARNING IN THE CLASSROOM

Similar to findings in children exposed to early trauma, children with RAD can also experience neurobiological changes that may affect behavior and learning (Embury et al., 2020). In fact, Corbin (2007) contends that neurobiological alterations associated with childhood neglect "equal and even surpass the impact of abuse and related trauma" (p. 539). Severe neglect, such as the absence of caregivers and disruption in the early caregiving environment, can significantly impact the hypothalamicpituitarya-drenal (HPA) axis, which regulates the response of the body and brain to stress. In addition, research has found reduced gray matter volume in the visual cortex of the brain of children with RAD in comparison to a control group (Shimada et al., 2015). According to Shimada and colleagues, the gray matter of the visual cortex is related to internalizing behaviors experienced by children with RAD and such alterations within this area may be related to impairment in emotion regulation.

In addition to social–emotional and behavioral difficulties that can impact classroom performance, school-aged children with RAD often experience learning difficulties in the classroom. Children who grow up in institutions, such as orphanages, typically have fewer opportunities in which they are exposed to enriching, yet challenging learning environments and limited opportunities to practice new skills (Raaska et al., 2012). Although some scholars note that some children who are adopted after living in institutions may seem to catch up cognitively once they get adjusted to their new environment, other scholars have found that the adoptive children's academic performance tends to lag behind their non-adopted peers, which can lead to more referrals for special education services in comparison to children who are not adopted (Raaska et al., 2012; van Ijzendoorn & Juffer, 2006).

A research study on adopted children in Finland found that about a third of the adoptees had learning problems (Raaska et al., 2012). In addition, the results of the study conducted by Raaska and colleagues demonstrated that children who were adopted at younger ages had less severe learning problems, and boys experienced more learning difficulties than girls (2012). Regarding children with RAD symptoms at the time of adoption, an association was found between RAD and learning difficulties; children with several RAD symptoms were more at risk of having learning difficulties, particularly severe learning problems (2012). It is important to note that this study was published prior to the *DSM-5* and, hence, it is likely that the RAD symptoms assessed in this study were based on the *DSM-IV* diagnostic criteria, which relied on inhibited and disinhibited subtypes. The authors of the study did not indicate any distinction between the two subtypes when assessing for RAD behaviors among the participants of the study. Therefore, it is not clear whether similar results would be different had a distinction between the two subtypes been made.

Children with several RAD symptoms were more at risk of having learning difficulties, particularly severe learning problems (Raaska et al., 2012).

In addition to learning difficulties, the teacher–child relationship can influence a young child's performance in the classroom, and this is particularly true with children diagnosed with RAD. As seen earlier, research studies have found that children with RAD demonstrate a lack of trust in their teachers (Bosmans et al., 2019). Previous research on teacher–child relationships has indicated that typically developing children who are securely attached to their parents tend to have a positive relationship with their teachers in which they seek support from the teacher and engage in exploration away from the teacher (Verschueren & Spilt, 2020). On the other hand, children who are not securely attached to their parents tend to have less close relationships with their teachers (Sabol & Pianta, 2012). Some scholars contend that children with RAD are at risk of difficulties establishing relationships with their teachers, which could potentially enhance the likelihood that the child will experience more emotional and behavioral difficulties in the classroom (Bosmans et al., 2020). Bosmans and colleagues (2020) contend that it is important that teachers are aware of the importance of the relationship that they establish with children who have RAD so that the child with RAD can adapt positively to the classroom and feel safe within that environment.

Managing the problem behaviors exhibited by children with RAD can be challenging for teachers. Bosmans et al. (2020) provide a model of the insecure cycle in the teacher–child with RAD relationship and how the child's inability to seek support when they are feeling overwhelmed can lead to stress-related emotional reactions being manifested in their behavior—either becoming withdrawn as if to shield oneself from the interaction with the teacher or becoming aggressive. In an effort to respond to the child's behavior, the teacher may attempt to communicate or engage the child. Although these efforts by the teacher are well intentioned, the child with RAD may view these efforts as intrusive, which may lead the child to have negative expectations of support from the teacher. This may lead to the child being disappointed in the teacher, who may become frustrated with the child or stop interacting with the child (Bosmans et al., 2020). As noted by Bosmans and colleagues (2020), it is important that teachers have an understanding of the social–emotional and behavioral needs of children with RAD so that they can better help address these needs in the classroom so that the child can focus on learning. In addition, it is important that teachers receive support from school personnel, such as the school psychologist, in how to respond to the child's emotional and behavioral needs so that the child's potential to learn in the classroom can be achieved.

IMPLICATIONS FOR SCHOOL PSYCHOLOGISTS

Although RAD is not a disorder that school psychologists are likely to encounter often, it is possible that some students will have a history of multiple foster care placements or have been adopted through an international adoption agency that helps families adopt children living in orphanages. RAD can have a significant impact on a child's functioning in the classroom, which can subsequently require the services of school psychologists. School psychologists are in a unique position to help children with RAD by serving as an advocate for children with RAD and their families, consulting with teachers of students exhibiting RAD behaviors, assessing students who have been referred for a special education evaluation, and providing school-based mental health interventions.

Advocacy

Advocacy is an important service that school psychologists can provide for children with RAD and their families. Good (2016) has addressed several issues related to the adoption of children with disabilities that are applicable to families who have experienced the process of international adoption of children who may have early histories of institutional care or adoption of a child who has been placed in multiple foster homes in which the child did not have an opportunity to establish an attachment to a nurturing caregiver in a stable environment. These issues include a lack of being prepared to address the needs of children with disabilities, need for support after the adoption, support directly related to the child's disability, and educational support for their disabled child. School psychologists can work directly with families of children with RAD to provide information about the social–emotional and behavioral needs of children with RAD and specifically the needs of their own child. The parents may need support in addressing emotional and behavioral problems exhibited by the child at home as well as support in navigating the educational system to advocate for educational services. In addition, school psychologists may work with families of children who are placed in new foster homes in which the parent is attempting to provide a safe and supportive home environment for the child. School psychologists can play an important role in helping parents of children with RAD to advocate for educational and mental health services to address the needs of children with RAD.

In addition to advocating for educational services provided in the schools, school psychologists can help parents advocate for multisystem services with community agencies. As Losinski and colleagues (2016) contend, a multisystem approach could provide intensive wraparound services for the child and family through community-based services such as family therapy and psychiatric care alongside school-based mental health counseling for the child with RAD. Thus, support could be provided for the child and family in the school, community, and home. By establishing a solid partnership with community-based agencies, the school psychologist can serve as a liaison between the school and community agency to guide parents through the process involved in obtaining needed services such as psychological and psychiatric services as well as family therapy services. As recommended by Losinski and colleagues (2016), consideration may be given to developing a family service plan that focuses on the child and family's strengths and needs. Advocating for a family service plan with the community agencies may be a service that the school psychologist can help in obtaining for the family to ensure that, not only are the child's needs addressed, but the family's needs are also taken into consideration.

> By establishing a solid partnership with community-based agencies, the school psychologist can serve as a liaison between the school and community agency to guide parents through the process involved in obtaining needed services such as psychological and psychiatric services as well as family therapy services.

Consultation

As a consultant to the family of a child with RAD, it is important for school psychologists to assist the school in establishing a partnership between the school and the family. Taft and colleagues (2016) emphasize the need for effective communication between families of children with RAD and schools regarding school-related concerns and the need to encourage family involvement in the school. Family involvement and effective communication promote a positive partnership between the school and family, which, we hope, has positive outcomes for the child in school and at home (Taft and Schlein, 2017). Research studies have found that interviews with families of children with RAD revealed that their interactions with school personnel were frequently confrontational and unproductive (Taft & Schlein, 2017). For example, Taft and Schlein (2017) interviewed parents of children with RAD about their interactions with school personnel and found that parents reported frustration that educators working with their child tended to only communicate with them to complain about their child's misbehavior and did not seem to view them as a valued partner in making decisions about their child's education. Unfortunately, such interactions hinder an understanding of the concerns of the family and school and can impede the child's academic progress. Therefore, it is imperative that the family and school work together collaboratively to establish a partnership that is respectful, positive, sensitive to the families' concerns and child's needs, and encourages family involvement.

In working with parents of children with RAD, school psychologists can provide psychoeducation regarding the impact of RAD on a child's social–emotional, behavioral, and academic functioning and what the child's needs may be in each of these domains. Parents will need guidance on how to build a trusting relationship with the child and understand the importance of providing a consistent, stable home environment for the child. The school psychologist and family may want to consider developing a plan for how to address behavioral difficulties at home and take into consideration an approach that is sensitive to the needs of the child and addresses behavioral problems in a nonpunitive manner.

Along with providing psychoeducation about RAD to parents, school psychologists can provide support for teachers and will need to guide them in understanding the impact that RAD has on a child's development and how RAD might present in the classroom. Teachers will need to know what to expect in terms of how the child's emotions may be manifested in the child's behavior. It is important to inform the teacher of the types of struggles that the child may experience in the classroom. For example, a child with RAD might appear emotionally withdrawn but, if they begin to feel overwhelmed, may begin to exhibit behavioral problems. It would be important for the teacher to know that children with RAD may behave younger than their chronological age and may experience tantrums longer than expected (Embury et al., 2020). In addition, it would be helpful to let the teacher know that the child may not seek help or support when they become distressed because they do not feel safe and, thus, may be unable to soothe themselves when they become distressed (2020).

Understanding the importance of establishing a stable, predictable learning environment and developing a trusting relationship with the child is imperative for teachers as they help the child adapt to the classroom (Floyd et al., 2008; Schwartz & Davis, 2006). The school psychologist can provide guidance to the teacher and other school personnel in establishing ways that promote a sense of security and help the child to feel safe in the classroom (Schwartz & Davis, 2006; Losinski et al., 2016). Being sensitive to the child's needs and accepting them while maintaining boundaries regarding misbehaviors is critical in helping the child adapt to the classroom environment.

Embury and colleagues (2020) note that it is also important that teachers be aware of potential difficulties experienced by some children with RAD such as social skill deficits, difficulty learning if they do not feel safe in the classroom, limited positive emotions, and lack of social connectedness. The school psychologist and teacher can work together on promoting prosocial behaviors in the classroom through teaching appropriate ways to interact with others and modeling prosocial behaviors (Floyd et al., 2008). In addition, it is important for teachers to be aware that children with RAD often experience difficulty regulating their emotions so supports to help the child manage overwhelming emotions could be identified (Bosmans et al., 2020). It is important to point out that teachers will need to be supported by the school psychologist and other school personnel in their efforts to create a safe learning environment for the child (2020).

Assessment

Given that children with RAD often exhibit challenging emotional behaviors in the classroom, a decision may be made to refer the child with RAD for an evaluation for special education services if the child has not responded to supports that have been provided for the child. Consent for an evaluation must be obtained from the child's parents, and a multidisciplinary team will have 60 days to complete their evaluation. As noted earlier, the child must meet eligibility requirements for a disability under IDEA (2004) such as ED (or Emotional Behavioral Disorder) and be in need of special education services before services can be rendered. Hence, the assessment data must indicate that the child has a disability that is having an adverse impact on the child's academic performance and the child will most likely not be successful in the classroom without special education services. Once parental permission is obtained, the school psychologist can begin conducting an assessment of the child's emotional and behavioral needs.

Conducting a thorough interview with the parent, teacher, and child (if appropriate) can provide information about the child's psychosocial history, developmental history, medical history, current functioning, and concerns regarding the child. For a child with RAD who may have lived in several foster homes or been adopted internationally, obtaining information about their early development may be challenging as the parents may only have limited information. However, parents can share information about the child's functioning since being in the home. Important information to obtain would include information such as descriptions of the emotional–behavioral problems exhibited at home, the duration and frequency of these problems, what strategies or interventions have been used thus far to address the problems, whether the strategies were effective, and whether the child experiences any psychosomatic symptoms. In addition, obtaining information about the child's educational history would also be important, particularly if the child had attended different schools. Teacher interviews can provide information about the child's functioning in the classroom and concerns that the teacher may have about the child. Depending on the child's developmental level and level of insight, an interview with the child may provide information about concerns that they have and their perspective on issues that they may be struggling with at home and school.

Rating scales can be useful ways of gathering information about a child's emotional and behavioral functioning. For example, the Child Behavior Checklist for Ages 6–18 (Achenbach & Rescorla, 2001) assesses internalizing and externalizing behaviors and also provides information about a child's social competence. It would be important for school psychologists to use rating scales that have multi-rater versions so that data could be collected from the child's parents and teachers as well as self-report versions if available.

Conducting a behavioral assessment could provide helpful information about the child's behavior in the classroom. Observations can yield useful information about the child's behavior such as antecedents triggering problematic behaviors and consequences of the behavior, how the child interacts with the teacher and peers, how the teachers and peers respond to the child, the function of the behavior, and so forth. Floyd and colleagues (2008) recommend that observations of children with RAD occur in various settings and note that other scholars have utilized a "conditioned observation system that highlight the variety of anxiety and conditions that heightened typical RAD behavioral characteristics" (Shepehris et al., 2003, as cited in Floyd et al., 2008, p. 253). It should also be noted that an observation is required in some states if the child is being considered for the IDEA disability ED (or Emotional Behavioral Disorder). Regarding the use of behavioral assessment specifically for children with RAD, it should be noted that some scholars, such as Taft et al. (2016), emphasize that although behavioral assessments can be effective tools for many children with behavioral problems, this form of assessment may be challenging to use for children with RAD when attempting to identify antecedents and consequences. Taft and scholars (2016) also note that children with RAD frequently do not respond to behavioral intervention programs.

Other areas that the school psychologist would need to assess include the child's cognitive functioning and academic achievement. Given the early deprivation that some children with RAD may experience and, as noted earlier, neurodevelopmental alterations among children with RAD have been documented in the literature, an assessment of the child' cognitive functioning would provide information about the child's ability to solve problems, process visual and auditory information, ability to remember information, and so on. To determine the child's current level of academic functioning, the school psychologist conducts an assessment of the child's academic achievement. Data obtained from an assessment of the child's academic skills will aid the team in determining whether a disability is adversely impacting the child's academic performance.

Therapeutic Interventions

The role of school psychologists as mental health providers is endorsed by the National Association of School Psychologists (NASP) 2020 Professional Standards domain of Mental and Behavioral Health Services and Interventions (NASP, 2020), which supports school psychological services in addressing social–emotional and behavioral impacts on learning and implementing evidence-based strategies that support social–emotional well-being. Through school-based mental health services, school psychologists who have received training in play therapy and cognitive behavioral therapy (CBT) could use techniques from these two therapeutic fields to help children with RAD learn ways in which to regulate their emotions while they are in school. It should be pointed out that the mental health needs of some children with RAD exceed the types of services that school can provide, and a referral to an outside mental health provider may be needed depending on the child's social–emotional and behavioral needs.

EDUCATIONAL AND SOCIAL–EMOTIONAL SUPPORTS

Addressing the challenging behaviors of children with RAD is imperative in helping them be successful in the school environment. School personnel may not be aware of the child's history or have knowledge of any prior diagnosis, but it is evident that the child is struggling in managing their emotions and behavior. Given that a medical diagnosis is not required for a child to receive special education services under the IDEA (2004) disability category of Emotional Disturbance, Losinski and colleagues (2016) recommend that Multi-Tiered Systems of Support (MTSS) be utilized in order to identify students (such as those with RAD) who are struggling to function in the classroom and may be in need of services under this disability category. Through this framework, supports are provided to students through a process that involves screening, progress monitoring, and targeted interventions. MTSS that are designed to provide support for children with emotional–behavioral problems may be helpful in addressing the behavioral needs of children with RAD. As proposed by Losinski et al. (2016), Tier 1 supports would include research-based instruction and universal screening to identify students at risk of behavioral problems. An example of a screening scale that might be considered is the Student Risk Screening Scale-Internalizing and Externalizing (Lane et al., 2012), which is a modified version of Drummond's (1994) original version of the scale (Student Risk Screening Scale). According to Losinski and colleagues, Tier 2 supports might include a targeted intervention such as the Check-In Check-Out program (Everett et al., 2011) and progress monitoring of the child's daily behavior using a tool such as the Daily Behavior Rating Scale (Chafouleas et al., 2009). Suggested Tier 3 interventions include conducting a functional behavioral assessment and developing a behavioral intervention plan that focuses on specific behaviors exhibited by the child (Losinski et al., 2016). The provision of these supports may help address some of the challenging behaviors exhibited by children with RAD but will also provide data regarding their response to these supports that will be needed if the child is referred for an evaluation for special education services under the IDEA disability of ED.

In addition to MTSS, other suggested supports offered by professionals in the field include creating a stable environment in the classroom in which the child knows what is expected and feels safe and supported. It is important that the child's environment at both home and school is consistent and predictable and, if the daily routine is going to change, the child should be informed about the change prior to its occurrence (Losinski et al., 2016). For activities in the classroom, it is important to teach expectations for the activities and post them in the classroom so that the child with RAD will better understand what is expected of students within the classroom (Embury et al., 2020).

Efforts should also be made to ensure that the child has a safe place to go to if they become emotionally overwhelmed (Losinski et al., 2016). As noted earlier, the school psychologist and teacher can work together with the child to determine the location of this safe space within the classroom or school. Other types of school-based support offered by Floyd and colleagues (2008) include the presence of caring, nurturing adults who are patient and understand the connection between the child's emotions and their behavior prior to disciplining the child for disruptive behaviors. This helps to establish the teacher as a safe, trustworthy attachment figure to whom the child can seek support when needed (Embury et al., 2020). Having a predictable environment and establishing an emotional bond with the teacher, the child with RAD begins to feel safe in the classroom and may be better able to manage their emotions and behaviors, which can enhance their ability to pay attention and follow instructions (Embury et al., 2020). When inappropriate behaviors are manifested in the classroom, clear consequences should be established that take into consideration the child's social–emotional and behavioral skills and deficits (Embury et al., 2020). Alongside these efforts, the child will benefit from the teacher's modeling and teaching appropriate play and social behaviors (Floyd et al., 2008).

> Having a predictable environment and establishing an emotional bond with the teacher, the child with RAD begins to feel safe in the classroom and may be better able to manage their emotions and behaviors, which can enhance their ability to pay attention and follow instructions (Embury et al., 2020).

Embury and colleagues (2020) proposed instructional supports that may help children with RAD to be successful in the classroom. These strategies include breaking up information into smaller units so that the child is better able to manage the amount of content to which the child is exposed at a time, potentially reducing anxiety. Offering step-by-step instruction on academic tasks can also be an effective strategy in helping children with RAD to be successful and learn to self-regulate. In addition, using daily agendas for older students and visual schedules for younger children helps the child know what activities will occur throughout the day, which promotes a sense of predictability (Embury et al., 2020).

SCHOOL-BASED MENTAL HEALTH INTERVENTIONS AND SUPPORTS

Regarding mental health treatment for children with RAD, scholars note the lack of evidence-based treatment protocols specifically used for RAD (Embury et al., 2020; Losinski et al., 2016; Schwartz & Davis, 2006), particularly school-based interventions. Possible explanations include the individualized history and symptom presentation among children with RAD (Ritchie, 2013). However, it is clear within the literature that children with RAD benefit from establishing a positive relationship with an adult with whom they feel safe and learning ways in which to regulate their emotions.

To build a positive relationship between the teacher and child with RAD and address inappropriate behaviors in the classroom, Embury and colleagues (2020) recommend that the school psychologist and teacher work together to utilize the principles of Playfulness, Acceptance, Curiosity, and Empathy (PACE), which have been used successfully by parents and caregivers in addressing inappropriate behaviors (Hughes & Golding, 2012). The PACE approach was developed by Hughes (2007), and the PACE approach is incorporated in dynamic developmental psychotherapy (Hughes et al., 2015). Using the PACE principles in communicating with children with RAD, a trusting relationship with an attachment figure (caregiver or teacher) can be established and emotional–behavioral difficulties addressed. Given that children with RAD exhibit little positive emotion, the use of playfulness can help the child experience positive emotions, participate in reciprocal enjoyment, and build confidence. Through understanding and acceptance of the child's thoughts and emotions, a sense of psychological safety is created while still communicating boundaries about behavior. Curiosity provides an opportunity to demonstrate an interest in the child and get to know the child on a deeper level, which, in turn, helps the child to be more responsive to the teacher. The final PACE principle, empathy, better enables the teacher to understand how the child's past experiences impact current functioning and to become more aware of the child's social–emotional and behavioral needs (Hughes & Golding, 2012). Through the use of PACE principles in communicating with the child, it is hoped that the teacher–child relationship is characterized by trust and sensitivity such that the child learns to trust the teacher and feels safe in the classroom environment, which, we hope, encourages positive social interactions with others in the classroom, thus helping the child to gain more self-confidence.

School-based play therapy may be an option for school psychologists who are trained in play therapy to consider when working with a child with RAD. Play therapy as a school-based intervention has been recommended by some scholars (Ritchie, 2013). As noted by Ritchie (2013), child-centered play therapy (CCPT) is guided by eight principles, which include (a) creating a positive, nurturing relationship with the play therapist; (b) accepting the child for who they are; (c) creating an environment in which the child feels safe to express their emotions; (d) recognizing the child's feelings; (e) providing opportunities for the child to develop responsibility to internally solve difficulties; (f) permitting the child to lead the play therapy sessions; (g) understanding that the therapeutic process occurs gradually; and (h) providing therapeutic limits when needed. Although CCPT is nondirective in nature, it should be emphasized that boundaries provide predictability and help the child to feel safe within the therapeutic environment so that they learn to be self-accepting (Ritchie, 2013). Through this process, the child also learns to be accepting of others, such as teachers.

Incorporating play therapy techniques with CBT is another school-based intervention that could be provided for children with RAD. The focus of CBT is to understand that cognitions can impact one's feelings and that distorted cognitions can lead to emotional difficulties. Although components of play therapy such as creating a safe environment for the child are maintained, features of CBT such as relaxation techniques and connecting thoughts to behaviors are integrated into the sessions (Ritchie, 2013). According to Ritchie (2013), a CBT approach paired with play therapy techniques can be used to address the emotional regulation difficulties that children with RAD often experience. By learning to recognize their emotions, the child can better understand the link between emotions and how emotions may be manifested in their behavior. This therapeutic approach also includes teaching the child coping skills, such as relaxation techniques, which can be used when they begin to become overwhelmed by their emotions (Ritchie, 2013).

In conclusion, children with RAD pose many challenges for schools as evidenced in the previous discussions. School psychologists can guide educators within their schools as to how to address their learning, social–emotional, and behavioral needs.

CASE STUDY 18.1 CRINA: A YOUNG ADOPTED GIRL DIAGNOSED WITH REACTIVE ATTACHMENT DISORDER

Background

Crina is a 6-year-old girl who was adopted by Mr. and Mrs. Collins 2 years ago through an international adoption agency that provided adoption services for children living in eastern European countries. The adoptive parents had no children of their own and decided to pursue an international adoption, which took 1 year to complete. According to her adoptive mother, Crina's biological parents abandoned their child when she was 2 months old because they could not afford to provide for her and their other four children. They left her at an orphanage and never attempted to visit her. The orphanage was located in a community marked by poverty and poor living conditions. The orphanage was overcrowded, and staff members were overwhelmed with the number of children in their care. Once the adoption was approved, Mr. and Mrs. Collins flew overseas to get Crina. The adoptive parents described their surprise at the level of deprivation and poverty within the community where the orphanage was located and the poor living conditions within the orphanage. When they first saw Crina, she was in a small room sitting on the floor with other children, but none of the children seemed to interact with one another. The adoptive mother stated that when she first attempted to interact with Crina, the child glanced at her and moved away. They spent a week in the country and visited Crina every day to attempt to help her become more comfortable with them before bringing her back home with them. Mr. and Mrs. Collins also acknowledged that the adoption agency provided little information about Crina and had not followed up with them since they returned to the United States.

Mrs. Collins stated that they were not prepared for how to manage Crina's emotional and behavioral problems once they brought her to their home in the United States. Her adoptive mother indicated that Crina was emotionally withdrawn and did not reciprocate any attempts they made to interact with her, oftentimes just looking at them as if she were frozen. Mrs. Collins also noted that her daughter, at times, seemed to get overwhelmed being in a new environment but did not seek comfort even though she was obviously distressed. Outbursts and crying for long periods of time when it was not obvious why she was upset were also noted by Mrs. Collins. At times, Crina became aggressive toward the adoptive parents, throwing things at them and attempting to bite them. She also reportedly would leave feces in her closet and sometimes urinated on the floor. In addition to not seeking comfort when distressed, Crina also did not respond to their attempts to show affection toward her and would tense up if they tried to hug her. She also reportedly broke toys, ripping some of her stuffed animals. Although Crina had a bed with pillows and a comforter, she would often sleep on the hardwood floor in her bedroom. Mrs. Collins also stated that she attempted to set up playdates with other children in their neighborhood, but Crina would either not interact with the other children or attempt to bite them if she became overwhelmed. After about 8 months, the parents sought the help of a mental health professional who has been working with the family to address Crina's emotional and behavioral difficulties.

Despite her initial reluctance to interact with them, Crina now interacts with the adoptive parents at a level with which she seems comfortable at the present time. She responds to them sometimes but does not typically initiate interaction with them. She has learned English and will communicate with them when she feels comfortable doing so. Although she still does not show affection, Crina will sometimes display a little more positive emotion and smile once in a while. The adoptive parents placed Crina in preschool and kindergarten for a few hours

(continued)

CASE STUDY 18.1 CRINA: A YOUNG ADOPTED GIRL DIAGNOSED WITH REACTIVE ATTACHMENT DISORDER (*continued*)

each day, but she often kept away from the other children in the classroom and would have outbursts if children or the teacher made frequent attempts to engage her in activities. She has struggled in both settings, and the adoptive parents are worried that she will continue to struggle in the first grade when more demands are placed on her. The adoptive parents have made arrangements with the school to let Crina visit the school before the academic year begins so that they can meet her teacher and give Crina an opportunity to be around the teacher and in the classroom prior to the first day of school.

Discussion

As evident from the case history, Crina exhibits symptoms associated with RAD. She has a history of institutional care living under conditions of social neglect and inadequate caregiving. She displays signs of emotional withdrawal and does not engage in social reciprocity or seek support when distressed. Moreover, she has difficulty regulating her emotions as evident in her outbursts of crying for long periods of time and aggressive behaviors that included throwing things at the adoptive parents and biting them. The decision to give her an opportunity to visit the school and meet her teacher prior to the beginning of the school year was wise in that it provides Crina a chance to see her classroom and meet her teacher so that she has a sense of what to expect.

It is important for the school psychologist to work with the teacher and parents to help Crina adjust to the new school environment. Providing psychoeducation about RAD to the teacher and parents will give them a better understanding of the social–emotional and behavioral difficulties experienced by children with RAD, which enables the teacher and parents to develop a sensitivity to Crina's social–emotional and behavioral needs. It is critical that they focus on helping Crina build a relationship with the teacher so that Crina can learn to trust the teacher. Consideration may be given to using the principles of PACE as a means of creating a stable environment in which Crina feels safe and begins to form a relationship with the teacher. It is important that Crina understands the routine of the school day and is aware of the expectations for behavior and participation in the classroom. If there are any changes to the routine, it will be important to inform Crina ahead of time so that she is expecting the change. The teacher must ensure consistency in her interactions with Crina. It is also important that there be clear and frequent communication between the teacher and the parents so that the parents know how Crina is adjusting to the new school environment and the teacher is aware of any changes in the home environment that might impact Crina's functioning in the classroom.

In addition to consulting with the parents and teacher, the school psychologist can also work with the parents to advocate for any additional types of services that might be helpful for Crina and her family. If wraparound services are needed, the school psychologist can help the parents advocate for those services. Serving as a liaison between community-based agencies that might become involved in Crina's care and the therapist who currently works with the family would be a role in which the school psychologist could be involved. Serving in this role, the school psychologist can help to ensure that there is open communication among all parties involved in providing services to Crina and her family.

If the school implements MTSS, social–emotional supports could be provided to Crina. As discussed earlier, Tier 1 supports could include a screening scale that assesses internalizing and externalizing behaviors. This would help identify specific emotional–behavioral struggles that Crina may be experiencing. Tier 2 supports could involve using Check-In Check-Out (Everett et al., 2011) so that Crina can check in each morning and afternoon with someone with whom she is comfortable to go over what her goals are for the day and which goals were met by the end of the school day. Daily progress monitoring of any emotional and behavioral problems could also be used at Tier 2. If Tier 3 supports are needed, the school psychologist may consider conducting a behavioral assessment and developing a behavioral intervention

(*continued*)

> **CASE STUDY 18.1 CRINA: A YOUNG ADOPTED GIRL DIAGNOSED WITH REACTIVE ATTACHMENT DISORDER** *(continued)*
>
> plan. It is important that the plan be sensitive to Crina's social–emotional and behavioral needs and her unique history.
>
> To address Crina's mental health needs, consideration may be given to providing school-based mental health services. If the school psychologist has been trained in play therapy and CBT techniques, this approach might be an appropriate choice for an intervention. It is important for the school psychologist to discuss this intervention, not only with the parents, but also with the therapist who is working with the family (with the parents' permission) to ensure that all parties support the implementation of this approach and not to duplicate services that the therapist may already be providing. Through this approach, the play therapy could help to create a safe environment in which a level of trust is established between Crina and the school psychologist. The use of play most likely will be helpful in helping Crina to feel comfortable with the school psychologist. Relaxation techniques and other CBT techniques could be implemented. It is hoped that this approach will help address difficulties in emotional regulation.
>
> As the year progresses, a decision may perhaps be made to refer Crina for a special education evaluation. If this is the case, the evaluation will need to be conducted within 60 days after the parents provide consent for the evaluation. Hearing and vision will first need to be assessed by the school nurse. Through a series of tests, the school psychologist will assess Crina's intellectual ability, academic achievement, adaptive behaviors, and social–emotional behaviors. Based on the assessment data, a determination will be made with regard to whether Crina is a student with a disability whose difficulties adversely impact her academic performance and whether there is a need for special education services. The multidisciplinary team will review the data and determine whether she meets eligibility criteria for one of the disability categories under IDEA (2004) such as ED. If the data indicate that Crina meets eligibility criteria for an IDEA disability and that she will not make academic progress without special education services, the team will determine her to be a student with a disability and will develop an Individual Education Program (IEP) for her.

SUMMARY POINTS

- RAD is a rare disorder related to an early history of social neglect that results in the child not having a selective attachment to a caregiver.
- RAD can significantly impair a child's social–emotional and behavioral functioning, particularly the ability to regulate emotions and connect to others on a social and emotional level.
- One of the most important interventions to help children with RAD is establishing a trusting relationship with a caregiver who is consistent and committed to providing a safe, stable environment.
- School psychologists can play a pivotal role in helping a child with RAD through advocacy, consultation, assessment, and mental health interventions.

TEST YOUR KNOWLEDGE

1. RAD symptoms must be present prior to what age?
   a. Two months of age
   b. Five months of age
   c. Two years of age
   d. Five years of age

2. A diagnosis of RAD can be made if the child has a diagnosis of ASD.
   a. True
   b. False

3. Establishing a trusting relationship with a teacher can help create a stable classroom environment in which the child with RAD can feel safe.
   a. True
   b. False

4. For a child with RAD, maladaptive behaviors, such as aggression, may be used when seeking social proximity and can serve as a means of _____.
   a. Retaliation for being misunderstood
   b. Self-protection against social rejection
   c. Adjustment to others
   d. Reducing sad feelings

5. Emotional dysregulation is experienced by many children with RAD.
   a. True
   b. False

Answers: (1) d, (2) b, (3) a, (4) b, (5) a.

DISCUSSION QUESTIONS

1. Describe the *DSM-5* diagnostic features of RAD.

2. Discuss how RAD can impact a child's social–emotional and behavioral functioning.

3. Identify five educational and social–emotional supports that may be useful for a child with RAD.

4. Discuss the PACE principles and how they can be used by a teacher of a child with RAD to build a trusting relationship.

5. Discuss how play therapy techniques can be used by a school-based mental health professional to address the emotional and behavioral needs of a child with RAD.

CHAPTER RESOURCES

Basic Information Websites

American Academy of Child and Adolescent Psychiatry *Attachment Disorders*: www.aacap.org/AACAP/Families_and_Youth/Facts_for_Families/FFF-Guide/Attachment-Disorders-085.aspx

Mayo Clinic *Reactive Attachment Disorder*: www.mayoclinic.org/diseases-conditions/reactive-attachment-disorder/symptoms-causes/syc-20352939

Resources for School Psychologists

National Association of School Psychologists DSM-5 *and School Psychology: Reactive Attachment Disorder and Disinhibited Social Engagement Disorder*: www.nasponline.org/publications/periodicals/communique/issues/volume-42-issue-8

RAD Advocates Factsheet *An Educator's Guide to RAD*: https://ec1409ca-cfb8-44d4-9ded-17ed84478048
.filesusr.com/ugd/980054_307ceaec0e484649ad057c4e5a4b4b97.pdf
RAD Advocates Factsheet *5 Ways to Support Parents of Kids With RAD*: https://ec1409ca-cfb8-44d4-9ded
-17ed84478048.filesusr.com/ugd/c30adf_c8d437ae45be48c7afb955d42b9e7fd8.pdf

Resources for Families

RAD Advocates Factsheet *How RAD Impacts a Family*: https://ec1409ca-cfb8-44d4-9ded-17ed84478048
.filesusr.com/ugd/c30adf_8d2a67db1a944a3591286da88e1d2ad0.pdf
RAD Advocates Factsheet *6 Lesser-Known Symptoms of RAD*: https://ec1409ca-cfb8-44d4-9ded-17ed84478048
.filesusr.com/ugd/980054_f48f22adf9e44f52b3b98a13393973bf.pdf

Fact Sheets on RAD

American Academy of Child and Adolescent Psychiatry *Attachment Disorders Fact Sheet*: www.aacap.org/
AACAP/Families_and_Youth/Facts_for_Families/FFF-Guide/Attachment-Disorders-085.aspx
Child Mind Institute *Quick Facts on Reactive Attachment Disorder*: https://childmind.org/article/quick
-facts-on-reactive-attachment-disorder/
Minnesota Association for Children's Mental Health *Reactive Attachment Fact Sheet*: www.aecsd.education/
tfiles/folder1488/Fact%20Sheet_RAD14.pdf

KEY REFERENCES

Only key references appear in the print edition. The full reference list appears in the digital product on Springer Publishing Connect: connect.springerpub.com/content/book/978-0-8261-3587-2/part/part07/chapter/ch18

American Psychiatric Association. (2013). *Diagnostic and statistical manual of mental disorders* (5th ed.). https://doi.org/10.1176/appi.books.9780890425596
Cuyvers, B., Vervoort, E., & Bosmans, G. (2020). Reactive attachment disorder symptoms and prosocial behavior in middle childhood: The role of Secure Base Script knowledge. *BMC Psychiatry*, 20(1), 1–13. https://doi.org/10.1186/s12888-020-02931-3
Embury, C.D., Clarke, L. S., & Leaver, C. (2020). Reactive attachment disorder in the classroom. *Preventing School Failure: Alternative Education for Children and Youth*, 64(3), 240–248. https://doi.org/10.1080/1045988X.2020.1732281
Floyd, K. K., Hester, P., Griffin, H. C., Golden, J., & Canter, L. L. S. (2008). Reactive attachment disorder: Challenges for early identification and intervention within the schools. *International Journal of Special Education*, 23(2), 47–55. https://files.eric.ed.gov/fulltext/EJ814399.pdf
Guyon-Harris, K. L., Humphreys, K. L., Fox, N. A., Nelson, C. A., & Zeanah, C. H. (2019). Signs of attachment disorders and social functioning among early adolescents with a history of institutional care. *Child Abuse & Neglect*, 88, 96–106. https://doi.org/10.1016/j.chiabu.2018.11.005
Lehmann, S., Breivik, K., Heiervang, E. R., Havik, T., & Havik, O. E. (2016). Reactive attachment disorder and disinhibited social engagement disorder in school-aged foster children-A confirmatory approach to dimensional measures. *Journal of Abnormal Child Psychology*, 44(3), 445–457. https://doi.org/10.1007/s10802-015-0045-4
Lehmann, S., Havik, O. E., Havik, T., & Heiervang, E. R. (2013). Mental disorders in foster children: a study of prevalence, comorbidity and risk factors. *Child and Adolescent Psychiatry and Mental Health*, 7(1), 1–12. https://doi.org/10.1186/1753-2000-7-39
Losinski, M., Katsiyannis, A., White, S., & Wiseman, N. (2016). Addressing the complex needs of students with attachment disorders. *Intervention in School and Clinic*, 51(3), 184–187. https://doi.org/10.1177/1053451215585800
Seim, A. R., Jozefiak, T., Wichstrøm, L., Lydersen, S., & Kayed, N. S. (2020). Reactive attachment disorder and disinhibited social engagement disorder in adolescence: Co-occurring psychopathology and psychosocial problems. *European Child & Adolescent Psychiatry*, 1–14. https://doi.org/10.1007/s00787-020-01673-7
Spilt, J. L., Vervoort, E., Koenen, A. K., Bosmans, G., & Verschueren, K. (2016). The socio-behavioral development of children with symptoms of attachment disorder: An observational study of teacher sensitivity in special education. *Research in Developmental Disabilities*, 56, 71–82. https://doi.org/10.1016/j.ridd.2016.05.014
Zeanah, C. H., Chesher, T., Boris, N. W., Walter, H. J., Bukstein, O. G., Bellonci, C., Scott Benson, R., Bussing, R., Chrisman, A., Hamilton, J., Hayek, M., Keable, H., Rockhill, C., Siegel, M., & Stock, S. (2016). Practice parameter for the assessment and treatment of children and adolescents with reactive attachment disorder and

disinhibited social engagement disorder. *Journal of the American Academy of Child & Adolescent Psychiatry*, 55(11), 990–1003. https://doi.org/10.1016/j.jaac.2016.08.004

Zeanah, C. H., Egger, H. L., Smyke, A. T., Nelson, C. A., Fox, N. A., Marshall, P. J., & Guthrie, D. (2009). Institutional rearing and psychiatric disorders in Romanian preschool children. *American Journal of Psychiatry*, 166(7), 777–785. https://doi.org/10.1176/appi.ajp.2009.08091438

Zeanah, C. H., & Gleason, M. M. (2010). *Reactive attachment disorder: A review for* DSM-V. American Psychiatric Association. https://www.researchgate.net/profile/Charles-Zeanah/publication/228683818_Reactive_Attachment_Disorder_a_review_for_DSM-V/links/0deec51e86576d1e8c000000/Reactive-Attachment-Disorder-a-review-for-DSM-V.pdf

Zeanah, C. H., & Gleason, M. M. (2015). Annual research review: Attachment disorders in early childhood–clinical presentation, causes, correlates, and treatment. *Journal of Child Psychology and Psychiatry*, 56(3), 207–222. https://doi.org/10.1111/jcpp.12347

CHAPTER 19

Disinhibited Social Engagement Disorder

LEARNING OBJECTIVES

- Summarize the *Diagnostic and Statistical Manual of Mental Disorders* (5th ed.; *DSM-5*; American Psychiatric Association [APA], 2013) diagnostic criteria of Disinhibited Social Engagement Disorder (DSED).
- Understand the social–emotional and behavioral concerns related to DSED.
- Identify the implications of DSED in the classroom.
- Describe the ways in which school psychologists can address the needs of children with DSED.
- Identify educational supports and school-based mental health interventions that may be effective in addressing education, social–emotional, and behavioral needs of children with DSED.

INTRODUCTION

Disinhibited social engagement disorder (DSED) is a mental health disorder that is characterized by aberrant social behavior in children whose early lives were marked by inadequate caregiving and social neglect. It is considered a rare disorder and little is known about the prevalence within the general population. In high-risk groups, such as children living in orphanages, the disorder is found in approximately 20% of the population (American Psychiatric Association [APA], 2013).

Research studies have demonstrated that children with DSED exhibit inappropriate social and physical boundaries and demonstrate little if any hesitation about approaching an adult stranger (APA, 2013; Zeanah & Gleason, 2015a, 2015b). Unlike children with reactive attachment disorder (RAD) who exhibit little positive emotions and are emotionally withdrawn, children with DSED generally have a more positive affect and are more engaging (Zeanah et al., 2016). They often seek the attention of adults with whom they are unfamiliar (APA, 2013; Zeanah et al., 2016). In fact, children with DSED will even venture off with a stranger without coming back to their caregiver. Although they present with a friendly disposition and may seek comfort from unfamiliar adults, their attention seeking can be aggressive (Guyon-Harris, Humphreys, Fox, et al., 2019; Zeanah et al., 2016). Their interactions may be viewed as intrusive by adults from whom they seek attention because they cross physical and social boundaries (Guyon-Harris, Humphreys, Fox, et al., 2019). This chapter examines diagnostic and cultural issues related to DSED. Social–emotional, behavioral, and learning difficulties are often experienced by children with this disorder. Consideration is also given to ways in which school psychologists can guide schools in addressing the needs of children with DSED and the types of supports needed to meet their social–emotional, behavioral, and learning needs.

DIAGNOSTIC ISSUES RELATED TO DISINHIBITED SOCIAL ENGAGEMENT DISORDER

Etiology and Course

Research on DSED stems from studies examining the influence of inadequate caregiving and is primarily focused on infants and young children in institutions. The Bucharest Early Intervention Project (Zeanah et al., 2005) was one of the earliest studies to examine the impact of institutional care on young children. In this research project, Zeanah and colleagues (2005) assessed children living in the institution with RAD and DSED symptoms at baseline. The findings indicated that more signs of RAD and DSED were found in children living in the institution compared to children with no history of institutional care (Zeanah et al., 2002). Assessments were conducted in each group of children again at 30, 42, and 54 months. The findings of the assessment at each of these time points revealed that children in foster care exhibited fewer signs of RAD in comparison to children living in the institution (Smyke et al., 2012). At 42 and 54 months, children in foster care had fewer signs of DSED than children in institutional care. A follow-up study done when the children were 8 years old revealed that children in foster care continued to show fewer signs of both disorders in comparison to children living in the institution (Smyke et al., 2012). The researchers conducted another follow-up study when the children were 12 years old which revealed that children living in the institution displayed more symptoms of RAD and DSED than children with no prior history of institutional care. In addition, at this point in time the study revealed that the foster care group showed significantly fewer symptoms of RAD and DSED (Humphreys et al., 2017).

In regard to the course of DSED, longitudinal studies research indicates that clinical symptoms of DSED are relatively stable over time in children raised in institutions and those who were later placed in foster care or adopted (APA, 2013; Zeanah et al., 2016). Zeanah and colleagues (2016) emphasize that research has consistently indicated that children in institutional care who were assessed at baseline continued to exhibit indiscriminate behavior whether they remained in institutional care or were placed in alternative living conditions. In addition, Gleason et al. (2011) found that, in children living in institutional care who were assessed at approximately 30, 42 and 54 months, DSED was predictive of psychiatric symptoms at 54 months. Other scholars have found that symptoms of DSED can continue to persist in children adopted after initially living in institutions even though they have already established a relationship with their adoptive parents (O'Connor et al., 2003).

DSM-5 Diagnostic Issues Related to Disinhibited Social Engagement Disorder

In the *Diagnostic and Statistical Manual of Mental Disorders*, Third Edition (*DSM-III*; APA, 1987), DSED was first conceptualized as one of two subtypes of RAD. At that time, RAD was considered to have a disinhibited subtype that was characterized by externalizing behaviors that included indiscriminate sociability and an inhibited subtype that was characterized by internalizing behaviors such as sadness, emotional withdrawal, and fearfulness (Zeanah & Gleason, 2010). As noted by Zeanah and Gleason (2010), children with the indiscriminate subtype demonstrate a lack of guardedness around unfamiliar adults and will inappropriately approach strangers, whereas children with the inhibited subtype are emotionally withdrawn and do not seek help or support from others. According to Zeanah and Gleason (2015a), the conceptualization of RAD as two subtypes of a single disorder was based on the view that the "phenotypes intended to describe a lack of attachment in children who had experienced adverse caregiving—in inhibited RAD, attachment behaviors were not expressed, and in disinhibited RAD, attachment behaviors were expressed nonselectively" (p. 208). The two subtypes remained part of the diagnostic criteria for RAD until the *DSM-5*, which conceptualized the two subtypes as two separate disorders, DSED and RAD under the category of Trauma- and Stressor-Related Disorders (APA, 2013). As noted by Zeanah and Smyke (2014), the reason for this change in conceptualization was that, although both RAD and DSED arise under conditions of severe social neglect, there are differences in their symptom presentation, psychiatric comorbidities, and response to interventions. For example, children with DSED demonstrate no hesitancy in approaching a stranger, whereas children with RAD are emotionally withdrawn from their caregivers and do not seek help from their caregivers (APA, 2013; Zeanah & Smyke, 2014; Zeanah et al., 2016). In addition, comorbid conditions in RAD include depression, whereas attention deficit hyperactivity behaviors often coexist with DSED (APA, 2013; Zeanah & Smyke, 2014; Zeanah et al., 2016). In regard to differences in how RAD and DSED respond to intervention, research data has demonstrated that children with RAD typically demonstrate a substantial reduction in symptoms once they are removed from conditions marked by deprivation and neglect and placed with a nurturing caregiver (Zeanah & Gleason, 2010, 2015a, 2015b). On the other hand, children with DSED show little reduction in symptoms once they are removed from inadequate caregiving and placed in a more nurturing environment (Zeanah & Gleason, 2010, 2015a, 2015b). According to Zeanah and Gleason (2015a), the decision to establish the disinhibited subtype of RAD as a separate disorder was also based on data from research studies on institutionalized children that indicated that the "core deficit of the disorder is not nonselective attachment behaviors, but more about unmodulated and indiscriminate social behavior, especially initial approaches to and interaction with unfamiliar adults" (p. 208). Hence with this new conceptualization of DSED, the emphasis is on social engagement rather than attachment (Zeanah & Gleason, 2015a).

Children with DSED show little reduction in symptoms once they are removed from inadequate caregiving and placed in a more nurturing environment (Zeanah & Gleason, 2010, 2015a, 2015b).

This change in the conceptualization of DSED and the focus from attachment to abnormal social behavior has been challenged by some scholars. For example, Lyons-Ruth and colleagues (2015) contend that this change raises the issue of whether DSED should be considered "a disorder of attachment or a disorder with a nonattachment-related etiology" (p. 223). Challenging the concept of DSED as no longer an attachment disorder, Lyons-Ruth and colleagues (2015) propose that a disruption in a youngster's primary attachment is ample evidence that DSED should still be considered an attachment disorder. According to Lyons-Ruth and colleagues (2015), children with secure attachments who exhibit indiscriminate behaviors are, in fact, securely attached as demonstrated by their indiscriminate behavior. However, Zeanah and Gleason (2015a, 2015b) contend that, in regard to DSED, the emphasis on social engagement rather than attachment is based on three issues evidenced in prior research on children raised in institutional care. One issue is that social neglect is a requirement for DSED, but it alone does not cause DSED (Zeanah & Gleason, 2015b). As Zeanah and Gleason point out, this is evident in the findings that most children living in deprived and neglectful conditions during infancy do not develop DSED. Another issue is that attachment behaviors aimed toward caregivers are not involved with DSED; the disorder involves socially inappropriate behaviors targeted toward people who are unfamiliar and essentially nonattachment figures (Zeanah & Gleason, 2015b). Finally, Zeanah and Gleason (2015b) point out that DSED can be present in youngsters who have no attachment figures, children who exhibit insecure or disorganized attachments to their caregivers, or children with secure attachments to caregivers. Furthermore, they emphasize that social engagement, although linked to attachment, differs from attachment and acknowledge that more research needs to be conducted to fully understand the etiology of DSED.

The *DSM-5* conceptualization of RAD and DSED as two separate constructs is supported by recent research studies of children living in foster care and residential youth centers. To determine whether there was support for RAD and DSED as individual constructs, Lehmann and colleagues (2016) used a sample of school-aged children living in foster care who had no previous history of institutional care. The results of their study revealed that RAD and DSED were statistically and conceptually two separate constructs that can be distinguished from more common mental health problems (Lehmann et al., 2016). Support for RAD and DSED as individual constructs was also found in a study conducted by Seim, Jozefiak, Wichstrøm, and Kayed (2020). The sample of participants consisted of Norwegian adolescents between the ages of 12 and 23 years old who lived in a residential youth center. The authors interviewed the adolescents using the Child and Adolescent Psychiatric Assessment (CAPA) to determine RAD and DSED symptoms/diagnoses and symptoms related to other psychiatric disorders. The findings of their study provided evidence to support RAD and DSED as individual disorders that were distinct from common psychiatric disorders (Seim, Jozefiak, Wichstrøm, & Kayed, 2020).

Based on the *DSM-5* diagnostic criteria, children with DSED exhibit a pattern of behavior that involves approaching and engaging with adults who are unfamiliar to them. This disturbed behavior is marked by at least two of the following features: (a) little to no reservation when approaching and engaging the stranger; (b) inappropriate, overly familiar behavior (verbal or physical) that breaches the social boundaries of the child's culture; (c) little to no checking back with their caregivers once they wander off with the stranger; and (d) little to no hesitation when wandering off with an adult who is unfamiliar (APA, 2013). The *DSM-5* criteria also note that this pattern of behavior is not limited to impulsivity that is associated with attention deficit hyperactivity disorder (ADHD) but is marked by socially disinhibited behavior (APA, 2013).

Similar to RAD, the *DSM-5* (APA, 2013) indicates that there must have been exposure to inadequate, neglectful care in the early development that is marked by one of the following (a) social neglect in which the child's basic emotional needs were not met by caregivers; (b) multiple changes in caregivers that limit the child's ability to establish a stable attachment; and (c) being raised in settings, such as orphanages, that have high child-caregiver ratios that limit opportunities to establish a selective attachment to a caregiver. The *DSM-5* also notes that this inadequate caregiving is responsible for the pattern of overly familiar behavior in which the child approaches and engages adults who are unfamiliar to them. It is important to note that a diagnosis of DSED cannot be made until the child has reached a developmental age of at least 9 months. The rationale for this stipulation is to ensure that the child has reached a developmental level in which selective attachment to a caregiver is possible. Symptoms of DSED are considered persistent if they last longer than 12 months and severe when all symptoms are present and occur at a high level.

Regarding differential diagnosis, the *DSM-5* indicates that a distinction between DSED and ADHD needs to be made. As Zeanah and colleagues (2016) note, social impulsivity is sometimes evident in children with ADHD, but usually the impulsivity associated with ADHD is related more to cognitive and behavioral aspects of functioning, whereas impulsivity related to DSED is clearly social.

Throughout the literature on DSED, few studies focus on comorbidity in children with DSED (APA, 2013). According to the *DSM-5* (APA, 2013), some conditions linked to neglect, such as cognitive and language delays, may coexist with DSED in some children. However, it should be noted that the findings of some studies indicate that in addition to disinhibited behavior, social deprivation is linked to inattention and hyperactivity (Roy et al., 2004; Zeanah et al., 2016). The *DSM-5* (APA, 2013) indicates that children with DSED can be concurrently diagnosed with ADHD. Research studies have found comorbidity of DSED and ADHD in preschoolers (Gleason et al., 2011) and in school-aged children (Rutter et al., 2007). Studies conducted by Roy et al. (2004) and Gleason and colleagues (2011) found moderately strong correlations between these two symptom presentations.

School-Based Eligibility

Although the *DSM-5* is used for diagnostic purposes and to guide psychological and psychiatric services in the clinical/medical field, a different type of classification system is used to determine whether a child is a student with a disability and eligible for special educational services. The educational classification of disabilities falls under the federal legislation known as the *Individuals with Disabilities Education Improvement Act* (IDEA) of 2004. In order to be found eligible for one of the 13 disability categories under IDEA (2004), a multidisciplinary team must determine (a) whether the child meets eligibility criteria to be identified as a student with a disability and (b) if there is a need for special educational services (Salvia et al., 2016). If the child is found to be a student with a disability, there must be evidence from the assessment data that the disability has an adverse impact on the child's academic functioning.

One of the 13 disability categories that would most likely be considered for a child exhibiting signs of DSED is Emotional Disturbance (which is known as *Emotional Behavioral Disorder* in some states). Section 300.8 (c) (4) of IDEA (2004) defines an *Emotional Disturbance* as a condition that has persisted for a substantial amount of time and one that has an adverse impact on the child's academic performance in the classroom. The federal definition stipulates that the child must be experiencing one or more of the characteristics to be eligible for an emotional disturbance: (a) an inability to learn in the classroom that is not due to an intellectual, sensory, or health factors; (b) an inability to establish and maintain relationships with teachers and peers; (c) atypical feelings and behaviors displayed under ordinary situations; (d) a persistent state of sadness; and (e) a tendency to develop physical symptoms or fear related to personal or school difficulties. In addition, Emotional Disturbance includes youth with schizophrenia. However, this disability excludes children and adolescents with social maladjustment unless there is evidence that the child or adolescent also has an emotional disturbance.

If the team reviews all of the assessment data and determines that the child's difficulties do not seem to negatively impact the child's educational performance and, hence, the child does not need special education services, a team may decide to consider a 504 plan for the child if the child would benefit from accommodations. The Rehabilitation Act of 1973 was established to protect the civil rights of individuals with a disability or suspected disability. Under the civil rights legislation Section 504 of the Rehabilitation Act of 1973, this Act was established to protect the civil rights of individuals with a disability or suspected disability. Under Section 504 of this legislation, there must be evidence that the person's disability has a negative impact on at least one or more major life functions. Therefore, if DSED is impacting a particular area of the child's life, a 504 plan may be considered so that the child can receive accommodations that may be needed.

CULTURAL ISSUES RELATED TO DISINHIBITED SOCIAL ENGAGEMENT DISORDER IN YOUTH

As noted earlier, the *DSM-5* denotes severe social neglect as a diagnostic criterion for DSED (APA, 2013). Severe social neglect is associated with institutional care or foster care (APA, 2013; Zeanah et al., 2016). Institutional care for children has been studied by Dozier and colleagues (2012), who note that young children are usually placed in this type of setting because of poverty and unstable home environments. The authors note that institutional care is typically unsuited to meet the needs of young children. Factors that contribute to conditions of social neglect in residential institutions include high child-to-caregiver ratios, untrained and uneducated staff, low salaries, rotating shifts, and a lack of emotional investment in the children living in the institution (Dozier et al., 2012). Estimates of the number of children living in institutions worldwide range from 2 to 4 million (Dozier et al., 2012). Although some areas of the world have made efforts to use alternative types of placement, such as foster care, there are many regions of the world in which institutional care is frequently used such as countries in Eastern Europe, Central America, South America, Africa, Asia, and the Middle East (Dozier et al., 2012).

> Factors that contribute to conditions of social neglect in residential institutions include high child-to-caregiver ratios, untrained and uneducated staff, low salaries, rotating shifts, and a lack of emotional investment in the children living in the institution (Dozier et al., 2012).

Research studies have documented symptoms of DSED in children living in institutional or foster care in various countries across the world. These include Norway (Lehmann et al., 2016; Seim, Jozefiak, Wichstrøm, & Kayed, 2020; Seim, Jozefiak, Wichstrøm, Lydersen, et al., 2020), Finland (Elovainio et al., 2015), Romania (Gleason et al., 2011; Humphreys et al., 2017), and Korea (Hong et al., 2018). However, there is a lack of research that has systematically examined cross-cultural differences among children with DSED. We hope that scholars will pursue future research that focuses on cultural differences in children diagnosed with DSED, particularly in countries that still utilize institutional care.

IMPACT ON DISINHIBITED SOCIAL ENGAGEMENT DISORDER ON SOCIAL–EMOTIONAL AND BEHAVIORAL FUNCTIONING IN SCHOOL AND HOME ENVIRONMENTS

Given the rarity of DSED, research studies on the social–emotional and behavioral functioning of children with a diagnosis based on *DSM-5* criteria are scant. Studies that use small sample sizes and combined samples of children with DSED and RAD complicate the interpretation in terms of which specific social–emotional and behavioral problems are unique to DSED.

Social–Emotional and Behavioral Functioning in School

The effects of severe social neglect and inadequate caregiving early in life can render a young child vulnerable socially, emotionally, and behaviorally. Research findings indicate that DSED is associated with functional impairment in young children (Gleason et al., 2011) and higher rates of psychopathology (Rutter et al., 2007). Children with DSED may exhibit challenging behaviors when they begin school. Therefore, it is important for the school psychologist to have an understanding of the psychological impact that deprived living conditions can have on a young child's development so that they can guide school personnel in how to best address the social–emotional and behavioral needs of a child with DSED.

COMPETENCE AND SELF-ESTEEM

Given that children with DSED exhibit challenging behaviors, competence in different areas of functioning has been explored by some scholars. Guyon-Harris, Humphreys, Miron, and colleagues (2019) examine competence in early adolescence in preteens with DSED. The study was part of the Bucharest Early Intervention Project, which was a longitudinal study of children who initially lived in institutions in Romania. The sample consisted of participants with disinhibited behaviors who were assessed at ages 30, 42, 54 months, and 12 years of age. Guyon-Harris, Humphreys, Miron, and colleagues (2019) examined competent functioning across seven domains, which included family relationships, peer relationships, academic performance, physical health, mental health, substance use, and risk-taking behavior. The findings of the study revealed that DSED was associated with reduced competence in preteens and that children with DSED in early childhood demonstrated less competence in early adolescence compared to a control group of children with no history of DSED (Guyon-Harris, Humphreys, Miron, et al., 2019). The authors also found that negative associations between early DSED and later competent functioning continued even if symptoms of DSED were reduced over the course of time (Guyon-Harris, Humphreys, Miron, et al., 2019).

To gain an understanding of self-esteem in adolescents with DSED, Seim, Jozefiak, Wichstrøm, and Kayed (2020) examined global and specific domains of self-esteem among adolescents between the ages of 12 and 20 who were living in a youth residential center. Youths were assessed for DSED. Results of the study indicated that, in comparison to a control group of youths from the general population, those with DSED had lower self-esteem for scholastic competence, social acceptance, athletic competence, physical appearance, and self-worth (Seim, Jozefiak, Wichstrøm, & Kayed, 2020). The findings also revealed that, in comparison to youths from the residential youth center who did not exhibit DSED, youths with DSED were found to have lower social acceptance and self-worth (Seim, Jozefiak, Wichstrøm, & Kayed, 2020).

EMOTIONAL–BEHAVIORAL PROBLEMS

Research studies have found that externalizing behaviors are associated with DSED, but the findings have not been consistent. For example, studies examining aggressive behavior in toddlers living in institutions indicated that there was no association between the toddlers' caregiver reports of indiscriminate behavior and global ratings of aggression (Zeanah et al., 2002). Similar findings were evident in studies related to the Bucharest Early Intervention Project in children ages 42 months and younger who exhibited DSED behaviors (Gleason et al., 2011; Zeanah et al., 2005). Although externalizing behaviors in young institutionalized children with indiscriminate behaviors were not indicated in these studies, there have been findings of externalizing behaviors as children with DSED got older. For example, Lyons-Ruth and colleagues (2009) found that toddlers who exhibited indiscriminate behaviors toward unfamiliar adults demonstrated more aggressive and hyperactive behaviors at age 5.

Other studies have found similar results as evidenced in Gleason and colleagues' (2011) findings that indiscriminate behaviors in institutionalized children at 54 months were associated with inattention, hyperactivity, and disruptive behaviors. A study conducted by Moran et al. (2017) examined the association of DSED and RAD symptoms and mental health problems among adolescent juvenile offenders between the ages of 12 and 17 who had been maltreated. The findings revealed an association between DSED and RAD symptoms and hyperactive behaviors (Moran et al., 2017). It should be noted that the symptoms of DSED and RAD among the sample of offenders were combined and, hence, the specific association of DSED is unclear.

The relationship between DSED and later behavioral problems among children was studied by Elovainio et al. (2015). The sample for the study consisted of a total of 1,359 internationally adopted children between the ages of 6 and 15 who were living in Finland. The authors assessed the children for DSED and RAD symptoms as well as emotional–behavioral problems and behaviors related to ADHD. The results of the study revealed that DSED and RAD were associated with behavioral problems and ADHD-related behaviors in the sample of international adoptees (Elovainio et al., 2015). To be specific, children with RAD symptoms were found to have more internalizing, externalizing, and total problem behaviors than the DSED group and a comparison group with no RAD or DSED symptoms. It is interesting to note that children with DSED symptoms had more externalizing behaviors and total problem behaviors than the comparison group. In regard to ADHD-related behaviors, symptoms of DSED and RAD were found to be associated with hyperactivity but not inattention.

Given that many of the research studies focusing on DSED have been conducted in young children, more studies examining DSED in adolescence are needed. Seim, Jozefiak, Wichstrøm, Lydersen, and colleagues (2020) examined emotional–behavioral problems in Norwegian adolescents with DSED who were between the ages of 12 and 20 who were living in a residential youth center. The results of the study indicated that some youths with DSED also experienced coexisting symptoms of conduct and oppositional defiant disorder as well as behaviors related to ADHD. Interestingly, Seim, Jozefiak, Wichstrøm, Lydersen, and colleagues (2020) reported that emotional problems were more prevalent in this sample of adolescents than in school-aged children who were adopted after being in institutional care as reported by Rutter et al. (2007). In addition, suicidal thoughts and attempts were reported by adolescents with DSED (Seim, Jozefiak, Wichstrøm, Lydersen, et al., 2020).

INTERPERSONAL RELATIONSHIPS

Given that children with DSED have early exposure to inadequate caregiving and lack opportunities to have learned appropriate social behaviors through modeling, it is important for scholars to examine social functioning and socio-behavioral problems among children with DSED. Research findings have indicated that DSED is predictive of difficulties with close relationships (Gleason et al., 2011; Rutter et al., 2007). In the Bucharest Early Intervention Project longitudinal study, Gleason and colleagues (2011) examined social–emotional competence at several different time points—approximately 20 months, which was baseline, 30, 42, and 54 months. The results of their study indicated that DSED behaviors were associated with a lack of social–emotional competence at 30 and 42 months and that there was a large association at 54 months of age, which reflected functional impairments. Rutter and colleagues (2007) similarly found that children between the ages of 6 and 11 who had initially lived in institutional care and were later adopted exhibited problems with peers.

> Research findings have indicated that DSED is predictive of difficulties with close relationships (Gleason et al., 2011; Rutter et al., 2007).

As indicated earlier, DSED can persist in children over time so it is important to gain an understanding of a child's social functioning as they get older. Guyon-Harris, Humphreys, Fox, and colleagues (2019) examined social functioning among children with DSED who were participants in the Bucharest Early Intervention Project at age 12. They used several instruments to assess various aspects of social functioning from the parent and teacher perspectives. Their findings revealed that DSED predicted higher scores on caregiver views of the child as victim in conflict resolution and lower scores on social competence (Guyon-Harris, Humphreys, Fox, et al., 2019). Other scholars have studied DSED and RAD symptoms and peer problems in a sample of juvenile offenders between the ages of 12 and 17 who had histories of maltreatment (Moran et al., 2017). The findings of this research indicated that DSED and RAD behaviors were moderately associated with parent-rated, but not teacher-rated peer relationship problems. However, the association specifically from DSED is not clear as DSED and RAD symptoms were combined.

An interesting study was conducted by Spilt et al. (2016) which explored the influence of teacher sensitivity on the socio-behavioral development of children exhibiting DSED and RAD behaviors over the course of 1 academic year. The sample consisted of Belgian children and teachers from various special education schools. Prior to conducting observations of teachers' sensitivity, Spilt and colleagues (2016) had teachers complete the teacher version of the Relationship Problem Questionnaire which is considered to be a valid and reliable instrument. This questionnaire assesses for disinhibited and inhibited behaviors of school-aged children. Over the course of the year, the researchers observed interactions of teachers with the targeted students across different types of tasks outside of the classroom. The results of the study revealed that no effects of teacher sensitivity on prosocial behavior or overt and relational aggression (Spilt et al., 2016). Spilt and colleagues (2016) concluded that the findings supported the concept that DSED was a social engagement disorder rather than an attachment disorder.

Social–Emotional and Behavioral Functioning at Home

Whether a child with RAD or DSED has lived in an institution or experienced multiple foster care placements, the transition to an adoptive home or a new foster home placement can be challenging for the family. Adoptive parents and foster care parents may not be prepared to manage the child's emotional and behavioral problems. It is important for school psychologists to have an understanding of emotional and behavioral problems experienced in the home and how these problems impact the home environment.

In a qualitative study, Vasquez and Miller (2018) interviewed adopted children and family members. Five families of adopted children participated in the study. The children had been previously diagnosed with RAD prior to their adoption so the diagnosis was not based on *DSM-5* diagnostic criteria, thus it's unclear whether the symptoms were related more to the disinhibited or inhibited subtypes among the children. During the interviews, a common concern among the children and family members was the extreme temper tantrums experienced by the children. Family members described these outbursts as uncontrollable rages. It was also noted that the tantrums tended to be targeted at the caregiver with whom the child was close. According to Vasquez and Miller (2018), difficulty in controlling the outbursts may reflect inhibitory control despite the children reporting that the rages were out of their control. As the researchers noted, inhibitory control of such rages reflects the possibility that the child may be able to suppress such intense feelings while they are in school or other situations and then release those feelings later on with the caregiver with whom they feel safe.

> Inhibitory control of such rages reflects the possibility that the child may be able to suppress such intense feelings while they are in school or other situations and then release those feelings later on with the caregiver with whom they feel safe.

As noted earlier, most studies on children with DSED include samples of children with histories of institutional and foster care placements. Zephyr and colleagues (2021) conducted an interesting study that examined dysfunctional behaviors of biological parents of children between the ages of 1 and 5 with a history of maltreatment and foster care placements who exhibited DSED behaviors. The researchers conducted observations of parent–child interactions and reviewed Child Protective Services files. The findings indicated that only a few children with histories of neglect exhibited high levels of DSED behaviors. Most of the children had an insecure attachment to their parent with just over half of the children exhibiting a disorganized type of attachment. Zephyr and colleagues (2021) found that the more parents exhibited disconnected and insensitive behaviors in their interactions with the child, the more DSED behaviors were exhibited by the child. The authors concluded that the quality of parental behavior may influence children's development and recovery of behaviors related to DSED (Zephyr et al., 2021).

> The quality of parental behavior may influence children's development and recovery of behaviors related to DSED (Zephyr et al., 2021).

Another unique study was conducted by Scheper et al. (2016). The researchers examined inhibited behaviors and disinhibited social engagement behaviors in home-reared children who had been referred for treatment of emotional and behavioral problems. The purpose of the study was to assess the clinical significance of inhibited and disinhibited social engagement behaviors in home-reared children in comparison to maltreated children with foster care. Scheper and colleagues (2016) found that, although inhibited behaviors were found less often in the referred home-reared group than the foster group, disinhibited social engagement behaviors were found in just over 40% of home-reared children, which was similar to the foster care group. The results also indicated that inhibited and disinhibited social engagement behaviors were not associated with child maltreatment. In addition, the findings revealed more inhibited behavior was linked with clinical levels of internalizing and externalizing behaviors in the home-reared group in comparison to the foster care group. Scheper et al. (2016) also found that more disinhibited social engagement behaviors were associated with externalizing behaviors and more parental stress in both groups.

IMPACT OF DISINHIBITED SOCIAL ENGAGEMENT DISORDER ON LEARNING IN THE CLASSROOM

The amount of research studies on how DSED impacts a child's learning in the classroom and how to address learning difficulties children with DSED may encounter is scant. There is research evidence indicating that DSED is predictive of more need for special education services (Rutter et al., 2007), but little more is evident in the literature. It is clear, however, that rich learning opportunities most likely are not associated with living environments characteristic of deprivation and social neglect such as institutional care and multiple foster care placements (Raaska et al., 2012). Given these circumstances, it would not be surprising if a child with a history of living in an institution or multiple foster homes struggled to learn in the classroom.

Raaska et al. (2012) examined learning issues among a sample of 395 internationally adopted youth between the ages of 9 and 15 who lived in Finland. The sample was assessed for RAD based on characteristics of the *DSM-IV* (APA, 1994) criteria so both inhibited and disinhibited subtypes were included. Although no distinction is made in regard to specific learning difficulties associated with the disinhibited subtype, which is now known as DSED, the findings are still relevant and provide a picture of learning issues that may be experienced by children with DSED. The findings of the study conducted by Raaska and colleagues (2012) revealed that children adopted at younger ages tended to have fewer severe learning difficulties in comparison to those who were adopted at older ages. The findings also indicated that boys, more than girls, experienced more learning problems (Raaska et al., 2012).

Given the challenging social–emotional and behavioral difficulties associated with DSED, one must take these difficulties into consideration when examining factors that can influence a child's performance in the classroom. As seen earlier, DSED in early childhood was associated with less competence in adolescence (Guyon-Harris, Humphreys, Fox, et al., 2019), which could potentially impact learning if someone does not feel competent in their abilities. In addition, DSED's association with a lack of social–emotional competence as reported by Gleason et al. (2011) and lower social competence as reported by Guyon-Harris, Humphreys, Fox, et al. (2019) would potentially impact learning as seen in the research by Wight and Chapparo (2008), which indicated that social competence was linked to academic performance. Lower self-esteem in areas such as scholastic competence, self-worth, and social acceptance was associated with DSED (Seim, Jozefiak, Wichstrøm, & Kayed, 2020), which could also potentially impact learning in the classroom if one has low self-esteem given the previous work of Trautwein et al. (2006) indicating the connection among self-esteem, academic self-esteem, and achievement. In addition, externalizing behaviors of hyperactivity (Elovaino et al., 2015; Seim, Jozefiak, Wichstrøm, Lydersen, et al., 2020) and disruptive behaviors (Seim, Jozefiak, Wichstrøm, & Kayed, 2020) have the potential to influence learning based on the previous work of McGee and Share (1988), which focused on ADHD and academic failure. Finally, emotional difficulties, such as suicidal thoughts and attempts, as reported by Seim, Jozefiak, Wichstrøm, Lydersen, et al. (2020) also may potentially influence the child's performance in the classroom based on the previous findings of Pate and colleagues (2017), which demonstrate a connection between emotional problems and academic outcomes.

IMPLICATIONS FOR SCHOOL PSYCHOLOGISTS

Advocacy

School psychologists can play an important advocacy role when working with families of a child with DSED. Establishing a partnership with the family is important and learning about the concerns and areas of need of the family as well as the child better enables the school to serve the child. If the family has undergone an international adoption, they most likely will have had an experience similar to other families who have gone through an adoption process in that they may feel that they were unprepared to manage the challenges associated with a child with a disability and were unsupported in their attempts to help address their child's needs after the adoption (Good, 2016). In many ways, foster families with whom a child with DSED may be placed may also feel unprepared to meet the child's needs. Therefore, it is imperative that school psychologists guide the family through the educational system and encourage them to become advocates for the child.

In addition to addressing the child's educational needs through the school system, some children with DSED and their families may need outside therapeutic services. Losinski et al. (2016) encourage school practitioners to consider a multisystem approach when working with children who have DSED or RAD. Given that family therapy, individual therapy for the child, and perhaps psychiatric services are often needed by families with children with DSED, a multisystem approach using wraparound services may be an effective tool in addressing the complex needs of children with DSED and their families (Losinski et al., 2016). Such an approach would involve the coordination of services through the school and community. School psychologists could advocate for wraparound services for the child and family and guide them through the process of seeking these types of services.

Consultation

Engaging parents of children with DSED as partners and seeking their involvement in their child's education is a vital task for school psychologists. Taft and colleagues (2016) indicate that a principle of IDEA (2004) is collaboration between schools and parents of students with disabilities and that this is particularly important for students with emotional–behavioral disorders. Therefore, to promote effective communication and enhance parental involvement with families of children with DSED, school psychologists need to develop a collaborative partnership with the parents of children with DSED. Scholars have noted that in their interactions with their child's school, parents of children with RAD in their interactions with their child's school, often feel as though their input is not valued and that they are sometimes blamed by the school for their child's behavior (Taft et al., 2016). Parents of children with DSED may also have similar experiences with school personnel so it would be important for the school psychologist to be a liaison between the parent and school personnel.

Some parents may have questions about DSED and how the disorder impacts their child as the child develops. School psychologists could gather information about this disorder that addresses the types of social, emotional, behavioral, and learning challenges experienced by some children with DSED and how best to address the child's needs in these areas. Parents may have questions about how they can help their child and how to manage behaviors related to DSED at home. The school psychologist could be a valuable resource for the parents and a trusted, supportive individual to whom they can go to learn how to maneuver through the educational system as they attempt to advocate for their child.

In addition to consulting with parents, school psychologists need to consult with the child's teacher and work collaboratively with the teacher to determine how best to meet the social–emotional, behavioral, and learning needs of the child and guide the teacher in understanding how DSED may manifest in the classroom. Sharing information about the disorder and how it impacts a child's development and functioning can help the teacher gain a better understanding of the challenges associated with DSED. It could be helpful to inform the teacher about some of the difficulties experienced by children with DSED that have been found in research studies such as hyperactive behaviors (Elovaino et al., 2015; Seim, Jozefiak, Wichstrøm, Lydersen, et al., 2020), disruptive behaviors (Seim, Jozefiak, Wichstrøm, Lydersen, et al., 2020), low self-esteem (Seim, Jozefiak, Wichstrøm, & Kayed, 2020), and a lack of socio-emotional confidence (Gleason et al., 2011). In addition, it is important to emphasize to the teacher the child's need to have stability and consistency in the classroom.

Assessment

Addressing the needs of children with DSED can be challenging and even though supports may have been provided in the classroom, a multidisciplinary team may decide that it is best to refer the child for a special education evaluation if the child has not made substantial progress. If this is the case, the school will need to seek consent from the parents to conduct an evaluation. After consent is obtained, the multidisciplinary team will have 60 days to complete their evaluation of the child. If an outside agency provides services to the child, permission from the parents needs to be obtained before requesting to review those records. Prior to beginning the evaluation, the school nurse conducts a vision and hearing screening.

As part of the assessment process, a review of relevant information needs to occur. The school psychologists and/or multidisciplinary team reviews information from the child's academic record such as state tests results, disciplinary referral, attendance, educational history, psychosocial history, and medical history. It might also be helpful to review work samples and progress-monitoring data.

Interviews provide a means of gathering information about the child's functioning from the parent, teacher, and child (depending on age). Given the challenging behaviors exhibited by children with DSED, it is important to gather information related to these behavioral problems such as onset of the behavior, frequency, and duration of the behavior and strategies used thus far to address the behavioral problems. Information about the child's developmental history could also be obtained, though if the child was adopted or has been in foster care, the parent may not have knowledge of the child's early history. Rating scales are frequently used to gather information about the child's emotional and behavioral functioning and typically there are multi-rater versions available so that information can be obtained from multiple sources.

Observations of the child's behavior can shed light on antecedents and consequences of behavior. It is generally recommended to conduct observation in more than one location (Floyd et al., 2008). Some scholars recommend the use of an observation system, which involves observing under conditions that are likely to elicit the problem behavior (Sheperis et al., 2003). In some states, an observation is a required component to determine the IDEA (2004) disability category of Emotional Disturbance.

School psychologists may also conduct assessment of the child's cognitive functioning, achievement, and social–emotional functioning. Assessment data can be reviewed by the multidisciplinary team to determine whether a disability is adversely impacting the child's academic performance.

Counseling/Therapeutic Services

Based on their training, school psychologists are in a unique position to serve as a provider of mental health services. School psychologists can provide school-based mental health interventions that address the social–emotional and/or behavioral needs of a child with DSED. Although there are no interventions identified in the literature that are specific for DSED, some interventions that have been applicable to RAD (Floyd et al., 2008; Schwartz & Davis, 2006) would be relevant for DSED. Also, scholars have emphasized that interventions for students with RAD and DSED in the schools should (a) be specific to the individual child, (b) be developmentally appropriate, and (c) involve no negative practices or emotional pressure (Zeanah, 1999 as cited in Floyd et al., 2008). Other scholars have recommended that school-based interventions address self-esteem and self-efficacy so that the child's overall functioning could improve (Haugaard & Hazan, 2004).

> Scholars have emphasized that interventions for students with RAD and DSED in the schools should (a) be specific to the individual child, (b) be developmentally appropriate, and (c) involve no negative practices or emotional pressure (Zeanah, 1999 as cited in Floyd et al., 2008).

School psychologists could provide cognitive behavioral therapy (CBT) techniques to address self-regulation difficulties and hyperactive behaviors that some children with DSED experience. Given that social competence and low self-esteem have been found to be areas of concern in children with DSED, the school psychologist could provide social skill interventions to address the child's social impulsivity and teach the child appropriate ways of interacting with others (Floyd et al., 2008). In addition, play therapy techniques may also be useful when addressing some of these issues with the child. School psychologists should have received training in the use of CBT and play therapy techniques prior to providing interventions. It is also important to remember that the child may be receiving mental health services from an outside agency so the school psychologist should collaborate with the outside therapist in determining what type of services might be provided in the school.

As noted earlier, scholars have reported suicidal thoughts and attempts among youths with DSED. Therefore, screening for suicidality may be needed to determine whether a child is experiencing suicidal ideation so that appropriate therapeutic services could be delivered. If a child acknowledges suicidal thoughts or suicidal attempts, the school psychologist should conduct a threat assessment to determine whether the child has current suicidal thoughts or plans to harm themself. If it is determined that the risk of suicide is high, crisis planning may be needed.

EDUCATIONAL SUPPORTS

Although few studies in the literature address school-related needs of children with DSED, it is imperative that school readiness be examined. Floyd and colleagues (2008) emphasize the need to provide teachers and school administrators with psychoeducation about the social–emotional and behavioral needs of children with RAD (which also applied to DSED at the time). Supportive approaches used for maltreated children have been recommended for children with RAD (or DSED; Schwartz & Davis, 2006). These suggestions include the need to understand the child's behavior, nurture the child, interact with the child at the child's emotional level, ensure consistency and maintain an environment that is predictable, and model appropriate social interactions (Perry, 2001). This approach could be used by teachers in the classroom and other school personnel who work with the child.

To address challenging behaviors exhibited by children with DSED and RAD, some scholars have recommended use of Multi-Tiered Systems of Support (MTSS; Losinski et al., 2016). This model is used to provide students with supports and involves screening, progress monitoring, and targeted interventions. It is used in schools to provide supports to address a child's emotional and behavioral needs. Losinski and colleagues (2016) contend that this model would benefit students with RAD and DSED. According to Losinski et al. (2016), Tier 1 supports include evidence-based instruction and screening to identify emotional and behavioral concerns. Tier 2 supports would address targeted behaviors and are sometimes provided in small groups. For a child with DSED, strategies that are designed to address social skills in a small-group setting might be considered. In addition, daily monitoring of the child's behavior may be helpful. Tier 3 supports would be targeted toward the child's individual needs and include a more intensive intervention. This type of intervention might perhaps be a one-on-one intervention with the school psychologist that addresses social competence and self-esteem.

As with supports for children with RAD (Losinki et al., 2016), children with DSED may benefit from supports that help the child feel safe in the classroom. The teacher and school psychologist could work together to determine how to best help the child feel safe in the learning environment, which might include having a special corner in the room where the child can go if they become overwhelmed. Predictability in the environment is key for children with DSED and RAD so make sure the child knows what is expected and is informed if there will be a change in routine (Losinki et al., 2016).

SCHOOL-BASED MENTAL HEALTH INTERVENTIONS AND SUPPORTS

Much work is needed in developing therapeutic approaches for children with DSED, particularly school-based mental health interventions. However, there are some scholars who report the use of school-based play therapy for children with RAD, which may be relevant to DSED. Ritchie (2013) recommends three types of play therapy that could benefit children with RAD (which included DSED). Given that children with DSED exhibit social disinhibition and hyperactivity, play therapy utilizing CBT might be an effective approach in addressing these issues. Through the use of CBT techniques, the school psychologist could help the child link thoughts to behavior, learn relaxation techniques to use when overwhelmed, use strategies to reduce impulsivity, and model appropriate social behaviors. Ritchie (2013) points out that a CBT approach paired with play therapy techniques can help address emotion regulation difficulties. Another play therapy approach recommended by Ritchie (2013) is child-centered play therapy (CCPT). The principles that guide this therapeutic approach include a positive relationship with the play therapist, acceptance of the child by the play therapist, a safe environment in which to explore feelings, helping the child to recognize feelings, helping the child to internally solve difficulties on their own, letting the child guide the play therapy sessions, understanding that the therapeutic process occurs over time, and setting limits when needed (Ritchie, 2013).

Another therapeutic technique that has been used with children with RAD is behavior management training (BMT). Buckner et al. (2008) acknowledges that there is a lack of evidence-based treatment for RAD (including DSED). However, parent training programs, such as BMT, use evidence-based treatment that focuses on working with parents to enhance parent–child interactions, communicate behavioral expectation, and provide appropriate consequences for misbehaviors. It is an approach that could be considered to help manage behavioral problems that children with RAD/DSED may experience. BMT is a structured program, consisting of 10 sessions as well as a manual to follow for each session. The program is designed to help caregivers of school-age children address externalizing behaviors and difficulties with attention and concentration. Psychoeducation is provided to the parent/caregiver, which focuses on misbehavior and parenting skills that can be utilized to reduce disruptive behaviors, increase compliance, develop appropriate discipline, and improve school behavior with a home-based reward. According to Buckner and colleagues (2008), it has been found to be effective in managing behavioral problems in children between the ages of 6 and 11. A type of BMT, Parent–Child Interaction Therapy, is a valid program in the treatment of externalizing behaviors (Dickmann & Allen, 2017). Dickmann and Allen (2017) indicated that it may be an appropriate treatment for children with DSED with adaptations, integrating CBT techniques, and an instrument to assess DSED behaviors.

Although there are no specific school-based interventions or treatments for DSED, these are approaches school psychologists could consider. It is important that school psychologists be trained in these therapeutic approaches of play therapy, CBT, and BMT.

CASE STUDY 19.1 LYLA: THE CASE OF A 4-YEAR-OLD GIRL WITH DISINHIBITED SOCIAL ENGAGEMENT DISORDER

Background

Lyla is a 4-year-old girl who recently started preschool. She currently lives in a foster home with her foster parents and foster brother, who is 10 years old. Lyla has been living with the family for about 6 months. Prior to living with this foster family, Lyla had been placed in four different foster homes since she was an infant. The foster mother reported that she did not have much information about Lyla's early history. However, she had been informed that the biological mother was unable to care for Lyla and, hence, placed her into foster care as there were no relatives able to take care of her.

The current foster mother also reported that the foster care agency had reported that some of the foster homes did not provide a nurturing environment for Lyla. While she was living in the first foster home, Lyla was often left in the crib for hours in a soiled diaper. A social worker came to visit and found that the first foster mother was using drugs and did not provide appropriate care for a baby. The second foster home had several other foster care children in the home. The foster mother tended to withhold food when the foster children, including Lyla, were misbehaving. Lyla learned to hide food at a young age. On one occasion when she was 3, Lyla walked away from the rest of the foster family while they were in a park so that she could talk to a teenage boy. She talked to the boy for a while and then was later found looking for food in the trash can at the park. She also has exhibited some aggressive and hyperactive behaviors. The foster mother reported that she had been told that Lyla is a "friendly girl" but can be "too friendly sometimes." According to the foster mother, Lyla

(continued)

> **CASE STUDY 19.1 LYLA: THE CASE OF A 4-YEAR-OLD GIRL WITH DISINHIBITED SOCIAL ENGAGEMENT DISORDER (continued)**
>
> approaches strangers readily and seems to be comfortable walking up to someone and starting a conversion with that person. She has even tried to hold the hand of a stranger with whom she talked and asked to sit in the lap of a male stranger. In the current foster home, she appears overly concerned about food even though food is provided for her. She continues to approach strangers and even asks intrusive questions. Sometimes the strangers look uncomfortable when she is so friendly toward them. Recently, Lyla was overly friendly with a male visitor whom she had never met. The foster mother and father were present and observed her interactions, which they believed were inappropriate for her age. The parents kept an eye on her the entire time. They noted that the male visitor stayed away from her after she tried to get physically close to him. She became upset and threw a small object on the floor. She exhibits similar behaviors at school, and her teacher and foster parents are concerned about her behaviors and worried that she will walk off with a stranger. In school, she is reportedly doing fine with academic tasks, but her teachers are not sure about how best to help Lyla. Both the parents and teacher report that she is overly active at times and can be aggressive in her interactions with others, particularly other children.
>
> ## Discussion
>
> It is clear that Lyla meets the criteria of DSED as is evident in the behaviors described by the foster mother. Lyla actively approaches unfamiliar adults and interacts with them. She shows no hesitation about approaching a stranger and can be overly physical toward people whom she does not know. She has a history of social neglect and inadequate living conditions as evidenced by being left alone in a soiled diaper for long periods of time. She also has been in situations in which food was withheld from her, which has led her to now hoarding food. In addition, she has had multiple foster homes even though she is only 4 years old. She is older than 9 months old so the time period to form a selective attachment to an adult has passed.
>
> Both the foster mother and the teacher are concerned about Lyla and understand the potentially risky situations she may place herself in as she grows older. To address their concerns, the school psychologist could work with them individually in a consultative role to provide psychoeducation about DSED. This provides the opportunity for the parent and teacher to learn about the impact of DSED on children's learning and social–emotional–behavioral functioning. With the parent, the school psychologist could determine whether additional services, such as mental health support outside the school, are needed. Helping the parents advocate for needed services would be an important role for the school psychologist. The school psychologist can be a supportive resource for the teacher and help guide the teacher in developing ways in which to address Lyla's behavior problems in the classroom.
>
> Educational supports may be provided in the classroom to address Lyla's social–emotional and behavioral needs. Educational supports could be provided through MTSS. At each tier of the system, supports could be provided. If Lyla does not respond to these supports, a multidisciplinary team may make a referral for an evaluation for special education services. The school psychologist will conduct a series of tests, and the team will review the results of the assessment to decide whether Lyla is a child with a disability and whether there is a need for special education services. If Lyla is determined to be a student with a disability, it must be evident that the disability is having an adverse impact on her academic performance.
>
> School-based mental health services may be an option to address Lyla's behavioral problems. Play therapy integrated with CBT may be an effective intervention for Lyla in that it provides a safe opportunity for her to explore her feelings and learn ways in which to manage her behavior. Through the play, she could also learn appropriate ways to communicate and interact socially. An alternative approach to consider may be BMT, which teaches the parent how to manage behavior. Lyla and her family will clearly need much support, and the school psychologist can serve as a valuable resource for the parents and teacher.

SUMMARY POINTS

- DSED is a disorder distinct from RAD in the *DSM-5*.
- Although children with DSED have a history of social neglect or inadequate care, DSED is now considered a disorder of social engagement rather than attachment.
- The quality of parental behavior may influence children's development and recovery of behaviors related to DSED.
- Inhibitory control of rage reflects the possibility that the child may be able to suppress such intense feelings while they are in school or other situations and then release those feelings later on with the caregiver with whom they feel safe.

TEST YOUR KNOWLEDGE

1. Social–emotional difficulties experience by children with DSED include all of the following EXCEPT:
   a. Hyperactive behaviors
   b. Schizophrenia
   c. Low self-esteem
   d. Interpersonal problems

2. Children with DSED present as emotionally withdrawn and sad.
   a. True
   b. False

3. When in a new situation with an unfamiliar adult, which of the following behaviors would be expected of a child with DSED?
   a. Cling to the caregiver
   b. Withdraw and hide from the unfamiliar adult
   c. Approach the unfamiliar adult with no reservation
   d. Run away from the unfamiliar adult

4. DSED is still considered by all scholars to be an attachment disorder.
   a. True
   b. False

5. An IDEA disability category that might be considered for a child with DSED is Emotional Disturbance.
   a. True
   b. False

Answers: (1) b, (2) b, (3) c, (4) b, (5) a.

DISCUSSION QUESTIONS

1. Describe the *DSM-5* diagnostic features of DSED.
2. Identify reasons why DSED is no longer considered an attachment disorder.
3. Discuss how DSED can impact a child's social–emotional and behavioral functioning.
4. Identify factors that may influence the learning of a child with DSED.
5. Identify educational and social–emotional supports that may be useful for a child with DSED.

CHAPTER RESOURCES

Resources for School Psychologists

American Academy of Child and Adolescent Psychiatry *Attachment Disorders*: www.aacap.org/AACAP/Families_and_Youth/Facts_for_Families/FFF-Guide/Attachment-Disorders-085.aspx

American Association of Child and Adolescent Mental Health *Disinhibited Social Engagement Behaviour Is Not Unique to Children Exposed to Inadequate Caregiving*: www.acamh.org/app/uploads/2020/01/RD_Disinhibited-social.pdf

KEY REFERENCES

Only key references appear in the print edition. The full reference list appears in the digital product on Springer Publishing Connect: connect.springerpub.com/content/book/978-0-8261-3587-2/part/part07/chapter/ch19

American Psychiatric Association. (2013). *Diagnostic and statistical manual of mental disorders* (5th ed.). https://doi.org/10.1176/appi.books.9780890425596

Floyd, K. K., Hester, P., Griffin, H. C., Golden, J., & Canter, L. L. S. (2008). Reactive attachment disorder: Challenges for early identification and intervention within the schools. *International Journal of Special Education*, 23(2), 47–55. https://files.eric.ed.gov/fulltext/EJ814399.pdf

Individuals with Disabilities Education Improvement Act. (2004). 20 U.S.C. § 1400.

Losinski, M., Katsiyannis, A., White, S., & Wiseman, N. (2016). Addressing the complex needs of students with attachment disorders. *Intervention in School & Clinic*, 51(3), 184–187. https://doi.org/10.1177/1053451215585800

Perry, B. D. (2001). *Bonding and attachment in maltreated children: Consequences of emotional neglect in childhood.* Child Trauma Academy Press. https://7079168e-705a-4dc7-be05-2218087aa989.filesusr.com/ugd/aa51c7_a9e562d294864796bdd5b3096a8d8c86.pdf

Rutter, M., Colvert, E., Kreppner, J., Beckett, C., Castle, J., Groothues, C., Hawkins, A., O'Connor, T. G., Stevens, S. E., & Sonuga-Barke, E. J. (2007). Early adolescent outcomes for institutionally-deprived and non-deprived adoptees. I: Disinhibited attachment. *Journal of Child Psychology and Psychiatry*, 48(1), 17–30. https://doi.org/10.1111/j.1469-7610.2006.01688.x

Scheper, F. Y., Abrahamse, M. E., Jonkman, C. S., Schuengel, C., Lindauer, R. J. L., Vries, A. L. C., Doreleijers, T. A. H., & Jansen, L. M. C. (2016). Inhibited attachment behaviour and disinhibited social engagement behaviour as relevant concepts in referred home reared children. *Child: Care, Health & Development*, 42(4), 544–552. https://doi.org/10.1111/cch.12319

Schwartz, E., & Davis, A. S. (2006). Reactive attachment disorder: Implications for school readiness and school functioning. *Psychology in the Schools*, 43(4), 471–479. https://doi.org/10.1002/pits.20161

Seim, A. R., Jozefiak, T., Wichstrøm, L., Lydersen, S., & Kayed, N. S. (2020). Reactive attachment disorder and disinhibited social engagement disorder in adolescence: Co-occurring psychopathology and psychosocial problems. *European Child & Adolescent Psychiatry*, 1–14. https://doi.org/10.1007/s00787-020-01673-7

Spilt, J. L., Vervoort, E., Koenen, A. K., Bosmans, G., & Verschueren, K. (2016). The socio-behavioral development of children with symptoms of attachment disorder: An observational study of teacher sensitivity in special education. *Research in Developmental Disabilities*, 56, 71–82. https://doi.org/10.1016/j.ridd.2016.05.014

Zeanah, C. H., & Gleason, M. M. (2010). *Reactive attachment disorder: A review for DSM-V.* American Psychiatric Association. https://www.researchgate.net/profile/Charles-Zeanah/publication/228683818_Reactive_Attachment_Disorder_a_review_for_DSM-V/links/0deec51e86576d1e8c000000/Reactive-Attachment-Disorder-a-review-for-DSM-V.pdf

Zeanah, C. H., & Gleason, M. M. (2015a). Annual research review: Attachment disorders in early childhood – Clinical presentation, causes, correlates, and treatment. *Journal of Child Psychology and Psychiatry*, 56, 207–222. https://doi.org/10.1111/jcpp.12347

Index

AAP. *See* American Academy of Pediatrics
ACEs. *See* adverse childhood experiences
ADHD. *See* attention deficit hyperactivity disorder
ADIS-IV-C/P. *See* Anxiety Disorders Interview Schedule for Children for *DSM-IV* Child/Parent Version
ADIS-IV-L. *See* Anxiety Disorder Interview Schedule for *DSM-IV* Lifetime
adolescents. *See also specific mental conditions*
  anxiety disorders, 5
  cyberbullying, 5
  impact of racism, 4
  living in poverty, 4
  mental health, 3
  racial stress, 4
  school violence, 4–5
  social media, 5
adverse childhood experiences (ACEs), 3, 4
aggressive behaviors, 310, 312, 314–315, 317, 319, 323
American Academy of Pediatrics (AAP), 4, 31, 161
American Psychiatric Association, 9
American Psychological Association, 3
antisocial personality disorder, 79, 81, 86, 90, 96
Anxiety Disorder Interview Schedule for *DSM-IV* Lifetime (ADIS-IV-L), 159
Anxiety Disorders Interview Schedule for Children for *DSM-IV* Child/Parent Version (ADIS-IV-C/P), 164–165
anxiety, 5, 6, 137–139, 214, 245, 263, 268–269, 274, 282–283, 312–313, 322. *See also specific anxiety conditions*
ASD. *See* autism spectrum disorder
attention deficit hyperactivity disorder (ADHD), 4, 5, 9, 17–35, 63, 65–67, 81–82, 86, 101, 107, 141, 179, 293, 294, 309, 358, 361
  adverse school experiences, 24–25
  case study, 33–34
  cultural considerations, 23–24
  DSM-5 diagnosis, 17–20
  educational supports, 30–32
  inattention symptoms, 17–18, 25–26
  intervention strategies, 32–33
  learning impairment, 26–28
  parenting difficulties, 25–26
  risk factors, 22–23
  school-based eligibility, 21
  stimulant medication, 27, 29, 33–34
  symptomatology, 18–19, 23, 25, 28
autism spectrum disorder (ASD), 9, 61–72, 194, 204, 332–333
  behavioral problems at school, 65–66
  case study, 71–72
  cultural considerations, 64–65
  DSM-5 diagnosis, 61–63
  educational supports, 69–70
  learning issues, 66–67
  parenting issues, 66
  risk factors, 64
  school psychologists
    advocacy, 67
    assessment, 68–69
    consultation, 68
  school-based eligibility, 63–64
  school-based interventions, 70–71
  social communication and interaction, 61–62, 67, 70–72

behavior management training (BMT), 367
behavioral intervention plan (BIP), 67, 70
Behavioral Rating Scale for Children-3, 321
BIP. *See* behavioral intervention plan
BMT. *See* behavior management training
brain development, and trauma, 309, 314, 319–320

Camp Cope-A-Lot (CCAL), 167
CAPA. *See* Child and Adolescent Psychiatric Assessment
CBITS. *See* Cognitive Behavioral Interventions for Trauma in Schools
CBT. *See* cognitive behavioral therapy
CCAL. *See* Camp Cope-A-Lot
CCPT. *See* child-centered play therapy

Centers for Disease Control and Prevention's Youth Risk Behavior Survey, 4, 5
Child and Adolescent Psychiatric Assessment (CAPA), 357
Child PTSD Symptom Scale, 318
Child Report of Post-Traumatic Symptoms, 318
Child Stress Disorder Checklist, 318
child-centered play therapy (CCPT), 347, 367
Childhood Trauma Questionnaire, 318
children. *See also specific mental conditions*
  ADHD disorders, 5
  behavior problems, 5, 6
  impact of racism, 4
  living in poverty, 4
  mental health, 3
  school violence, 4–5
Children's Saving Inventory (CSI), 297
Child's Reactions to Traumatic Events Scale-Revised, 318
Clinician-Administered PTSD Scale for DSM-5, 321
Cognitive Behavioral Interventions for Trauma in Schools (CBITS), 321–322
cognitive behavioral therapy (CBT), 71, 109, 111, 114, 153, 167–168, 173, 183, 186–187, 189, 201, 203, 205, 252–253, 265, 281, 298, 300, 302, 345, 347, 365–368
complex trauma, 309–310, 314, 319, 323
conduct disorder
  case study, 93–95
  cultural considerations, 85
  DSM-5 diagnosis, 79–80
  educational supports, 91–92
  home life, 86–87
  IDEA eligibility, 81–83
  learning issues, 87–88
  prevalence and comorbidity, 80–81
  risk factors, 84–85
  peers, 80–81, 84–87, 89, 91–93, 96
  school psychologists
    advocacy role, 90
    assessment role, 88–90
    consultation role, 90
    counseling and therapy role, 90–91
  school setting, 85–86
  school-based eligibility, 81–84
  school-based interventions, 92–93
  Section 504 eligibility, 83–84
COVID-19, 183–184, 187–189, 293, 307
CSI. *See* Children's Saving Inventory
cyberbullying, 5

Developmental and Ecological Model of Youth Racial Trauma, 311
developmental trauma disorder (DTD), 309–310, 324

Diagnostic and Statistical Manual of Mental Disorders (DSM), 9–10
  Fifth Edition (*DSM-5*)
    attention deficit hyperactivity disorder, 17–20
    autism spectrum disorder, 61–63
    conduct disorder, 79–80
    disinhibited social engagement disorder, 356–358
    disruptive mood dysregulation disorder, 227–230
    generalized anxiety disorder, 137–139
    hoarding disorder, 289–291
    intellectual disability, 39–41
    intermittent explosive disorder, 117–120
    major depressive disorder, 211–214
    obsessive-compulsive disorder, 263–264
    oppositional defiant disorder, 99–101
    persistent depressive disorder, 243–245
    posttraumatic stress disorder, 308–309
    reactive attachment disorder, 331–332
    selective mutism, 193–196
    separation anxiety disorder, 153–154
    social anxiety disorder, 173–174
  Fourth Edition (*DSM-IV*), 156–159, 164, 167, 179–180, 184, 331, 333, 336, 341
  Fourth Edition, Text Revision (*DSM-IV-TR*), 174, 177–179, 184, 194, 331
  Third Edition (*DSM-III*), 331
  Third Edition, Revised (*DSM-III-R*), 158
disinhibited social engagement disorder (DSED), 329–331, 333–339
  case study, 367–368
  characteristics, 355
  competence and self-esteem, 360
  DSM-5 diagnosis, 356–358
  educational supports, 366
  emotional–behavioral problems, 360–361
  etiology and course, 355–356
  functioning in school and home, 359–360, 362–363
  IDEA eligibility, 358
  interpersonal relationships, 361–362
  learning issues, 363
  school psychologists
    advocacy, 363–364
    assessment, 364–365
    consultation, 364
    counseling/therapeutic services, 365–366
  school-based interventions, 366–367
  Section 504 eligibility, 359
  symptoms, 356–358, 360–362
disruptive behaviors, 309, 312, 314–315, 317, 319, 323, 360, 363–364, 367
disruptive mood dysregulation disorder (DMDD)
  case study, 237–238
  cultural considerations, 232
  dialectical behavioral therapy, 235–237

DSM-5 classification and diagnosis, 227–230
educational supports, 235–236
functional behavioral assessment, 234–235, 238
IDEA eligibility, 230–231
irritability, 228–229, 231–236, 238
learning issues, 233
outbursts, 228–229, 231–236, 238
prevalence, 229
risk factors, 231–232
school and home functioning, 232–233
school psychologists
  advocacy role, 234–235
  assessment role, 233–234
  consultation role, 235
  counseling/therapy role, 235
school-based interventions, 236–237
Section 504 eligibility, 231
symptomatology, 227, 229, 230–232, 234, 237
treatment, 228, 232, 234, 236, 238
DMDD. *See* disruptive mood dysregulation disorder
DSED. *See* disinhibited social engagement disorder
DSM. *See* Diagnostic and Statistical Manual of Mental Disorders
DTD. *See* developmental trauma disorder

Emotional Disturbance, IDEA disability category, 10, 81–82, 88–89, 102, 108, 120, 139, 155, 175, 195–196, 215, 230, 245–246, 265, 291–292, 296, 311, 334–335, 344, 345–346, 358
ESSA. *See* Every Student Succeeds Act
Every Student Succeeds Act (ESSA), 8

face-to-face instruction, 183, 187–189
FAPE. *See* free and appropriate public education
FBA/BIP. *See* functional analysis of behavior/ behavior intervention plan
free and appropriate public education (FAPE), 10, 21, 42, 83, 102, 120, 139, 140, 156, 214, 292
Fun FRIENDS, 251
functional analysis of behavior (FBA)/behavior intervention plan (BIP), 182

GAD. *See* generalized anxiety disorder
generalized anxiety disorder (GAD), 137–147, 149, 154, 178–180, 268, 273
  case study, 148–149
  cultural consideration, 141–142
  DSM-5 diagnosis, 137–139
  educational supports, 146
  IDEA eligibility, 139–140
  learning issues, 143–144
  risk factors, 140–141
  school psychologists
    advocacy role, 145
    assessment role, 144
    consultation role, 145
    counseling/therapy role, 145–146
  school-based interventions, 146–147
  Section 504 eligibility, 140
  sleeping issues, 142–143
  social relationships, 142
  symptomatology, 138, 144–146
GPAs. *See* grade point averages
grade point averages (GPAs), depression, 218

hoarding disorder
  behavior, 290–291, 293–295, 297–298, 300, 302
  case study, 301–302
  cultural consideration, 294
  development, 293, 295, 302
  DSM classification and diagnosis, 289–291
  educational supports, 299
  executive functioning deficits, 296, 299
  functioning at school and home, 294–295
  IDEA eligibility, 291–292
  learning issues, 295–296
  risk factors, 293
  school psychologists
    advocacy role, 297
    assessment role, 296–297
    consultation role, 297–298
    counseling and therapy role, 298–299
  school-based interventions, 299–300
  Section 504 eligibility, 292
  symptoms, 290–291, 293–295, 297–298, 302

ID. *See* intellectual disability
IDEA. *See* Individuals with Disabilities Education Improvement Act
IEP. *See* Individual Education Program
Individual Education Program (IEP), 10, 47, 56, 63, 67, 72, 83, 154–155, 214, 279, 350
Individuals with Disabilities Education Improvement Act (IDEA), 10–11, 21, 28, 34, 39–40, 42, 47, 49, 51–52, 55–57, 63–65, 101–103, 108, 110, 139–140, 144, 154

intellectual disability (ID)
  behavioral challenges (school and home), 46–49
  caregiving considerations, 44–46
  case study, 54–56
  cultural sensitivity, 43
  DSM-5 classification, 39–41
  educational supports, 52–53
  IDEA eligibility, 41–42
  learning issues, 49–50
  negative connotations, 43–44
  occupational therapy, 54, 56
  risk factors, 42–43
  school-based interventions, 53–54
  school psychologists
    advocacy role, 51
    assessment role, 50–51
    consultation role, 51
    counseling and therapy role, 51–52
interconnected systems framework (ISF), 222
intermittent explosive disorder
  case study, 130–132
  cultural considerations, 123
  DSM-5 classification and diagnosis, 117–120
  educational supports, 128–129
  home environment, 124–125
  IDEA eligibility, 120–121
  learning issues, 125–126
  risk factors, 121–123
  school functioning and academic environment, 123–124
  school psychologists
    advocacy role, 127
    assessment role, 126–127
    consultation role, 127–128
    counseling/therapy role, 128
  school-based interventions, 129–130
  Section 504 eligibility, 121
International Classification of Diseases, 157, 194, 228, 336
International OCD Foundation (IOCDF), 275
IOCDF. *See* International OCD Foundation
ISF. *See* interconnected systems framework

Japanese psychiatric classification system, 181

Kiddie Schedule for Affective Disorders and Schizophrenia Present and Lifetime (K-SADS-PL), 157, 178
K-SADS-PL. *See* Kiddie Schedule for Affective Disorders and Schizophrenia Present and Lifetime

LEA. *See* local education agency
Liebowitz Social Anxiety Scale for Children and Adolescents (LSAC-CA), 185
lifetime morbid risk (LMR) ratio, separation anxiety disorder, 157
LMR ratio. *See* lifetime morbid risk ratio
local education agency (LEA), 42, 47, 56
LSAC-CA. *See* Liebowitz Social Anxiety Scale for Children and Adolescents

major depressive disorder (MDD), 211–224, 243–244
  case study, 223–224
  cultural consideration, 216–217
  DSM-5 classification and diagnosis, 211–214
  educational supports, 221
  functioning in school and home, 217–218
  IDEA eligibility, 214–215
  learning issues, 218–219
  prevention efforts, 212, 222–223
  risk factors, 215–216
  school psychologists
    advocacy role, 219–220
    assessment role, 219
    consultation role, 220
    counseling/therapy role, 220–221
  school-based interventions, 221–223
  Section 504 eligibility, 215
  suicide risk, 214, 220–221
  symptoms, 211–216, 219–220, 222
MASC. *See* Multidimensional Anxiety Scale for Children
MDD. *See* major depressive disorder
MTSS. *See* Multi-Tiered Systems of Support
Multidimensional Anxiety Scale for Children (MASC), 165, 167, 184, 278
Multi-Tiered Systems of Support (MTSS), 8–9, 33, 112, 166, 173, 176, 177, 182, 185, 186, 187, 219, 222, 234, 237, 249–250, 317, 320–322, 346, 366

NASP. *See* National Association of School Psychologists
National Association of School Psychologists (NASP), 7, 43, 176, 274, 276, 345
  Practice Model, 7–9
National Child Traumatic Stress Network (NCTSN), 316, 317, 318, 321
National Comorbidity Survey Replication (NCS-R), 156, 180
National Comorbidity Survey Replication Adolescent Supplement (NCS-A), 19, 118, 156, 174, 177
National Epidemiological Survey, 179

National Survey of Children's Health (NSCH), 19, 212, 213, 215, 216
National Survey of Student Health, 5
NCS-A. *See* National Comorbidity Survey Replication Adolescent Supplement
NCS-R. *See* National Comorbidity Survey Replication
NCTSN. *See* National Child Traumatic Stress Network
nonverbal behaviors, 204
NSCH. *See* National Survey of Children's Health

obsessive-compulsive disorder (OCD), 195, 289–291, 293–295, 297
 anxiety-management techniques, 282–283
 behavioral functioning, 270–271
 case study, 283–284
 characteristics, 259–260
 cognitive behavioral therapy, 281–282
 comorbidity, 265
 cultural issues, 265–267
 diagnostic issues, 260–261
 DSM-5 diagnosis, 263–265
 educational supports, 279–280
 emotional distress, 268–269
 etiological considerations, 261–263
 family functioning at home, 271–272
 IDEA eligibility, 265
 learning issues, 272–274
 level of insight, 264–265
 neuropsychological impairments, 273–274
 noncompliant behavior, 274
 Response to Intervention, 281
 school and home functioning, 267–270
 school psychologists
  assessment role, 277–278
  behavioral observations, 277–278
  consultation issues, 277
  educator awareness and knowledge, 276
  promoting awareness and knowledge, 274–276
 school-based interventions, 281–283
 Section 504 eligibility, 265
 social–emotional support, 280
 social functioning impairment, 269–270
 symptom dimensions, 264
 symptoms, difficulties related to, 272
OCD. *See* obsessive-compulsive disorder
Office of Special Education Programs (OSEP), 155
OHI. *See* Other Health Impairment
oppositional defiant disorder
 case study, 111–114
 cultural considerations, 105
 DSM-5 classification and diagnosis, 99–101
 educational supports, 110
 IDEA eligibility, 101–103
 learning issues, 107–108
 parenting issues, 106–107
 risk factors, 104–105
 school psychologists
  advocacy role, 109
  assessment role, 108
  consultation role, 109
  counseling/therapy role, 109–110
 school-based interventions, 111–112
 Section 504 eligibility, 103–104
 symptoms, 99–101, 103–107, 111–112, 114
 teacher and peer relationship, 105–106
oppositional behavior, 105, 106, 194, 199, 205, 233, 270
OSEP. *See* Office of Special Education Programs
Other Health Impairment (OHI), IDEA disability category, 10, 21, 82, 88–89, 103, 108, 120–121, 139–140, 175–176, 230–231, 265, 291–292, 296

PACE. *See* Playfulness, Acceptance, Curiosity, and Empathy
PBS. *See* positive behavioral supports
PDD. *See* persistent depressive disorder; Pervasive Developmental Disorders
PEERS. *See* Program for the Education and Enrichment of Relational Skills
persistent depressive disorder (PDD)
 case study, 252–253
 DSM-5 classification and diagnosis, 243–245
 educational supports, 251
 IDEA eligibility, 245–246
 learning issues, 248–249
 risk factors, 246–247
 school and home functioning, 247–248
 school psychologists
  advocacy role, 250
  assessment role, 249–250
  consultation role, 250
  counseling/therapy role, 250
 school-based interventions, 251–252
 Section 504 eligibility, 246
 symptomatology, 244, 246
Pervasive Developmental Disorders (PDD), 61
Play Skills for Shy Children, 251
Playfulness, Acceptance, Curiosity, and Empathy (PACE), 347, 349
positive behavioral supports (PBS), 54, 87, 121, 124, 300, 320–321
posttraumatic stress disorder (PTSD)
 behavioral functioning, 313–314
 Bounce Back program, 322
 case study, 322–324
 CBITS program, 321–322
 cultural issues, 310–311

posttraumatic stress disorder (*continued*)
   DSM-5 diagnosis, 308–309
   educational supports, 320–321
   learning issues, 314–315
   prevalence in United States, 307, 309
   protective factors, 311–312
   risk factors, 311–312
   school psychologists
      awareness among parents, 317
      in-service workshops for educators, 316
      raising awareness, 315–317
   school-based assessment practices, 317
   school-based evaluations, 318–320
   school-based interventions, 321–322
   single and multiple traumatic events, 309–310
   social–emotional functioning, 312–313
   SSET program, 322
   trauma screening in schools, 317–318
poverty, 4
Preschool PATHS Program, 251
Program for the Education and Enrichment of Relational Skills (PEERS), 70
psychoeducation, 29, 32, 145, 166, 203, 220, 236, 252, 321, 343, 366, 367
psychiatric disorders, 229, 232-233
psychosocial development theory (Erikson), 182–183
PTSD. *See* posttraumatic stress disorder

racial discrimination, 4, 24, 310–311
racial stress, 4, 310–311
RAD. *See* reactive attachment disorder
reactive attachment disorder (RAD)
   case study, 348–350
   characteristics, 329–330
   comorbidity, 333–334
   cultural issues, 335–336
   differential diagnosis, 332–333
   DSM-5 diagnosis, 331–332
   educational supports, 345–346
   emotional and behavioral difficulties, 338–339
   emotional dysregulation, 339
   etiological considerations, 330–331
   IDEA eligibility, 334–335
   interpersonal relationships, 339–340
   learning issues, 341–342
   school and home functioning, 336–341
   school psychologists
      advocacy, 342–343
      assessment, 344–345
      consultation, 343–344
      therapeutic interventions, 345
   school-based interventions, 347–348
   Section 504 eligibility, 335
   self-esteem, 336–338
   symptoms, 329, 331–332, 334–335, 338, 349
Rehabilitation Act of 1973, 11, 21, 64, 83, 89, 103–104, 121, 140, 144, 155–156, 176–177, 196, 215, 231, 246, 292, 335, 359
Response to Intervention (RtI), 176, 281
RtI. *See* Response to Intervention

SAAS-C. *See* Separation Anxiety Assessment Scale Children and Adolescent Version
SAAS-P. *See* Separation Anxiety Assessment Scale Parent Version
SAD. *See* separation anxiety disorder
SCARED. *See* Screen for Child Anxiety Related Emotional Disorders
schizophrenia, 292, 358
school-based mental health services, 6–9
school psychologists
   DSM-5 classification, use of, 9–10
   IDEA disability classification, 10–11
   National Association of School Psychologists Practice Model, 7–9
   need for mental health services, 6–9
   critical role in psychoeducation, 29–30
   psychosocial treatments, 30
school violence, 4–5
Screen for Child Anxiety Related Emotional Disorders (SCARED), 165, 184
   Child Version, 180
selective mutism
   case study, 203–205
   cultural considerations, 196–197
   DSM-5 classification and diagnosis, 193–195
   educational supports, 201–202
   functioning in school and home, 197–198
   IDEA eligibility, 195–196
   learning issues, 198–199
   risk factors, 196
   school psychologists
      advocacy role, 200–201
      assessment role, 199–200
      consultation role, 201
      counseling/therapy role, 201
   school-based interventions, 202–203
   Section 504 eligibility, 196
selective serotonin uptake inhibitors (SSRIs), 167–168, 187, 189, 200, 220
self-esteem, 360, 363, 365–366
Separation Anxiety Assessment Scale Children and Adolescent Version (SAAS-C), 165
Separation Anxiety Assessment Scale Parent Version (SAAS-P), 165
separation anxiety disorder (SAD)
   behavior at school and home, 163–164
   case study, 168–169
   comorbidities, 158–159

cultural issues, 161–162
DSM-5 category and diagnosis, 153–154
educational supports, 166
IDEA eligibility, 154–155
impact on child development, 163
international studies, 157–158
learning issues, 164
prevalence and onset, 156
risk factors, 160
school psychologists
  advocacy role, 166
  as consultants with parents, 166
  assessment, 164–165
school-based interventions, 166–168
Section 504 eligibility, 155–156
U.S. studies, 156–157
SOC. *See* social anxiety disorder
social anxiety disorder (SOC)
  academic interventions, 186
  case study, 188–189
  comorbidity, 178–180
  cultural issues, 181
  DSM-5 classification and diagnosis, 173, 174–175
  DSM-IV TR, 174–175
  educational supports, 185–186
  IDEA eligibility, 175–176
  impact on child social development, 182–183
  international studies, 178
  learning issues, 183–184
  prevalence and onset, 177
  risk factors, 180–181
  school and home functioning, 182–183
  school psychologists
    advocacy, 185
    assessment, 184–185
    consulting with parents and teachers, 185
  school-based interventions, 186–187
  Section 504 eligibility, 176–177
  U.S. studies, 177–178
social competence, 47, 111, 142, 264, 319, 339, 361, 363, 365, 366
social learning theory, 111
social media, 5
social skills training (SST), 70, 72, 109, 111, 114
socioeconomic status, 103–105
somatic symptoms, common, 249
SP. *See* specific phobias
specific phobias (SP), 141
SSET. *See* Support for Students Exposed to Trauma
SSRIs. *See* selective serotonin uptake inhibitors
SST. *See* social skills training
suicide, 5, 6–7, 214, 220–221, 230, 245, 250, 252, 366

Support for Students Exposed to Trauma (SSET), 321–322
  SSET Group Leader Training Manual, 322

TBI. *See* traumatic brain injury
trauma screenings, 317–318
  Child PTSD Symptom Scale, 318
  Child Report of Post-Traumatic Symptoms, 318
  Child Stress Disorder Checklist, 318
  Child's Reactions to Traumatic Events Scale-Revised, 318
  Childhood Trauma Questionnaire, 318
  Trauma Symptom Checklist for Children-PTSD Subscale, 318
  Traumatic Events Screening Inventory for Children: Brief Form, 318
  UCLA Posttraumatic Stress Disorder Reaction Index, 318
Trauma Symptom Checklist for Children-PTSD Subscale, 318
traumatic brain injury (TBI), 262
Traumatic Events Screening Inventory for Children: Brief Form, 318
traumatic stress symptoms, 308–310, 321–322

UCLA Posttraumatic Stress Disorder Reaction Index. *See* University of California at Los Angeles Posttraumatic Stress Disorder Reaction Index
UCLA PEERS. *See* University of California Los Angeles Program for the Education and Enrichment of Relational Skills
University of California at Los Angeles (UCLA) Posttraumatic Stress Disorder Reaction Index, 318
University of California Los Angeles (UCLA) Program for the Education and Enrichment of Relational Skills (PEERS), 70

violence, 4–5, 23, 48, 84, 85, 125, 128–129, 162, 307, 310, 314

WHO. *See* World Health Organization
World Health Organization (WHO), 157, 212
  World Mental Health Survey Initiative, 157

Youth Risk Behavior Survey, Center for Disease Control and Prevention's, 4, 5

www.ingramcontent.com/pod-product-compliance
Ingram Content Group UK Ltd.
Pitfield, Milton Keynes, MK11 3LW, UK
UKHW051849210426
5322IPUK00024B/619